Techniques in extracorporeal circulation

Techniques in extracorporeal circulation

FOURTH EDITION

Edited by

PHILIP H KAY MA DM FRCS

Consultant Cardiothoracic Surgeon,
Yorkshire Heart Centre,
The General Infirmary,
Leeds, UK

and

CHRISTOPHER M MUNSCH ChM FRCS (C/Th)

Consultant Cardiothoracic Surgeon,
Yorkshire Heart Centre,
The General Infirmary,
Leeds, UK

ARNOLD

A member of the Hodder Headline Group
LONDON

First published in 1976 by Butterworth-Heinemann Ltd,
Linacre House, Jordan Hill, Oxford, OX2 8DP.
This edition published in Great Britain in 2004 by
Arnold, a member of the Hodder Headline Group,
338 Euston Road, London NW1 3BH

http://www.arnoldpublishers.com

First published 1976
Second edition 1981
Reprinted 1982
Third edition 1992
Reprinted 1993
Fourth edition 2004

Distributed in the United States of America by
Oxford University Press Inc.,
198 Madison Avenue, New York, NY10016
Oxford is a registered trademark of Oxford University Press

Whilst the advice and information in this book are believed to be true and
accurate at the date of going to press, neither the author[s] nor the publisher
can accept any legal responsibility or liability for any errors or omissions
that may be made. In particular (but without limiting the generality of the
preceding disclaimer) every effort has been made to check drug dosages;
however, it is still possible that errors have been missed. Furthermore, dosage
schedules are constantly being revised and new side-effects recognized.
For these reasons the reader is strongly urged to consult the drug companies'
printed instructions before administering any of the drugs recommended in
this book.

British Library Cataloguing in Publication Data
A catalogue record for this book is available from the British Library

Library of Congress Cataloging-in-Publication Data
A catalog record for this book is available from the Library of Congress

ISBN 0 340 80723 7

1 2 3 4 5 6 7 8 9 10

Commissioning Editor: Joanna Koster
Development Editor: Sarah Burrows
Project Editor: Zelah Pengilley
Production Controller: Deborah Smith
Cover Design: Lee-May Lim
Indexer: Laurence Errington

Typeset in 10/12 pt Minion by Charon Tec Pvt Ltd, Chennai, India
Printed and bound in Great Britain by Butler & Tanner Ltd

What do you think about this book? Or any other Arnold title?
Please send your comments to **feedback.arnold@hodder.co.uk**

Contents

Contributors

Scott K Alpard MD
Surgical Research Fellow,
Division of Cardiothoracic Surgery,
University of Texas Medical Branch,
Galveston, TX, USA

Saeed Ashraf FRCS(CTh) MD
Consultant Cardiothoracic Surgeon,
Regional Cardiothoracic Centre,
The Morriston Hospital, and Honorary Senior Lecturer,
University of Swansea,
Swansea, UK

Farah NK Bhatti
Specialist Registrar in Cardiothoracic Surgery,
Wythenshawe Hospital,
Manchester, UK

Piet W Boonstra
Department of Cardiothoracic Surgery,
University Hospital,
Groningen, The Netherlands

Walt Carpenter
Director of Cardiopulmonary R&D,
Medtronic Perfusion Systems,
Minneapolis, MN, USA

W Randolph Chitwood Jr MD
Senior Associate Vice Chancellor and Director,
North Carolina Cardiovascular Institute,
Professor and Chairman,
Professor of Surgery,
Chief, Division of Cardiothoracic and Vascular Surgery,
The Brody School of Medicine,
East Carolina University,
Greenville, NC, USA

Dai H Chung MD
Assistant Professor of Surgery,
Chief, Section of Pediatric Surgery,
Department of Surgery,
University of Texas Medical Branch,
Galveston, TX, USA

Mike Cross
Consultant Anaesthetist,
Yorkshire Heart Centre,
The General Infirmary at Leeds,
Leeds, UK

Ralph E Delius MD
Children's Hospital of Michigan,
Detroit, MI, US

Carin van Doorn
Senior Lecturer in Cardiothoracic Surgery,
University College London,
and Honorary Consultant Cardiothoracic Surgeon,
Cardiothoracic Unit,
Great Ormond Street Hospital for Children,
London, UK

Martin Elliott
Consultant Cardiothoracic Surgeon,
Cardiothoracic Unit,
Great Ormond Street Hospital for Children,
London, UK

John WC Entwistle III MD PhD
Assistant Professor of Cardiothoracic Surgery,
Department of Cardiothoracic Surgery,
Drexel University College of Medicine,
Philadelphia, PA, USA

John WW Gothard FRCA
Consultant Anaesthetist,
Royal Brompton Hospital,
London, UK

Terry Gourlay PhD BSc (Hons) CBiol MIBiol ILTHE FRSH
British Heart Foundation Perfusion Specialist,
Department of Cardiothoracic Surgery,
NHLI,
Imperial College Medical School,
Hammersmith Hospital Campus,
London, UK

Hilary P Grocott MD FRCPC
Associate Professor,
Department of Anesthesiology,
Duke Heart Center,
Duke University Medical Center,
Durham, NC, USA

Y John Gu
Department of Cardiothoracic Surgery,
University Hospital,
Groningen, The Netherlands

Stephen D Hansbro
Department of Clinical Perfusion,
Leeds General Infirmary,
Leeds, UK

Timothy L Hooper
Consultant Cardiac Surgeon,
Wythenshawe Hospital,
Manchester, UK

Kieran Horgan
Department of General Surgery,
Leeds General Infirmary,
Leeds, UK

Jonathan AJ Hyde MD FRCS(CTh)
Consultant Cardiac Surgeon,
Royal Sussex County Hospital,
Brighton, UK

Jonathan M Johnson BSc ACP
Chief Clinical Perfusionist,
Royal Sussex County Hospital,
Brighton, UK

Bruce Jones
Cardiopulmonary Product Manager,
Medtronic Perfusion Systems,
Minneapolis, MN, USA

Philip H Kay MA DM FRCS
Consultant Cardiothoracic Surgeon,
The Yorkshire Heart Centre,
The General Infirmary,
Leeds, UK

Alan P Kypson MD
Assistant Professor of Surgery,
Division of Cardiothoracic Surgery,
Brody School of Medicine,
East Carolina University,
Greenville, NC, USA

G Burkhard Mackensen MD
Assistant Professor,
Klinik für Anaesthesiologie,
Technische Universität München,
Klinikum rechts der Isar,
München, Germany

Joseph P McGoldrick MD FRCS
Consultant Cardiothoracic Surgeon,
The Yorkshire Heart Centre,
The General Infirmary at Leeds,
Leeds, UK

Anil Kumar Mulpur MS MCh FRCS (Edin)
FRCS (Glasgow) FRCS C/Th (Edin) FETCS
Consultant Cardiothoracic Surgeon,
Sri Sathya Sai Institute of Higher Medical Sciences,
Whitefield, Bangalore, India

Christopher M Munsch ChM FRCS (C/Th)
Consultant Cardiothoracic Surgeon,
Department of Cardiothoracic Surgery,
The Yorkshire Heart Centre,
The General Infirmary,
Leeds, UK

Linda Nel FRCA
Consultant Anaesthetist,
Southampton University Hospitals Trust,
Southampton, UK

Mark F Newman MD
Professor and Chairman,
Department of Anesthesiology,
Duke Heart Center,
Duke University Medical Center,
Durham, NC, USA

Dumbor Ngaage
Department of Cardiothoracic Surgery,
Leeds General Infirmary,
Leeds, UK

John Pollitt
Department of General Surgery,
Leeds General Infirmary,
Leeds, UK

Stephen Robins PgDip AACP
Chief Clinical Perfusionist,
New Cross Hospital,
Wolverhampton, UK

Satoshi Saito MD PhD
Senior Clinical Research Fellow,
Department of Cardiothoracic Surgery,
Oxford Heart Centre,
John Radcliffe Hospital,
Oxford, UK

Ludwig K Von Segesser
Service de Chirurgie Cardio-Vasculaire,
Centre Hospitalier Universitaire Vaudois (CHUV),
Lausanne, Switzerland

Samir Shah
Department of Cardiothoracic Surgery,
Leeds General Infirmary,
Leeds, UK

Alfred H Stammers MSA CCP
Chief Perfusionist,
Department of Surgery,
Geisinger Medical Center,
Danville, PA, USA

Editor, Journal of Extracorporeal Technology

Jeanne Stanislawski
Cardiopulmonary Product Manager,
Medtronic Perfusion Systems,
Minneapolis, MN, USA

Wendy Svee
Cardiopulmonary Product Manager,
Medtronic Perfusion Systems,
Minneapolis, MN, USA

Kenneth M Taylor
Professor of Cardiac Surgery,
Department of Cardiothoracic Surgery,
NHLI,
Imperial College Medical School,
Hammersmith Hospital Campus,
London, UK

Andrew S Wechsler MD
Professor and Chairman,
Department of Cardiothoracic Surgery,
Drexel University College of Medicine,
Philadelphia, PA, USA

Stuart Welland
European Marketing Manager,
Medtronic Europe Sàrl,
Tolochenaz, Switzerland

Stephen Westaby PhD FETCS MS
Consultant Cardiac Surgeon,
Department of Cardiothoracic Surgery,
Oxford Heart Centre,
John Radcliffe Hospital,
Oxford, UK

Michael Whitehorne MSC ACP FCCPS
Consultant Clinical Perfusion Scientist,
Department of Cardiothoracic Surgery,
King's College Hospital,
London, UK

Joseph B Zwischenberger MD
Professor of Surgery, Medicine, and Radiology,
Director, General Thoracic Surgery and ECMO Programs,
Division of Cardiothoracic Surgery,
University of Texas Medical Branch,
Galveston, TX, USA

Foreword

I am most grateful to the editors for their invitation to write the foreword for this – the fourth edition of *Techniques of Extracorporeal Circulation*. My office bookcase currently contains the three previous editions, and if I am not considered presumptuous, I look forward to adding a copy of this fourth edition.

John Gibbon received international acclaim for his courage and determination on the 50th anniversary of that historic open-heart operation in Philadelphia on May 5th 1953 when the heart–lung machine was used successfully in a patient for the first time. Fifty years does not seem to me to be that long, although when I was younger (i.e. not over 50) my opinions were different. It is always fascinating to hear graphic personal accounts of those early days of cardiopulmonary bypass where the challenges seemed almost insuperable.

Things are very different 50 years on. The technology and the practice of cardiopulmonary bypass have been refined to an exceptional degree. The benefits to the cardiac surgical patients and the cardiac team of surgeons, anaesthetists, perfusionists and nursing staff have been incalculable. I was asked a few years ago to give a talk on the topic: 'Can cardiopulmonary bypass become more patient friendly?' I observed at the start of the talk that cardiopulmonary bypass had been a *great* friend to cardiac surgical patients and to cardiac surgeons and their colleagues, and that John Gibbon would be turning over in his grave at the very thought of the topic I had been given.

I was exaggerating of course, and Gibbon and his fellow pioneers would be the very last to encourage complacency regarding cardiopulmonary bypass. As it so happened, the following year I was asked to speak to another question: 'Is cardiopulmonary bypass in 2001 as good as it gets?' I trust you will already have worked out that I was somewhat negative in my response to that proposition!

They say that things come along in threes – and it fell to me to address another cardiopulmonary bypass related question in 2002. 'Would you invest in cardiopulmonary bypass in 2002?' was the title. I found this exercise particularly interesting. By then, cardiac surgery and cardiopulmonary bypass were each facing major challenges to their future importance. For cardiac surgery, the challenge – indeed the threat – was the increasing preference for medical revascularisation (percutaneous transluminal coronary angioplasty, stents, the expanding range of percutaneous coronary interventions) at the expense of what we used to consider the unassailable gold standard: conventional coronary artery bypass graft surgery.

For cardiopulmonary bypass and the perfusion professionals, the challenge was different, but no less daunting: would off-pump coronary bypass render the use of cardiopulmonary bypass in coronary surgery obsolete? One might reasonably assume that now is *not* the time to invest in cardiopulmonary bypass – far too risky! I beg to differ, however. I would suggest that now is precisely the time for investment in cardiopulmonary bypass. It should, however, be specifically targeted investment, a balanced investment portfolio.

First, the further continual refinement of cardiopulmonary bypass remains as great a challenge and an opportunity now as it was in the 1950s. Developments in medicine in general (particularly including molecular science and genetics/genomics) offer great potential to increase our understanding of the fundamental pathophysiological mechanisms of cardiopulmonary bypass and consequently introduce more effective preventative and therapeutic strategies.

Second, we need to broaden our horizons as far as extracorporeal circulation is concerned. Its potential roles in other forms of surgery (both in cardiac and non-cardiac) in local circulations and in systemic circulatory and respiratory support present a wealth of opportunities.

Third and finally, to quote the UK Prime Minister Tony Blair (who interestingly was born on May 5th 1953 – Gibbon's historic day) '... education, education, education'. We need to apply ourselves, both individually and in the medical and perfusion schools of the future. New science brings with it new terminologies – we need to learn the languages. Then we can communicate with the basic scientists, with molecular experts, with geneticists and who knows who else!

It may be a daunting prospect for us, but spare a thought also for the basic scientists – when have they ever before been visited by an enthusiastic perfusionist or cardiac surgical trainee?

So these are the challenges, and the opportunities. This textbook will help considerably. Philip Kay and Chris Munsch have brought into this book the right subjects and the right authors. This book contains a lot of information, which can be a launch pad for new ideas and new questions.

Are there risks? Of course there are! We must never forget, however, that in cardiac surgery we come from an honourable tradition of risk-takers. As one of the North American insurance corporations proclaims in its advertising: 'the only risk is not to take one'.

John Gibbon would profoundly agree with that.

Professor Kenneth M Taylor MD FRCS
FRCSE FESC FETCS FSA
BHF Professor of Cardiac Surgery

Preface to Fourth Edition — 50 years on

In May 1953 Edmund Hilary and Sherpa Tensing became the first men to stand on the summit of Mount Everest. In that same month came John Gibbon's moment of triumph, with the first successful use of mechanical cardiopulmonary bypass in a human patient.

The seed had been sown and it subsequently fell to other pioneers to develop the science of extracorporeal circulation.

Leeds was at the forefront of this exciting development and, in 1957, Geoffrey Wooler used cardiopulmonary bypass to repair a mitral valve. He then went on to edit the first edition of *Techniques in Extracorporeal Circulation*, published in 1976. The change in authorship and content of the subsequent three editions reflects the evolution of the speciality over a generation of cardiac surgery.

Who, reading the first edition, would have predicted that the fourth edition, 27 years later, would contain chapters on robotic surgery and off-pump surgery? Will the combined threat of increasing angioplasty and off-pump surgery make the clinical perfusionist obsolete? Whatever happens there is no doubt that clinical perfusion will continue to evolve and develop. We believe that this fourth edition of *Techniques in Extracorporeal Circulation* deserves a place on the bookshelves of all healthcare professionals working in the cardiac surgical operating room. We suspect, in an era of electronic communication, that the bookshelf may well be the first to become obsolete.

Progress in surgery is often compared with mountaineering and exploration (and contributors to this book have themselves used the analogy). A lot has happened in both spheres in the past 50 years. With that in mind, we would like to follow in John Hunt's illustrious footsteps and, as he did in *The Ascent of Everest*, dedicate this book … 'To those who made it possible'.

Philip Kay and Chris Munsch
Leeds
2003

Preface to Third Edition

The heart is a unique organ, simple in concept as a muscle pump, but complex in design and function. Heart failure, from whatever cause, remains the commonest cause of death in the western world.

It is now almost 100 years since von Reyn contravened the dictates of Billroth, risked 'loosing the esteme of his colleagues' and successfully operated on the heart. However, cardiac surgery proceeded at a slow pace until the development of the extracorporeal circuit. Thereafter the understanding of the complex anatomy, biochemistry, pharmacology and physiology of the heart has enabled us to take great strides in the complex repair work that is now so common place in the operating room. Concomitantly, advances in rheology and material science have provided a wider safety margin and therefore expanded the number of patients able to benefit from cardiac surgery. It is these advances that form the basis of the third edition of *Techniques in Extracorporeal Circulation*.

The first edition of this book, edited by Mr M. Ionescu and Mr G. Wooller 16 years ago, laid a solid foundation for the student of extracorporeal circulation. It was followed by a second edition five years later and, after a further 11 years, by this edition. Yet progress in this field is so fast that many of the new developments in this book were not even contemplated in the final 'future developments' chapter of the second edition, and so I am sure will be the case for the fourth edition. Similarly, much progress has been made during the three years it has taken to produce this book. Nevertheless, this edition, like the original, provides a firm basis for doctors, nurses, perfusionists and physicians' assistants alike, all students of the extracorporeal circulation and its ever increasing number of applications.

I hope that it will stimulate its readers to continuing the pioneering interface between the lone surgeon and the increasingly complex machinery that surrounds him.

P.H. Kay

Preface to Second Edition

The preface to the first edition of this book was preceded by Michelangelo's humble remark 'ancora imparo'. Even for the contents of this small book on techniques in extracorporeal circulation it proved its timeless veracity as we 'continue to learn'.

The first edition, however, despite many short-comings, has fulfilled its role.

During the past few years the energetic clinical and research activities have led to many advances and have further broadened the concept of artificial circulation and oxygenation so that an increasing number of sub-specialties are now attaining a certain contour.

In recent years, several areas of extracorporeal circulation have assumed increasing importance. The progress made in the field of ischaemic heart disease and the major impact of myocardial protection through cardioplegia are only two of the most obvious examples. Refinements in the construction and performance of bubble oxygenators and the introduction of disposable membrane oxygenating systems have changed the techniques of heart–lung bypass and broadened its scope.

Many pioneers in these fields have discovered and rediscovered noteworthy features of great clinical significance.

This second edition attempts to summarize the major technical problems and touches on some of the more theoretical aspects of extracorporeal circulation but does not necessarily provide final answers.

In an effort to keep abreast of the many advances which have occurred, a number of additional topics have been included in this present edition. Several new, outstanding contributors have participated, whilst the great majority of those chapters which appeared in the first edition have been updated or augmented.

Despite the awareness of discontinuity and reiteration, this second edition of *Techniques in Extracorporeal Circulation* retains the structure of most modern books by being comprised of a series of individual chapters.

I wish to express my enthusiasm for the privilege of editing this text and gratefully acknowledge the outstanding contributions of the authors who have joined in this endeavour.

I should like to thank Miss Wendy Lawrence for the complex and seemingly endless secretarial work.

My sincere appreciation is extended to Messrs Butterworths for their unfailing attention to detail and for the maintenance of the high standards for which they are known.

Marian I. Ionescu

Preface to First Edition

ancora imparo
Michelangelo Buonarotti

Extracorporeal circulation with an artificial heart-lung machine has established itself as the routine adjunct to intracardiac and vascular surgery. Since its introduction in 1953, this method has been progressively improved by development and simplification of the equipment and by better understanding of the body response to the alterations induced by the use of artificial perfusions.

The method, established in the experimental laboratory, has been perfected by clinical use. For many poorly understood aspects the method has continued to be investigated in the laboratory, where answers and solutions have been found for innumerable bewildering and knotty clinical problems.

A superficial look at today's methods would give the uninformed the general impression that no substantial progress has been made in the past ten years. For example, the same principle of bubble oxygenation used at the beginning of the open-heart surgery era is almost universally employed today. The same may be said for metallic prosthetic valves with a ball or disc occluder mechanism. The best method for 'myocardial preservation' during open-heart surgery is yet to be established and the Montagues of hypothermia still have to convince the Capulets of coronary perfusion of the veracity and superiority of their principle just as much as they had to ten years ago.

On closer examination, one realizes that during the past ten years an enormous wealth of data and knowledge has been accumulated and the application of this knowledge has made clinical perfusions incomparably better and safer. The results of cardiovascular surgery obtained today, whether in the newborn or the elderly, for great arteries or coronary arteries, in routine cases or in emergencies, when compared with the results obtained only ten years ago, are the best proof of progress and continuous improvement in extracorporeal circulation.

During the past few years many new and exciting principles and techniques based on extracorporeal circulation have been brought into clinical use. Deep hypothermia for heart surgery in the newborn, prolonged extracorporeal oxygenation-perfusion for pulmonary insufficiency and intra-aortic balloon pumping for circulatory assistance are some of the major achievements of the past decade.

The paucity of books devoted exclusively to extracorporeal circulation has prompted us to bring together in a single volume standard *current techniques in extracorporeal circulation* along with the more recent developments in this field. This is an attempt to answer some of the innumerable practical problems associated with the routine use of artificial circulation and oxygenation and to present some models of standardized techniques.

A major problem with such a book is to decide what to include and what to omit. We are aware that omissions have been made, but we have aimed to keep the subject matter strictly circumscribed in the interest of text size and readability. The esoteric has been omitted on purpose and emphasis is placed on the current practical methodology.

Advances in modern surgical and perfusion techniques have been developed to such a degree that an entirely new spectrum of problems evolves with each new development. Such rapid changes and improvements will certainly call for another publication in the near future, and this is another reason for limiting the size of this book.

Since this is a multi-authored book and the chapters are designed to be read separately, some reiteration has been inevitable, although an attempt was made to avoid repetition.

Major attention has been focused on the cardio-vascular system, the lung, the renal function and haematological changes. Clearly the brain, liver, gut, muscle masses and reticuloendothelial system are of great importance in the body response to extracorporeal circulation, but the measurement of their function in the cardiovascular patient is at the moment largely in the realm of the investigator. Although the principles and techniques described have become routine for practical purposes, they are by no means beyond challenge. As William Hazlitt put it 'when a thing ceases to be a subject of controversy, it ceases to be a subject of interest'.

The Editors join the contributors in hoping that this volume will be of interest to those active in the field of cardiovascular surgery.

We take great pleasure in expressing our thanks to Dr Frank Gerbode for kindly writing the Foreword of this work. We are grateful to Miss Nancy Evans for her continuous and enthusiastic help.

Completion of this book within a few months was promised, but it has taken almost two years and we appreciate the forbearance and continuous help of our publishers, Butterworth and Co. Ltd.

M.I. Ionescu

Acknowledgements

Philip H Kay and Christopher M Munsch would like to thank the individual chapter authors for their skilful and patient contributions to this beautifully crafted book.

We are also indebted to everyone at Hodder Arnold who worked so hard to make it happen.

A brief history of bypass

ANIL KUMAR MULPUR AND CHRISTOPHER M MUNSCH

INTRODUCTION

The history of cardiopulmonary bypass is, in many ways, a miniature representation of the history of all surgery. The discoveries and the experiments, the longed-for triumphs and the all too frequent disasters, the blood (especially the blood), the sweat and the tears of years of surgical endeavour are all mirrored in the evolution of cardiac surgery. In 1880 Billroth stated that 'any surgeon who wishes to preserve the respect of his colleagues, would never attempt to suture the heart'. What was once considered hazardous, outrageous or even sacrilegious has now become routine and commonplace. There is no doubt that the bravery and determination of the pioneers (both doctors and patients) has seen bypass develop rapidly. Most cardiac surgeons these days prefer their heart surgery to be, if not boring, then at least not too exciting.

Much has been written about the history of cardiopulmonary bypass and the development of cardiac surgery. The interested reader, particularly one with an eye for the flamboyant, is recommended to study *Landmarks in Cardiac Surgery* (Westaby and Bosher, 1997). This chapter could never compete in such exalted company and, in fact, subsequent chapters in the current book will cover the historical background to specific areas of bypass in greater detail. Therefore, this introductory chapter will simply document some of the major milestones in the (relatively short) journey from impossible to mundane.

THE FIRST HEART–LUNG MACHINE

The concept of cardiopulmonary bypass is rightly credited to Dr John Heysham Gibbon Jr (1903–1973). Dr Gibbon came from a family of doctors and was working with Dr Churchill at Harvard Medical School. In October 1930 a female patient, who had undergone a cholecystectomy two weeks before, collapsed due to pulmonary thrombo-embolism. Dr Churchill did undertake a pulmonary embolectomy on her, but in that era there were no survivors of this procedure in the USA. Dr Gibbon looked after this patient in her last stages. This led to the genesis of an idea that Dr Gibbon outlined (Gibbon, 1970):

> During that long night, helplessly watching the patient struggle for life as her blood became darker and veins more distended, the idea naturally occurred to me that if it were possible to remove continuously some of the blue blood from the patient's swollen veins, put oxygen into that blood and allow carbon dioxide to escape from it, and then to inject continuously the now-red blood back into the patient's arteries, we might have saved her life. We would have bypassed the obstructing embolus and performed part of the work of the patient's heart and lungs outside the body.

Dr Gibbon set out to devise a mechanical pump oxygenator and, with his wife Mary Hopkinson, spent the next 20 years in pursuit of his goal. The heart–lung machine Model I was built by International Business Machines (IBM) laboratories in 1949, by which time Gibbon was able to keep small dogs on bypass with only 10 per cent mortality, and by 1951 a machine for clinical use was built. In 1953, using Model II, an atrial septal defect was closed successfully on cardiopulmonary bypass, for the first time in history.

However, this momentous occasion had much of the feel of a false dawn. Gibbon operated on four further patients, all of whom died. He became disillusioned with the technique and critical of his own surgical abilities, and called a halt to the programme.

All was not lost though, and John Kirklin, using a modified Model II, operated on eight patients with intra-cardiac defects, with just four deaths, only one of which he attributed directly to complications of bypass. The impetus had been regained and further progress in mechanical cardiopulmonary bypass was stimulated.

OXYGENATION

The historical development of oxygenators is summarized in Fig. 1.1. Many methods of oxygenating the blood have been investigated over the years. Early experiments involved actually injecting oxygen directly into the blood stream, whilst other equally inventive techniques of oxygenation were attempted and soon abandoned. These early experiments focused purely on artificial oxygenation, without concerning themselves with the need for carbon dioxide removal. It seemed that what was actually needed was in fact a lung, either natural or artificial.

The lungs

In 1956, Campbell reported successful cardiac surgical procedures in humans on bypass, by use of dog lungs (Campbell *et al.*, 1956), and Mustard and co-workers reported the use of scrupulously washed monkey lungs for oxygenation in human cardiac surgery in 1954. These experiments, although seemingly moderately successful, were extremely complicated and soon abandoned (Mustard *et al.*, 1954; Mustard and Thomson, 1957). In 1958 Drew used patients' own lungs as the oxygenator, with a combination of right and left heart bypass and profound hypothermia (Drew and Anderson, 1959). With this technique, the time available for surgical repair was increased and more complex abnormalities could be addressed (Westaby and Bosher, 1997).

Cross-circulation

Andreasen and Watson conducted some canine experiments in Kent, England and published their results in 1952. If the superior vena caval entry into the heart was snared at the cavo-atrial junction, no dog survived beyond 10 minutes. If the snare was distal to azygos vein, allowing azygos venous flow into the right atrium, there

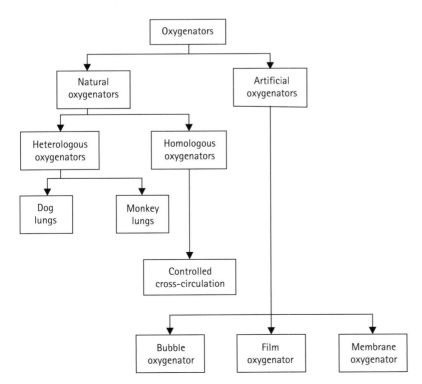

Figure 1.1 *Development of oxygenators for cardiopulmonary bypass.*

was adequate flow to prevent cerebral damage for up to 40 minutes. This finding challenged the existing notion that flows equivalent to normal cardiac output were necessary to prevent damage to vital centres, and suggested that in fact only eight to nine per cent of normal flow was needed (Andreasen and Watson, 1952).

Lillehei, at the University of Minnesota, recognized the significance of these findings for cardiac surgery (Lillehei, 2000). After a series of careful experiments (Cohen and Lillehei, 1954), he introduced the technique of 'controlled cross-circulation'. As the name suggests, the technique used an adult whose circulation was connected to a child patient, the adult subject acting as the oxygenator. In Lillehei's own words, 'controlled' refers to the use of a pump to precisely control the balance of the volume of blood flowing into and out of the donor and the patient.

This was a daring and innovative idea. These operations carried a theoretical 200 per cent mortality. In fact, there was no donor mortality in 45 operations. Of 45 patients, 28 survived and were discharged from hospital, many surviving for as long as 30 years (Lillehei et al., 1986). Controlled cross-circulation, however, was limited in its use and could not fully support the circulation. At the same time, more conventional forms of extracorporeal circulation were being developed, and before long Lillihei himself went on to develop a new pump oxygenator.

Bubble oxygenators

Simple measures to bubble oxygen into the blood met with disastrous results because of air embolism. Clark and co-workers had a breakthrough in 1950, when they started to use small glass beads or rods coated with DC Antifoam A, made by the Dow Corning Company in Michigan (Clark et al., 1950). This concept was further developed by Lillehei and DeWall, who used a spiral settling tube with a helical system that largely eliminated bubbles. The initial models were sterilized and re-used. Later on, disposable bubble oxygenators were developed. The first clinical use of the DeWall–Lillehei bubble oxygenator was on 13 May 1955, for a three-year-old child with a ventricular septal defect and pulmonary hypertension. By use of normothermia, a Sigmamotor pump and flows of 25–30 mL/kg, Lillehei reported the first success story with the bubble oxygenator (Lillehei et al., 1956).

Bubble oxygenators were later refined to serve adult patients. The Rygg–Kyvsgaard bag (Rygg and Kyvsgaard, 1956) combined the bubbling and settling chambers with a reservoir, all in one plastic bag. Sponges made of polyethylene and coated with antifoam agent were used for bubble removal. This model was manufactured in Denmark. Up to 3 L/min flows were possible. Gott and co-workers developed a self-contained unitized plastic sheet oxygenator, and improved the DeWall–Lillehei bubble oxygenator further, which meant that the bubble oxygenator became available as a sterile sealed unit. This development played a significant role in expanding cardiac surgery beyond Minnesota (Gott et al., 1957a,b).

Naef (1990) wrote:

> the home made helix reservoir bubble oxygenator of DeWall and Lillehei, first used clinically on May 13, 1955, went to conquer the world and helped many teams to embark on the correction of malformations inside the heart in a precise and unhurried manner. The road to open-heart surgery had been opened.

DeWall went on to develop the bubble oxygenator further and introduced the oxygenator and omnithermic heat exchanger in a disposable and pre-sterilized polycarbonate unit (DeWall et al., 1966). With the advent of better technology, and safer operations under more controlled circumstances, surgeons were, for the first time, appreciating the intricacies of pathologic anatomy in congenital and acquired heart disease, and leading to the development of surgical techniques in the present form.

Film oxygenators

Gibbon developed a film oxygenator with a rapidly revolving vertical cylinder. The film itself was a thin film of blood on the metal plate, where the oxygenation took place. In the first model, there was no reservoir. Gas flow included a 95 per cent oxygen and five per cent carbon dioxide mixture at 5 L/min. The venous and arterial sides of the oxygenators had roller pumps and blood passed through tubing, which was immersed in a waterbath to maintain a constant temperature throughout the perfusion. Flows of up to 500 mL/min were generated with the initial model (Gibbon, 1937). Next, a wire mesh was introduced to produce a turbulent blood–gas interface to improve oxygenation (Gibbon, 1954). This was further improvised at the Mayo Clinic, with 14 wire meshes enclosed in a lucite case. Blood flowed onto the screens through a series of 0.6 micron slots. Gas flow was 10 L of oxygen, and the carbon dioxide flow was varied depending on the pH of the blood (Kirklin et al., 1955). However, compared with the DeWall–Lillehei bubble oxygenator, the Mayo Clinic Gibbon film oxygenator, although impressive, was handcrafted and expensive, and difficult to use and maintain.

Kay and Cross developed a rotating disk film oxygenator in Cleveland, USA. Although this device did become commercially available, it had serious drawbacks in terms of ease of use, massive priming volumes, and difficulty in cleaning and sterilizing (Cross et al., 1956; Kay et al., 1956).

Membrane oxygenators

By 1944, Kolff had refined a cellophane membrane apparatus for dialysis as an artificial kidney. He later tried to use this as a membrane oxygenator, but found it to be inefficient (Kolff and Berk, 1944; Kolff and Balzer, 1955). However, Clowes and Neville developed a teflon membrane oxygenator for human usage in 1957. The membrane area was 25 m^2, but the oxygenator was bulky with problems of sterilization and assembly (Clowes and Neville, 1957). Once silicone became available as a membrane with satisfactory permeability to both oxygen and carbon dioxide, Bramson and colleagues (Bramson *et al.*, 1965) reported a new disposable membrane oxygenator with integral heat exchanger. This model had 14 cells, each having a silicone rubber membrane across which diffusion took place. Bodell *et al.* (1963) proposed the use of tubular capillary membranes instead of film, and this notion led to the hollow-fibre membrane oxygenators. Not to be outdone, Lillehei was also associated with the availability of the first compact, disposable and commercially manufactured membrane oxygenator for clinical use (Lande *et al.*, 1967).

PUMPING THE BLOOD

A critical component of the heart bypass apparatus is some form of efficient atraumatic mechanical pump. A variety of pumping devices was developed before the double roller pump became widely used. Dale and Schuster (1928) developed a diaphragm pump with valved inlet and outlet ports, but a single pump could not generate sufficient flow, so Jongbloed used six pumps of this type in parallel to conduct cardiopulmonary bypass (Jongbloed, 1949). In Minnesota, Lillehei's group initially used a multicam activated sigmamotor pump.

However, as early as 1934, DeBakey had modified a previously available Porter–Bradley roller pump for rapid blood transfusion (DeBakey, 1934). This pump was applied to cardiopulmonary bypass, and rapidly became – and remains – the most common type of pump in use for clinical perfusion.

HAEMODILUTION

Two major problems were identified in patients after cardiopulmonary bypass, namely 'post-perfusion syndrome' and 'homologous blood syndrome'. In the early days the oxygenators and the circuit were primed with donor blood. Zuhdi *et al.* (1961a, 1961b), however, developed the concept of haemodilution with five per cent dextrose and thus began the usage of clear priming or crystalloid

priming of the cardiopulmonary bypass circuits. DeWall and Lillehei subsequently confirmed the benefits of haemodilution on cardiopulmonary bypass (DeWall and Lillehei, 1962; DeWall *et al.*, 1962; Lillehei, 1962). Despite abundant literature, the actual degree of acceptable haemodilution remains controversial even today.

HYPOTHERMIA

Historically, it is interesting to note that hypothermia usage in cardiac surgery precedes the development of cardiopulmonary bypass. Following his earlier work on the treatment of frostbite, William Bigelow had already done extensive experimental work on dogs on the physiological effects of hypothermia (Bigelow *et al.*, 1950). He predicted the possible use of hypothermia in cardiac surgery thus:

> The use of hypothermia as a form of anesthetic could conceivably extend the scope of surgery in many new directions. A state in which the body temperature is lowered and the oxygen requirements of tissue are reduced to a small fraction of normal would allow exclusion of organs from the circulation for prolonged periods. Such a technic might permit surgeons to operate upon the 'bloodless heart' without recourse to extra corporal pumps, and perhaps allow transplantation of organs.

These experiments soon led to the use of hypothermia alone, with inflow occlusion but without cardiopulmonary bypass, for the treatment of atrial septal defects. On 2 September, 1952 Dr F. John Lewis and his team closed an ostium secundum atrial septal defect in a five-year-old girl on inflow occlusion and moderate total body hypothermia.

Gollan should be given the credit of working on the concept of combining hypothermia and cardiopulmonary bypass, before either actually became clinically applicable (Gollan *et al.*, 1955). Sealy, of Duke University, North Carolina, USA, subsequently employed a combination of cardiopulmonary bypass and hypothermia for the first time in a clinical situation for closure of atrial septal defect and this operation lasted for seven hours and 15 minutes! By 1958, Sealy reported a series of 49 patients operated on by the combined technique (Sealy *et al.*, 1958). As mentioned previously, Drew took the temperature down to 12–15°C and pioneered the concept of circulatory arrest for cardiac surgery (Drew and Anderson, 1959).

HEPARIN

It is almost impossible to imagine the conduct of cardiopulmonary bypass without the use of heparin.

The discovery of heparin is an interesting story (Jaques, 1978), and in the history of medicine is quoted as a classical example of 'serendipity'. Horace Well coined this term in 1754; 'The Three Princes of Serendip', was the title of a fairy tale in which the heroes were always making fortunate discoveries (Concise OED, 2002). McLean was a medical student working with W. H. Howell in 1916, on the nature of ether soluble procoagulants, and by chance discovered a phospholipid anti-coagulant. Some years later a water-soluble mucopolysaccharide was identified by Howell, and this proved to be heparin (McLean, 1959). Even today, except in very rare circumstances, where it cannot be used, because of genuine hypersensitivity or heparin-induced thrombocytopenias, heparin and cardiopulmonary bypass are inseparable.

SUMMARY

The history of cardiopulmonary bypass is a truly fascinating story. Against many difficulties, with a combination of perseverance, intellect and skill, the early pioneers developed the art of cardiopulmonary bypass as we see it today. A large range of congenital and acquired heart diseases can be treated surgically with the aid of cardiopulmonary bypass. With advancing technology, cardiopulmonary bypass continues to develop. Advances such as heparin-bonded circuits, methods minimizing systemic inflammatory response, percutaneous applications of bypass, port access surgery, continued improvement in oxygenators and ventricular assist devices; all these and others will change the picture of cardiopulmonary bypass beyond recognition, and the present day will then become the history.

Key early events in the development of extracorporeal circulation

- 1916: McLean; discovery of heparin.
- 1930: Gibbon; initial idea of cardiopulmonary bypass.
- 1934: DeBakey; concept of roller pump for extracorporeal circulation.
- 1950: Bigelow; profound hypothermia for open-heart surgery.
- 1953: Gibbon; first successful clinical use of cardiopulmonary bypass.
- 1954: Lillehei; use of controlled cross-circulation.

FURTHER READING

- General reading: Westaby, S., Bosher, C. 1997: *Landmarks in cardiac surgery*. Oxford: ISIS Medical Media, 1997. A very well-written book on the history of cardiac surgery.

REFERENCES

Andreasen, A.T., Watson, F. 1952: Experimental cardiovascular surgery. *British Journal of Surgery* **39**, 548–51.

Bigelow, W.G., Lindsay, W.K., Greenwood, W.F. 1950: Hypothermia: its possible role in cardiac surgery. An investigation of factors governing survival in dogs at low body temperatures. *Annals of Surgery* **132**, 849–66.

Bodell, B.R., Head, J.M., Head, L.R. 1963: A capillary membrane oxygenator. *Journal of Thoracic and Cardiovascular Surgery* **46**, 639–50.

Bramson, M.L., Osborn, J.J., Main, F.B. *et al.* 1965: A new disposable membrane oxygenator with integral heat exchanger. *Journal of Thoracic and Cardiovascular Surgery* **50**, 391–400.

Campbell, G.S., Crisp, N.W., Brown, E.B. Jr. 1956: Total cardiac bypass in humans utilising a pump and heterologous lung oxygenator (dog lung). *Surgery* **40**, 364–71.

Clark, L.C., Gollan, F., Gupta, V.B. 1950: The oxygenation of blood by gas dispersion. *Science* **III**, 85–7.

Clowes, G.H.S., Neville, W.E. 1957: Further development of a blood oxygenator dependent upon the diffusion of gases through plastic membranes. *Transactions of the American Society for Artificial Internal Organs* **3**, 53–8.

Cohen, M., Lillehei, C.W. 1954: A quantitative study of the 'azygos factor' during vena caval occlusion in the dog. *Surgery, Gynecology and Obstetrics* **98**, 225–32.

Concise Oxford English Dictionary (Tenth edition). 2002: Oxford: Oxford University Press.

Cross, F.S., Berne, R.M., Hirose, Y. *et al.* 1956: Description and evaluation of a rotating disc type reservoir oxygenator. *Surgical Forum* **7**, 274–8.

Dale, H.H., Schuster, E.A. 1928: A double perfusion pump. *Journal of Physiology* **64**, 356–64.

DeBakey, M.E. 1934: A simple continuous flow blood transfusion instrument. *New Orleans Med Surg J* **87**, 386–9.

DeWall, R., Lillehei, C.W. 1962: Simplified total body perfusion-reduced flows, moderate hypothermia and hemodilution. *Journal of the American Medical Association* **179**, 430–4.

DeWall, R., Lillehei, C.W., Sellers, R. 1962: Hemodilution perfusion for open heart surgery. *New England Journal of Medicine* **266**, 1078–84.

DeWall, R.A., Bentley, D.J., Hirose, M. *et al.* 1966: A temperature controlling (omnithermic) disposable bubble oxygenator for total body perfusion. *Diseases of the Chest* **49**, 207–11.

Drew, C., Anderson, I.M. 1959: Profound hypothermia in cardiac surgery. *Lancet* April 11: 748–50.

Gibbon, J.H. Jr. 1937: Artificial maintenance of circulation during experimental occlusion of pulmonary artery. *Archives of Surgery* **34**, 1105–31.

Gibbon, J.H. Jr. 1954: Application of mechanical heart and lung apparatus to cardiac surgery. *Minnesota Medicine* **37**, 171–80.

Gibbon, J.H. Jr. 1970: The development of the heart–lung apparatus. *Rev Surg* **27**, 231–44.

Gollan, F., Phillips, R., Grace, J.T. *et al.* 1955: Open left heart surgery in dogs during hypothermic asystole with and without extracorporeal circulation. *Journal of Thoracic Surgery* **30**, 626–30.

Gott, V.L., DeWall, R.A., Paneth, M. *et al.* 1957a: A self contained, disposable oxygenator of plastic sheet for intracardiac surgery. *Thorax* **12**, 1–9.

Gott, V.L., Sellers, R.D., DeWall, R.A. *et al.* 1957b: A disposable unitized plastic sheet oxygenator for open heart surgery. *Diseases of the Chest* **32**, 615–25.

Jaques, L.B. 1978: Addendum: the discovery of heparin. *Seminars in Thrombosis and Hemostasis* **4**, 350–3.

Jongbloed, J. 1949: The mechanical heart/lung system. *Surgery, Gynecology and Obstetrics* **89**, 684–91.

Kay, E.B., Zimmerman, H.A., Berne, R.M. *et al.* 1956: Certain clinical aspects in the use of the pump oxygenator. *Journal of the American Medical Association* **162**, 639–41.

Kirklin, J.W., Dushane, J.W., Patrick, R.T. *et al.* 1955: Intracardiac surgery with the aid of a mechanical pump oxygenator system (Gibbon type): report of eight cases. *Proceedings of Staff Meetings of the Mayo Clinic* **30**, 201–7.

Kolff, W.J., Balzer, R. 1955: The artificial coil lung. *Transactions of the American Society for Artificial Internal Organs* **1**, 39–42.

Kolff, W.J., Berk, H.T.J. 1944: Artificial kidney: dialyser with a great area. *Acta Medica Scandinavica* **117**, 121–34.

Lande, A.J., Dos, S.J., Carlson, R.G. *et al.* 1967: A new membrane oxygenator–dialyser. *Surgical Clinics of North America* **47**, 1461–70.

Lillehei, C.W. 1962: Hemodilution perfusion for open heart surgery. Use of low molecular weight dextran and five per cent dextrose. *Surgery* **52**, 30–31.

Lillehei, C.W. 2000: Historical development of cardiopulmonary bypass in Minnesota. In: G.P. Gravlee *et al.* (eds), *Cardiopulmonary bypass: principles and practice* (second edition). Baltimore, MD: Lippincott Williams & Wilkins, 3–21.

Lillehei, C.W., DeWall, R.A., Read, R.C. *et al.* 1956: Direct vision intracardiac surgery in man using a simple, disposable artificial oxygenator. *Diseases of the Chest* **29**, 1–8.

Lillehei, C.W., Varco, R.L., Cohen, M. *et al.* 1986: The first open heart repairs of ventricular septal defect, atrioventricular communis, and tetralogy of Fallot using extracorporeal circulation by cross circulation: a 30 year follow up. *Annals of Thoracic Surgery* **41**, 4–21.

McLean, J. 1959: The discovery of heparin. *Circulation* **XIX**, 75–78.

Mustard, W.T., Thomson, J.A. 1957: Clinical experience with the artificial heart–lung preparation. *Journal of the Canadian Medical Association* **76**, 265–9.

Mustard, W.T., Chute, A.L., Keith, J.D. *et al.* 1954: A surgical approach to transposition of the great vessels with extracorporeal circuit. *Surgery* **36**, 39–51.

Naef, A.P. 1990: *The story of thoracic surgery*. Toronto: Hografe & Huber, 113–19.

Rygg, H., Kyvsgaard, E. 1956: A disposable polyethylene oxygenator system applied in the heart/lung machine. *Acta Chirurgica Scandinavica* **112**, 433–7.

Sealy, W.C., Brown, I.W., Young, W.G. 1958: A report on the use of both extracorporeal circulation and hypothermia for open-heart surgery. *Annals of Surgery* **147**, 603–13.

Westaby, S., Bosher, C. 1997: *Landmarks in cardiac surgery*. Oxford: ISIS Medical Media.

Zuhdi, N., McCollough, B., Carey, J. *et al.* 1961a: Hypothermic perfusion for open heart surgical procedures – report of the use of a heart–lung machine primed with five per cent dextrose in water inducing hemodilution. *J Int Coll Surg* **35**, 319–26.

Zuhdi, N., McCollough, B., Carey, J. *et al.* 1961b: Double helical reservoir heart–lung machine designed for hypothermic perfusion primed with five per cent glucose in water inducing hemodilution. *Archives of Surgery* **82**, 320–5.

2

Design and principles of the extracorporeal circuit

MEDTRONIC, INC., A MANUFACTURER OF TECHNOLOGIES FOR EXTRACORPOREAL CIRCULATION

KEY POINTS

- The essential components of the clinical extracorporeal circuit are a pump (artificial heart), an oxygenator (artificial lung), a reservoir and the tubing to connect these devices, although systems are now emerging without traditional reservoirs.
- Additional components include a heat exchanger, a system for myocardial protection, and gas and emboli filters. Secondary suction circuits may be added for salvaging shed blood, and venting the heart.
- The current generation of membrane oxygenators incorporating reservoirs and heat exchangers provide safety, efficacy and ease of use.
- Centrifugal pumps are compact, durable, easy to set up and cause minimal haemolysis compared with roller pumps. While their cost is certainly higher than a simple length of roller pump tubing, it may be more than offset by savings in ventilatory and ICU time, as well as overall hospital stay.
- A body of published evidence, as well as extensive clinical experience by surgeons and perfusionists, supports the value of heparin-based biosurfaces for thrombo-resistance and biocompatibility during extracorporeal circulation.
- It is the responsibility of the perfusionist to ensure that the organs of the body supported by

the extracorporeal circuit are adequately perfused with oxygenated blood by continual monitoring of blood flow rate, perfusion pressure, acid/base state, oxygen consumption, coagulation and renal function.

HISTORY OF CARDIOPULMONARY BYPASS

The first proposal for artificial circulation was put forward by Le Gallois in 1812 when he perfused rabbit brains through carotid arteries. Between 1848 and 1853 Brown Sequard showed that dark venous blood, when exposed to air and shaken, turned bright red. He further demonstrated the feasability of perfusing isolated brain specimens with this 'arterialized' blood. The first bubble oxygenator, utilizing the same principle of mixing venous blood with air, was assembled by Shroder in 1882. And then, two years later, von Frey and Gruber created the first membrane oxygenator, in which the direct blood–air interface of the bubbler design was avoided.

In 1900, Howell and colleagues discovered the anticoagulant properties of heparin. Without the risk of catastrophic clotting within the bypass circuit, it was now possible to expose the blood to extended periods of extracorporeal circulation.

The first clinical application of extracorporeal circulation was performed by Dr John Gibbon, Massachusetts

Table 2.1 *Developmental history of oxygenators*

Non-membrane oxygenators

1937	Gibbon	Blood filter – pulmonary embolus
1951	Dennis/Bjork	Rotating screen and cardiopulmonary bypass rotating disk
1955	Lillehei/DeWall	First bubble oxygenator with helix reservoir
1956	Kay/Cross	Refind disk oxygenator for up to 4000 mL of venous blood
1956	Rygg/Kyvsgaard	First disposable plastic bag oxygenator, Polystan (Rygg Bag)
1962	Cooley/Beall	Proposed use of commercially available disposable bubble oxygenators (Travenol Bag)
1966	DeWall/Najafe/Roden	First disposable hard shell oxygenator (polycarbonate) with built-in heat exchanger (Bentley Labs)

Membrane oxygenators

1955	Kolff/Balzfer	Oxygenated blood through polyethylene membrane (animals)
1956	Kolff	First coiled polyethylene tube oxygenator
1958	Clowes	First to test Teflon as membrane plate oxygenator
1968	Lande	Methyl silicone folded plate membrane oxygenator (Lande/Edwards)
1969	Pierce	Co-polymer of dimethyl siloxan and polycarbonate
1969	Pierce	Pierce-GE
1971	Kolobow	Silicone rubber reinforced by nylon mesh rolled or coiled (SciMed–Kolobow)
1972	Eiseman/Spencer	Expanded (Teflon) membrane sheets (Travenol/TMO)
1975	Travenol Labs	Polypropylene (expanded) plate or sheets (TMO)
1985	J&J Cardiopulmonary	First hollowfibre polypropylene oxygenator (Maxima)

General Hospital who, in 1953, successfully repaired an atrial septal defect in a young female. Despite subsequent setbacks, Dr C Walton Lillehei of the University of Minnesota and several others persevered in further developing the techniques and equipment, with Lillehei using the first bubble oxygenator in 1955.

The bubble oxygenator, first developed by Rygg, was produced commercially by 1956. The years since have seen myriad refinements and improvements in oxygenator and other component designs, which unlike the early systems are now completely disposable. A brief history of the development of oxygenators is summarized in Table 2.1.

BUBBLE OXYGENATORS

Bubble oxygenators were the first design to be commercially available in completely disposable form, and were in wide use throughout the world for more than 46 years. A 'bubbler' usually consists of an integrated design, incorporating the oxygenator, heat exchanger, arterial reservoir and cardiotomy filter in one unit. The unit functions by passing incoming venous blood over a perforated or porous sparger plate, through which oxygen is passed, turning the venous blood into a foam of variously sized bubbles. As oxygen diffuses across the bubble surfaces into the blood, and conversely, as excess carbon dioxide diffuses from the blood into the bubbles, the blood is arterialized. The blood is then passed through a silicone-based defoaming medium, collects in an arterial reservoir section and is returned to the patient. The heat exchanger in most bubble oxygenators was incorporated

into the bubble chamber. The early Bentley model has the heat exchanger located within the arterial reservoir.

Bubble oxygenators are efficient and easy to use. Unfortunately, the nature of the foaming/defoaming process causes significant haemolysis, which becomes clinically significant after only a few hours. Bubble oxygenators also present a higher risk of micro- and macro-air embolism: the defoaming process is imperfect, and inadvertent emptying of the arterial reservoir can lead to massive amounts of air being pumped directly to the patient, at least when roller pumps are used. Further, because of the bubbling process, it is not considered safe to blend oxygen with air (since nitrogen bubbles would be so much less soluble) making independent control of pO_2 and pCO_2 impossible. This would also necessitate the mixing of small amounts of carbon dioxide with the oxygen to prevent the pCO_2 from falling too far. For these reasons, bubblers are rarely used today. Several safe, efficient membrane oxygenators currently dominate the market.

MEMBRANE OXYGENATORS

Membrane oxygenators of various designs have been used sporadically since the mid-1950s, but it was not until 19 years ago that relatively low-prime volume, easy-to-use units became commercially available. In the membrane oxygenator, the ventilating gas is separated from the blood by a semi-permeable membrane fabricated from polypropylene, or in one case, silicone rubber. Unlike bubble oxygenators, there is no direct contact between the blood and ventilating gas. Gas exchange is accomplished

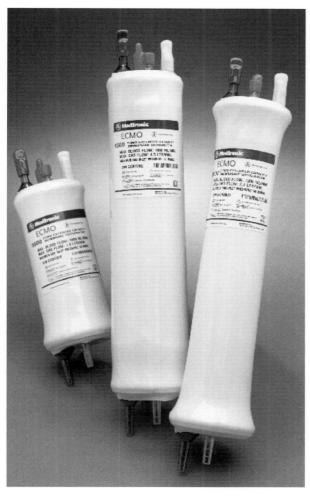

Figure 2.1 *Kolobow/SciMed/Medtronic paediatric membrane oxygenators. Photo © copyright Medtronic, Inc.*

by diffusion across the membrane, driven by the partial pressure gradients of dissolved gases between the blood side of the membrane and the gas side. This same mechanism drives respiration in the natural lung, making the membrane oxygenator a much more physiologic substitute than the bubbler for artificial ventilation. Since there is no foaming/defoaming process, it is safe to blend air with the oxygen, making independent control of pO_2 and pCO_2 possible.

Most commercially available membrane oxygenators use silicone rubber or micro-porous polypropylene. The best-known example of a silicone device is the Medtronic/Kolobow design, in which a long narrow sheet of silicone rubber is wound spirally along with spacer/support material to form two independent pathways for blood and gas. These devices are available in various sizes to accommodate different patients, from small neonates to large adults (Fig. 2.1). They are biocompatible, minimize damage to the blood and are the membrane of choice for long-term ventilatory assistance.

For routine use, the micro-porous polypropylene membrane, with its lower blood volume, is considered to be more versatile and easier to prime and use. In this design, the material is manufactured with tiny holes, too small for blood to pass through but large enough to allow gas transfer. The material can be fabricated in sheet form or more commonly, in tubular or 'microfibre' form. In most cases, the micro-fibres are arranged – much like the relationship between blood and gas in the alveoli – to allow blood to flow around the outside of the tubes while the ventilating gas passes through the lumen of the tubes. Although the arrangement has been reversed in some units, this configuration is by far the most common and considered by most practitioners to be more physiological and less damaging to the formed elements of the blood.

Modern membrane oxygenators often incorporate an integral heat exchanger where blood can be cooled or warmed before being ventilated. The Medtronic AFFINITY® oxygenator is an example of the latest in membrane/heat exchanger design and can be used with or without the integral cardiotomy/venous reservoir (Fig. 2.2).

COMPONENTS OF THE EXTRACORPOREAL CIRCUIT

The extracorporeal system consists of interconnected devices for the oxygenation and circulation of the blood, temporarily replacing the function of the heart and lungs. The main components of the circuit (Fig. 2.3) are a pump (artificial heart), an oxygenator (artificial lung), venous and cardiotomy reservoirs (sometimes integrated), a heat exchanger (usually integrated with the oxygenator), a system for myocardial protection (cardioplegia), gas and emboli filters, and the tubing to connect these devices. Typical secondary circuits include suction, provided by roller pumps or a vacuum source, for salvaging shed blood, and venting to prevent distension of the left ventricle.

PUMPS

While the oxygenator performs the ventilatory task of the lungs on cardiopulmonary bypass, the arterial pump takes over for the heart. Its sole function is to provide an adequate flow of oxygenated blood to the patient's arterial circulation. The main technical requirements of an arterial pump are as follows:

1 Wide flow range (up to 7+ L/min).
2 Low haemolytic effect.
3 Minimum turbulence and blood stagnation.
4 Simplicity and safety of use.
5 Cost-effectiveness.

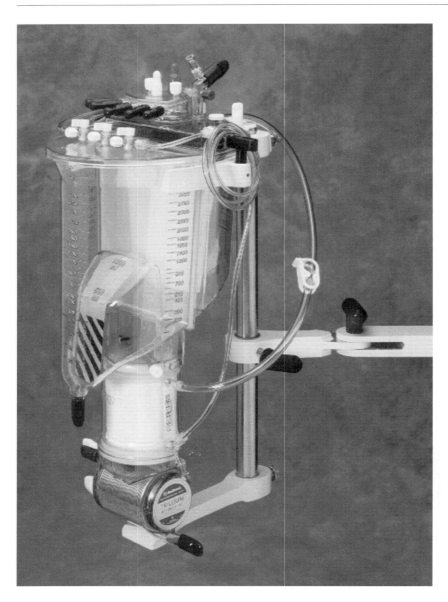

Figure 2.2 *AFFINITY® adult hollow fibre oxygenator with integrated CVR. Photo © copyright Medtronic, Inc.*

Of the myriad arterial pump designs that were applied to extracorporeal circulation in the early years, only two are in widespread use today. Worldwide, just over half of cardiopulmonary bypass procedures are performed with roller pumps, the remainder use centrifugal pumps.

Roller pumps

The roller pump (Fig. 2.4) consists of a semi-circular stator, within which is mounted a rotor with twin rollers placed at 180° to each other. The blood tubing is compressed between the stator and the rotor. Since one roller is engaged with the stator just before the other roller leaves the semi-circle, flow is unidirectional. In

order to minimize the inevitable resultant haemolysis, the rollers are adjusted axially so that the pump is slightly underocclusive. (This is defined as allowing a 1 cm/min drop along a 1 m high saline column in 3/8-inch tubing.) Flow rate in a roller pump is a derived value, calculated from the stroke volume multiplied by the revolutions per minute (RPM).

The roller pump is a simple, inexpensive, easy-to-use mechanism. One must keep in mind, however, that it is a positive-displacement pump. A line restriction upstream will create an excessive vacuum, leading to degassing of the blood and generation of a 'bubble train' inside the tubing. Conversely, a line restriction downstream will lead to immediate pressure build-up, with possible dire consequences depending on the source of the obstruction.

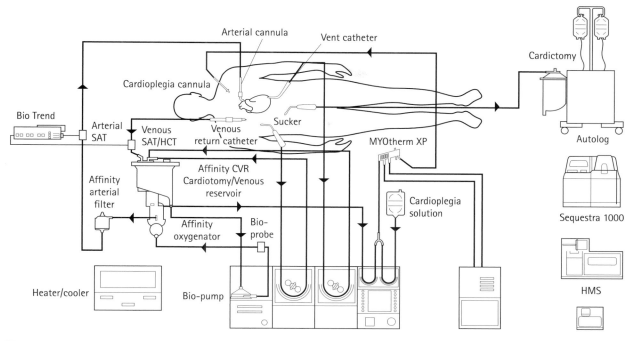

Figure 2.3 *Components of the extracorporeal circuit. Schematic © copyright Medtronic, Inc.*

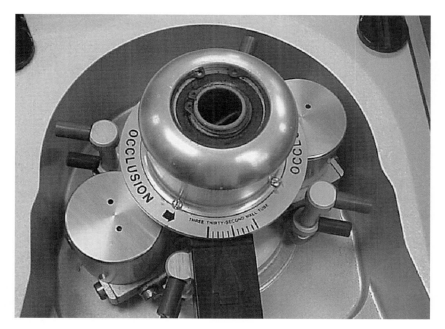

Figure 2.4 *Roller pump head. Photo © copyright Medtronic, Inc.*

A roller pump displaces air as effectively as blood, so that it is possible, for instance in the event of inadvertent emptying of a hard shell venous reservoir, to pass massive amounts of air downstream towards the patient. Several techniques and systems are utilized to mitigate against such a disaster, such as reservoir level sensors, in-line air detectors, membrane oxygenators and arterial filters.

Centrifugal pumps

The centrifugal pump is essentially a vortex generator. By spinning an impeller (which may consist of vanes or, in the case of the Medtronic Bio-Pump® Centrifugal Blood Pump, nested cones) within a housing at high speed, an area of low pressure is created in the centre, and higher

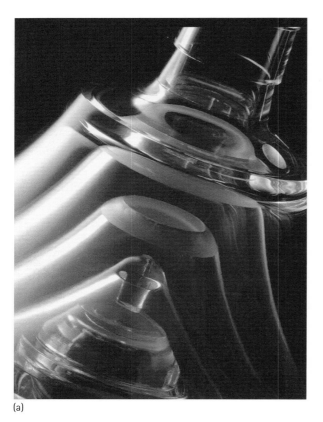

(a)

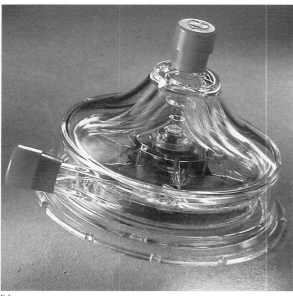

(b)

Figure 2.5 *(a) The nested cones design within the Medtronic Bio-Pump®; (b) BPX-80 adult Bio-Pump®. Photos © copyright Medtronic, Inc.*

pressure is generated along the outside circumference. Blood is drawn axially into the centre by the vortex and expelled under pressure through a port oriented tangential to the axis of rotation. With the vane design, energy is imparted to the blood by the hydrofoil configuration of the vanes. This is efficient, but can create turbulence on the trailing edges of these vanes. In the Medtronic Bio-Pump® design (Fig. 2.5 (a) and (b)) energy is imparted strictly by viscous drag inherent in the blood itself, minimizing turbulence. An inherent safety feature of centrifugal pumps is their inability to pump very large amounts of air. When air fills the pump chamber, the pump is not able to develop sufficient pressure to expel it against the backpressure of the extracorporeal circuit.

Whatever the impeller design, centrifugal pumps are all classified as non-positive displacement pumps – they will respond to changes in both pre-load and after-load with changes in flow rate, much as the native heart does.

Centrifugal pumps require in-line monitoring of the flow rate that is accomplished in the Medtronic system, for example, by electromagnetic induction. Other systems use an ultrasonic probe to detect flow. The in-line flow measurement allows accurate adjustment of the pump speed when necessary to regulate flow in the case of changes in pre-load and after-load.

Centrifugal pumps are very practical. They are compact, durable, easy to set up, and cause minimal haemolysis compared with roller pumps. While their cost is certainly higher than a simple length of roller pump tubing, it may be more than offset by savings in ventilatory and ICU time, as well as overall hospital stays that have been demonstrated in numerous clinical studies (Morgan *et al.*, 1998).

VENOUS RESERVOIR

The general functions of the venous reservoir are to accumulate blood from the patient's venous system and to remove both air and microaggregates present in venous blood. Venous reservoirs may be either rigid (hard shell) or soft (bag).

Rigid reservoir

A rigid reservoir consists of a clear plastic shell, vented to the atmosphere either by basic design or integral valve, with a provision for defoaming and gross-filtering (100– 200 μ) of incoming venous blood. Typical reservoir capacity may range from 1 L to 4.5 L (Fig. 2.6).

Soft reservoir

The soft or 'bag' reservoir is constructed of soft PVC with a 100–200 μ filtering screen. Typical reservoir capacity ranges between 200 mL and 3.0 L (Fig. 2.7).

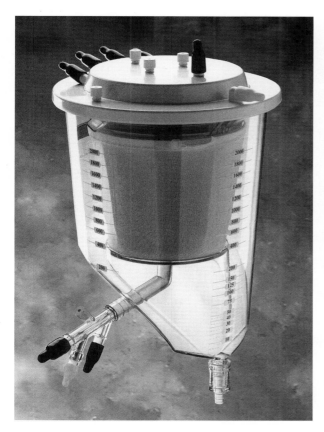

Figure 2.6 *Hard shell reservoir. Photo © copyright Medtronic, Inc.*

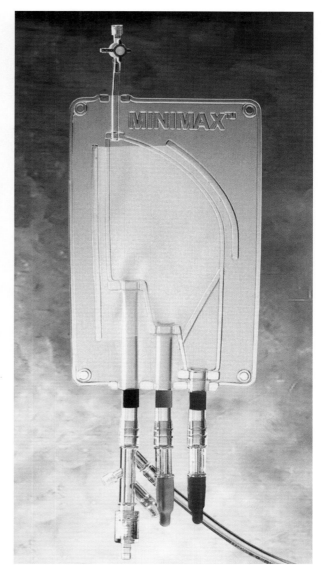

Figure 2.7 *Soft reservoir bag. Photo © copyright Medtronic, Inc.*

Hard shell reservoirs are easy to use and offer the advantage of integration with the cardiotomy function, simplifying the circuit. They can handle incoming venous air with ease. With simple modifications, hard shell reservoirs can be used for vacuum-assisted venous drainage. Their principal disadvantage is that it is very possible to empty the reservoir and pass air to the arterial pump, which, if it is a roller pump, will pass the air downstream. This risk can be mitigated somewhat with the use of reservoir level sensors and in-line air detectors, which may or may not shut the arterial pump off automatically.

Bag reservoirs can be slightly more cumbersome to use since incoming venous air does not vent automatically and must be actively aspirated from the bag. Also, they require a separate hard shell cardiotomy reservoir to handle returning cardiotomy suction blood and left ventricle vent return. Many practitioners consider them safer than hard shell reservoirs since, when maintained properly air-free, bag reservoirs will not allow massive air embolism, because the soft bag simply collapses upon emptying, presenting nothing for the arterial pump to pass. The soft shell system also may be preferable because of the elimination of the air–blood interface found in open, hard shell systems.

CARDIOTOMY RESERVOIRS

Blood from the cardiotomy suckers and vents is most often delivered to the cardiotomy reservoir. This serves as a storage area and also filters the large number of solid and gaseous micro-emboli. The rigid reservoir is made of polycarbonate, with ports that direct incoming blood through both defoaming layers and micro-aggregate filters of between 20 μ and 40 μ (Fig. 2.8).

Another option with growing acceptance is to deliver suction blood to a cell-saving device (Fig. 2.9). Here, the red cells can be separated from the activated platelets, white cells and plasma before returning them to the patient. It is common practice today to integrate

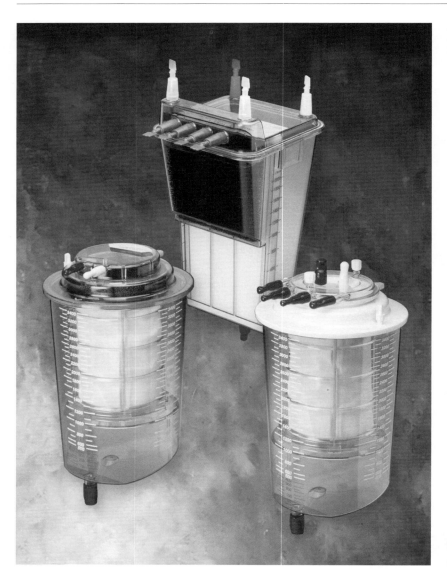

Figure 2.8 *Cardiotomy reservoirs. Photo © copyright Medtronic, Inc.*

these cardiotomy functions with a hard shell venous reservoir.

HEAT EXCHANGERS

During cardiopulmonary bypass the temperature of the perfusate may be adjusted to improve myocardial protection and optimize the operating conditions for the patient. This is accomplished within the extracorporeal circuit by one or more heat exchangers that are composed of two pathways, one for the perfusate and one for water. These pathways are separated by material that allows efficient thermal exchange between the fluids. The material may be plastic, aluminum or stainless steel, all of which have their strengths and weaknesses. Aluminum has by far the best heat exchange performance, but is not biocompatible unless coated, which degrades its performance somewhat. Plastic is inexpensive, but has relatively poor heat transfer properties and requires large surface areas. Stainless steel seems to be the most popular because of its combination of good heat exchange coefficient, ease of fabrication in either pleated or tubular form, and biocompatibility.

To adjust the temperature of the perfusate, water of variable temperatures is circulated through the heat exchanger, cooling or warming the perfusate as the clinical situation dictates. To further enhance efficiency, the water flows in the opposite direction relative to the perfusate, maximizing the temperature differential throughout the transit.

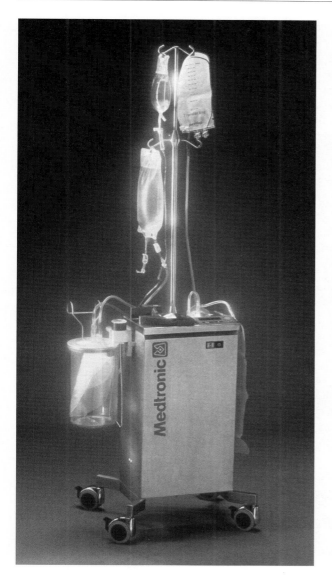

Figure 2.9 *autoLog™ autotransfusion system. Photo © copyright Medtronic, Inc.*

Heat exchangers are rated with regard to a performance factor, which may be calculated by use of the following formula:

$$\text{Performance factor} = \frac{Tbo - Tbi}{Twi - Tbi}$$

where Tbo = blood outlet temperature; Tbi = blood inlet temperature; Twi = water inlet temperature.

The theoretically perfect performance factor is therefore 1.0, with most systemic heat exchangers falling in the 0.4–0.5 range. However, the factor is heavily influenced by the flow rate, so that at the low flows (<1 L/min) typically found in cardioplegia delivery, performance factors exceeding 0.9 are attainable with some units.

TUBING

Although most research has focused on the principal components of the extracorporeal circuit, the tubing system remains a vital component. Several metres of tubing of different size and rigidity, linked by multidirectional connectors, form the pathway between the patient's venous system, through the extracorporeal circuit and back to the patient's arterial system (Fig. 2.10).

Latex rubber tubing was used in the early years because of its favourable elastic characteristics, making it especially useful for roller pumps. For some time now, however, various formulations of silicone rubber have found favour as a replacement for latex, but early formulations of silicone exhibited problems with spallation in roller heads. Polyvinyl chloride, or PVC, is the tubing of choice for most circuit applications today. It offers the advantages of greater durability, minimal spallation, availability in a wide variety of sizes and durometers (degrees of stiffness), biocompatibility and transparency. Problems with long-term leaching of plasticizers to the surface have been improved with more recent formulations.

MYOCARDIAL PROTECTION

Currently, most procedures involving cardiopulmonary bypass require cross-clamping of the aorta to isolate the heart from the circulation. This produces an ischaemic state in the myocardium that must be addressed. Historically, many practitioners used an intermittent ischaemia technique, in which the aortic cross-clamp is removed periodically to give the myocardium a chance to be reperfused with oxygenated blood. While still seen occasionally, this practice has largely been supplanted by various forms of cardioplegia – literally, paralysing of the heart. This is accomplished immediately after cross-clamping by an infusion of potassium chloride, which initiates diastolic arrest in the heart, providing a motionless field in which the surgeon can operate. Buffers are added to the solution to maintain a more favourable alkalotic environment during ischaemia, as well as osmotic agents, such as Mannitol, to prevent myocardial oedema. More recently, blood from the main circuit has been mixed with the cardioplegic solution to help support myocardial metabolism and provide natural plasma buffering against ischaemic acidosis. Metabolic substrates, such as aspartate and glutamate, are also used to better preserve cell metabolism. The cardioplegia can be administered cold or warm, intermittently or continuously, antegrade from the aortic root or retrograde through the coronary sinus. The possible variations in dosing regimen and cardioplegia composition are almost limitless, but they all share a common goal – preservation of cardiac function.

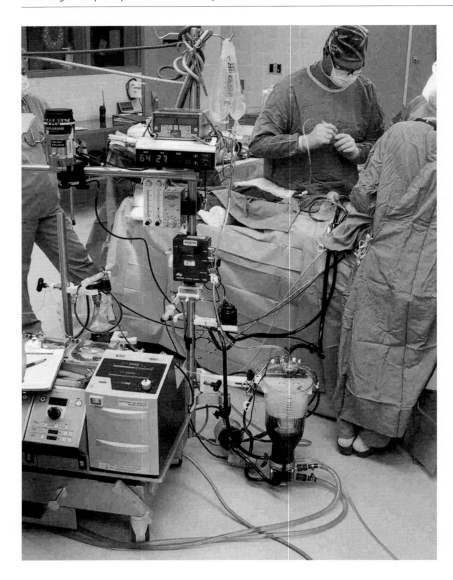

Figure 2.10 *Typical operating room set-up. Photo courtesy of Tom McDonough, CCP.*

Modern units for cardioplegia administration, such as the Medtronic MYOtherm® cardioplegia delivery system (Fig. 2.11), incorporate an integral bubble trap and heat exchanger, and the tubing necessary for adding the cardioplegia solution and mixing at a fixed ratio with the patient's blood (when used for blood cardioplegia). Cardioplegia has greatly increased the time available to the surgeon for even the most complex procedures.

BIOCOMPATIBILITY

Heparin–based biocompatible surfaces

The dilemma during cardiopulmonary bypass is that while blood in the human body is compatible with the vascular endothelium, blood outside the human body is not compatible with the large artificial surface area of extracorporeal circuits, including the air interface in open systems. The artificial surface lacks the active role normally played by endothelium in maintaining the checks and balances between the defensive systems. The foreign surface interaction may initiate multiple biological reactions involving whole defensive systems in the human body, such as the coagulation, fibrinolytic, complement, kallikrein and kinin systems. These systems may lead to the activation and consumption of platelets, the activation of leukocytes and the destruction of red blood cells. They may also lead to other inter-related reactions and substances, such as destructive enzymes released from certain blood cells, anaphylactic reactions, oxygen free radicals and endotoxins. Not only do these systems act simultaneously, they can cross-activate each other. Ultimately, these biological reactions may affect the heart, lungs, brain and other organs to cause conditions known as 'systemic inflammatory response', 'post-perfusion syndrome' or 'whole-body inflammatory response'.

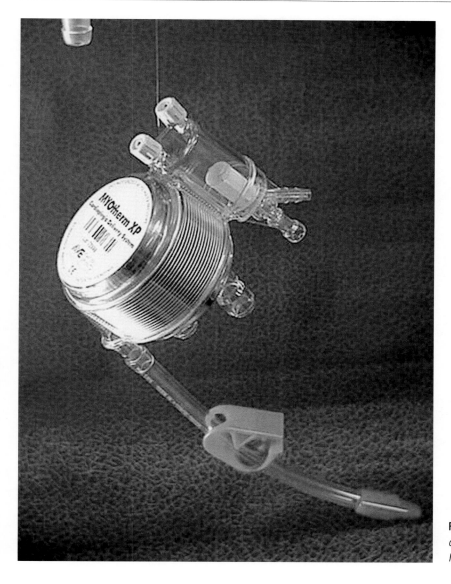

Figure 2.11 *MYOtherm® cardioplegia delivery system. Photo © copyright Medtronic, Inc.*

Healthy vascular endothelium is the ultimate biocompatible surface. Complex hemostatic mechanisms within the vascular endothelium maintain blood within the vessels without causing thrombosis. These systems initiate haemostasis to maintain vessel integrity, stimulate fibrinolysis to dispose of fibrin and clots, attack foreign bodies, activate the immune systems, and perform other roles to maintain or restore the balance between these systems. The endothelium inhibits blood coagulation by synthesizing and secreting onto its surface thrombomodulin and heparan sulfate (Coleman *et al.*, 2001), a heparin-like substance. Heparan sulfate activates antithrombin (AT), catalysing the inhibition of thrombin and factor Xa (Marcum *et al.*, 1984; Coleman *et al.*, 2001). Also, vascular endothelial cells are highly negatively charged, a feature that may repel the negatively charged platelets (Coleman *et al.*, 2001).

Heparin biosurfaces for extracorporeal circuits mimic critical characteristics of healthy endothelium for thrombo-resistance and biocompatibility during cardiopulmonary bypass. Heparin biosurfaces imitate the heparan sulfate of the vascular endothelium by inhibiting thrombin and by preventing activation of the coagulation cascade at multiple points in the coagulation cascade, including activation of Factor Xa and XIIa (Elgue *et al.*, 1993a, b; Sanchez *et al.*, 1995; Hsu, 2001). Heparin biosurfaces also limit interaction between blood and the artificial surface, and resist protein and cell deposition. Heparin biosurfaces are well-known for their role in heparin binding to antithrombin, mediating the inhibition of thrombin (Fig. 2.12).

Published clinical and scientific research indicates that heparin biosurfaces have additional mitigating effects across several human body defensive systems and at multiple points in the coagulation cascade (Fig. 2.13). Therefore,

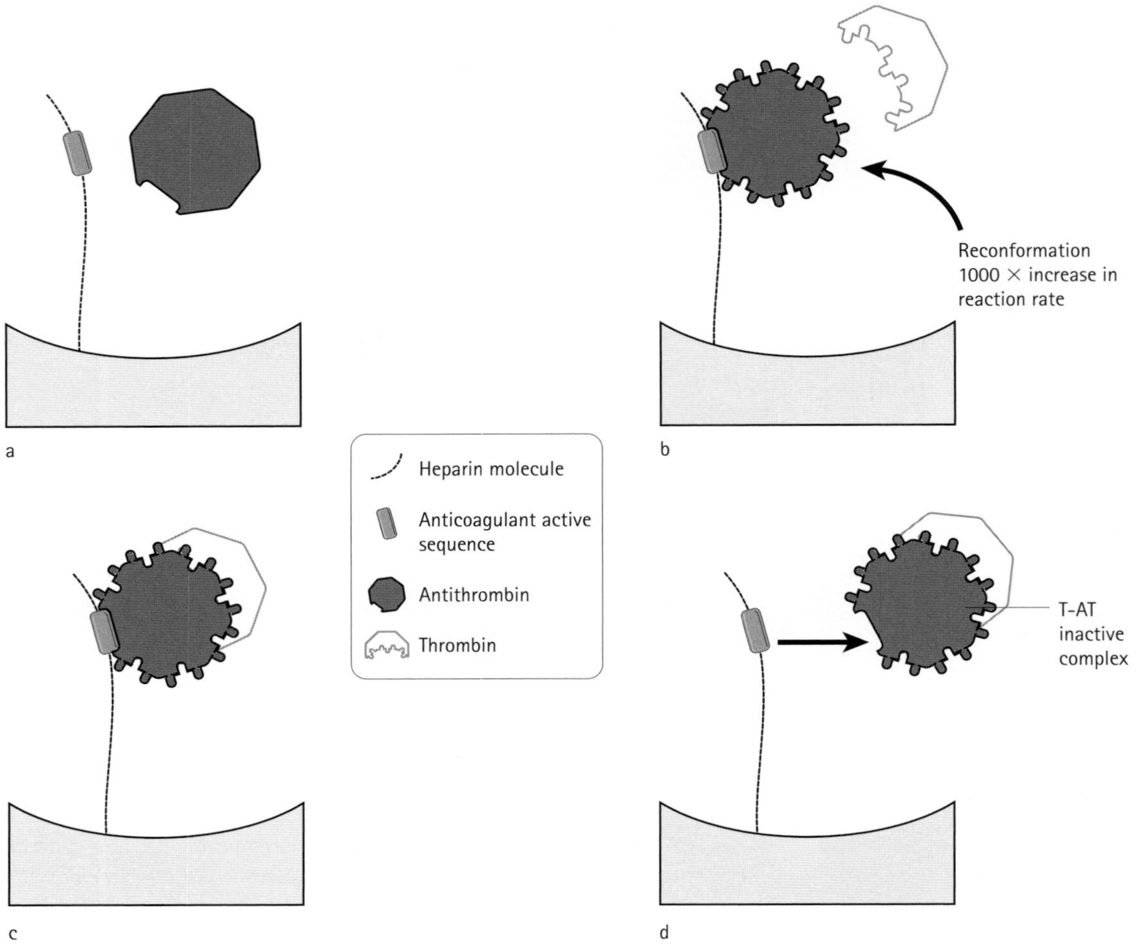

Heparin molecule

Anticoagulant active sequence

Antithrombin

Thrombin

Reconformation 1000 × increase in reaction rate

T-AT inactive complex

Figure 2.12 *(a) Shows an antithrombin molecule in close proximity to an immobilized heparin module with an available anticoagulant active site; (b) antithrombin is bound to the heparin's anticoagulant active sequence. Upon binding to heparin, the antithrombin undergoes a conformational change that increases its affinity for most of the coagulation factors in the coagulation cascade at least 1000 times; (c) heparin–antithrombin complex attaches to thrombin in the blood. Once attached to antithrombin, thrombin can no longer work to produce thrombi; (d) thrombin–antithrombin complex detaches from the heparin anticoagulant active sequence of the heparin molecule, leaving the anticoagulant active sequence intact and free to begin the bonding process over and over again. Schematic © copyright Medtronic, Inc.*

increasing numbers of cardiovascular surgeons and perfusionists are adopting the routine use of heparin biosurfaces as one component of a systems approach to reduce the deleterious effects of extracorporeal circulation.

Both Carmeda® BioActive Surface (Fig. 2.14) and Trillium™ Biosurface incorporate immobilized heparin, which provides thrombo-resistance and biocompatibility. However, Carmeda® and Trillium™ differ with respect to their heparin characteristics and other features that mimic healthy vascular endothelium. Both heparin biosurfaces provide:

- covalently bonded heparin,
- hydrophilicity,
- negative charge,
- complete coverage.

The Carmeda® BioActive Surface End-Point Attached heparin bonding process mimics the orientation of heparan sulfate on the plasma membrane of natural vascular endothelial cells to provide a stable, non-leaching, bioactive surface. With this process, an aldehyde of each heparin molecule is covalently bound to the prepared artificial surface while the remainder of the molecule, including the active binding sites, remains free to participate in biological reactions, similar to heparan sulfate molecules attached to natural endothelium. The End-Point Attachment heparin bonding process uses a stable covalent bond. Therefore, heparin does not leach from the surface into systemic circulation and remains available on the artificial surface to provide thrombo-resistance and biocompatibility. Engineering research demonstrates that Carmeda®-coated

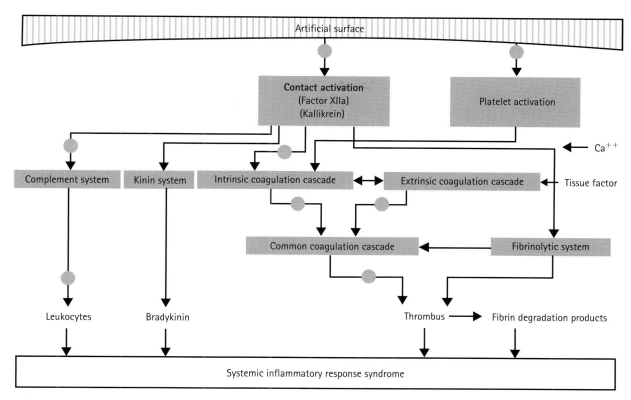

Research indicates mitigating effects by heparin biosurfaces.

Figure 2.13 *Clinical and scientific evidence supports the conclusion that heparin biosurfaces may reduce contact activation and platelet activation. Heparin biosurfaces are also found to mitigate activation of the coagulation cascade and complement systems. Graphic © copyright Medtronic, Inc.*

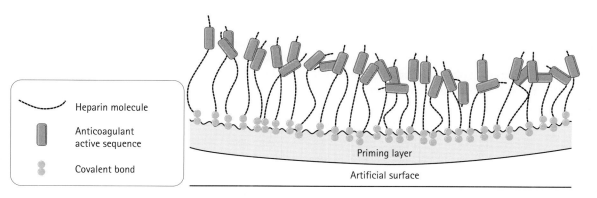

Figure 2.14 *Carmeda® BioActive Surface® helps fulfil the clinical need to mimic natural endothelium and minimize detrimental effects generated by extracorporeal circulation of blood with the following vascular endothelium-like properties: (1) heparin, for thrombo-resistance and biocompatibility; (2) end-point attached heparin bonding process that leaves the heparin's anticoagulant active sequence binding sites free to participate in biological reactions such as binding to antithrombin, similar to the orientation of heparan sulfate on the vascular endothelium; (3) hydrophilicity to repel cells and prevent protein deposition; (4) negative charge, a natural characteristic of heparin molecules and similar to the negative charge of vascular endothelium that repels the negatively charged platelet cell membrane. Schematic © copyright Medtronic, Inc.*

components have complete coverage on blood contacting surfaces (Medtronic Inc., 2000). This ensures that the entire blood contact surface is consistently non-thrombogenic and bioactive.

Carmeda® BioActive Surface is the most extensively researched biosurface for cardiopulmonary bypass circuits to date. Clinical and scientific findings published in peer-reviewed cardiovascular surgery and perfusion literature include:

- Reduced the risk of bleeding through maintenance of natural hemostatic system (Larm *et al.*, 1982).
- Reduced blood transfusion requirements (Mahoney and Lemole, 1999; Svenmarker *et al.*, 2001).
- Prevents activation of the coagulation cascade at Factor XIIa (Elgue *et al.*, 1993b).
- Maintenance of platelet function normally compromised during extracorporeal circulation (Larsson *et al.*, 1987; Olsson, 1990).
- Thrombin inactivation, minimizing surface activation of the coagulation cascade and the whole-body inflammatory response (Larm *et al.*, 1986; Videm *et al.*, 1991a).
- Less leukocytosis (Belboul and Najib, 1997) less granulocyte activation (Borowiec *et al.*, 1997; Kagisaki *et al.*, 1997; Lundblad *et al.*, 1997) and reduced granular release by neutrophils (Videm *et al.*, 1991b; Borowiec *et al.*, 1992) for reduced immune response to cardiopulmonary bypass.
- Significantly less complement activation (Mollnes *et al.*, 1991; Videm *et al.*, 1991a; Fukutomi *et al.*, 1996; Kagisaki *et al.*, 1997).
- Cost savings related to improved clinical outcomes (Mahoney, 1998).

Trillium™ Biosurface (Fig. 2.15), a second Medtronic heparin biosurface, is designed to mimic the endothelium in three ways:

1 Non-leaching heparin is covalently bound into the biosurface, affording the same beneficial natural anticoagulatory effects as heparan sulfate does in the endothelium.
2 Due to the high content of its sulphate and sulphonate groups, Trillium™ Biosurface, like the vascular

endothelium, carries a strong negative charge to repel the negatively charged cell membranes of platelets.
3 Polyethylene oxide (PEO) chains in the polymer are strongly hydrophilic. This creates a stable water layer structure to repel cell adhesion and protein deposition.

Trillium™ Biosurface is applied to the artificial surface using manufacturing processes that ensure complete coverage on blood contacting surfaces.

Published scientific research demonstrates the heparin-like anticoagulant activity of negatively charged sulphonated polymers. Sulphonated polymers, with negatively charged groups resembling sulphonated functional groups of heparin, bind to antithrombin in a heparin-like manner, accelerating thrombin inhibition (Silver *et al.*, 1992; Han *et al.*, 1995; Charef *et al.*, 1996). Sulphonated polymers have been shown to complex through electrostatic interactions with fibrin monomers, preventing fibrin from the proper alignment necessary to form protofibrils and thrombi (Silver *et al.*, 1992). Sulphonated polymers impair the ability of fibrinogen to attract additional protein, thus impairing thrombus formation (Santerre *et al.*, 1992). Also, negatively charged sulphonated polymers repel the negatively charged platelets (Lelah *et al.*, 1985; Grasel and Cooper, 1989; Okkema *et al.*, 1991).

PEO polymers are extremely hydrophilic along their entire chain, providing cell and protein resistance to artificial surfaces (Lee *et al.*, 1995). Proteins begin to adsorb on artificial surfaces during the first few minutes of contact with the blood. Protein adsorption results in platelet adhesion and the activation of coagulation pathways, leading to thrombus formation (Lee and Oh, 2002). PEO creates an 'insulating' hydrated layer at the interface between the blood and artificial surface. The PEO–water interface has very low free energy and therefore a low driving force for protein adsorption or platelet adhesion

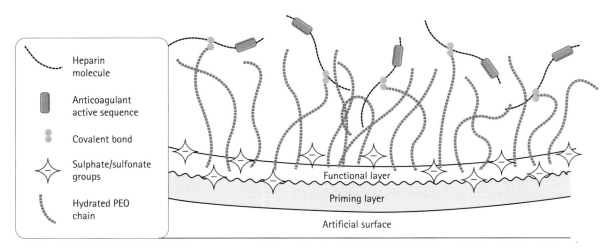

Figure 2.15 *Trillium™ Biosurface. Schematic © copyright Medtronic, Inc.*

(Lee *et al.*, 1995, 2000). PEO chains are in continuous motion (Lee *et al.*, 1995), due to their flexible molecular structure. The dynamic hydrated surface created by PEO chains is believed to repel proteins or platelets (Lee *et al.*, 1995, 2000).

Peer-reviewed published clinical and scientific research in perfusion literature suggest that Trillium™ Biosurface may provide beneficial effects for circulating platelet count preservation (Baksaas *et al.*, 1999; Palanzo *et al.*, 1999; Tevaearai *et al.*, 1999; Cazzaniga *et al.*, 2000; Palanzo *et al.*, 2001) and affords the AFFINITY® NT oxygenator the same protective effects on circulating platelet counts as adding albumin to the prime (Palanzo *et al.*, 1999). Additional published findings include reduced likelihood to require blood product transfusion (Dickinson *et al.*, 2002), reduced leukocytosis at the end of surgery (Cazzaniga *et al.*, 2000), less granulocyte and platelet activation (Baksaas *et al.*, 1999), and reduced clotting (Tevaearai *et al.*, 1999).

Heparin coatings for cardiopulmonary bypass have the most extensive published scientific and clinical data supporting their benefits. The body of published evidence, as well as extensive clinical experience by surgeons and perfusionists, supports the value of heparin-based biosurfaces for thrombo-resistance and biocompatibility during extracorporeal circulation.

ADEQUACY OF PERFUSION

During cardiopulmonary bypass the main responsibility of the perfusionist is to ensure that all the organs of the body supported by the extracorporeal circuit are adequately perfused with oxygenated blood. In order to achieve this the perfusionist continually monitors the following parameters:

- Acid–base status (metabolic/respiratory).
- Blood flow rate.
- Oxygen consumption rates (oxygen delivery/oxygen demand).
- Peripheral vascular resistance (perfusion pressure).
- Renal function.
- Coagulatory status.

ACKNOWLEDGEMENTS

This chapter is based on Chapter 3 in the third edition of *Techniques in Extracorporeal Circulation* and was originally written by L. Bigi, N. Ghelli, A. Menghini and I. Panzani of Dideco SpA, Italy.

Medtronic, AFFINITY, autoLog, Bio-Pump, MYOtherm and Trillium are trademarks of Medtronic, Inc. Carmeda is a registered trademark of Carmeda AB, Sweden.

REFERENCES

Baksaas, S.T., Videm, V., Fosse, E. *et al.* 1999: *In vitro* evaluation of new surface coatings for extracorporeal circulation. *Perfusion* **14**, 11–19.

Belboul, A., Najib, A-K. 1997: Does heparin coating improve biocompatibility? A study on complement, blood cells and postoperative morbidity during cardiac surgery. *Perfusion* **12**, 385–91.

Borowiec, J., Thelin, S., Bagge, L., Hultman, J., Hansson, H.E. 1992: Heparin-coated circuits reduce activation of granulocytes during cardiopulmonary bypass – a clinical study. *Journal of Thoracic and Cardiovascular Surgery* **104**, 642–7.

Borowiec, J., Jaramillo, A., Venge, P., Nilsson, L., Thelin, S. 1997: Effects of heparin-coating of cardiopulmonary bypass circuits on leukocytes during simulated extracorporeal circulation. *Cardiovascular Surgery* **5**, 568–73.

Cazzaniga, A., Ranucci, M., Igsgrò, G. *et al.* 2000: Trillium Biopassive Surface: a new biocompatible treatment for extracorporeal circulation circuits. *International Journal of Artificial Organs* **23**, 319–24.

Charef, S., Tapon-Bretaudière, J., Fischer, A.M. *et al.* 1996: Heparin-like functionalized polymer surfaces: discrimination between catalytic and adsorption processes during the course of thrombin inhibition. *Biomaterials* **17**, 903–12.

Coleman, R.W., Clowes, A.W., George, J.N., Hirsch, J., Marder, V. 2001: Overview of hemostasis. In: R.W. Coleman, A.W. Clowes, J.N. George, J. Hirsch, V. Marder (eds), *Hemostasis and thrombosis: basic principles and clinical practice* (fourth edition). Philadelphia, PA: Lippincott Williams & Wilkins, 3–16.

Dickinson, T., Mahoney, C.B., Simmons, M. *et al.* 2002: Trillium™-coated oxygenators in adult open-heart surgery: a prospective randomized trial. *Journal of Extracorporeal Technology* **34**, 248–53.

Elgue, G., Blombäck, M., Olsson, P., Riesenfeld, J. 1993a: On the mechanism of coagulation inhibition on surfaces with end point immobilized heparin. *Thrombosis and Haemostasis* **70**, 289–93.

Elgue, G., Sanchez, J., Egberg, N., Olsson, P., Riesenfeld, J. 1993b: Effect of surface-immobilized heparin on the activation of adsorbed Factor XII. *Artificial Organs* **17**, 721–6.

Fukutomi, M., Kobayashi, S., Hamada, Y., Kitamura, S. 1996: Changes in platelet, granulocyte, and complement activation during cardiopulmonary bypass using heparin-coated equipment. *Artificial Organs* **20**, 767–76.

Grasel, T.G., Cooper, S. 1989: Properties and biological interactions of polyurethane aniomers: effect of sulfonate incorporation. *Journal of Biomedical Materials Research* **23**, 311–38.

Han, D.K., Lee, N.Y., Park, K.I. *et al.* 1995: Heparin-like anticoagulant activity of sulphonated poly(ethelene oxide) and sulphonated poly(ethylene oxide)-grafted polyurethane. *Biomaterials* **16**, 467–71.

Hsu, L.C. 2001: Heparin-coated cardiopulmonary bypass circuits: current status. *Perfusion* **16**, 417–28.

Kagisaki, K., Masai, T., Kadoba, K. *et al.* 1997: Biocompatibility of heparin-coated circuits in pediatric cardiopulmonary bypass. *Artificial Organs* **21**, 836–40.

Larm, O., Larson, R., Olsson, P. 1982: A new non-thrombogenic surface prepared by selective covalent binding of heparin via a modified reducing terminal residue. *Biomat Med Dev Art Org* **11**, 161–8.

Larm, O., Lins, L.E., Olsson, P. 1986: An approach to anti-thrombosis by surface modification. In: C. Kjellstrand, Y. Nose (eds), *Progress in artificial organs 1985*. Cleveland, OH: ISAIO Press, 313–18.

Larsson, R., Larm, O., Olsson, P. 1987: The search for thromboresistance using immobilized heparin. Blood in contact with natural and artificial surfaces. *Annals of the New York Academy of Sciences* **516**, 102–15.

Lee, J.H., Oh, S.E. 2002: MMA/MPEOMA/VSA copolymer as a novel blood-compatible material: effect of PEO and the negatively charged side chains on protein adsorption and platelet adhesion. *Journal of Biomaterials Research* **60**, 44–52.

Lee, J.H., Lee, H.B., Andrade, J.D. 1995: Blood compatibility of polyethylene oxide surfaces. *Progress in Polymer Science* **20**, 1043–79.

Lee, J.H., Ju, Y.M., Kim, D.M. 2000: Platelet adhesion onto segmented polyurethane film surfaces modified by addition and crosslinking of PEO-containing block copolymers. *Biomaterials* **21**, 683–91.

Lelah, M.D., Pierce, J.A., Lambrecht, L.K., Cooper, S.I. 1985: Polyether–urethan ionomers: surface property/*ex vivo* blood compatibility relationships. *Journal of Colloid Interface Science* **104**, 422–39.

Lundblad, R., Moen, O., Fosse, E. 1997: Endothelin-1 and neutrophil activation during heparin-coated cardiopulmonary bypass. *Annals of Thoracic Surgery* **63**, 1361–7.

Mahoney CB. 1998: Heparin-bonded circuits: clinical outcomes and costs. *Perfusion* **13**, 192–204.

Mahoney, C.B., Lemole, G.M. 1999: Transfusion after coronary artery bypass surgery: the impact of heparin bonded circuits. *European Journal of Cardiothoracic Surgery* **16**, 206–10.

Marcum, J.A., McKenny, J.B., Rosenberg, R.D. 1984: Acceleration of thrombin–antithrombin complex formation in rat hind quarters via heparin-like molecules bound to the endothelium. *Journal of Clinical Investigation* **74**, 341–50.

Medtronic, Inc. 2000: *Carmeda® BioActive Surface compendium II: clinical and scientific information*, 8–10.

Mollnes, T.E., Videm, V., Götze, O., Harboe, M., Oppermann, M. 1991: Formation of C5a during cardiopulmonary bypass: inhibition by precoating with heparin. *Annals of Thoracic Surgery* **52**, 92–7.

Morgan, I.S., Codispoti, M., Sanger, K., Mankad, P.S. 1998: Superiority of centrifugal pump over roller pump in paediatric cardiac surgery; prospective randomized trial. *European Journal of Cardiothoracic Surgery* **13**, 526–32.

Okkema, A.Z., Yu, X.H., Cooper, S.L. 1991: Physical and blood contacting characteristics of propyl sulphonate grafted biomer. *Biomaterials* **12**, 3–12.

Olsson, P. 1990: Non-thrombogenic systems for extracorporeal gas exchange. *International Journal of Artificial Organs* **13**, 9.

Palanzo, D.A., Zarro, D.L., Montesano, R.M. *et al.* 1999: Effect of Trillium Biopassive Surface coating of the oxygenator on platelet count during cardiopulmonary bypass. *Perfusion* **14**, 473–9.

Palanzo, D.A., Zarro, D.L., Manley, N.J. *et al.* 2001: Effect of Carmeda BioActive Surface coating versus Trillium Biopassive Surface coating of the oxygenator on circulating platelet count drop during cardiopulmonary bypass. *Perfusion* **16**, 279–83.

Sanchez, J., Elgue, G., Riesenfeld, J., Olsson, P. 1995: Control of contact activation on end-point immobilized heparin: the role of antithrombin and the specific antithrombin-binding sequence. *Journal of Biomedical Materials Research* **29**, 655–61.

Santerre, J.P., Van der Kamp, N.H., Brash, J.L. 1992: Effect of sulfonation of segmented polyurethanes on the transient adsorption of fibrinogen from plasma: possible correlation with anticoagulant behaviour. *Journal of Biomedical Materials Research* **26**, 39–57.

Silver, J.H., Hart, A.P., Williams, E.C. *et al.* 1992: Anticoagulant effects of sulphonated polyurethanes. *Biomaterials* **13**, 339–43.

Svenmarker, S., Sandström, E., Karlsson, T. *et al.* 2001: Neurological and general outcome in low-risk coronary artery bypass patients using heparin coated circuits. *European Journal of Cardiothoracic Surgery* **19**, 47–53.

Tevaearai, H.T., Mueller, X.M., Seigneul, I. *et al.* 1999: Trillium coating of cardiopulmonary bypass circuits improves biocompatibility. *International Journal of Artificial Organs* **22**, 629–34.

Videm, V., Mollnes, T.E., Garred, P., Svennevig, J.L., Videm, V. 1991a: Biocompatibility of extracorporeal circulation. *In vitro* comparison of heparin-coated and uncoated oxygenator circuits. *Journal of Thoracic and Cardiovascular Surgery* **101**, 654–60.

Videm, V., Nilsson, L., Venge, P., Svennevig, J.L. 1991b: Reduced granulocyte activation with heparin coated device in an *in vitro* model of cardiopulmonary bypass. *Artificial Organs* **15**, 90–5.

3

Physiology and pathophysiology of extracorporeal circulation

JONATHAN AJ HYDE AND RALPH E DELIUS

KEY POINTS

- The major pathophysiological alterations caused by extracorporeal circulation are related to surface contact with artificial material, with resultant blood damage and mediator activation.
- Other factors producing abnormal physiological responses include abnormal flow generation, hypothermia and haemodilution.
- Although there are demonstrable changes in intestinal permeability and function after cardiopulmonary bypass, most gastrointestinal complications are actually related to post-operative low output state.
- A degree of renal dysfunction after cardiopulmonary bypass is relatively common, and is related to a combination of pre-operative function, length of bypass and post-operative cardiac output.
- Pulmonary function is invariably impaired by cardiopulmonary bypass, but the clinical impact of this is generally less severe than it used to be.
- Neurological and neuropsychological dysfunction are important consequences of cardiopulmonary bypass and, depending on the criteria used, have an incidence of between one per cent and 80 per cent.

INTRODUCTION

Extracorporeal circulation, by definition, implies the maintenance of full support of the normal physiological circulation by means of artificial devices. Although its development, most of which has occurred in the last half-century, has allowed enormous advances in medical treatment, the fact remains that it is unphysiological. Cardiac surgery as we know it would not have been possible without cardiopulmonary bypass, by far the most common type of extracorporeal circulation in current use. Its application allows the heart and lungs to be arrested for increasing periods of time in order to facilitate a range of cardiac procedures. Other less common types of extracorporeal circulation in current use include extracorporeal membrane oxygenation, extracorporeal carbon dioxide removal and ventricular assist devices. The latter are precursors of attempts to create a total artificial heart, or at least a device that can support the circulation for extended periods of time as a bridge to transplantation. Huge amounts of research and money are being invested in such programmes and some very promising breakthroughs have been made in the past five years, with encouraging clinical applications.

Although the applications of the different types of extracorporeal circulation mentioned above are widely varied, they all employ many similar basic principles. For the purposes of this chapter, we shall concentrate on cardiopulmonary bypass, but it should be clear to the reader that the majority of pathophysiological sequelae are shared by them all.

Historical background

Although the earliest records of attempts to create an artificial circulation date back to the early nineteenth century, the clinical introduction of cardiopulmonary bypass was by Gibbon in 1953 (Brown-Sequard, 1858; von Frey and Gruber, 1885; Galletti and Mora, 1995). At this time Gibbon successfully used total extracorporeal circulation whilst closing an atrial septal defect in a young woman (Gibbon, 1954). His work originated in 1937 with artificial circulation during temporary occlusion of the pulmonary artery in cases of massive pulmonary embolus (Gibbon, 1937, 1939). Soon after Gibbon's initial clinical application, several other milestones were passed to enable current practices to exist. One of these was the work of Lillehei, who brought about the concept of cross-circulation (Lillehei, 1955). In 1954, Lillehei established a support circulation from a compatible adult to a child that needed congenital cardiac surgery. In this instance, the adult was effectively acting as the cardiopulmonary bypass machine. Lillehei performed similar support procedures on 47 patients over the next two years with a survival rate of more than 50 per cent for the patients, and 100 per cent for the support adults. This work established the real potential for artificial extracorporeal circulation, and it was only a matter of time before appropriate machines were developed. Other milestones included the development of adequate applications of hypothermia, and a greater understanding of the effect of artificial surfaces on blood components, and the generalized inflammatory response associated with cardiopulmonary bypass (Senning, 1954; Gollan, 1959; Swan and Paton, 1960; van Oeveren et al., 1990).

Within the last 25 years, cardiopulmonary bypass has become an easily performed, safe and practical option for the facilitation of cardiac surgery. A great deal of research continues to be carried out on all aspects of cardiopulmonary bypass with the goal of making it even safer. However, it remains unphysiological and its detrimental effects will never be eliminated entirely. It is for this reason that the recent concept of off-pump surgery has gained in popularity, and there are many surgeons who perform nearly 100 per cent of their cases of coronary artery surgery without the use of cardiopulmonary bypass. For the majority, however, it remains a valuable tool but it is of paramount importance that the possible pathophysiological sequelae are well understood.

Physiology versus pathophysiology

Some would argue that extracorporeal circulation alters most aspects of physiology to such an extent that it is pathophysiological itself. The term 'physiology' was coined by the great Dutch physician Boerhaave to describe the study of interdependent organ function under normal conditions. Pathophysiology is defined as the derangement or alteration of normal physiological function seen in disease. Extracorporeal circulation imposes several conditions that lead to a series of changes in normal organ function, and in this instance represents 'disease'. The physiology of extracorporeal circulation, as mentioned above, refers to interdependent organ function during the conditions imposed by veno-arterial cardiopulmonary bypass. The changes occurring with extracorporeal circulation are outlined in Table 3.1. Physiological function under these conditions differs considerably from normal physiology, and could, therefore, be said to be pathophysiological per se. The normal functions of blood flow, gas exchange, blood surface interface effects and reticulo-endothelial function are the physiological functions that are replaced in total or in part by the extracorporeal device. Subsequent changes in individual organ function are secondary to these substitutions. The mechanical and pharmacological factors which are inherent in the design of the device (and hence responsible for physiological changes) are also listed in Table 3.1.

Abnormal, deteriorating or inadequate organ function associated with extracorporeal circulation is the pathophysiology of extracorporeal circulation. It is difficult, if not impossible, to separate the uniform and ubiquitous changes in organ function that are associated with extracorporeal circulation from specific organ damage or deteriorating function that can occur when a mechanical device is used to substitute for the heart and lungs. In addition, all clinical studies of extracorporeal circulation are conducted on patients with underlying intrinsic disease, usually in conjunction with a cardiac operation.

Therefore, 'physiology' and 'pathophysiology' are defined from an abnormal baseline, and for the purposes of this chapter should be grouped together. Although some aspects of extracorporeal circulation can be clearly identified as pathophysiology (gross air embolism, for example), others cannot be separated from normal function of the apparatus (platelet aggregation, for example). In this sense Table 3.1 represents both the physiology of extracorporeal circulation and the inherent pathophysiology.

Component-related factors

Mechanical failure should be avoided by a preventative maintenance programme of replacing elements of the

Table 3.1 *Physiology and pharmacology of extracorporeal circulation compared with normal circulation and pulmonary function*

Normal function	Physiological changes with ECC	Mechanical factors	Pharmacological factors
Blood flow	↓ Total flow negative venous pressure	Venous cannula size	Steroids
	↑ Adrenergic response		Adrenergic blockers
	↑ Renin-angiotensin	Arterial cannula site	Diuretics
	Abnormal distribution		
	Non-pulsatile	Pump characteristics	
	Non-servo		Volume expanders
	↓ Tissue washout		
	↓ Oxygen delivery	Heat exchanger	Hypothermia buffers-tris HCO_3
	Acidosis		
Gas exchange	O_2–CO_2 exchange requires large blood volume	Oxygenator: disk, bubble, membrane	Defoamer
	Microbubbles		
	Emboli and aggregates	Reservoir: connectors, tubing	? Platelet-active drugs
	Stagnant zones		
Blood–endothelial interface	Anticoagulation	Surface coating	Heparin priming solutions
	↑ Fibrinolytic activity		
	↓ Platelet function	Coronary suction	
	Blood dilution		Haemodilution
Reticulo-endothelial function	Tissue histiocytes loaded	Filters	
	Phagocytosis ↓		

bypass circuit at regular intervals. The use of single-use, disposable, pre-sterilized items for all blood contact has largely eliminated failures in this area. Careful attention to roller pump settings and continuous monitoring of flow and pressure in the arterial line during bypass will minimize complications. The pump team should rehearse rapid replacement of any part of the bypass circuit as well as procedures to deal with man-made problems of air embolism, thrombosis in the oxygenator, aortic dissection, improper venous cannulation, etc. Attention to these details in avoiding pathophysiological function of the extracorporeal circuit will be discussed in other chapters in this book.

The components of the extracorporeal circuit must be absolutely clean, inert, sterile and non-toxic. Mechanical cleaning may not be adequate to remove all foreign proteins and pyrogens from reused portions of the circuit. Such a foreign protein was implicated as acting as a plasminogen activator and causing abnormal bleeding in open-heart patients in one study. Cleaning in 20 per cent sodium hydroxide removed the offending material (Brooks and Bahnson, 1971). Pre-packaged single-use components should be clean but may not be necessarily so. Systemic emboli of particles of Dacron and nylon thread, antifoam or other materials may originate from components that are allegedly clean for single use. Some extracorporeal components may contain plasticizers or solvents which could leak out into the circulating blood during extracorporeal circulation. All plastic materials which are used for contact with human blood must meet government standards for biomedical plastics. These standards involve injecting extracts of the material into animals and subcutaneous implantation of the material in animals. All medical plastics undergo this testing procedure. Designations such as 'medical grade' or 'implant tested' do not connote any specific standard or unique characteristic.

The fact that plastic raw materials have successfully undergone conventional government testing does not mean that the finished product will be non-toxic. Adhesive used in construction, heat sealing, radiation or gas sterilization may alter the characteristics of the material or add new materials that are potentially damaging to patients. A tragic experience with toxicity of ethylene oxide sterilization of an extracorporeal circuit resulting in a fatality and clearly identified later in dogs was reported by Stanley *et al.* (1971).

This lethal toxicity associated with ethylene oxide has now been described from several sources; however, little is known of the interactions of drugs such as halothane, penthrane, nitrous oxide, narcotics, antibiotics and analgesics with prolonged exposure to various plastic surfaces. Clinical experience indicates that minimal interaction takes place, although we have all seen clear polyvinyl chloride tubing become turbid and white silicone tubing become yellow with prolonged blood exposure. The interrelationships of these types of plastics with blood components for long periods of time deserve further study.

Antifoam is coated on some part of all gas interface oxygenators. When present in excessive amounts, or when incompletely adhered to the surface, particles of this material may break loose and embolize (Reed and Kittle, 1959). The plastic material itself can erode on the inside of the extracorporeal circuit. Polyvinyl chloride tubing in the roller pump usually deteriorates by cracking and breaking from the outer edge in; however, prolonged pumping with a roller pump on silicone rubber tubing results in crumbling away from the inside out.

If air is trapped in the extracorporeal circuit and suddenly enters the arterial perfusion line, systemic air embolism will result. The possibility of this occurring from the arterial line filters has been demonstrated by Wellons and Nolan (1973), who showed that air could be trapped in the arterial line filter. This problem was solved by ventilating the filter with carbon dioxide before priming. Carbon dioxide is much more soluble than oxygen or nitrogen in priming solution and bubbles can be completely removed in this fashion. The same procedure is helpful in priming membrane oxygenators. Prevention of air embolism from intracardiac chambers has been emphasized by many authors (Lawrence *et al.*, 1971; Gomes *et al.*, 1973). Techniques to avoid air embolism from cardiac chambers while extracorporeal circulation is turned on and off for various manoeuvres are described in other chapters.

Lastly, infection occurring as a result of contamination of the extracorporeal circuit is another form of pathophysiology associated with extracorporeal circulation. Blakemore *et al.* (1971) showed that the extracorporeal circuit becomes contaminated from the coronary suction line, although the ventilation gas fed to the oxygenator itself may be contaminated from the tubing or from nebulizing or humidification devices. Appropriate use of air filters wherever possible and meticulous attention to avoiding air contamination in the field of the coronary suction will help minimize this contamination. However, bloodstream contamination, in particular in the face of decreased phagocytic and bactericidal recticuloendothelial function, as mentioned previously, predisposes extracorporeal circulation patients to infection. The possibility of infection and contamination during extracorporeal circulation has prompted most surgeons to add prophylactic antibiotics to the perfusion system or to patients during extracorporeal circulation, although their value is difficult to demonstrate (Benner, 1969; Conte *et al.*, 1972; Rosendorf *et al.*, 1974).

THE ARTIFICIAL ENVIRONMENT CREATED BY EXTRACORPOREAL CIRCULATION

Extracorporeal circulations such as cardiopulmonary bypass confer an unphysiological environment upon the body in a number of ways. It is the disruption of normal homeostasis and exposure to unfamiliar conditions and materials that result in unwanted effects. Although most patients undergoing cardiopulmonary bypass make a full recovery, with no signs of harmful effects, everybody is subjected to the physiological changes that occur. Cardiopulmonary bypass, as with the other forms of extracorporeal circulation, confers a shock-like state upon the body. The organs must tolerate an extended period of lower perfusion pressures and are exposed to a range of other unphysiological conditions, such as haemodilution, hypothermia and non-pulsatile flow.

Haemodilution

The pump circuit, consisting of all tubing components, reservoirs, oxygenator and filters, must be primed with fluid before cardiopulmonary bypass is established. The priming volume of the circuit depends on the gas exchange device, the venous reservoir volume and the blood volume of the patient. It is feasible to avoid blood transfusion altogether at the expense of oxygen-carrying capacity. Recent caution with blood-borne diseases, among other reasons, has resulted in the priming solution of the pump being non-haemic in the majority of adult cases. A high haematocrit and excellent oxygen-carrying capacity can certainly be achieved with an all-blood prime, but at the expense of increased viscosity, haemolysis, potential for transfusion reaction, and transmission of infections such as hepatitis and HIV. These factors generally balance out at a bypass haematocrit of 25–30 per cent of normal, which generally requires 500–1000 mL of blood in the prime or to be infused during bypass. This figure, of course, is dependent on the co-existence of other factors, such as hypothermia, or else the oxygen-carrying capacity of the blood may be compromised (Kawashima *et al.*, 1974; Utley *et al.*, 1976). Haemodilution counters the increased viscosity and tendency to sludging caused by hypothermia.

Blood should be less than 24 hours old to maintain adequate levels of active blood platelets; otherwise fresh components should be used. The remainder of the prime can be isotonic saline or a colloid solution. Haemodilution is the main cause of the fluid retention associated with cardiopulmonary bypass by decreasing the plasma colloid oncotic pressure, and this needs to be compensated for (Utley *et al.*, 1981). When non-blood prime is used the resultant exchange transfusion and rapid haemodilution will result in equilibration of priming solution into the appropriate body fluid space, causing hypovolaemia as referred to earlier in this chapter. Saline or saline-like crystalloid solutions will equilibrate into the extracellular fluid, requiring volume supplement to return blood volume to normal. Priming with crystalloid solutions necessarily expands the total body water and the extracellular fluid compartments. Some studies have found no difference between crystalloid and colloid primes (Ohgrist et al., 1981; Gallagher et al., 1985), whereas others have found colloid preferable (Sade et al., 1985). Colloid solutions containing albumin or hydroxyethyl starch appear to work equally well (Sade et al., 1985; Lumb, 1987). One other prime solution that received attention was Fluosol-DA, an oxygen-carrying fluorocarbon solution. This solution was found to be comparable to saline and blood as a priming solution in experimental studies (Rousou et al., 1985; Stone et al., 1986). However, clinical application of fluorocarbons has been disappointing and they have not been widely adopted.

Several investigators have studied the effect of eliminating blood transfusion for the cardiac surgical patient altogether. The reasons for wishing to do this include cost, simplicity, saving vital blood bank stores, avoiding the possible effects of microembolism from platelet fibrin aggregates in stored blood as well as possible damage to lung and other organs from transfused white blood cells, and most importantly, avoiding the risk of diseases transmitted through transfusion, such as hepatitis and human immunodeficiency virus. Successful major open heart operations performed without the use of blood products have been described in adult and paediatric patients of the Jehovah Witness faith (Gombotz et al., 1985; Hening, 1988). The use of blood salvage and autologous transfusion before and after extracorporeal circulation (Kaplan et al., 1977; Schaff et al., 1978) and reinfusion of washed cells from the used circuit (Moran et al., 1978) are major advances that save blood bank resources.

Hypothermia

Controlled hypothermia is a major issue in cardiac surgery, and is utilized to some degree in most procedures. Oxygen consumption has been shown to fall by about 50 per cent for each 10°C drop in temperature over the range 0–42°C (median 36°C). The more common applications of this technique range from moderate hypothermia (34°C) allowing intermittent aortic cross-clamping with fibrillation, to complete circulatory arrest which at 10°C can be safely carried out for over an hour (Kirklin and Barratt-Boyes, 1988).

Aside from the moderate low-flow state imposed by most cardiac operations, there are no specific metabolic sequelae of extracorporeal circulation. One appropriate method to compensate for the moderate low flow is the use of moderate hypothermia, which decreases oxygen requirement and carbon dioxide production, so that the lower flow can be matched to specific metabolic requirements. The use of moderate hypothermia (to 30°C) is widely carried out, although the effects of skin and perhaps muscle ischaemia related to this cold temperature and the increased sympathetic effects may balance out any

potential advantages. Moreover, shivering during rewarming has been associated with increased oxygen consumption (Chiara et al., 1980; Zwischenberger et al., 1986). Paralytic agents which prevent shivering have been shown to decrease oxygen consumption and improve haemodynamic stability during rewarming (Zwischenberger et al., 1986). Another effect of hypothermia is that the blood viscosity increases as the temperature drops so that use of haemodilution to lower the haematocrit is required in order to decrease blood viscosity.

One major advantage of hypothermia is to allow a safety factor to the surgeon. Faced with excessive bleeding or a disastrous scenario, the entire bypass circuit can be turned off safely and the brain protected by hypothermia for periods from 10 minutes at 30°C to 60 minutes at 10°C.

Flow generation

The goal of producing an artificial blood pump began in earnest at the beginning of the twentieth century. The ideal qualities of a blood pump are to produce a predictable and adjustable rate and volume of flow. It should also keep haemolysis to a minimum, so blood handling needs to be carefully considered, and stagnation, cavitation and turbulence must be avoided where possible (Trocchio and Sketel, 1995). Other important features include disposable tubing, manual back-up in case of power failure, temperature control, and monitoring. The work of De Bakey with the application of blood displacement devices led to the use of roller pumps as the main method for flow generation in early cardiopulmonary bypass (Clark et al., 1950), and laminar roller pumping remains the most commonly used method of cardiopulmonary bypass to this day. The three main types of flow generation employed in all forms of extracorporeal circulation are:

- non-pulsatile flow with a roller pump
- pulsatile flow with a roller pump
- non-pulsatile flow with a centrifugal pump.

The issue of pulsatility is a controversial one and has been the focus of much research. It would seem logical that the reproduction of normal physiological pulsatility should confer benefits on the patient, but this has not necessarily been shown to be the case. This will be discussed in more detail later. At present, centrifugal flow is increasing in popularity all the time and is actually becoming more widely used than roller flow for routine cases in many cardiac centres. In addition, centrifugal pumps can now deliver pulsatile flow if required.

Non–pulsatile roller flow

Roller flow became popular initially because of its ease of use and set-up, better control and acceptable haemolysis.

It also had the advantage (very important initially) of hand-cranking in the case of power malfunction. The basic design has retained the principles of the early pumps of the 1920s and 1930s, although many modifications such as number of rollers (single, double or more) and pump housing have been made. They do not rely on valves, and output depends on speed of rotation and volume displaced per compression. Further refinements include pressure dependent shut-off systems, as well as automatic shut-off to low reservoir levels and gaseous emboli.

The output of the pump depends upon the speed of the pump and the stroke volume, in much the same way as the human heart. The mechanism of action is one or more rollers compressing a segment of blood-filled tubing against a semi-circular backing plate, thus propelling a column of blood forwards. 'Pump occlusion' is the term applied when the roller causes maximal compression of the tubing against the backing plate. This is usually adjustable, and the degree of pump occlusion directly affects the degree of blood component damage. Perhaps surprisingly, non-occlusive pumps are associated with high rates of haemolysis as well as fully occlusive ones. This is due to turbulence, back-flow, and the build-up of kinetic energy within the tubing, as well as the need for faster revolutions, since less volume is displaced in each cycle. The best form of occlusion has been shown to be 'just non-occlusive', exhibiting the lowest rates of haemolysis. Blood cell trauma has been associated with increased speed and increased number of rollers, mainly because of their effects on shear stress, kinetic energy, friction heat and direct compressive action. The accepted compromise, in use in the majority of roller pumps now, is wider bore tubing (inner diameter) and two diametrically opposed rollers. The two-roller pump has a 210° arc backing plate, and the diametric opposition of the rollers means that as one finishes its compression, the other starts.

PULSATILE ROLLER FLOW

One of the earliest pulsatile devices to be used clinically was the Sigmamotor pump. This had occlusive 'fingers' that rhythmically compressed the tubing to propel the blood in a forward direction (Castillo et al., 1991). These pumps produced a pulsatile waveform, which satisfied the researchers of the time as being most physiological. Problems were soon discovered, and it was difficult to control and synchronize such pumps, particularly at high flow rates. This, and the extensive haemolysis seen, precluded their use and non-pulsatile pumps were favoured for many years.

The use of pulsatile pumps for routine cardiopulmonary bypass remains a controversial subject. There have been numerous studies in both animals and humans comparing various aspects of physiology and clinical response to pulsatile flow, but its benefits are still the subject of considerable debate. The advantages ascribed to pulsatile flow are: increased urine volume; normal stress response; less metabolic acidosis; lower peripheral resistance; smaller transfusion volumes; increased oxygen consumption; and better myocardial perfusion and reperfusion (Mitchell and Casthely, 1991). These advantages are contested, with evidence to the contrary (Frater et al., 1980; Kono et al., 1983). There are concerns about the disruptive effects of a high pressure pulsatile jet on the inside of the aorta, and the possibility of embolic shedding (Finlayson, 1987). The benefits mentioned above are for the duration of cardiopulmonary bypass only, and any long-term differences remain unclear.

CENTRIFUGAL FLOW

Although the first experimental use of a centrifugal pump was reported by Saxton and Andrews (1960), the centrifugal pump came into favour in the early 1970s during the quest for an artificial implantable heart. A joint enterprise between the universities of Minnesota, California and San Diego, and Medtronic Inc., in 1964 had created the first magnetically coupled centrifugal pump appropriate for implantation. Although abandoned early on for implantation as an artificial heart, the centrifugal pump retained popularity as the drive for external ventricular assist devices. It produces flow by imparting kinetic energy to blood inside a rapidly rotating head. Centrifugal pumps are surprisingly simple in concept, and have very few moving parts – factors that have contributed to their popularity.

There are two broad types of centrifugal blood pump: the inverted cone and the vaned impellar (fin). The cone type has a series of concentric cones that spin within the housing and create a large negative pressure at the apex, pulling blood into it. Once inside, the spinning cones impart kinetic energy to the blood, and a vortex is established. This vortex is constrained by the rigid housing and creates pressure to force the blood out of the exit port at the base. The vaned impellar type has a number of impellar blades that rotate and generate pressure within the housing. The fins rely on friction and shear to impart kinetic energy to the blood, and also have a direct lifting effect within the pump housing. There has been a lot of work to evaluate the optimal fin size, curvature and angle, in order to minimize turbulence, cavitation and other factors associated with blood cell damage. The advantage of the impellar pumps is that they are more efficient at moving given quantities of blood at given speeds, but which type causes the least blood damage is still disputed (Edelman et al., 1992).

Centrifugal pumps have no valves between the inflow and outflow ports, and are thus heavily dependent on pre-load and after-load pressures. If the cones are not spinning, blood can easily flow in both directions, which is a potential source of danger (Landis et al., 1979). Pump heads are disposable, but sit inside a permanent drive console, which contains a magnet. When the drive rotates this magnet, it couples to a magnet in the head, which therefore spins at an equal rate.

PULSATILE VERSUS NON-PULSATILE FLOW

This is perhaps one of the longest-running debates in the field of cardiopulmonary bypass, with evidence in favour of both types of flow. Nonetheless, pulsatility remains a little-used technique. It is perhaps the apparent contradictory scientific evidence that tends to discourage the majority of cardiac surgeons from the adoption of this technique (Taylor, 1995). Pulsatile blood flow is a natural and physiological concept, and has effects far beyond the simple delivery of blood to tissues.

The key issue in favour of pulsatility over non-pulsatile flow is that of systemic vasoconstriction. It has been shown that the systemic vascular resistance generally rises immediately after the onset of extracorporeal circulation, and may remain high for up to several days afterwards (Jacobs et al., 1969; Dunn et al., 1974; Taylor et al., 1980; Hickey et al., 1983; Taylor, 1995). Excessive vasoconstriction will cause inadequate blood flow to selected areas, with the potential for organ failure. It also results in an increase in left ventricular work to counter the resistance (Taylor, 1995). In patients undergoing cardiac surgery with impaired ventricular function, this may have a deleterious effect. The mechanisms behind vasoconstriction during cardiopulmonary bypass are multifactorial and involve a combination of catecholamine release, activation of the renin-angiotensin system, vasopressin release, and local tissue factor release. All of these are known to be increased when pulsatility is withdrawn from the circulation (Many et al., 1967; Taylor et al., 1979a,b, 1980). In addition, carotid baroreceptors have been studied through alternating pulsatile and non-pulsatile flow, and found to discharge significantly more when pulsatility is withdrawn (Angell, 1971), which will also increase peripheral vasoconstriction. This has prompted the development of perfusion systems that reproduce physiological pulsatility for cardiopulmonary bypass.

When assessing the effects of pulsatility on organ function, it is still possible to find much evidence showing its beneficial effects. It has been shown to preserve the microcirculation and improve tissue metabolism, and transfusion requirements post-operatively have been reported lower. Renal metabolism and urine output are also apparently improved with pulsatility (Pacquet, 1969; Angell, 1971), particularly for longer perfusion runs. Many studies to investigate left ventricular function and other myocardial parameters have demonstrated improvement with pulsatile perfusion; however, the evidence has not been unanimous (Levine et al., 1980). The cerebral consequences of pulsatility versus non-pulsatility have

been investigated, but to date no clear advantage has been demonstrated. This is also the case with pulmonary function, which has the least number of reported studies relating to this issue.

There is equipment available that will convert roller pumps into machines capable of generating pulsatile flow. It involves the addition of a pulsatile flow controller into the system, which sequentially accelerates and decelerates the pump head at a controllable rate. There are sections of the cardiopulmonary bypass circuit where some degree of damping of the pulsatility will take place. Most current oxygenators will damp the pulsatile wave form up to 20 per cent, which still provides sufficient pulsatility of blood flow at the point of entry into the aorta.

Although the issue of increased vasoconstriction with non-pulsatile flow is generally accepted, most patients do not suffer from related post-operative problems because of the use of vasodilators such as glycerol trinitrate (GTN) and anaesthetic agents.

CENTRIFUGAL VERSUS ROLLER FLOW

Comparisons of roller and centrifugal pumps in both the laboratory and clinical settings have produced conflicting results. The potential advantages of centrifugal flow are mainly pressure-related. If the after-load increases, such as in an occluded or kinked arterial line, a catastrophic high pressure build-up in the pump head is avoided. Also, in the constrained vortex of the centrifugal pump, there is high pressure at the periphery and low pressure at the centre. This tends to annex air that may enter the pump head, and it will not be expelled through the arterial line. A massive bolus of air into the pump will effectively deprime it and stop flow all together. There remains some debate about the issue of prevention of air emboli from blood pumps (Stoney et al., 1980; Wheeldon et al., 1990). One potential danger of the lack of valves within the centrifugal head is the passage of blood in both directions. When the pump stops there is no protection against retrograde flow back out of the aorta if a siphoning phenomenon occurs. This can be prevented in practice by either clamping of the arterial line, or fitting a valve into the outflow line.

Temperature does not affect the centrifugal pump in the way it affects roller pumps, which is a distinct advantage. Decreasing temperatures in roller pumps results in stiffer tubing and decreased compliance, resulting in an overall reduction in flow (Kuo and Graham, 1995). However, centrifugal flow is more dependent on viscosity than the roller pump, which results in reduced flow if the outflow blood viscosity increases (Landis et al., 1979).

Particulate microembolization, consisting of blood components or foreign materials from spallation of the tubing, is a potential problem with extracorporeal circulation. Studies to compare the incidence of microembolization in roller and centrifugal pumps have all shown an enormous difference. Spallation is commonplace with roller flow, mainly at the interface of the backing plate and roller heads, but is minimal with centrifugal flow (Orenstein *et al.*, 1982; Uretzky *et al.*, 1987).

Another major area in which centrifugal pumps have been postulated to have advantages over roller pumps is blood handling (Horton and Butt, 1992). Manufacturers of both types of centrifugal pump claim that platelet damage and haemolysis are lower with their machines than with roller flow, and can quote supportive evidence in their favour. Although this may be so, its significance in the short bypass times seen with simple cardiac procedures may not outweigh the increased cost implications. Centrifugal pumps are now used for more than 50 per cent of routine cardiopulmonary bypass cases in the USA, and are increasing in popularity in the UK and Europe.

Mechanical considerations of extracorporeal circulation

Even with conditions of alpha-blockade and volume loading, can normal peripheral blood flow of 3.21 m^2/min be achieved with an artificial device? Probably so, but at the expense of some loss of safety caused by increased flow in the extracorporeal circuit. High arterial line pressure, more surface exposure per minute, increased cavitation, and possibly a greater chance of aggregate embolism are present at high flow rates (Kirklin and Barratt-Boyes, 1986). With the current state of the art, bypass flows of 2.2–2.4 L/min/m^2 are generally considered a reasonable compromise (Replogle and Gross, 1961; Tarhan and Moffitt, 1971; Kirklin and Barratt-Boyes, 1986). The resulting moderate flow is well tolerated for the one to two hours required for most intracardiac operations and usually does not result in any permanent sequelae. Hence, flow levels of 2.4 L/min/m^2 have come to be considered the 'normal' physiology of extracorporeal circulation, although this is not necessarily the case. Mechanical factors affecting bypass flow rates include the size and position of venous and arterial cannulae, the nature of the pump and type of oxygenator. The flow obtained in total bypass is a function of the blood volume and the diameter of the tubing used for the venous lines. Assuming that 100 cmH$_2$O of siphon suction is applied to the venous cannulae, the maximal possible flow increases linearly with tubing size until high flow rates are achieved (Peirce, 1969). Under conditions of inadequate venous return, whether due to low blood volume or low arterial perfusion with sequestration, the flow through the venous line is regulated by the collapsing of the vena cavae around the venous cannula. Under conditions of adequate venous return the bypass flow is limited by the size and length of the venous drainage lines. The resistance to flow is directly related to the length of tubing and inversely related to the fourth power of the radius of the tubing (Holloway *et al.*, 1988).

Theoretically, the size of the arterial cannula is not a major consideration during non-pulsatile flow. If 5 L/min is pumped then 5 L/min will flow through the arterial cannula. However, the flow rate will be maintained only at the expense of higher pressures and greater turbulence in the perfusion system. These factors may lead to haemolysis (Blacksheer *et al.*, 1965) and also increase the risk of tubing separation or rupture. Arterial cannulae which are capable of providing adequate flow with a pressure gradient across the cannula of less than 100 mmHg and arterial line pressures of less than 250 mmHg have been recommended (Brodman *et al.*, 1985; Kirklin and Kirklin, 1990). Brodman *et al.* (1985) found that there is poor correlation between the pressure flow characteristics of arterial cannulae and French designation, which is a measure of the outside diameter of the tip of the cannulae. Therefore, comparison of performance characteristics between similarly sized cannulae is difficult. Montoya *et al.* (1990) devised a numerical designation based on a Reynolds number friction factor correlation that can allow easy comparison of pressure flow characteristics between different cannulae.

Normally, blood flow is approximately 110 mL/kg body weight with a pulse amplitude of 20–40 mmHg (with some species variation). The studies that demonstrated acidosis and organ failure during non-pulsatile flow were conducted at flow rates ranging from 60 mL/kg to 100 mL/kg. Those investigators who found no difference between pulsatile and non-pulsatile flow used total perfusion rates between 130 mL/kg and 200 mL/kg (Rudy *et al.*, 1970a; Boucher *et al.*, 1974; Harker *et al.*, 1980). This relationship could have been predicted from the studies of Harrison (Harrison *et al.*, 1970; Harrison and Seton, 1973), which showed that adrenal catecholamine secretion is regulated in part by carotid sinus baroreceptors. Decreased pulse amplitude caused maximal catecholamine output when total flow was less than normal, but minimal catecholamine output during normal and above normal flow rates. From Harrison's findings, one might expect no difference between pulsatile perfusion and non-pulsatile perfusion at flow rates over 110 mL/kg. High vascular resistance and metabolic acidosis would occur during non-pulsatile perfusion only at flow rates of 80–110 mL/kg and would occur during both pulsatile and non-pulsatile perfusion at flow rates less than 70 mL/kg (Fig. 3.1). This corresponds closely to the reports listed above.

The implications of these studies for total cardiopulmonary bypass in cardiac surgery are significant as total perfusion is usually carried out at flow rates of 70–100 mL/kg. At this abnormally low flow rate the adrenal catecholamine secretion is increased by the decreased

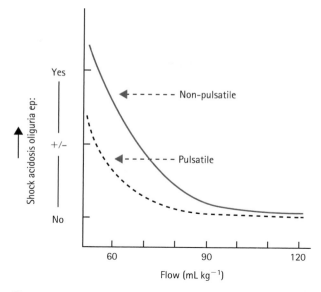

Figure 3.1 *Low-flow syndrome related to total perfusion, with and without pulsation.*

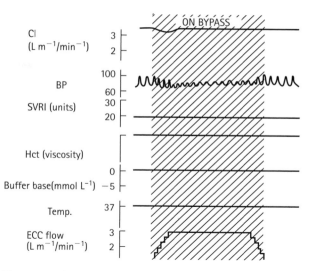

Figure 3.2 *Typical haemodynamic changes during veno-arterial bypass in an infant on prolonged bypass (ECMO) with normal haematocrit, temperature and flow. CI = cardiac index; BP = blood pressure; SVRI = systemic vascular resistance index; Hct = haematocrit; Temp. = temperature; ECC = extracorporeal circulation.*

pulse amplitude, hence pulsatile flow (Bregman, 1976) or alpha-blockade should be used to ameliorate the systemic effects of the altered flow pattern. During partial pulmonary bypass for life support, total flow should be maintained as near normal as possible and should be regulated by whatever means necessary to assure a pulse amplitude of 15 mmHg or more.

THE PATHOPHYSIOLOGICAL RESPONSE TO EXTRACORPOREAL CIRCULATION

Haemodynamic

Both systemic and pulmonary haemodynamics are wildly deranged in response to extracorporeal circulation, and only start to return to normal after its discontinuation. Low cardiac output after cardiopulmonary bypass is initially organ-threatening, and if not addressed promptly, will soon become life-threatening. It can be classified into reversible or non-reversible, but the majority of patients who develop a low cardiac output syndrome after coronary artery surgery fall into the reversible category and are therefore amenable to pharmacological and haemodynamic manipulation (Emmi and Jacobs, 1992).

A common factor involved in the production of low cardiac output after elective coronary artery surgery is low volume state. Intravascular dehydration is a reflection of plasma volume loss, which may be related to excessive diuresis, insensible losses peri-operatively and the third space phenomenon. The latter is seen in patients with altered vascular permeability caused by cardiopulmonary bypass. The majority of the original studies on the effects

of cardiopulmonary bypass used the standard non-pulsatile roller pump for their investigations, and it was clearly shown that haemodynamic parameters were distorted, along with major metabolic and hormonal changes (Uozumi *et al.*, 1972; Taylor *et al.*, 1978a,b,c).

The large increase in peripheral resistance (systemic vascular resistance) normally associated with cardiopulmonary bypass has been shown in many studies to be ameliorated by the incorporation of pulsatile flow. This is largely thought to be due to the fact that the addition of pulsatility prevents excessive activation of the renin-angiotensin system, thereby causing less release of the powerful vasoconstrictor angiotensin II (Taylor *et al.*, 1979a,b). There are great concerns that an elevated systemic vascular resistance is a hazardous situation in the post-operative period because of its sequelae on other haemodynamic parameters. High systemic vascular resistance states increase left ventricular work, and consequently sub-endocardial perfusion may be compromised (Taylor *et al.*, 1982).

Physiological studies of prolonged normothermic extracorporeal circulation have demonstrated that changes in haemodynamic measurements and other physiological parameters are present (Fig. 3.2). The only substantial deviations from normal physiology during normothermic extracorporeal circulation are the anticoagulation required and the non-pulsatile flow imposed by the system. Hence, much of the 'normal' physiology of extracorporeal circulation is probably best defined in patients requiring veno-arterial bypass for respiratory failure. In contrast, cardiopulmonary bypass during cardiac surgery

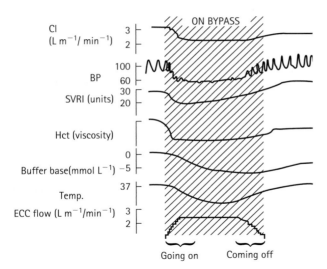

Figure 3.3 *Typical haemodynamic changes during conventional veno-arterial bypass with haemodilution, hypothermia and low-flow. CI = cardiac index; BP = blood pressure; SVRI = systemic vascular resistance index; Hct = haematocrit; Temp. = temperature; ECC = extracorporeal circulation.*

superimposes several other conditions that can alter normal physiology, including haemodilution, hypothermia, and relative hypoperfusion. Figure 3.2 illustrates that during normothermic extracorporeal circulation we can go from total bypass to normal cardiac function and back to total bypass without significant changes in oxygen kinetics or metabolic changes, whereas Fig. 3.3 shows that several haemodynamic functions are altered during conventional bypass with haemodilution, hypothermia and low flow. Hypotension is common after initiation of bypass and has been attributed to several factors. First of all, flow is usually initiated at 2.4 L/min/m², which is less than normal, physiological perfusion. In addition, elevated histamine levels have been documented in the circuit prime and have been shown to be elevated when extracorporeal circulation is initiated (Marath *et al.*, 1987, 1988). Hypotension caused by vasodilation is a known response to histamine. Another factor that may contribute to hypotension is activation of the alternative complement pathways, with resultant formation of anaphylatoxins such as C3a (Chenoworth, 1986; Reigel *et al.*, 1988). Complement activation, in turn, has been associated with neutrophil activation and granule release (Cavarocchi *et al.*, 1986b; Wachtfogel *et al.*, 1987), which may also adversely affect haemodynamics. A sudden decrease in systemic vascular resistance due to abrupt haemodilution, which affects blood viscosity, appears to be a significant cause of hypotension after initiation of extracorporeal circulation (Robicsek *et al.*, 1983).

If the total flow remains constant with the increase in pressure, blood is preferentially directed to organs that are more responsive to increased perfusion pressure and

least dependent on arteriolar tone. This includes the two most important organs – the brain and the heart. At the same time blood flow is most decreased in organs such as skin and skeletal muscle, in which the vasculature is the least sensitive to increased perfusion pressure. The resulting redistribution of blood flow under these circumstances has been studied by several investigators (Lees *et al.*, 1970; Rudy *et al.*, 1970a, b). The results indicate that during cardiopulmonary bypass there is a redistribution of blood flow that is caused by factors other than the alterations in pulse pressure that occur when non-pulsatile perfusion is used. The factors include anaesthesia, peripheral emboli, amount of haemodilution, effects on blood elements, etc. This neuroendocrine response and redistribution phenomenon may be diminished by alpha-adrenergic blocking anaesthetic drugs, such as halothane, in which case the arterial pressure remains relatively low under conditions of constant flow. Occasionally, the neuroendocrine sympathetic response will dominate the haemodynamics, creating the syndrome of hypertension at constant flow with poor organ perfusion which may be serious enough to require definitive alpha-adrenergic blockade (Maxwell *et al.*, 1958; Lemieux *et al.*, 1967; Gomes and McGoon, 1969; Burack *et al.*, 1972; Mannucci, 1988).

These haemodynamic effects of extracorporeal circulation have been evaluated by Gazzaniga *et al.* (1970) and Gazzaniga *et al.* (1972), who utilized the method of skeletal muscle surface pH measurement to evaluate the perfusion metabolism relationship in that specific tissue. Since the arterial blood under conditions of anaesthesia or bypass is completely saturated with oxygen, decreasing muscle surface pH is a direct reflection of decreasing capillary flow. An initial decrease in muscle surface pH occurs with the induction of anaesthesia and its attendant minor myocardial depressant effects, demonstrating the sensitivity of the measurement. With the institution of cardiopulmonary bypass, muscle surface pH drops remarkably and then gradually continues to fall during the period of extracorporeal circulation, indicating inadequate tissue perfusion. The addition of blood volume can result in an increase in arterial pressure at constant flow and minimize decreased organ perfusion to some extent, leading to a low plateau of muscle surface pH rather than a continuing fall. Pre-loading with volume can further minimize the low flow. The addition of alpha-adrenergic blockade reverses or nearly eliminates the muscle surface acidosis, indicating the major role of alpha-adrenergic stimulation during extracorporeal circulation (Gazzaniga *et al.*, 1972). Venous pH, as a more general and less sensitive measure of organ perfusion, falls during bypass at a constant PCO_2. More specifically, a condition of metabolic acidosis can be detected by measurement of pH and PCO_2. Urine output usually falls during bypass, although the concomitant effects of antidiuretic endocrine stimuli and pharmacologically induced diuresis by mannitol or diuretics make observation of the urine output a questionable indicator of perfusion in a clinical situation. Similarly, Del Canale *et al.* (1988) showed that hypothermic, low flow extracorporeal circulation leads to increased anaerobic metabolism in skeletal muscle, with a concurrent increase in lactate and decrease in phosphocreatine levels and intracellular pH. Fantini *et al.* (1987) found that low-flow hypothermic extracorporeal circulation leads to a decrease in skeletal muscle transmembrane potential and an increase in intracellular sodium and selective membrane permeability to sodium and potassium. These findings are similar to that found in haemorrhagic shock, and support the studies of Gazzaniga demonstrating inadequate tissue perfusion during extracorporeal circulation as usually performed for cardiac surgery.

Blood volume

If blood flow is held constant during perfusion, transfusion of blood and fluid will be necessary to maintain constant intravascular volume. Although blood loss at the surgical site accounts for some of the loss of volume, other factors also appear to be involved. Several groups have demonstrated a significant increase in extracellular fluid following cardiopulmonary bypass (Breckenridge *et al.*, 1969; Cohn *et al.*, 1971). One mechanism for this may be related to the decreased plasma oncotic pressure that occurs as a result of haemodilution. However, an eventual increase in interstitial pressure and decrease in interstitial oncotic pressure leads to an equilibrium that appears to ultimately limit oedema formation (Rein *et al.*, 1988). A primary increase in capillary permeability has been demonstrated by Smith *et al.* (1987). The factors responsible for this increase in capillary permeability are uncertain, but activated neutrophils have been shown to increase capillary permeability (Henney *et al.*, 1971). This corresponds nicely with *in vitro* studies demonstrating disruption of the cytoskeleton in endothelial cells exposed to hydrogen peroxide, with resultant loss of cell shape (Hind *et al.*, 1988). Taken together, these studies suggest that activated neutrophils may injure endothelial cells and subsequently lead to an increase in micro-vascular permeability. Plasma volume loss may also result from diuresis induced by adding mannitol or a potent diuretic to the oxygenator priming solution. Venous return to the extracorporeal device is impaired if blood volume is not adequately replaced, which in turn results in a decreased arterial flow rate. Tissue perfusion is not optimal if this occurs and can lead to metabolic acidosis.

Endocrine

Changes in blood hormone levels and their release have been associated with extracorporeal circulation for some time. If these changes could be ameliorated or controlled, there is the potential to preserve remote organ function. Many of the changes can be attributed to the stress response to the shock-like state conferred by cardiopulmonary bypass. Antidiuretic hormone has been shown to rise significantly during cardiopulmonary bypass, but return to baseline by 24 hours. The increase during extracorporeal circulation is probably due to the decreased stimulation of baroreceptors that occurs during bypass (Fedderson *et al.*, 1985; Viinamaki *et al.*, 1986). No untoward effects can be attributed to this alone, but in certain susceptible environments it may have undesired consequences.

The gonadotrophic hormones are all affected by cardiopulmonary bypass, but the significance is uncertain. Adrenocorticotrophic hormone (ACTH) levels increase with the surgical incision, but decrease on non-pulsatile cardiopulmonary bypass (Taylor *et al.*, 1976). Growth hormone levels rise on incision and continue to rise throughout cardiopulmonary bypass, peaking at two hours (MacDonald *et al.*, 1975). Several investigators have shown that ACTH and cortisol are elevated in response to extracorporeal circulation (Kono *et al.*, 1983; Pollack *et al.*, 1988). Cortisol secretion does not appear to be influenced by non-pulsatile flow. The secretion of cortisol and growth hormone during extracorporeal circulation contributes to the changes in glucose metabolism seen during cardiopulmonary bypass. A mild hyperglycaemia is seen during normothermic cardiopulmonary bypass, which is caused by increased gluconeogenesis and peripheral insulin resistance in response to the elevated levels of stress hormones (Kuntschen *et al.*, 1986). Glucose levels are normal during hypothermic extracorporeal circulation, probably because of the inhibition of hepatic gluconeogenesis during hypothermia. However, glucose levels rise during rewarming and glucose metabolism becomes similar to that seen during normothermic extracorporeal circulation (Kuntschen *et al.*, 1985).

Anaesthesia and surgery alone are both known to elicit the stress response, which is characterized by raised ADH, renin, cortisol and catecholamine levels. Cardiopulmonary bypass only further exaggerates the response, and is also responsible for the widespread release of a number of vasoactive substances into the circulation. These include prostaglandins and serotonin, and the levels of endogenous adrenaline and noradrenaline released are equivalent to those released during a myocardial infarct or strenuous exercise (Replogle *et al.*, 1962). The generalized factors mentioned earlier (hypothermia, haemodilution, low perfusion) are all responsible for a metabolic or endocrine response.

Operations requiring cardiopulmonary bypass display a generalized increase in serum catecholamine levels in excess of that seen during operations not requiring extracorporeal circulation (Replogle *et al.*, 1962; Tan *et al.*, 1976; Fedderson *et al.*, 1985). This release of catecholamines results from stimulation of both the carotid sinus and aortic baroreceptors (Harrison and Seton, 1973). These receptors appear to respond to low pulse amplitude, which occurs during non-pulsatile perfusion (Stein and Ferris, 1973), when total flow is decreased. Hypothermia also appears to be a major stimulus for catecholamine release and can adversely affect post-operative haemodynamics and increase oxygen consumption during rewarming. These adverse effects can be ameliorated by neuromuscular paralysis during the rewarming period (Zwischenberger *et al.*, 1987).

Renin secretion from the kidney is also increased in response to the decrease in mean arterial pressure and reduction of left atrial pressure, which in turn leads to angiotensin activation and subsequent aldosterone secretion (Kono *et al.*, 1983). The increase in catecholamines, vasopressin and angiotensin II combine to increase arteriolar constriction, which returns the blood pressure towards normal.

Several other important endocrine changes occur in response to extracorporeal circulation. Atrial natriuretic factor (ANF) is a peptide hormone secreted by atrial cardiocytes in response to stretching of the atrial wall (Needleman and Greenwald, 1986). This hormone has a wide variety of actions, including an increase in glomerular filtration rate and pronounced natriuresis, inhibition of aldosterone secretion, attenuation of the vasopressin release (that occurs in response to hypovolaemia), suppression of renin release and direct relaxation of blood vessels, resulting in a decrease in systemic vascular resistance. Since extracorporeal circulation involves emptying of the atria for several hours it would be anticipated that ANF levels would decrease because the primary stimulus for ANF release, atrial stretch, would not be present. However, Dewar *et al.* (1988) surprisingly found a paradoxical increase in ANF during cardiopulmonary bypass and a decrease after termination of bypass. Furthermore, these workers found a lack of correlation between atrial filling pressure and ANF release in the early post-operative period. Two subsequent studies, however, did not show any significant change in ANF levels during extracorporeal circulation but found that ANF levels increased markedly early after bypass (Asari *et al.*, 1989; Schaff *et al.*, 1989). Although the clinical significance of these findings is uncertain, the peri-operative changes in ANF release which are unique to operations performed during extracorporeal circulation may play a role in post-operative diuresis (Schaff *et al.*, 1989).

Fluid and electrolytes

Fluid and electrolyte disorders after extracorporeal circulation for cardiac surgery are major clinical considerations.

Sodium retention, expanded extracellular fluid and decreased total body potassium are characteristic of patients with some degree of cardiac failure pre-operatively, particularly if they had been treated with diuretics. Inadequate post-operative myocardial function as a result of hypothermia, anoxia or the cardiac lesion itself may cause similar problems. A sophisticated study of fluid compartment composition and electrolyte status was reported by Pacifico and colleagues (1970). These workers used moderate haemodilution and found a significant increase in extracellular fluid and exchangeable sodium with a significant decrease in total body potassium in response to extracorporeal circulation. The increased expanded extracellular fluid would be expected from the equilibrium of a saline type of haemodilution priming solution, plus the effects of exposure of platelets, white cells and proteins to a gas interface, which might result in increased capillary permeability. The decreased total body potassium is explained on the basis of kaliuresis and anticipated maximal aldosterone response associated with maximum stress. Similar changes in blood potassium were reported by Dieter *et al.* (1969). Hypokalaemia is the only major electrolyte abnormality of significance and is important because of the potential of developing digitalis-induced dysrhythmias. Hypokalaemia may be avoided by including potassium chloride in the priming solution (Pacifico *et al.*, 1970; Henling *et al.*, 1985). Extensive studies on calcium (Pedersen and Juhl, 1983; Chambers *et al.*, 1984) and magnesium (Turnier *et al.*, 1972; Romero *et al.*, 1973) show that these cations decrease initially with dilution at the onset of bypass and remain somewhat low throughout the course of extracorporeal circulation. The normal feedback loop between parathyroid hormone and calcium does not appear to function normally during cardiopulmonary bypass (Chambers *et al.*, 1984). Therefore, levels must be maintained at normal by supplementing calcium at the end of extracorporeal circulation. Although it has been suggested that hypomagnesaemia may predispose to dyrhythmias in extracorporeal circulation patients (Turnier *et al.*, 1972), it appears that these minor variations in calcium and magnesium do not commonly cause significant clinical abnormalities.

GAS EXCHANGE DURING EXTRACORPOREAL CIRCULATION

Gas exchange for extracorporeal circulation has proved to be the easiest problem to overcome. Flowing blood is exposed to oxygen either directly or through a gas-permeable membrane. Oxygen diffuses into the blood plasma because of a gradient between high PO_2 in the gas phase and the low PO_2 in mixed venous blood. Oxygen then diffuses from the plasma through the red cell membrane to combine with unsaturated haemoglobin. The binding of oxygen to haemoglobin proceeds very rapidly and the limiting factor in oxygenation of flowing blood is the rate of oxygen diffusion through plasma (Bartlett, 1971). Hence, the thickness of the blood film between gas bubbles or surfaces, or between gas exchange membranes becomes the rate limiting factor. Carbon dioxide diffuses out of the flowing blood in the gas exchange device because of the gradient between the PCO_2 in mixed venous blood and the partial pressure of CO_2 in the ventilating gas. Although the gradient of CO_2 exchange is relatively low and can never be greater than the mixed venous PCO_2, the rate of diffusion through plasma is so rapid that CO_2 removal always proceeds more efficiently than oxygenation. Therefore, to avoid excess CO_2 removal with its attendant alkalosis, the gradient is diminished by adding CO_2 to the ventilating gas or by reducing the gas flow to the oxygenator.

Oxygenator performance

The performance characteristics of the gas exchange device must be thoroughly documented to plan the best extracorporeal circuit for any given patient. Since CO_2 removal is almost invariably greater than oxygenation, it is sufficient to describe the performance of gas exchange devices in terms of their oxygenating efficiency. The following factors must be known about the gas exchange device. How much oxygen can actually be supplied per minute? How much oxygen can be supplied under conditions of variable blood flow and variable mixed venous saturation? How much oxygen can be supplied at flow rates which are compatible with adequate perfusion for the patient in question (that is, at least $2.4\,L/min/m^2$)? What flow of ventilating gas is required? How much foreign surface is exposed to the flowing blood (this number is easy to derive for membrane oxygenators, but much more difficult for gas interface oxygenators)? What effects, if any, does the gas exchange device have on the components of flowing blood?

Many of these factors have been conveniently combined into a single expression of oxygenator performance defined as rated flow (Galletti et al., 1972). The rated flow is the flow at which blood leaving the oxygenator is 95 per cent saturated, under the conditions of mixed venous blood inflow. In other words, when venous blood (haemoglobin $15\,g/100\,mL$, PO_2 $40\,mmHg$, saturation 65 per cent, O_2 content $15\,mL/100\,mL$) is pumped through a gas exchange device at $200\,mL/min$, the outflow blood will be 100 per cent saturated (PO_2 $150\,mmHg$, O_2 content $20\,mL/100\,mL$). The amount of O_2 actually delivered by the device is determined by the flow rate and the arterio-venous difference. As blood

flow through the device is increased, a point is reached at which the limiting factor is the thickness of the blood film and the rate at which O_2 diffuses through that particular film. When that point is exceeded, the outflow blood will exit at less than 100 per cent saturation. The rated flow for a given device is that flow at which this limitation is reached. The rated O_2 delivery is the amount of O_2 that can be taken up by the blood at the rated flow. The upper limit of O_2 delivery is related to the flow and to the amount of unsaturated haemoglobin presented to the oxygenator per minute. If total bypass flow is decreased at a constant level of tissue oxygen consumption, venous saturation must decrease as more oxygen is extracted from the flowing blood. As long as this does not exceed the oxygenating capability of the gas exchange device, the oxygenator will compensate and function at a wider arterio-venous difference. Some of these variables are outlined in Fig. 3.4, in which oxygen delivery per minute is related to the flow in litres per minute for different levels of venous saturation or arterio-venous difference. Notice that oxygen delivery is entirely dependent on flow. Decreasing flow severely decreases oxygen delivery, although fully saturated blood with a high PO_2 will be perfused into the arterial system.

Reports on oxygenation performance of gas exchange devices must include at least enough data to calculate inflow and outflow O_2 content and rated flow. In planning

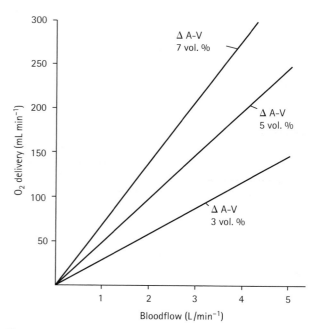

Figure 3.4 *Oxygen delivery is directly related to blood flow and arterio-venous difference. The maximum oxygen that can be delivered for a given blood flow at a given venous saturation is shown here. This represents the maximum amount of oxygen delivery that could be accomplished by a gas exchange device under a given set of flow and inlet conditions.*

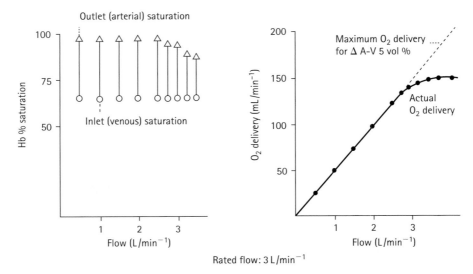

Figure 3.5 *The concept of rated flow. A hypothetical gas exchange device has a maximum oxygen transfer capability of 150 mL/min⁻¹, based on the surface area and blood flow characteristics. As long as the oxygen transport capability of flowing blood is less than 150 mL/min⁻¹, fully saturated blood leaves the oxygenator. When the oxygen transport capability of flowing blood exceeds this amount, a desaturated blood results. Under normal venous blood conditions this occurs at a flow rate of 3 L/min⁻¹, the rated flow of this device. At flow rates in excess of 3 L/min⁻¹, the outlet blood is desaturated, the arterio-venous difference is narrow and the actual oxygen transferred reaches a plateau.*

the components of an extracorporeal circuit the oxygen requirement of the patient at normothermia is calculated ($150 \, \text{mL/min/m}^2$). The blood flow which will deliver this amount of oxygen with an arterio-venous difference of $5 \, \text{mL}/100 \, \text{mL}$ is calculated or determined from a graph (Fig. 3.5). The cannulae, tubing and pump are chosen to provide the desired flow.

The concept of rated flow is demonstrated again in Fig. 3.5, and the rated flow for several oxygenators is outlined in Fig. 3.6. If a gas exchange device is operated at flow rates higher than its rated flow, desaturated blood will be perfused and the actual O_2 delivery per minute reaches a fairly level plateau regardless of flow rate.

Types of oxygenator

Assuming that the oxygenator will be used at appropriate flow rates below the rated flow, the choice of an oxygenator must be related to the ease of use and possible damage to blood components. Two basic types of gas exchange devices are used in extracorporeal circuits: a direct gas interface oxygenator in which O_2 is bubbled, filmed or foamed directly through blood, which is then defoamed or debubbled through some type of settling or filtering chamber, or a membrane oxygenator in which a gas exchange membrane is interposed between the gas phase and the blood phase. Older membrane oxygenators used silicone 'rubber', whereas the new generation of

membrane oxygenators utilize micro-porous materials such as polypropylene. These new oxygenators with either micro-porous hollow fibres or sheet membranes have much greater gas transfer capacities than membrane oxygenators used in the past (Bjork *et al.*, 1985). Gas interface oxygenators have the advantage of simplicity, disposability and relatively low cost. Disadvantages include the possibility of gross or microscopic air embolism, relatively large priming volumes (although if the priming volume remains constant the exact volume is not important), variable reservoir level resulting in potential shifts in blood volume between the intracorporeal and extracorporeal circuit and the effects of direct gas interface, including protein denaturation (Lee *et al.*, 1961; Dobell *et al.*, 1965), increased haemolysis, platelet dysfunction and thrombocytopenia (van Oeveren *et al.*, 1985; Boonstra *et al.*, 1986). One group also found greater complement activation with bubble oxygenators (Cavarocchi *et al.*, 1986), although van Oeveren *et al.* (1985) were not able to demonstrate any difference in complement activation between membrane and bubble oxygenators. Membrane oxygenators have the advantages of eliminating blood–gas interface effects, ease of operation, less haemolysis, less platelet and neutrophil activation, better platelet preservation and less microemboli (van Oeveren *et al.*, 1985; Boonstra *et al.*, 1986; Cavarocchi *et al.*, 1986; Blauth *et al.*, 1990). The disadvantages of membrane oxygenators include expense, potential difficulty in eliminating all bubbles during priming and moderately

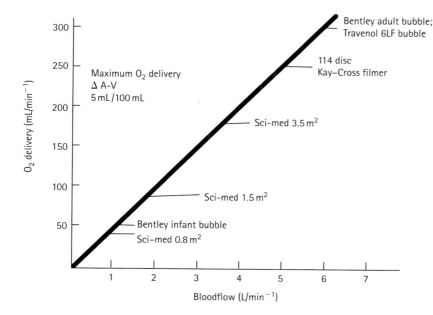

Figure 3.6 *Rated flow under normal venous inlet conditions for a variety of commercial oxygenators. (Data based on publications cited in text or manufacturers' data sheet.) When modular units are used in parallel the rated flow becomes the sum of rated flows of all units in the circuit.*

large, although constant, priming volumes in some instances.

Many of the published reports on pump or membrane oxygenator characteristics have included an open gas interface reservoir in the experimental design (Bernstein and Gleason, 1967; Dutton and Edmunds, 1973). Data from these studies are applicable to extracorporeal circulation for cardiac surgery, as coronary suction, which has been to shown to injure platelets (Boonstra et al., 1985), will always require some of the blood exposed to a direct gas interface. However, characterization of physiological changes of extracorporeal circulation or blood surface exposure should be done in experimental models that specifically exclude any gas interface to eliminate any variations caused by this factor.

Microporous membranes are made of non-wettable substances, such as Teflon®, perforated with multiple small holes that permit gas transfer but preclude blood leakage because of surface tension effects. Oxygen and CO_2 transfer in a gas-to-gas test system are virtually unlimited with this type of membrane, but the plasma oxygen diffusion limitations still exist when blood is applied to the membrane. Hence, microporous membranes have oxygen transfer characteristics similar to other membrane oxygenators of similar flow design. Carbon dioxide transfer will be significantly better, however. The latter consideration is important only in oxygenators where mixing is intense (Bartlett et al., 1974) and CO_2 transfer is the limiting design variable. Haemotological studies indicate that microporous membrane oxygenators cause less haemolysis and platelet dysfunction than bubble oxygenators (van Oeveren et al., 1985; Boonstra et al., 1986; Calafiore et al., 1987). Specific types of gas interface and membrane oxygenators and performance data are discussed in subsequent chapters in this book.

Oxygen delivery

An understanding of the relationship between oxygen delivery and consumption is necessary before the physiology of extracorporeal circulation can be fully appreciated. Systemic oxygen delivery during extracorporeal circulation is dependent on the flow supplied by the extracorporeal support device and the oxygen content of the blood, which in turn is affected by the haemoglobin content, degree of saturation and factors which affect the haemoglobin–oxygen dissociation curve, such as temperature, PCO_2, level of 2, 3 diphosphoglycerate, etc. Oxygen consumption during extracorporeal circulation is normally influenced by factors such as body temperature and catecholamine release but may be modified by other circumstances, such as sepsis. Normally, systemic oxygen delivery is five times systemic oxygen consumption.

Measurement of mixed venous blood oxygen saturation provides a quick estimation of the relationship between oxygen delivery and consumption. If the arterial haemoglobin saturation is 100 per cent, and 20 per cent of the delivered oxygen is required for metabolic processes, then the saturation of the mixed venous blood will be approximately 80 per cent (Zwischenberger et al., 1986). If systemic oxygen delivery is reduced, or if the systemic consumption of oxygen is increased, then the delivery: consumption ratio falls. For example, if the delivery:consumption ratio is 2:1 then one-half of the oxygen supplied by the arterial blood is consumed. If the arterial

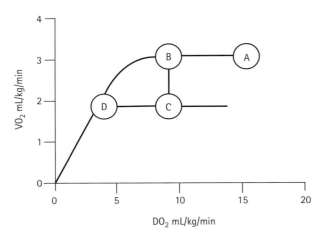

Figure 3.7 *Relationship between oxygen consumption and oxygen delivery. (See text for explanation.)*

saturation was 100 per cent then the mixed venous saturation would be 50 per cent. Hence, the measurement of mixed venous saturation provides a reasonably accurate approximation of the ratio between oxygen delivery and consumption. Organ function will be normal as long as the ratio between systemic oxygen delivery and consumption is 2.5 or greater. However, oxygen consumption will be impaired if the ratio is below this level. This can result in anaerobic metabolism, with resulting lactic acidosis and subsequent organ dysfunction and failure. These relationships are shown diagramatically in Fig. 3.7, in which (A) represents normal physiological conditions and (B) represents the systemic oxygen delivery that occurs during low-flow veno-arterial bypass with haemodilution. This point is very close to the critical ratio at which anaerobic metabolism occurs. To compensate for this, oxygen consumption is decreased by lowering the metabolic rate through the use of hypothermia (C). The segment between (D) and (C) represents the margin of safety afforded by the use of flows that are in excess of that required by the hypothermic patient. This is reflected by an abnormally elevated mixed venous saturation, which demonstrates less systemic oxygen consumption at a given flow due to hypothermia. During rewarming the metabolic rate increases, so oxygen delivery must be increased to maintain the proper relationship between oxygen delivery and consumption.

BLOOD COMPONENT DYSFUNCTION DURING EXTRACORPOREAL CIRCULATION

Normally, flowing blood is continuously exposed to endothelial cells. Fibrin formation takes place at a continuous rate on the endothelial surface balanced exactly by plasmin formation and concomitant fibrinolysis.

Both of these reactions proceed at a slow and balanced rate so that the end effect is a slow but definitely measurable gradual conversion of fibrinogen to fibrin, counterbalanced by an identical rate of fibrin degradation and elimination of fibrin degradation products. This delicate balance is abruptly upset by exposure of blood to collagen fibres underlying endothelial cells, tissue collagen, tissue thromboplastin, air, necrotic tissue or disrupted cells, and to some extent foreign material in the bloodstream itself, such as endotoxin. Under these circumstances the rate of conversion of fibrinogen to fibrin is greatly enhanced and proceeds to clotting at a much faster rate than fibrinolysis takes place. Concomitantly, platelet surfaces are altered, platelet adhesion and aggregation occurs, and platelets release factors that further stimulate the formation of fibrin clot. This chain of events occurs during normal haemostasis. If any deficiencies occur in any of the factors required for coagulation or if any of the steps are inhibited by a drug or lack of a catalyst such as calcium, or if platelet numbers or function are severely decreased, then haemostasis is severely disordered. The effects of extracorporeal circulation on the constituent elements of the coagulation system, as well as platelet function and the physiology of the fibrinolytic system, have been the subject of a great deal of recent research.

Fibrin formation and fibrinolysis

Extracorporeal circulation exposes the blood to a wide variety of surface textures and materials. During cardiac surgery, blood is aspirated from the field (cardiotomy suction) and mixed with the perfusate. This aspirated blood may include tissue thromboplastin, clots, serum, gross particles of fat, muscle and bone, suture and other foreign material (Okies *et al.*, 1977). In addition, the extracorporeal circuit contains innumerable flat edges, right-angled turns, stagnant zones, recirculating zones, jet zones and other flow characteristics not typically found in the normal circulatory system. All of these factors have the effect of gross stimulation of platelet function, the coagulation cascade and the fibrinolytic system. Until recently, heparin has been an absolutely indispensable drug in controlling these systems during extracorporeal circulation. At present heparin still plays a major role in the management of blood coagulation during extracorporeal circulation, but other drugs and devices as well as partially heparinized or heparin-free bypass systems have being studied intensively and have been used in clinical practice (Whittlesey *et al.*, 1988; Bidstrup *et al.*, 1989; Von Segesser and Turina, 1989).

Heparin has several pharmacokinetic properties that make it an ideal anticoagulant for extracorporeal circulation, including maximal effect within minutes of intravenous administration. It also has a very short, dose-dependent half-life and a safe and effective reversal agent in protamine sulphate (Bjornsson *et al.*, 1982; Tollefsen and Blinder, 1995). Monitoring systems such as the activated clotting time are accurate and widely used in practice both before, during and after cardiopulmonary bypass (Despotis *et al.*, 1995). Unfortunately, it also has some features that make it unattractive for use which has prompted the research into the heparin-free systems mentioned above. It can cause platelet aggregation by both immune and non-immune mediated mechanisms (Hirsch *et al.*, 1995), which may result in potentially catastrophic thrombocytopenia and intravascular coagulation. In addition, studies suggest that it may inhibit neutrophil activation and raise hepatic transaminases, and both antithrombin III deficiency and protamine sensitivity may cause serious problems in affected individuals.

Currently, the physiological changes associated with extracorporeal circulation must include those associated with heparinization as part of the normal baseline. To measure clotting accurately by any of the many tests which require a fibrin clot as an end-point, the amount of heparin in the blood must be measured or estimated and inactivated with an appropriate agent. For cardiac surgery it is desirable to maintain a prolonged clotting time with excessive amounts of heparin during the period of bypass. This requires at least 200 units/kg^{-1} of patient weight and 200 units/L^{-1} of blood in the priming solution. To provide an extra margin of safety most teams infuse 300 units/kg^{-1} into the patient and 150 units/kg^{-1} at 30-minute intervals during the entire period of bypass. (Since heparin activity is measured by bioassay, activity is standardized in units of anticoagulant activity. Most heparin preparations are considered to contain 100 units/mg^{-1}, although this may be technically incorrect.) Heparin carries a very strong negative charge and will become bonded to positive charges wherever they occur on glass or plastic surfaces, therefore care must be taken when adding small amounts of heparin to fluids that are exposed to a large surface area.

Changes that occur in the coagulation system during prolonged extracorporeal circulation (24–48 hours) in a system without a direct gas interface are outlined in Figs 3.8 and 3.9. These studies are used as examples of extensive contact between blood and foreign surfaces. Changes during the first few hours are typical of those seen during cardiac surgery. In these studies partial (60–80 per cent) veno-arterial bypass was carried out in awake lambs and the heparin dose regulated at a low level. The initial drop in the levels of factors V and VIII after initiation of bypass is largely caused by haemodilution. This has been corroborated in several clinical studies which have demonstrated that the drop in most clotting factors, as well as antithrombin III, plasminogen, and alpha-2antiplasmin, correlates with the drop in haematocrit and is therefore

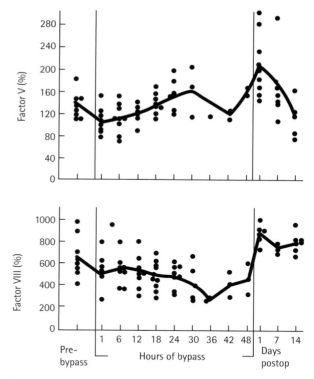

Figure 3.8 *Changes in clotting factors during prolonged extracorporeal circulation in sheep. Reprinted from Fong et al., (1974).*

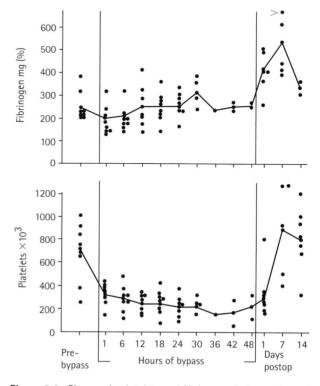

Figure 3.9 *Changes in platelets and fibrinogen during prolonged extracorporeal circulation in sheep. Reprinted from Fong et al., (1974).*

caused by haemodilution (Mammen *et al.*, 1985; Wolk *et al.*, 1985). One study has noted diminished factor VIII coagulant activity during bypass which does not correlate with the drop in haematocrit, suggesting consumption of this factor during extracorporeal circulation (Jones *et al.*, 1988). Desmopressin, a synthetic derivative of arginine-vasopressin, has been shown to increase the synthesis of von Willebrand factor and VIII:C (Mannucci, 1988). Administration of this agent to patients undergoing cardiac surgery has been shown to decrease blood loss (Salzman *et al.*, 1986). During prolonged bypass, a subsequent increase in fibrinogen and most other clotting factors is noted, owing to synthesis by the liver. The concentration of these proteins returns to pre-bypass level within a period of hours and remains normal throughout the bypass period. However, during the one to three hours of extracorporeal circulation required for most intracardiac operations this compensation has not had time to proceed to completion and levels of most protein clotting factors are slightly decreased at the time bypass is discontinued and heparin is inactivated (Gans *et al.*, 1967). Clinical studies have also demonstrated a decrease in the levels of factors II and V as well as antithrombin III after termination of bypass (Mammen *et al.*, 1985; Wolk *et al.*, 1985).

Activation of circulating plasminogen to plasmin invariably occurs as fibrinogen is activated to fibrin; hence, any clot contains the enzymatic means for its own destruction. Evidence of active circulating plasmin can be detected whenever gross clotting is present. Tissue plasminogen activating factor, which is in part responsible for plasminogen activation, has been shown to be increased during extracorporeal circulation (Stibbe *et al.*, 1984). Numerous other factors are also responsible for plasmin activation, including proteases such as kallikrein. A correlation between protease activity and postoperative bleeding has been demonstrated (Hinshaw *et al.*, 1988). Aprotinin is a recently described protease inactivator that inhibits plasmin activation (von Oeveren *et al.*, 1987). A European double-blinded prospective clinical study with aprotinin demonstrated markedly less blood loss during cardiac surgery (Bidstrup *et al.*, 1989). Tranexamic acid, which binds to plasminogen and plasmin and blocks fibrinolysis, has also been shown to reduce post-operative blood loss (Horrow *et al.*, 1990). Agents such as aprotinin and tranexamic acid are already gaining wide acceptance in clinical practice.

Platelets

Platelet dysfunction, activation and loss have all been attributed to cardiopulmonary bypass and, as mentioned previously, heparin probably contributes to the effect. Post-cardiopulmonary bypass bleeding problems are well-recognized, and platelets have been shown to be a major contributing factor. There is a dramatic fall in platelet count and loss of function immediately after the onset of cardiopulmonary bypass known as a 'first pass effect', which is generally held to be attributable to exposure of the blood to artificial surfaces. Platelet physiology during extracorporeal circulation has been an area of intense interest over the past 15 years. It is of such importance that Chapter 10 of this book is devoted in large part to this subject. Studies have consistently shown that the concentration of platelets drops with the initiation of bypass and remains depressed as long as extracorporeal circulation continues. This has even been demonstrated in *in vitro* systems in which blood is circulated through a closed circuit (Addonizio and Colman, 1982). This suggests that interactions involving platelets and foreign surfaces are in large part responsible for the drop in platelet count during extracorporeal circulation. Fibrinogen is known to be absorbed to the circuit surface. Fibrinogen receptors on the surface of platelets appear to bind to the absorbed fibrinogen, resulting in adherence of platelets to the circuit surface as well as fragmentation of circulating platelets (Wenger *et al.*, 1989). Other factors also appear to influence the adhesion of platelets to foreign surfaces, including surface texture, wettability, flow rates and geometry of the blood flow through the circuit (Addonizio and Colman, 1982). Platelets also adhere to each other, forming aggregates. These platelet aggregates form microemboli and have been visualized in retinal vessels (Blauth *et al.*, 1990). The extent to which these microemboli cause damage and affect organ function is uncertain. Patients have been supported during prolonged extracorporeal circulation for periods of more than two weeks without evidence of embolization, infarcts or aggregates at autopsy. The platelet aggregates appear to disperse into individual platelet components in the microcirculation and reappear in the circulating blood (Hickey *et al.*, 1983).

Platelet function also appears to be transiently affected by extracorporeal circulation (Harken, 1975; Tamari *et al.*, 1975). Platelet granule release occurs, suggesting some degree of activation. Platelets also become less sensitive to agonists such as ADP and epinephrine (Addonizio and Colman, 1982). These alterations in platelet function are probably significant and may contribute to bleeding complications related to extracorporeal circulation. There has been considerable interest in the clinical use of agents that inhibit platelet activation during extracorporeal circulation. Prostaglandin E, dipyrimadole, prostacyclin (epoprostenol) and the stable prostacyclin analogue iloprost have been used experimentally and clinically in an attempt to preserve platelet numbers and function during the post-operative period (Addonizio *et al.*, 1978; Fish *et al.*, 1986; Cottrell *et al.*, 1988; Teoh *et al.*, 1988). Although potentially promising, a randomized, double blind clinical trial utilizing prostacyclin showed only minor clinical impact (Fish *et al.*, 1986). Use of this agent is also limited by hypotension, which is a significant side effect. An animal study with iloprost has demonstrated significant preservation of platelet number and function and suggests this agent may be clinically useful. Aprotinin, the serine protease inhibitor mentioned earlier, has not been shown to preserve platelet concentration but does appear to have beneficial effects on platelet function (Bidstrup *et al.*, 1989).

Erythrocytes and neutrophils

Extracorporeal circulation systems such as cardiopulmonary bypass have long been known to have a dramatic effect on other formed elements of the blood, specifically red and white blood cells. The forces applied to blood cells during cardiopulmonary bypass are pressure, shear stress, wall impact and surface phenomenon (Wright, 1986).

Experimental work has shown erythrocytes to be able to withstand very high pressures, but cardiopulmonary bypass causes a significant rate of haemolysis (Hirayama *et al.*, 1985). The aetiology is multifactorial, including blood pump, oxygenator type and suction rates. Haemolysis liberates large quantities of plasma free haemoglobin into the circulation, which may have serious nephrotoxic effects (Jaenike and Schneeberger, 1966). Damaged erythrocytes may also produce lipid membrane ghosts, which can occlude the microcirculation of remote organs. They also liberate substances such as ADP and potassium, which affect platelet activation and tendency to dysrhythmias respectively. The relatively non-deformable red cells are targeted by denatured proteins, adhered to and themselves made more adhesive. They then form aggregates and have a greater likelihood of sludging and blocking capillaries, resulting in reduced flow to those areas. Clinical studies have demonstrated that minimizing red cell trauma is associated with a shorter time on the ventilator (Hirayama *et al.*, 1988).

Damage to erythrocytes during extracorporeal circulation has largely been attributed to shear stresses (Kirklin and Barratt-Boyes, 1986). Most studies of this problem, however, have a blood–gas interface somewhere within the system. Bubble oxygenators cause a greater degree of haemolysis than membrane oxygenators (Clark and Mills, 1969). Cardiotomy suction systems in particular appear to injure red blood cells (Kirklin and Barratt-Boyes, 1986). In contrast, experiments involving systems without a blood–gas interface demonstrate minimal haemolysis (Hill *et al.*, 1969; Bartlett and Gazzaniga, 1978). Since extracorporeal circulation for cardiac surgery will usually involve a direct gas interface with cardiotomy suction, the haemolysis that occurs after the red cells have been exposed to a gas interface will probably always be a part of extracorporeal circulation for cardiac surgery. Factors other than mechanical or shear stresses have also been implicated in extracorporeal circulation-induced haemolysis. The deposition of terminal C5b-9 complement complexes on erythrocytes has been demonstrated during extracorporeal circulation. In this study, all red cell ghosts were found to have the terminal complement complex embedded in the plasma membranes, whereas intact cells did not carry this complex. This suggests that complement activation may play a role in haemolysis (Salama *et al.*, 1988). Indeglia *et al.* (1967) studied red cell lysis under controlled conditions and found that haemolysis increased dramatically in lipaemic plasma and decreased with decreasing temperature in normal and lipaemic plasma. They concluded that the factors which predispose sensitized red cells to haemolysis are more chemical than mechanical, and pointed out the importance of avoiding lipaemic blood for transfusion or priming for extracorporeal circulation.

In comparisons between different flow generation techniques and their effects on red cell trauma, it has been shown that the mean hourly increment of plasma free haemoglobin (PFH) in the roller pump is six times that of the centrifugal pump (Koja *et al.*, 1986). Other studies have shown an early higher haemolytic index in roller pumps when compared with centrifugal (Oku *et al.*, 1988) and significantly higher haemolysis occurring after 16 hours of pumping (Hoerr *et al.*, 1987).

In general, the haematocrit is reduced by about 30–50 per cent from haemodilution, and further trauma to the red cells and haemolysis only serves to worsen that. Cardiopulmonary bypass has been shown to be associated with an anaemia and a shortened red cell lifespan, and it is likely that red cell losses may exceed the erythropoietic capacity of the body.

The effects of extracorporeal circulation on leukocyte kinetics, function and activation have been an area of intense interest during the past two decades. Neutrophil activation is a recognized and accepted feature of cardiopulmonary bypass and represents part of the generalized inflammatory response (Butler *et al.*, 1993). However, although recognized, enormous amounts of research have been invested in attempting to both understand and minimise the sequelae of this phenomenon. Neutrophil activation with granule release results in the generation of superoxide anions, and the release of cytokines such as tumour necrosis factor alpha, proteinases such as elastase and Cathepsin G, and neutrophil adhesion molecules. The onset of cardiopulmonary bypass causes an immediate fall in circulating numbers of neutrophils, but unlike platelets, the levels then rise again during the pump run to actually increase to above pre-operative values. This latter event appears to be temperature-related and does not occur at hypothermia, but is initiated at the onset of rewarming to normothermia. Both animal and clinical studies suggest that oxygen free radicals and leukocyte-generated enzymes may be responsible for myocardial and pulmonary damage produced by cardiopulmonary bypass (Wilson *et al.*, 1993). The incorporation of leukocyte depletion systems into the extracorporeal circulation has been demonstrated by many groups to ameliorate this damaging effect (Wilson *et al.*, 1993). Other groups, however, have questioned this and have demonstrated minimal or no amelioration. There are definitely two schools of thought on this matter, but the question remains largely unanswered, and a greater understanding is required.

Complement activation, largely through the alternative pathway, has been demonstrated in several studies (Kirklin *et al.*, 1983; Fosse *et al.*, 1987). Stimulation of the complement pathway can activate neutrophils, which release toxic oxygen species such as hydrogen peroxide as well as potentially damaging enzymes such as elastase (Hill *et al.*, 1972; Antonesen *et al.*, 1987; Wachtfogel *et al.*, 1987). Elevated levels of hydrogen peroxide have been demonstrated in patients during extracorporeal circulation (Cavarocchi *et al.*, 1986a). Furthermore, increased levels of lipid peroxidation products have been found during cardiopulmonary bypass, suggesting significant oxidant activity (Royston *et al.*, 1986). Pulmonary leukocyte sequestration during extracorporeal circulation has been demonstrated and has been implicated as a possible cause of post-operative respiratory failure (Howard *et al.*, 1988; Utoh *et al.*, 1988). Neutrophil function during bypass will continue to be an active area of research during the next decade and interventions designed to limit the activation of neutrophils and to prevent damage from the oxidants released from these cells may come into clinical practice. Methylprednisolone and free radical scavengers such as superoxide dismutase have already been used in preliminary clinical studies (Tennenberg *et al.*, 1985).

Surface effects

Stagnant blood will clot even in undamaged surfaces lined with endothelium. Correspondingly, areas with very low flow in an extracorporeal circuit will form thrombi even when the patient is completely heparinized. Scientific validity was lent to this empirical observation by Spaeth *et al.* (1973), who demonstrated the formation of fibrin and platelet deposits on surfaces where flow was stagnant. It is equally important to avoid right-angled turns and eddy current areas in extracorporeal circuits. A 2-mm step-off between a connector and a piece of tubing in the bypass circuit seems insignificant with 5–6 L/min^{-1} of blood lavaging its surface. However, a stagnant area many microns in diameter will exist in the corner of such a junction, where platelets and white cells may lie relatively

still for long periods of time. Here, heparin may be metabolized and thrombus formation can occur. The fewer connections and access sites, and the simpler the extracorporeal circuit, the less the problem of thrombus formation and direct embolization will be.

Filters

Since platelet aggregation may not be detrimental to the microcirculation it appears unnecessary to attempt to filter out aggregates that form during a single pass through the extracorporeal circuit. The observation that significant amounts of material can be removed from the circulation by filters does not necessarily mean that filtration is clinically helpful (Gervin *et al.*, 1974). Aris *et al.* (1986) did not find any evidence that arterial line filters were beneficial in preventing subtle post-operative neuropsychiatric changes. The use of a 40 mm arterial line filter did not prevent microemboli from appearing in retina vessels after cardiopulmonary bypass (Blauth *et al.*, 1988). In contrast to arterial line filtration, careful filtration of the cardiotomy aspirate and of transfused blood is mandatory in order to filter out micro-aggregates that are glued together with fibrin, since these micro-aggregates will not break up when they arrive at a capillary bed. Total perfusion filtration may even be detrimental, as platelet aggregate will be removed from the circulation and may disaggregate more slowly in the prosthetic filter than in the spleen, liver or lymph nodes. These filters can also contribute to complement activation. It should be noted, however, that filters serve as excellent microbubble traps and may be particularly useful when a bubble oxygenator is used (Padayachee *et al.*, 1988). It is doubtful that arterial line filtration is necessary if a membrane oxygenator and gas-free reservoir is used. Filters are not generally included in extracorporeal life support systems that are likely to have a duration of days or weeks.

Clinical significance of blood surface interface effects

Currently, coagulation during bypass is prevented with heparin, although many surface effects occur. The important clinical problem is returning to normal haemostasis and prevention of bleeding after extracorporeal circulation. First, the heparin effect must be reversed. This is generally done by adding an appropriate dose of protamine sulphate. Clots in the operative field are evidence of adequate heparin reversal. If the heparin effect persists, more protamine is given and the measurements repeated. Reversal of heparin was studied by Jaberi *et al.* (1973), who reported better heparin control with accelerated blood recalcification time and more accurate protamine administration. These results were confirmed by Bull *et al.* (1975), Babka *et al.* (1977) and Friesen and Clement (1976). Activated clotting time must be measured in whole-blood (rather than plasma) because the heparin effect is inversely related to platelet count. We have found that kaolin-activated clotting (as in most commercial systems) is satisfactory when the platelet count is normal, but inadequate during thrombocytopenia. This may account for the erratic results reported by some (Arkin *et al.*, 1978). For measuring activated clotting time during bypass, therefore, the reagent should contain fresh thromboplastins (Mullin *et al.*, 1976). Routine use of whole-blood activated clotting time measurements when reversing heparin should be a routine aspect of extracorporeal circulation. Protamine is a moderate peripheral vasodilator and will cause-hypotension when infused rapidly. It has a positive isotropic effect and peripheral flow appears to increase with protamine (Gourin *et al.*, 1970). Despite evidence of increased fibrinolytic activity and altered platelet function with extracorporeal circulation, post-operative bleeding that requires re-operation is almost always related to specific bleeding vessels (Gomes and McGoon, 1969). If the patient is allowed to bleed, but transfused to the point of near total blood volume, then a coagulopathy associated with platelet-poor blood will be produced, requiring fresh platelet transfusion. The indication for re-operation should be precise and conservative (for example, cumulative chest drainage of 15 per cent of the blood volume any time within the first 12 hours after bypass requires re-operation). When a significant coagulopathy occurs, it is associated with prolonged bypass with gas interface oxygenation, low platelet count and multiple transfusions. The defect is largely caused by platelet quantity and quality, and must be treated by fresh platelet concentrate or fresh blood. A study has suggested that one unit of fresh whole-blood is more effective than platelet concentrates in improving haemostasis after cardiopulmonary bypass (Lavee *et al.*, 1989).

Patients with platelet function defects before bypass will present severe bleeding problems after operation despite normal 'screening' tests of coagulation. These rare disorders are suggested by a history of bleeding with minor trauma and are detected by bleeding time or *in vitro* platelet function tests. Children with cyanotic heart disease appear to have abnormally functioning platelets which improve their function after correction of the cardiac defect (Ekert and Sheers, 1974). This platelet abnormality has been related to polycythaemia (Ware *et al.*, 1983). This may explain the propensity for bleeding that occurs after bypass in cyanotic heart disease (Kevy *et al.*, 1966).

After extracorporeal circulation, clotting factors and platelets return to normal or above-normal levels (Fong *et al.*, 1974). In occasional cases where abnormal coagulation occurs 24 hours or more after bypass it is usually caused by consumption coagulopathy associated with low cardiac output (Boyd *et al.*, 1972).

ORGAN DYSFUNCTION DURING EXTRACORPOREAL CIRCULATION

As noted previously, cardiopulmonary bypass, as usually carried out, invokes a moderate low-flow state or 'shock-like' environment. Changes in organ function that occur after extracorporeal circulation are related to one to two hours of relatively inadequate perfusion for metabolic demands and preferential diversion of flow to 'important' organs, rather than the specific effects of the bypass. Studies of prolonged near-total bypass in awake alert animals and patients without significant metabolic or functional sequelae substantiate this observation. The changes that do occur in many of the remote organs as a consequence of cardiopulmonary bypass are discussed below.

Neurological

It has become clear that there is a significant incidence of neurological and neuropsychiatric symptoms after cardiopulmonary bypass. Both neurological and neuropsychological dysfunction after cardiopulmonary bypass remain significant contributors to post-cardiopulmonary bypass morbidity, with an incidence ranging from one per cent to 80 per cent, depending on the criteria applied and the method of evaluation. Completed neurological deficit, such as stroke, has an incidence of one to three per cent (Gardner *et al.*, 1985; Taggart *et al.*, 1987), whereas more subtle neuropsychological dysfunction is considerably more common (Shaw and Bates, 1986; Smith and Treasure, 1986; Murkin and Martzke, 1992). Shaw *et al.* (1987) found that at the time of discharge 17 per cent of patients had some degree of neurological disability and 38 per cent had neuropsychiatric symptoms. Most of these findings were subtle. The occurrence of brain dysfunction is related to the duration of extracorporeal circulation, as shown by Lee *et al.* (1970) and Goy *et al.* (1984). The percentage of patients with central nervous system damage was 10 per cent after one hour extracorporeal circulation, 25 per cent after two hours and 35 per cent after three hours. Similar data was reported by Gilman (1965), Tufo *et al.* (1970) and Kornfeld *et al.* (1978). Most of this central nervous system damage is manifested as delirium or disorientation and the disturbance usually returns to normal in one to four weeks. Some follow-up studies of intellectual functioning showed return to pre-operative levels (Frank *et al.*, 1972), but a recent study has shown that 25 per cent of patients had a diminished IQ score six months after cardiopulmonary bypass when compared with the pre-operative score (Goy *et al.*, 1984).

Risk factors for neurological deficit post-cardiopulmonary bypass are age, systemic hypertension and cerebrovascular disease. Intraoperative actors affecting cerebral blood flow and function include duration of bypass, mode of pH management, hypothermia, and the pump circuit and mechanics. Perfusion pressure is obviously important, and cerebral perfusion pressure has been measured under varying conditions of cardiopulmonary bypass (Govier *et al.*, 1984; Murkin *et al.*, 1987). It was recognized that during cardiopulmonary bypass, cerebral perfusion pressure does not necessarily equate to mean arterial pressure and this factor must be accounted for. The effects of pulsatility have been investigated, and found to be beneficial in terms of decreased vascular resistance and subsequent increased uniformity of tissue perfusion (Matsumo *et al.*, 1971; Henze *et al.*, 1990; Murkin and Lee, 1991, Murkin, 1993). Further controlled clinical studies are required to establish the optimal pump conditions for cerebroprotection.

The reversible delirium syndrome, which is related to the duration of bypass with gas interface oxygenators and minimized by the use of membrane oxygenators, may be caused by microbubble embolism. An earlier study by Carlson *et al.* (1973) reported results comparing bubble and membrane oxygenators combined with the ultrasonic detection of microbubbles in the arterial circuit. A high correlation was found between bubble oxygenator use, microbubble embolism and minor cerebral dysfunction after operation. Brain function by psychological testing was more nearly normal and returned to normal more quickly in patients perfused with the membrane oxygenator, in whom no microbubbles were present in the arterial circuit. The use of a filter as a microbubble trap diminished particles and improved central nervous system function with the bubble oxygenator. Blauth *et al.* (1988, 1990) recently studied cerebral microemboli by using fluorescein angiography to examine the retinal vessels. They were able to confirm the finding of Carlson *et al.* (1973) that membrane oxygenators produced less microemboli than bubble oxygenators. However, they found no benefit from the use of arterial filters in reducing the number of microemboli. These studies did not attempt to correlate post-operative cerebral function with the presence of microemboli. Aris *et al.* (1986) did not find arterial line filters useful in preventing neurological and neuropsychiatric disturbances when a bubble oxygenator was used.

Cerebral effects of extracorporeal circulation can also be major and permanent. Brain damage that is not reversible is often lethal (Hicks *et al.*, 1973; Witoszka *et al.*, 1973) and may be detectable during operations by electroencephalography (EEG) (Witoszka *et al.*, 1973). It can be caused by gross embolism of fat or other particles (Hicks *et al.*, 1973) or by hypotension during or after bypass in older patients, especially those with cerebrovascular disease (Tufo *et al.*, 1970). Neurologic sequelae after repair of congenital cardiac defects has also been documented (Ferry, 1987, 1990). Acute symptoms in these patients include seizures, diminished level of consciousness, focal motor deficits and movement disorders. Potential long term sequelae include language and learning disorders, mental retardation, seizures and cerebral palsy. These have been attributed to embolization, hypoxia, decreased cerebral perfusion and biochemical disturbances.

In summary, transient brain dysfunction is common and increases in incidence with the duration of bypass. It appears to be caused by microbubble embolism and is most common with bubble oxygenators, therefore it is hardly applicable to current practice. Major brain damage is usually caused by particulate embolism or hypotension superimposed on atherosclerosis. Scrupulous attention to cleaning the field before cardiotomy suction will help to prevent particulate embolism. Maintenance of adequate perfusion pressure before and after extracorporeal circulation is recommended in patients with atherosclerosis.

Gastrointestinal

The gastrointestinal system is one of the least-studied of all organ systems with relation to the effects sustained during cardiopulmonary bypass. This is surprising, as it has recently been postulated as the 'motor of multi-organ failure'. The basis behind this theory is that the shock-like state conferred by cardiopulmonary bypass results in preferential blood diversion to 'important' organs and the gut mucosa is left relatively ischaemic. This causes a progressive acidosis and subsequent increased permeability to larger molecules, including endotoxins. These are then able to traverse the broken-down barrier of the intestine and become absorbed into the blood stream. Clearly, in predisposed individuals, such as the immunosuppressed, this may have severe consequences, such as multiple organ failure and death.

Reviews of gastrointestinal complications after cardiopulmonary bypass suggest an incidence ranging from 0.6 per cent to 2 per cent (Desai and Ohri, 1990), of which the mortality rate is between 12 per cent and 67 per cent (Wallwork and Davidson, 1980; Hanks *et al.*, 1982; Pinson and Alberty, 1983; Moneta *et al.*, 1985; Welling *et al.*, 1986; Heikkinen and Ala-Kulju, 1987; Leitman *et al.*, 1987; Huddy *et al.*, 1991). Unlike predictable decreases in lung function, there appear to be no predictable changes in gastrointestinal function after cardiac surgery with bypass. Indeed, most patients are eating normally 24–48 hours after uncomplicated elective procedures (Ramsey, 1995). Fiddian-Green and Baker (1987) studied stomach wall pH by tonometry in patients during and after bypass. In one study, half the patients developed stomach wall acidosis, and all serious complications (eight of 85 patients) occurred in this group. Although duration of hypotension was the single best predictor of adverse outcome, the addition of degree and duration of stomach wall acidosis significantly improved predictive ability (Gaer *et al.*, 1994). This work, and previous work by the first group (Fiddian-Green *et al.*, 1986), suggests stomach wall acidosis is a sensitive indicator of gut hypoperfusion.

More recent work by Landow and colleagues (Landow *et al.*, 1991; Andersen *et al.*, 1993), using similar monitoring techniques, has documented a gradual reduction in gastric pH after routine bypass, the degree of which correlates with duration of the pump run. Associated with the decrease in gastric pH is the appearance of endotoxin in the circulation (Andersen *et al.*, 1987; Rocke *et al.*, 1987; Andersen *et al.*, 1988, 1993; Karlstad *et al.*, 1993). In these studies, the presence of endotoxin was not associated with infective complications, but it did confirm that intestinal barrier function was compromised. Rocke *et al.* (1987) reported that plasma endotoxin levels were increased transiently after release of the aortic cross-clamp. Their nine patients had an uneventful intraoperative and peri-operative course, therefore preventing an analysis of the role of endotoxin in subsequent development of post-operative sepsis. However, it is informative that the degree and time course of endotoxaemia in these patients closely resembles that of the effect of one hour of superior mesenteric artery occlusion in cats (Gathiram *et al.*, 1986). Furthermore, the magnitude of endotoxaemia was directly related to duration of cardiopulmonary bypass. More recently, methods have been described to measure plasma endotoxin (Bowles *et al.*, 1995), which are suitable for use during cardiopulmonary bypass.

Intestinal permeability to plasma proteins is also affected by cardiopulmonary bypass: extravasation of these proteins into the interstitial space is increased as much as fourfold during non-pulsatile normothermic cardiopulmonary bypass in dogs. This increased permeability was most pronounced for the larger molecules. Thus, cardiopulmonary bypass produces an intestinal mucosal injury characterized by abnormal permeation of macromolecules. The significance of increased endotoxin translocation into the circulation is that this may occur in patients with the longest cardiopulmonary bypass times, which already poses an increased risk of gastrointestinal and hepatic injury. These factors may all contribute to development of post-operative sepsis and multiple system organ failure.

It is known that intestinal permeability to 51-Chromium labelled EDTA increases enormously during cardiopulmonary bypass, and Ohri *et al.* (1993) has also demonstrated this quantitatively using sugar probes. Further trials by the same group have shown that the tendency towards intramucosal acidosis in the rewarming and immediate post-cardiopulmonary bypass phases following hypothermic non-pulsatile cardiopulmonary bypass, may impair the gut barrier and predispose patients to the absorption of luminal toxins (Ohri *et al.*, 1994). These studies help to verify the previously mentioned hypotheses. Although the incidence of gastrointestinal complications resulting from cardiopulmonary bypass is low, and probably attributable to low-output syndromes, the implications are far-reaching.

Hepatic

Liver damage is detectable by isoenzyme determination within minutes of the institution of bypass, but this is generally clinically insignificant. The incidence of hyperbilirubinaemia (>3 mg/dL) has been reported to be as high as 20–23 per cent (Collins *et al.*, 1983; Chu *et al.*, 1984). When liver damage does occur it usually appears as cholestatic jaundice which regresses spontaneously. However, 'post-pump jaundice' has been associated with a poor outcome, with a 25 per cent mortality rate reported by Collins *et al.* (1983). The factors which contribute to post-operative jaundice, such as hypoxia and hypotension, are usually responsible for the high mortality seen in these patients rather than the liver injury *per se* (Chu *et al.*, 1984). When massive liver injury does occur after cardiopulmonary bypass it is almost invariably associated with a fatal outcome.

Renal

The effects of cardiopulmonary bypass on renal function have been investigated extensively. Many studies have documented a very high incidence of post-operative 'renal failure' (as defined by increases in serum urea and creatinine, and clinically by decreased measured urine output). The problem with the interpretation of these studies is that they reveal an incidence of post-operative renal dysfunction of up to 30 per cent (Yeboah *et al.*, 1972; Abel *et al.*, 1974; Bhat *et al.*, 1976), but a relatively low incidence of severe renal impairment necessitating dialysis (one to five per cent) (Yeboah *et al.*, 1972; Abel *et al.*, 1974; Bhat *et al.*, 1976; Lange *et al.*, 1987; Corwin *et al.*, 1989). This would be expected from the effects of renin and angiotensin on renal cortical flow related, at least in part, to the non-pulsatile contour. When renal failure does occur it is usually a manifestation of acute tubular necrosis and is reversible. Acute renal failure has been associated with a high mortality rate (66–88 per cent), probably from factors associated with renal failure, and attempts must be made to prevent it (Abel *et al.*, 1976a, 1976b; Baxter *et al.*, 1985; Heikkinen *et al.*, 1985).

Acute renal failure results in several dangerous metabolic derangements, including hyperkalaemia, hypocalcaemia and progressive acidosis. In most cases, the renal failure is a consequence of post-operative hypoperfusion rather than a result of the period of bypass itself, but there are probably a significant number of patients whose renal injury is a direct consequence of cardiopulmonary bypass (Slogoff *et al.*, 1990). Among the factors that contribute to peri-operative renal dysfunction are diminished renal blood flow, the immunoinflammatory renal injury, nephrotoxic drugs and pre-existing renal disease. Most studies have established a direct link between duration of bypass and post-cardiopulmonary bypass renal dysfunction. This may be related to the increased levels of plasma free haemoglobin also found with cardiopulmonary bypass. PFH is certainly nephrotoxic in low perfusion situations, but the perfusion levels achieved during cardiopulmonary bypass would make this unlikely.

Postulated reasons for the reduction in function included renal artery vasoconstriction, hypothermia and loss of pulsatile perfusion, these factors being interdependent. Although flow generation does not appear to affect catecholamine levels, angiotensin II levels are higher with nonpulsatile flow. A comprehensive review of the subject by Hickey *et al.* (1983) concludes that the bulk of the evidence does support increased renal vasoconstriction with the loss of pulsatile perfusion. There are, however, few clinical studies comparing the incidence of post-operative renal dysfunction and renal failure with the use of pulsatile or non-pulsatile perfusion. Neither are there many studies investigating the effects of centrifugal flow on renal function.

For reasons that are not completely understood, it appears to be the tubular cells rather than the glomerular cells that are the most susceptible to acute reductions in renal perfusion, especially those of the proximal tubule. With ischaemia and necrosis of the cells lining the tubules, swelling occurs, with sloughing and tubular obstruction in the early stages. It appears to be the tubular injury that is responsible for the impaired renal function, whereas in the later stages, the rate and degree of recovery are determined by restoration of glomerular filtration rate (GFR). This depends on the maintenance of normal renal perfusion.

The Stanford group has investigated post-bypass renal dysfunction both prospectively and retrospectively (Hilberman *et al.*, 1980). They identified three typical courses of renal failure developing after cardiac surgery. The first shows a brief ischaemic insult, which is ameliorated by protective agents such as mannitol, and assuming reasonable cardiac output and blood pressure are maintained, makes a full recovery. The second type also succumbs to the initial insult, but poor cardiac output causes a slow recovery, with oliguric periods. In the third,

and most severe, type there is a prolonged period of poor cardiac output, and oliguria and dialysis ensue. It has been established that predictors for poor renal outcome are compromised cardiac or renal function pre-operatively, duration of bypass and peri-operative circulatory status.

Pulmonary

Pulmonary function is unavoidably changed in the majority of patients undergoing cardiopulmonary bypass. It has been attributed to many factors, including complement activation causing microvascular permeability, and ultimately atelectasis. Pulmonary insufficiency is now unusual after bypass of two hours or less, but often occurs to some degree when perfusion is carried out for a longer period of time. This effect is probably not related to lung perfusion (Abel *et al.*, 1976a) or lack of perfusion (Shah-Mirany *et al.*, 1970) via the pulmonary artery or to primary increased pulmonary extravascular water (O'Connor *et al.*, 1971). Once again, haemodilution seems to play a protective role. It reduces alveolar capillary damage and the associated capillary permeability changes. Dilute prime does not cause pulmonary oedema as the decreased serum colloid oncotic pressure is matched by a drop in the colloid osmotic pressure of the proteins in the interstitial fluid and a compensatory increase in pulmonary lymph flow.

Microembolic events are a large risk to the pulmonary circulation during cardiopulmonary bypass, and must be minimized as discussed in previous sections. There is a high incidence of alveolar collapse and intrapulmonary shunting with cardiopulmonary bypass. This can be attributed to increased capillary permeability and pressure, and decreased lung volume due to lowered compliance and altered chest wall mechanics.

The decrease in pulmonary insufficiency over the past two decades is related to at least two important factors:

- Pre-packaged, sterile, single-use, easily primed circuits that can be prepared immediately before instituting bypass rather than requiring long periods of recirculation and blood interface exposure prior to bypass.
- A better understanding of pulmonary physiology and management after operation.

There is ample evidence that the well-inflated alveolus is less susceptible to damage than the collapsed alveolus (Bartlett *et al.*, 1972). The same principle holds true during extracorporeal circulation. Weedn *et al.* (1970) demonstrated that lung dysfunction was least in a group of dogs managed with static inflation during extracorporeal circulation, rather than static deflation or conventional ventilation. The lungs should be managed by static inflation during extracorporeal circulation unless this interferes with cardiac exposure. As mentioned earlier in this chapter, complement and neutrophil activation occurs with cardiopulmonary bypass. In addition, sequestration of neutrophils in the lungs during extracorporeal circulation has been demonstrated (Utoh *et al.*, 1988). Neutrophil-mediated pulmonary endothelial cell injury can lead to increased capillary permeability and may contribute to the adverse effects of extracorporeal circulation on pulmonary function (Kirklin and Barratt-Boyes, 1986; Hernandez *et al.*, 1987).

A large amount of research has been directed at minimizing pulmonary injury on cardiopulmonary bypass. Factors already shown to be critical are cardiopulmonary bypass times greater than 120–150 minutes, the amount of leukosequestration in the alveolar vasculature and pre-morbid lung function (Kirklin *et al.*, 1983).

Cardiac

Cardiopulmonary bypass by itself does not affect myocardial function. Many changes occur in myocardial function after operation, related to the type of operation, the valve or cardiac chamber being repaired, or the 'constitution' of the coronary perfusate during bypass.

Following the institution of cardiopulmonary bypass, the natural perfusion of the heart is then stopped in most cases to facilitate appropriate surgical conditions. This is the concept of myocardial protection, of which there are several types. The effects of cardiopulmonary bypass on the heart have frequently been reported as a combined effect of cardiopulmonary bypass and myocardial protection, but for the purposes of this introduction, we shall concentrate on cardiopulmonary bypass effects alone.

By virtue of the need for surgery, most hearts subjected to cardiopulmonary bypass are dysfunctional to varying extents. Extremely diseased hearts, or ones with poor myocardial reserve, are prone to experience difficulties in discontinuation of cardiopulmonary bypass. These may require pharmacological or mechanical support for a period of time. There are some situations that may be dramatically compromised by cardiopulmonary bypass. Critical coronary stenoses may cause acute myocardial ischaemia upon induction of anaesthesia or initiation of cardiopulmonary bypass, since these are times of hypotension. Haemodilution may cause a coronary steal syndrome from vulnerable subendocardium in the presence of collateral vessels. Hypothermia may take away the ability of the heart to autoregulate local blood flow. Ventricular distension, particularly occurring when no venting is used, may cause a decreased blood flow to the inner layers of the heart, especially the subendocardium.

Ideally, cardiopulmonary bypass should be started and maintained with coronary perfusion equal to pre-cardiopulmonary bypass levels as cooling proceeds. The majority of detrimental myocardial effects after the institution of cardiopulmonary bypass are attributable to inadequate myocardial protection.

Reticulo–endothelial function changes

Silva *et al.* (1974) reported an elegant study of phagocytosis and bacterial killing capacity of circulating leucocytes during extracorporeal circulation. Using the nitroblue-tetrazolium test for phagocytosis, these workers found significantly decreased phagocytic activity in the circulating white cells of 12 patients undergoing cardiopulmonary bypass. They postulated that these changes were caused by derangements in oxidative metabolism of these circulating white cells and supported this hypothesis by demonstrating that the bactericidal activity was decreased in two of four patients in whom it was measured. This clinical study supported the laboratory work of Kusserow and Larrow (1968) in which decreased phagocytic activity during extracorporeal circulation in dogs was demonstrated. Decreased activity in fixed tissue phagocytes has been demonstrated by Subramanian *et al.* (1968). They conducted extracorporeal circulation and isolated liver perfusion in rats and demonstrated that the clearance of radioactive gold by Kupffer cells in the liver was significantly impaired with extracorporeal circulation. In a later study this same group demonstrated that blood which was recirculated *ex vivo* for 30 minutes caused the same effect when perfused through a rat liver. They concluded from these studies that the decreased recticulo-endothelial function was due to mechanical or chemical effects of the extracorporeal circuit on blood rather than the effect on the liver itself. The reason for this impaired recticulo-endothelial function of circulating and fixed phagocytes has not been identified, but these observations correlate very nicely with studies of platelet aggregation and uptake in recticulo-endothelial organs. If circulating and fixed phagocytes become loaded with platelet aggregates or other micro-particles and debris from coronary suction or the extracorporeal circuit, then the ability of these cells further to phagocytize radioactive gold or bacteria would be reduced. If this hypothesis is proven to be true, it affords further evidence that avoiding platelet aggregation by platelet active drugs or modification of the surface of the extracorporeal circuit may be important not only in haemostasis but in maintenance of normal recticulo-endothelial function after extracorporeal circulation.

CONCLUSION

Extracorporeal circulation involves the use of a prosthetic device totally to replace the function of the heart and lungs and partially replace the blood endothelial surface and recticulo-endothelial system. Properly used, it allows the function of the other organs of the body to remain unchanged during the conduct of the procedure. Moderate hypovolaemia caused by haemodilution and hypotension usually accompanies extracorporeal circulation, with systemic flow maintained at an adequate but barely normal level. Gas exchange is easily accomplished by any of a variety of devices. The major physiological alterations caused by extracorporeal circulation are related to prosthetic surface exposure, with resultant blood component damage and complement and other mediator activation.

ACKNOWLEDGEMENTS

This chapter is based on Chapter 2 in the third edition of *Techniques in Extracorporeal Circulation* and was originally written by Robert H. Barlett and Ralph E. Delius of the University of Michigan Medical Center, Ann Arbor, Michigan, USA.

REFERENCES

Abel, R.M., Wick, J., Beck, C.H. Jr., Buckley, M.J., Austen, W.G. 1974: Renal dysfunction following open-heart operations. *Archives of Surgery* **108**, 175–7.

Abel, R.M., Buckley, M.J., Austen, W.G. *et al.* 1976a: Acute postoperative renal failure in cardiac surgical patients. *Journal of Surgical Research* **20**, 341–8.

Abel, R.M., Buckley, M.J., Austen, W.G. *et al.* 1976b: Aetiology, incidence, and prognosis of renal failure following cardiac operations. Results of a prospective analysis of 500 consecutive patients. *Journal of Thoracic and Cardiovascular Surgery* **71**, 323–33.

Addonizio, V.P., Colman, R.W. 1982: Platelets and extracorporeal circulation. *Biomaterials* **3**, 9–15.

Addonizio, V.P., Strauss, J.F., Macarak, E.J. *et al.* 1978: Preservation of platelet number and function with prostaglandin E, during total cardiopulmonary bypass in rhesus monkeys. *Surgery* **83**, 619–25.

Andersen, L.W., Baek, L., Degn, H. 1987: Presence of circulating endotoxins during cardiac operations. *Journal of Thoracic and Cardiovascular Surgery* **93**, 115–19.

Andersen, L.W., Jensen, T.H., Jensen, F.M. 1988: Absorption of lipopolysaccaride from the intestine during aortic cross-clamping in humans. *Journal of Cardiothoracic Anesthesia* **2**, 861–3.

Andersen, L.W., Landow, L., Baek, L. 1993: Association between gastric intramucosal pH and splanchnic endotoxin, antibody to endotoxin and tumour necrosis factor concentrations in patients undergoing cardiopulmonary bypass. *Critical Care Medicine* **21**, 210–17.

Angell, J.J.E. 1971: The effects of altering mean pressure, pulse pressure and pulse frequency of the impulse activity in baroreceptor fibres from the aortic arch and right subclavian artery in the rabbit. *Journal of Physiology* (London) **214**, 65–88.

Antonesen, S., Brandslund, I., Clemensen, S. *et al.* 1987: Neutrophil lysosomal enzyme release and complement activation during cardiopulmonary bypass. *Scandinavian Journal of Thoracic and Cardiovascular Surgery* **21**, 47–52.

Aris, A., Solanes, H., Camara, M.L. *et al.* 1986: Arterial line filtration during cardiopulmonary bypass. Neurologic, neuropsychologic, and hematologic studies. *Journal of Thoracic and Cardiovascular Surgery* **91**, 526–33.

Arkin, C.F., Shahsavari, M., Copeland, B.E., Kim, A. 1978: Evaluation of the activated clotting time to control heparin and protamine dosage in open-heart surgery. *Journal of Thoracic and Cardiovascular Surgery* **75**, 790–2.

Asari, H., Kondo, H., Ishihara, A. *et al.* 1989: Extracorporeal circulation influence on plasma atrial natriuretic peptide concentration in cardiac surgery patients. *Chest* **5**, 757–60.

Babka, R., Colby, C., El-Etr, A., Pifarre, R. 1977: Monitoring of intra-operative heparinization and blood loss following cardiopulmonary bypass surgery. *Journal of Thoracic and Cardiovascular Surgery* **73**, 780–2.

Bartlett, R.H. 1971: Posttraumatic pulmonary insufficiency. In: P. Cooper, L. Nyhus (eds), *Surgery annual.* New York, NY: Appleton–Century–Crofts: 1–35.

Bartlett, R.H., Gazzaniga, A.B. 1978: Extracorporeal circulation for cardiopulmonary failure. *Current Problems in Surgery* **15**, 1–96.

Bartlett, R.H., Drinker, P.A., Burns, N.E. *et al.* 1972: The toroidal membrane oxygenator: design, performance and bypass testing of a clinical model. *Transactions of the American Society for Artificial Internal Organs* **18**, 369–73.

Bartlett, R.H., Fong, S.W., Burns, N.E., Gazziniga, A.E. 1974: Prolonged partial venoarterial bypass: physiologic, biochemical and hematologic responses. *Annals of Surgery* e. American Society Microbiology **92**, 373.

Baxter, P., Rigby, M.L., Jones, O.D. *et al.* 1985: Acute renal failure following cardiopulmonary bypass in children: results of treatment. *International Journal of Cardiology* **7**, 235–9.

Benner, J.E. 1969: Metabolism of antibiotics during cardiopulmonary bypass for open-heart surgery. *American Society for Microbiology* **92**, 373–8.

Bernstein, E.F., Gleason, L.R. 1967: Factors influencing haemolysis with roller pumps. *Surgery* **61**, 432–42.

Bhat, J.G., Gluck, M.C., Lowenstein, J. 1976: Renal failure after open heart surgery. *Annals of Internal Medicine* **84**, 677–82.

Bidstrup, B., Royston, D., Sapsford, R.N., Taylor, K.M. 1989: Reduction in blood loss and blood use after cardiopulmonary bypass with high dose aprotinin (Trasylol). *Journal of Thoracic and Cardiovascular Surgery* **97**, 364–72.

Bjork, V.O., Sternlieb, J.J., Davenport, C. 1985: From the spinning disc to the membrane oxygenator for open heart surgery. *Scandinavian Journal of Thoracic and Cardiovascular Surgery* **19**, 207–16.

Bjornsson, T.D., Wolfram, K.M., Kitchell, B.B. 1982: Heparin kinetics determined by three assay methods. *Clinical Pharmacology and Therapeutics* **31**, 104–13.

Blacksheer, P.L., Dorman, F.D., Steinback, J.H. 1965: Some mechanical effects that influence hemolysis. *Transactions of the American Society for Artificial Internal Organs* **11**, 112–17.

Blakemore, W.S., McGarrity, G.J., Thiurer, R.J. et al. 1971: Infection by air-borne bacteria with cardiopulmonary bypass. *Surgery* **70**, 830–8.

Blauth, C.I., Arnold, J.V., Schulenberg, W.E. et al. 1988: Cerebral microembolism during cardiopulmonary bypass. Retinal microvascular studies *in vivo* with fluorescein angiography. *Journal of Thoracic and Cardiovascular Surgery* **95**, 668–76.

Blauth, C.I., Smith, D.L., Arnold, J.V. et al. 1990: Influence of oxygenator type on the prevalence and extent of microembolic retinal ischemia during cardiopulmonary bypass. *Journal of Thoracic and Cardiovascular Surgery* **99**, 61–9.

Boonstra, P.W., van Imhoff, G.W., Eysman, L. et al. 1985: Reduced platelet activation and improved hemostasis after controlled cardiotomy suction during clinical membrane oxygenator perfusions. *Journal of Thoracic and Cardiovascular Surgery* **89**, 900–6.

Boonstra, P.W., Vermeulen, F.E., Leusink, J.A. et al. 1986: Hematological advantage of a membrane oxygenator over a bubble oxygenator in long perfusions. *Annals of Thoracic Surgery* **41**, 297–300.

Boucher, J.K., Rudy, L.W., Edmunds, L.H. 1974: Organ blood flow during pulsatile cardiopulmonary bypass. *Journal of Applied Physiology* **36**, 86–90.

Bowles, C.T., Ohri, S.K., Klangsuk, N., Keogh, B.E., Yacoub, M.H., Taylor, K.M. 1995: Endotoxaemia detected during cardiopulmonary bypass with a modified *Limulus* amoebic lysate assay. *Perfusion* **10**, 219–28.

Boyd, A.D., Engelman, R.M., Beaudet, R.L., Lackner, H. 1972: Disseminated intravascular coagulation following extracorporeal circulation. *Journal of Thoracic and Cardiovascular Surgery* **64**, 685–93.

Breckenridge, I.M., Digerness, S.B., Kirklin, J.W. 1969: Validity of concept of increased extracellular fluid after open-heart surgery. *Surgical Forum* **20**, 169–71.

Bregman, D. 1976. Mechanical support of the failing heart. *Current Problems in Surgery* **13**, 1–84.

Brodman, R., Siegel, H., Lesser, M., Frater, R. 1985: A comparison of flow gradients across disposable arterial perfusion cannulas. *Annals of Thoracic Surgery* **39**, 225–33.

Brooks, D.H., Bahnson, H.T. 1971: An outbreak of haemorrhage following cardiopulmonary bypass. Epidemiologic studies. *Journal of Thoracic and Cardiovascular Surgery* **63**, 449–52.

Brown-Sequard, E. 1858: Recherches experimentales sur les proprietes physiologiques et les usages du sang rouge et du sang noir et leurs principaux elements gazeux, l'oxygene et l'acide carbonique. *Journal de Physiologiques de l'homme* **1**, 95–122.

Bull, B.S., Korpman, R.A., Huse, W.M., Briggs, D.B. 1975: Heparin therapy during extracorporeal circulation. Problems inherent in existing heparin protocols. *Journal of Thoracic and Cardiovascular Surgery* **69**, 674–84.

Burack, B., Marcus, D., Miyamoto, A. et al. 1972: Response of class IV patients to alpha blockade prior to open-heart surgery. *American Heart Journal* **84**, 456–62.

Butler, J., Parker, D., Pillai, R. et al. 1993: Effect of cardiopulmonary bypass on systemic release of neutrophil elastase and tumour necrosis factor. *Journal of Thoracic and Cardiovascular Surgery* **228**, 123–32.

Calafiore, A.M., Glieca, F., Marchesani, F. et al. 1987: A comparative clinical assessment of a hollow fibre membrane oxygenator

(Capiox II) and bubble oxygenator (Harvey 1500). *Journal of Cardiovascular Surgery* **28**, 633–7.

Carlson, R.G., Lande, A.J., Landis, B. et al. 1973: The Lande–Edwards membrane oxygenator during heart surgery. *Journal of Thoracic and Cardiovascular Surgery* **66**, 894–905.

Castillo, J.E., Bocchieri, K.A., Fyman, P. et al. 1991: Historical aspects of cardiopulmonary surgery. In: P.A. Casthely, D. Bregman (eds), *Cardiopulmonary bypass: physiology, related complications and pharmacology.* Mount Kisco, NY: Futura.

Cavarocchi, N.C., England, M.D., Schaff, H.V. et al. 1986a: Oxygen free radical generation during cardiopulmonary bypass: correlation with complement activation. *Circulation* **74**, 111–30.

Cavarocchi, N.C., Pluth, J.R., Schaff, H.V. et al. 1986b: Complement activation during cardiopulmonary bypass. Comparison of bubble and membrane oxygenator. *Journal of Thoracic and Cardiovascular Surgery* **91**, 252–8.

Chambers, D.J., Karimzandi, N., Baimbridge, M.V. et al. 1984: Hormonal and electrolyte responses during and after open heart surgery. *Journal of Thoracic and Cardiovascular Surgery* **32**, 358–64.

Chenoworth, D.E. 1986: Anaphylatoxin formation in extracorporeal circuits. *Complement* **3**, 152–7.

Chiara, O., Giomarelli, P.P., Biagioli, B. et al. 1980: Hypermetabolic response after hypothermic cardiopulmonary bypass. *Critical Care Medicine* **15**, 995–1000.

Chu, C.M., Chang, C.H., Liaw, Y.F., Hsieh, M.J. 1984: Jaundice after open-heart surgery: a prospective study. *Thorax* **39**, 52–6.

Clark, R.E., Mills, M. 1969: The infant temptrol oxygenator. *Journal of Thoracic and Cardiovascular Surgery* **60**, 54–62.

Clark, L.C., Gollan, F., Gupta, V.B. 1950: The oxygenation of blood by gas dispersion. *Science* **111**, 85–7.

Cohn, L.H., Angell, W.W., Shumway, N.E. 1971: Body fluid shifts after cardiopulmonary bypass. Effects of congestive heart failure and haemodilution. *Journal of Thoracic and Cardiovascular Surgery* **62**, 423–30.

Collins, J.D., Bassendine, M.F., Ferner, R. et al. 1983: Incidence and prognostic importance of jaundice after cardiopulmonary bypass surgery. *Lancet* **i**, 1119–23.

Conte, J.E. Jr, Cohen, S.N., Roe, B.B., Elashoff, R.M. 1972: Antibiotic prophylaxis and cardiac surgery: a prospective double-blind comparison of single-dose versus multiple-dose regimens. *Annals of Internal Medicine* **76**, 943–9.

Corwin, H.L., Sprague, S.M., DeLaria, G.A., Norusis, M.J. 1989: Acute renal failure associated with cardiac operations. A case-control study. *Journal of Thoracic and Cardiovascular Surgery* **98**, 1107–12.

Cottrell, E.D., Kappa, J.R., Stenach, N. et al. 1988: Temporary inhibition of platelet function with iloprost (ZK36374) preserves canine platelets during extracorporeal membrane oxygenation. *Journal of Thoracic and Cardiovascular Surgery* **96**, 535–41.

Del Canale, S., Fiaccadori, E., Vezzani, A. et al. 1988: Cell metabolism response to cardiopulmonary bypass in patients undergoing aorto-coronary grafting. *Scandinavian Journal of Thoracic and Cardiovascular Surgery* **22**, 159–64.

Desai, J.B., Ohri, S.K. 1990: Gastrointestinal damage following cardiopulmonary bypass. *Perfusion* **5**, 161–8.

Despotis, G.J., Joist, J.H., Hogue, C.W.J. et al. 1995: The impact of heparin concentration and activated clotting time monitored on blood conservation. A prospective randomised evaluation in patients undergoing cardiac operation. *Journal of Thoracic and Cardiovascular Surgery* **110**, 46–54.

Dewar, M.L., Walsh, G., Chin, R.C.-J. *et al.* 1988: Atrial natriuretic factor: response to cardiac operation. *Journal of Thoracic and Cardiovascular Surgery* **96**, 266–70.

Dieter, R.A., Neville, W.E., Pifarro, R. 1969: Hypokalaemia following haemodilution cardiopulmonary bypass. *Annals of Surgery* **171**, 17–23.

Dobell, A.R.C., Mitri, M., Galva, R. *et al.* 1965: Biologic evaluation of blood after prolonged recirculation through film and membrane oxygenators. *Annals of Surgery* **161**, 617–22.

Dunn, J., Kirsch, M., Harness, J. *et al.* 1974: Haemodynamic, metabolic, and haematologic effects of pulsatile cardiopulmonary bypass. *Journal of Thoracic and Cardiovascular Surgery* **68**, 138–47.

Dutton, R.C., Edmunds, L.H. Jr. 1973: Measurement of emboli in extracorporeal perfusion system. *Journal of Thoracic and Cardiovascular Surgery* **65**, 523–30.

Edelman, W., Levendusky, J., Lichtenstein, I. 1992: Alternate views of hydraulics for an impellar centrifugal pump. *Perfusion* **13**, 70–2.

Emmi, R.P., Jacobs, L.E. 1992: The recognition and management of the patient with low cardiac output following open heart surgery. In: M.N. Kotler, A. Alfieri (eds), *Cardiac and non-cardiac complications of open heart surgery: prevention, diagnosis, and treatment.* Mount Kisco, NY: Futura, 107–43.

Ekert, H., Sheers, M. 1974: Pre-operative and post-operative platelet function in cyanotic congenital heart disease. *Journal of Thoracic and Cardiovascular Surgery* **68**, 184–90.

Fantini, G.A., Zadeh, B.J., Chiao, J. *et al.* 1987: Effect of hypothermia on cellular membrane function during low-flow extracorporeal circulation. *Surgery* **102**, 132–9.

Fedderson, K., Aurell, M., Delin, K. *et al.* 1985: Effects of cardiopulmonary bypass and prostacyclin on plasma catecholamines, angiotensin 11 and arginine-vasopressin. *Acta Anaesthesiologica Scandinavica* **29**, 224–30.

Ferry, P.C. 1987: Neurologic sequelae of cardiac surgery in children. *American Journal of Diseases of Children* **141**, 309–12.

Ferry, P.C. 1990: Neurologic sequelae of open-heart surgery in children. *American Journal of Diseases in Children* **144**, 369–73.

Fiddian-Green, R.G., Baker, S. 1987: The predictive value of measurements of pH in the wall of the stomach for complicatons after cardiac surgery: a comparison with other forms of monitoring. *Critical Care Medicine* **15**, 153–6.

Fiddian-Green, R.G., Amelin, P.M., Herrmann, J.B. *et al.* 1986: Prediction of the development of sigmoid ischaemia on the day of aortic operations. Indirect measurements of intramural pH in the colon. *Archives of Surgery* **121**, 654–60.

Finlayson, D.C. 1987: Non-pulsatile flow is preferable to pulsatile flow during cardiopulmonary bypass. *Journal of Cardiothoracic Anaesthesia* **1**, 169–70.

Fish, K.J., Sarnquist, F.H., van Steenis, C. *et al.* 1986: A prospective randomized study of the effects of prostacyclin on platelets and blood loss during coronary bypass operations. *Journal of Thoracic and Cardiovascular Surgery* **91**, 436–42.

Fong, S.W., Burns, N.E., Williams, G. *et al.* 1974: Changes in coagulation and platelet function during prolonged extracorporeal circulation (ECC) in sheep and man. *Transactions of the American Society for Artificial Internal Organs* **20**, 239–47.

Fosse, E., Mollnes, T.E., Ingvaldsen, B. 1987: Complement activation during major operations with or without cardiopulmonary bypass. *Journal of Thoracic and Cardiovascular Surgery* **93**, 860–6.

Frank, K.A., Heller, S.S., Kornfeld, D.S., Malm, J.R. 1972:Long-term effects of open-heart surgery on intellectual functioning. *Journal of Thoracic and Cardiovascular Surgery* **64**, 811–15.

Frater, R.W.M., Wakayama, S., Oka, V. 1980: Pulsatile cardiopulmonary bypass: failure to influence haemodynamics or hormones. *Circulation* **62**, 19–25.

von Frey, M., Gruber, M. 1885: Untersuchungen uber den stoffwechsel isolierter organe. Ein respirations-apparat fur isolierte organe. *Virchow's Achives of Physiology* **9**, 519–32.

Friesen, R.H., Clement, A.J. 1976: Individual responses to heparinization for extracorporeal circulation. *Journal of Thoracic and Cardiovascular Surgery* **72**, 875–9.

Gaer, J.A., Shaw, A.D., Wild, R. *et al.* 1994: Effect of cardiopulmonary bypass on gastrointestinal perfusion and function. *Annals of Thoracic Surgery* **57**, 371–5.

Gallagher, J.D., Moore, R.A., Kerns, D. *et al.* 1985: Effects of colloid or crystalloid administration on pulmonary extravascular water in the post-operative period after coronary artery bypass grafting. *Anesthesia and Analgesia* **64**, 753–8.

Galletti, P.M., Mora, C.T. 1995: Cardiopulmonary bypass: the historical foundation, the future promise. In: C.T. Mora (ed.), *Cardiopulmonary bypass: principles and techniques of extracorporeal circulation.* New York, NY: Springer-Verlag, 3–21.

Galletti, P.M., Richardson, P.D., Snider, M.T. 1972: A standardized method for defining the overall gas transfer performance of artificial lungs. *Transactions of the American Society for Artificial Internal Organs* **18**, 359–68.

Gans, H., Castaneda, A.R., Subramanian, V.A. 1967: Problems in haemostasis during open-heart surgery. IX. Changes observed in the plasminogen-plasma system and their significance for therapy. *Annals of Surgery* **166**, 980–6.

Gardner, T.J., Horneffer, P.J., Manolio, T.A. 1985: Stroke following coronary artery bypass grafting: a ten year study. *Annals of Thoracic Surgery* **40**, 574–81.

Gathiram, P., Gaffin, S.L., Wells, M.T. 1986: Superior mesenteric artery occlusion shock in cats: modification of the endotoxaemia by antilipopolysaccaride antibodies. *Circulatory Shock* **19**, 231–7.

Gazzaniga, A.B., Byrd, C.L., Gross, R.E. 1970: The use of skeletal muscle surface hydrogen ion concentration to monitor peripheral perfusion: experimental and clinical results. *Surgical Forum* **21**, 147–9.

Gazzaniga, A.B., Byrd, C.L., Stewart, D.R., Gross, R.E. 1972: Effects of dexamethasone and chlorpromazine on skeletal muscle surface hydrogen ion concentration during cardiopulmonary bypass. *Annals of Surgery* **176**, 757–60.

Gervin, A.S., McNeer, J.F., Wolfe, W.G. *et al.* 1974: Ultrapore haemofiltration during extracorporeal circulation. *Journal of Thoracic and Cardiovascular Surgery* **67**, 237–41.

Gibbon, J.H. 1937: Artificial maintenance of circulation during experimental occlusion of the pulmonary artery. *Archives of Surgery* **34**, 1105–31.

Gibbon, J.H. 1939: The maintenance of life during experimental occlusion of the pulmonary artery followed by survival. *Surgery, Gynecology and Obstetrics* **69**, 602–14.

Gibbon, J.H. 1954: Application of a mechanical heart and lung apparatus to cardiac surgery. *Minnesota Medicine* **37**, 171–85.

Gilman, S. 1965: Cerebral disorders after open-heart operations. *New England Journal of Medicine* **272**, 489–97.

Gollan, F. 1959: Physiology of deep hypothermia by total body perfusion. *Annals of the New York Academy of Science* **80**, 301–14.

Gombotz, H., Metzler, H., Hiotakis, K., Dacar, D. 1985: Open heart surgery in Jehovah's Witnesses. *Wiener Klinische Wochenschrift* **97**, 525–30.

Gomes, M.M.R., McGoon, D.C. 1969: Bleeding patterns after open-heart surgery. *Journal of Thoracic and Cardiovascular Surgery* **60**, 87–97.

Gomes, O.M., Pereira, S.N., Castagna, R.C. *et al.* 1973: The importance of the different sites of air injection in the tolerance of arterial air-embolism. *Journal of Thoracic and Cardiovascular Surgery* **65**, 563–8.

Gourin, A., Streisand, R.L., Stuckey, J.H. 1970: Total cardiopulmonary bypass, myocardial contractility, and the administration of protamine sulfate. *Journal of Thoracic and Cardiovascular Surgery* **61**, 160–6.

Govier, A.V., Reves, J.G., McKay, R.D. 1984: Factors and their influences on regional cerebral blood flow during non-pulsatile cardiopulmonary bypass. *Annals of Thoracic Surgery* **38**, 559–600.

Goy, M., Schmitt, R., Sabatier, M., Kreitmann, P. 1984: Effect of open heart surgery on intellectual efficiency. Prospective study apropos of 40 cases. *Archives des Maladies du Coeur et des Vaisseaux* **77**, 167–73.

Hanks, J.B., Curtis, S.E., Hanks, B.B. 1982: Gastrointestinal complications after cardiopulmonary bypass. *Surgery* **67**, 410–12.

Harken, A.H. 1975: The influence of pulsatile perfusion on oxygen uptake by the isolated canine hind limb. *Journal of Thoracic and Cardiovascular Surgery* **70**, 237–41.

Harker, L.A., Malpass, T.W., Branson, H.E. *et al.* 1980: Mechanism of abnormal bleeding in patients undergoing cardiopulmonary bypass: acquired transient platelet dysfunction associated with selective alpha granule release. *Blood* **56**, 824–34.

Harrison, T.S., Seton, J.F. 1973: An analysis of pulse frequency as an adrenergic excitant in pulsatile circulatory support. *Surgery* **73**, 868–72.

Harrison, T.S., Chawla, R.C., Seton, J.F., Robinson, B.H. 1970: Carotid sinus origin of adrenergic responses compromising the effectiveness of artificial circulatory support. *Surgery* **68**, 20–6.

Heikkinen, L.O., Ala-Kulju, K.V. 1987: Abdominal complications following cardiopulmonary bypass surgery. *American Journal of Surgery* **146**, 133–7.

Heikkinen, L., Hargula, A., Merikallio, E. 1985: Acute renal failure related to open heart surgery. *Annales Chirurgiae et Gynaecologiae* **74**, 203–9.

Hening, C.R. 1988: *Modern cardiovascular physiology.* Boston, MA: Little, Brown & Co.

Henling, C.E., Carmichael, M.J., Keats, A.S., Cooley, D.A. 1985: Cardiac operation for congenital heart disease in children of Jehovah's Witnesses. *Journal of Thoracic and Cardiovascular Surgery* **89**, 914–20.

Henney, P.R., Riemenschneider, T.A., DeLand, E.C., Maloney, J.V. Jr. 1971: Prevention of hypokalaemic cardiac arrhythmias associated with cardiopulmonary bypass and haemodilution. *Surgical Forum* **21**, 145–7.

Henze, T., Stephan, H., Sonntag, H. 1990: Cerebral dysfunction following extracorporeal circulation for aortocoronary bypass surgery: no differences in neurophysiological outcome after pulsatile versus non-pulsatile flow. *Thoracic and Cardiovascular Surgery* **38**, 65–8.

Hernandez, L.A., Grisham, M.B., Twohig, B. 1987: Role of neutrophils in ischemia-reperfusion induced microvascular injury. *American Journal of Physiology* **253**, 699–703.

Hickey, P.R., Buckley, M.J., Philbin, D.M. 1983: Pulsatile and nonpulsatile cardiopulmonary bypass: review of a counterproductive controversy. *Annals of Thoracic Surgery* **36**, 720–37.

Hicks, R.E., Dutton, R.C., Ries, C.A. *et al.* 1973: Production and fate of platelet aggregate emboli during venovenous perfusion. *Surgical Forum* **24**, 250–2.

Hilberman, M., Derby, G.C., Spencer, R.J., Stinson, E.B. 1980: Sequential pathological changes characterizing the progression from renal dysfunction to actual renal failure following cardiac operation. *Journal of Thoracic and Cardiovascular Surgery* **79**, 838–44.

Hill, J.D., Aguilar, M.J., Baranco, A., Gerbode, F. 1969: Neuropathological manifestations of cardiac surgery. *Annals of Thoracic Surgery* **7**, 409–19.

Hill, J.D., DeLeval, M.R., Fallat, R.J. *et al.* 1972: Acute respiratory insufficiency: treatment with prolonged extracorporeal oxygenation. *Journal of Thoracic and Cardiovascular Surgery* **64**, 551–62.

Hind, C.R., Griffin, J.F., Pack, S. *et al.* 1988: Effect of cardiopulmonary bypass on circulating concentrations of leucocyte elastase and free radical activity. *Cardiovascular Research* **22**, 37–41.

Hinshaw, D.B., Armstrong, B.C., Burger, J.M. *et al.* 1988: ATP and micro-filaments in cellular oxidant injury. *American Journal of Pathology* **132**, 479–88.

Hirayama, T., Yamaguchi, H., Allers, M., Roberts, D. 1985: Evaluation of red cell damage during cardiopulmonary bypass. *Journal of Thoracic and Cardiovascular Surgery* **19**, 263–5.

Hirayama, T., Roberts, D.G., Allers, M., Belboul, A., Al-Khaja, N., William-Olsson, G. 1988: Association between pulmonary dysfunction and reduced red cell deformity following. *Scandinavian Journal of Thoracic and Cardiovascular Surgery* **22**, 175–7.

Hirsch, J., Raschke, R., Warentin, T.E., Dalen, J.E., Deykin, D., Poller, L. 1995: Heparin: mechanism of action, pharmacokinetics, dosing considerations, monitoring, efficacy and safety. *Chest* **108**, 258–75.

Hoerr, H.R., Kraemer, M.F., Williams, J.L. 1987: *In vitro* comparison of the blood handling by the constrained vortex and twin roller blood pumps. *Journal of Extracorporeal Techniques* **19**, 316–20.

Holloway, D.S., Summaria, L., Sandesara, J. *et al.* 1988: Decreased platelet number and function and increased fibrinolysis contribute to post-operative bleeding in cardiopulmonary bypass patients. *Thrombosis and Haemostasis* **59**, 62–7.

Horrow, J.C., Hlavacek, J., Strong, M.D. *et al.* 1990: Prophylactic tranexamic acid decreases bleeding after cardiac operations. *Journal of Thoracic and Cardiovascular Surgery* **99**, 70–4.

Howard, R.J., Crain, C., Franzini, D.A. *et al.* 1988: Effects of cardiopulmonary bypass on pulmonary leukostasis and complement activation. *Archives of Surgery* **123**, 1496–1501.

Huddy, S.P.J., Joyce, W.P., Pepper, J.R. 1991: Gastrointestinal complications in 4473 patients who underwent cardiopulmonary bypass surgery. *British Journal of Surgery* **78**, 293–6.

Indeglia, R., Shea, M.A., Varco, R.L., Bernstein, E.F. 1967: Mechanical and biological considerations in erythrocyte damage. *Surgery* **62**, 47–53.

Jaberi, M., Bell, W.R., Benson, D.W. 1973: Control of heparin therapy in open-heart surgery. *Journal of Thoracic and Cardiovascular Surgery* **67**, 133–41.

Jacobs, L.A., Klopp, E.H., Seamone, W., Topaz, S.R., Gott, V.L. 1969: Improved organ function during cardiac bypass with a roller pump modified to deliver pulsatile flow. *Journal of Thoracic and Cardiovascular Surgery* **68**, 138–47.

Jaenike, J.R., Schneeberger, E.E. 1966: The renal lesion associated with haemoglobinaemia. II. Its structural characteristics in rats. *Journal of Experimental Medicine* **123**, 537–45.

Jones, D.K., Luddington, R., Higenbottam, T.W. *et al.* 1988: Changes in factor VIII proteins after cardiopulmonary bypass in man suggests endothelial damage. *Thrombosis and Haemostasis* **60**, 199–204.

Kaplan, J.A., Cannarella, C., Jones, E.L. *et al.* 1977: Autologous blood transfusion during cardiac surgery. A re-evaluation of three methods. *Journal of Thoracic and Cardiovascular Surgery* **74**, 4–10.

Karlstad, M.D., Patteson, S.K., Guszcza, J.A. 1993: Methylprednisolone does not influence endotoxin translocation during cardiopulmonary bypass. *Journal of Cardiothoracic and Vascular Anesthesia* **7**, 23–7.

Kawashima, Y., Yamamoto, Z., Manabe, H. 1974: Safe limits of hemodilution in cardiopulmonary bypass. *Surgery* **76**, 391–7.

Kevy, S.V., Glickman, R.M., Bernhard, W.F. 1966: The pathogenesis and control of the haemorrhagic defect in open-heart surgery. *Surgery, Gynecology, and Obstetrics* **126**, 313–18.

Kirklin, J.W., Barratt-Boyes, B.G. 1986: Hypothermia, circulatory arrest, and cardiopulmonary bypass. In: J.W. Kirklin, B.G. Barratt-Boyes (eds), *Cardiac surgery*. New York, NY: Wiley, 30–74.

Kirklin, J.K., Kirklin, J.W. 1990: Cardiopulmonary bypass for cardiac surgery. In: D.C. Sabiston, F.C. Spencer (eds), *Surgery of the chest* (fifth edition). Philadelphia, PA: WB Saunders, 1107–22.

Kirklin, J.K., Westaby, S., Blackstone, E.H. *et al.* 1983: Complement and the damaging effects of cardiopulmonary bypass. *Journal of Thoracic and Cardiovascular Surgery* **86**, 845–57.

Koja, K., Kunisyoshi, Y., Ikemura, F. 1986: Influence of the centrifugal pump (Bio-pump) on blood components. *Japanese Journal of Artificial Organs* **15**, 545–8.

Kono, K., Philbin, D.M., Coggins, C.H. *et al.* 1983: Adrenocortical hormone levels during cardiopulmonary bypass with and without pulsatile flow. *Journal of Thoracic and Cardiovascular Surgery* **85**, 129–33.

Kornfeld, D.S., Heller, S.S., Frank, K.A. *et al.* 1978: Delirium after coronary artery bypass surgery. *Journal of Thoracic and Cardiovascular Surgery* **76**, 93–6.

Kuntschen, F.R., Galletti, P.M., Hahn, C. *et al.* 1985: Alterations of insulin and glucose metabolism during cardiopulmonary bypass under normothermia. *Journal of Thoracic and Cardiovascular Surgery* **89**, 97–106.

Kuntschen, F.R., Galletti, P.M., Hahn, C. 1986: Glucose insulin interactions during cardiopulmonary bypass. Hypothermia versus normothermia. *Journal of Thoracic and Cardiovascular Surgery* **91**, 451–9.

Kuo, J., Graham, T.R. 1995: The choice of blood pump for cardiopulmonary bypass. In: T.R. Graham, C.T. Lewis (eds), *Mechanical circulatory support*. London: Edward Arnold, 118–29.

Kusserow, B.K., Larrow, R. 1968. Studies of leukocyte responses to prolonged blood pumping-effects upon phagocytic capability and total white cell count. *Transactions of the American Society for Artificial Internal Organs* **14**, 261–3.

Landis, G.H., Mandl, J.P., Holt, D. 1979: Pump flow dynamics of the roller pump and constrained vortex pump. *Journal of Extracorporeal Technology* **6**, 210–13.

Landow, L., Phillips, D.A., Heard, S.O. 1991: Gastric tonometry and venous oximetry in cardiac surgery patients. *Critical Care Medicine* **19**, 1226–33.

Lange, H.W., Aeppli, D.M., Brown, D.C. 1987: Survival of patients with acute renal failure requiring dialysis after open heart surgery: early prognostic indicators. *American Heart Journal* **113**, 1138–43.

Lavee, J., Martinowitz, U., Mohr, R. *et al.* 1989: The effect of transfusion of fresh whole blood versus platelet concentrates after cardiac operations. A scanning electron micro-scope study of platelet aggregation on extracellular matrix. *Journal of Thoracic and Cardiovascular Surgery* **97**, 204–12.

Lawrence, G.H., McKay, H.A., Sherensky, R.T. 1971: Effective measures in the prevention of intraoperative aeroembolus. *Journal of Thoracic and Cardiovascular Surgery* **62**, 731–5.

Lee, W.H. Jr, Krumhaar, D., Fonkalsrud, E.W. *et al.* 1961: Denaturation of plasma proteins as a cause of morbidity and death after intracardiac operations. *Surgery* **50**, 29–33.

Lee, W.H. Jr, Brady, M.P., Rowe, J.M., Miller, W.C. Jr. 1970: Effects of extracorporeal circulation upon behavior, personality, and brain function: Part II, Haemodynamic, metabolic and psychometric correlations. *Annals of Surgery* **173**, 1013–23.

Lees, M.H., Herr, R.H., Hill, J.D. *et al.* 1970: Distribution of systemic blood flow of the rhesus monkey during cardiopulmonary bypass. *Journal of Thoracic and Cardiovascular Surgery* **61**, 570–86.

Leitman, I.M., Paull, D.E., Barie, P.S., Isom, O.W., Shires, G.T. 1987: Intra-abdominal complications of cardiopulmonary bypass operations. *Surgery, Gynecology, and Obstetrics* **165**, 251–4.

Lemieux, M., Tice, D.A., Reed, G.E., Chauss, R.H. 1967: Chlorpromazine; adjunct to physiologic perfusion. *Journal of Thoracic and Cardiovascular Surgery* **53**, 425–9.

Levine, F.H., Grotte, G.J., Falon, J.T. 1980: Effects of pulsatile and nonpulsatile reperfusion on the postischemic myocardium. *American Journal of Cardiology* **45**, 394–8.

Lillehei, C.W. 1955: Controlled cross-circulation for direct vision intracardiac surgery: correction of ventricular septal defects, atrioventricularis communis and tetralogy of Fallot. *Postgraduate Medicine* **17**, 388–96.

Lumb, P.D. 1987: A comparison between 25% albumin and 6% hydroxyethyl starch solutions on lung water accumulation during and immediately after cardiopulmonary bypass. *Annals of Surgery* **206**, 210–13.

MacDonald, R.G., Buckler, J.M., Deverall, P.B. 1975: Growth hormone and blood glucose concentrations during cardiopulmonary bypass. *British Journal of Anaesthesia* **47**, 713–18.

Mammen, E.F., Koets, M.H., Washington, B.C. et al. 1985: Hemostasis changes during cardiopulmonary bypass surgery. *Seminars in Thrombosis and Hemostasis* **11**, 281–92.

Mannucci, P.M. 1988: Desmopressin: a nontransfusional form of treatment for congenital and acquired bleeding disorders. *Blood* **72**, 1449–55.

Many, M., Giron, F., Birtwell, W.C. et al., 1969: Effects of depulsation of renal blood flow upon renal function and renin secretion. *Surgery* **66**, 242–5.

Marath, A., Man, W., Taylor, K.M. 1987: Histamine release in paediatric cardiopulmonary bypass – a possible role in the capillary leak syndrome. *Agents and Actions* **20**, 299–302.

Marath, A., Man, W., Taylor, K.M. 1988: Plasma histamine profiles in paediatric cardiopulmonary bypass. *Agents and Actions* **23**, 339–42.

Matsumo, T., Wolferth, C.C., Perlmann, M.H. 1971: Effects of pulsatile and non-pulsatile perfusion upon cerebral and conjunctival microcirculation in dogs. *American Surgery* **37**, 61–4.

Maxwell, G.M., Rowe, C.G., Castillo, G. et al. 1958: Haemodynamic effects of chlorpromazine: including studies of cardiac work and coronary blood flow. *Anesthesiology* **19**, 64–7.

Mitchell, B.A., Casthely, P.A. 1991: Optimal flow during cardiopulmonary bypass. In: P.A. Casthely, D. Bregman (eds), *Cardiopulmonary bypass: physiology, related complications, and pharmacology*. Mount Kisco, NY: Futura.

Moneta, G.L., Misback, G.A., Ivey, T.D. 1985: Hypoperfusion as a possible factor in the development of gastrointestinal complications after cardiac surgery. *American Journal of Surgery* **149**, 648–50.

Montoya, J.P., Merz, S.I., Bartlett, R.H. 1990: A standardized system for describing flow/pressure relationships in vascular access devices. *Transactions of the American Society for Artificial Internal Organs* **37**, 4–8.

Moran, J.M., Babka, R., Silberman, S. et al. 1978: Immediate centrifugation of oxygenator contents after cardiopulmonary bypass. *Journal of Thoracic and Cardiovascular Surgery* **76**, 510–17.

Mullin, P., Lee, S., Burd, S. et al. 1976: A new device for the rapid automated determination of the activated clotting time for whole blood. *American Society of Extra-Corporeal Technology Proceedings,* 6–8.

Murkin, J.M. 1993: Anesthesia, the brain, and cardiopulmonary bypass. *Annals of Thoracic Surgery* **56**, 1461–3.

Murkin, J.M., Lee, D.H. 1991: Transcranial doppler verification of pulsatile cerebral blood flow during cardiopulmonary bypass. *Anesthesia and Analgesia* **72**, 194–7.

Murkin, J.M., Martzke, J.S. 1992: Cognitive and neurological function after coronary artery surgery. A prospective study. *Anesthesia and Analgesia* **74**, 215–21.

Murkin, J.M., Farrar, J.K., Tweed, W.A., McKenzie, F.N., Guiraudon, G. 1987: Cerebral autoregulation and flow/metabolism coupling during cardiopulmonary bypass: the influence of $PaCO_2$. *Anesthesia and Analgesia* **66**, 825–32.

Needleman, P., Greenwald, J.E. 1986: Atriopeptin: a cardiac hormone intimately involved in fluid, electrolyte, and blood pressure homeostasis. *New England Journal of Medicine* **314**, 828–34.

O'Connor, N.E., Sheh, J.M., Bartlett, R.H., Gazzaniga, A.B. 1971: Changes in pulmonary extravascular water volume following

mitral valve replacement. *Journal of Thoracic and Cardiovascular Surgery* **61**, 342–47.

van Oeveren, W., Kazatchkine, M.D., Descamps-Latscha, B. et al. 1985: Deleterious effects of cardiopulmonary bypass. A prospective study of bubble versus membrane oxygenation. *Journal of Thoracic and Cardiovascular Surgery* **89**, 888–99.

van Oeveren, W., Jansen, N.J., Bidstrup, B.P. et al. 1987: Effects of aprotinin on hemostatic mechanisms during cardiopulmonary bypass. *Annals of Thoracic Surgery* **44**, 640–5.

van Oeveren, W., Wildevuur, C.R.H., Kazatchkine, M.D. 1990: Biocompatibility of extracorporeal circuits in heart surgery. *Transactions in Science* **11**, 5–33.

Ohgrist, G., Settergren, G., Lundberg, S. 1981: Pulmonary oxygenation, central hemodynamics and glomerular filtration following cardiopulmonary bypass with colloid and non-colloid priming solution. *Scandinavian Journal of Thoracic and Cardiovascular Surgery* **15**, 257–62.

Ohri, S.K., Bjarnason, I., Pathi, V. 1993: Cardiopulmonary bypass impairs small intestine transport and impairs gut permeability. *Annals of Thoracic Surgery* **55**, 1080–6.

Ohri, S.K., Somasundaram, S., Koak Y. et al. 1994: The effect of intestinal hypoperfusion on intestinal absorption and permeability during cardiopulmonary bypass. *Gastroenterology* **106**, 318–23.

Okies, J.E., Goodnight, S.H., Kitchford, B. et al. 1977: Effect of infusion of cardiotomy suction blood during extracorporeal circulation for coronary artery bypass surgery. *Journal of Thoracic and Cardiovascular Surgery* **74**, 440–4.

Oku, T., Harasaki, H., Smith, W., Nose, Y. 1988: Haemolysis: a comparative study of four non-pulsatile pumps. *Transactions of the American Society of Artificial Organs* **34**, 500–4.

Orenstein, J.M., Sato, N., Aaron, B., Buchholz, B., Bloom, S. 1982: Microemboli observed in deaths following cardiopulmonary bypass surgery: silicone antifoam agents and polyvinyl chloride tubing as sources of emboli. *Human Pathology* **13**, 1082–90.

Pacifico, A.D., Digerness, S., Kirklin, J.W. 1970: Acute alterations of body composition after open intracardiac operations. *Circulation* **41**, 331–41.

Pacquet, K.J. 1969: Haemodynamic studies on normothermic perfusion of the isolated pig kidney with pulsatile and non-pulsatile flow. *Journal of Thoracic and Cardiovascular Surgery* **1**, 45–9.

Padayachee, T.S., Parsons, S., Theobold, R. et al. 1988: The effect of arterial filtration on reduction of gaseous microemboli in the middle cerebral artery during cardiopulmonary bypass. *Annals of Thoracic Surgery* **45**, 647–9.

Pedersen, K.O., Juhl, O. 1983: Blood ionized calcium measurements during aortocoronary bypass graft operations. *Scandinavian Journal of Clinical and Laboratory Investigation* (Supplement) **165**, 107–9.

Peirce, E.C. II. 1969: *Extracorporeal circulation for open-heart surgery*. Springfield, IL: Thomas.

Pinson, C.W., Alberty, R.E. 1983: General surgical complications after cardiopulmonary bypass surgery. *British Journal of Surgery* **146**, 133–7.

Pollack, E.M., Pollock, J.C., Jamieson, M.P. et al. 1988: Adrenocortical hormone concentrations in children during cardiopulmonary bypass with and without pulsatile flow. *British Journal of Anaesthesia* **60**, 536–41.

Ramsey, J.G. 1995: The respiratory, renal and hepatic systems: effects of cardiac surgery and cardiopulmonary bypass. In: C.T. Mora (ed.), *Cardiopulmonary bypass: principles and techniques of extracorporeal circulation.* New York, NY: Springer-Verlag, 147–69.

Reed, W.A., Kittle, C.F. 1959: Observations on toxicity and use of antifoam. *Archives of Surgery* **78**, 220–9.

Rein, K.A., Semb, G.K., Myhre, H.O. *et al.* 1988: Transcapillary fluid balance in subcutaneous tissue of patients undergoing aortocoronary bypass with extracorporeal circulation. *Scandinavian Journal of Thoracic and Cardiovascular Surgery* **22**, 267–70.

Replogle, R.L., Gross, R.E. 1961. Renal function during extracorporeal circulation. *Journal of Surgical Research* **1**, 91–104.

Replogle, R.L., Levy, M., DeWall, R.A., Lillehei, R.C. 1962: Catecholamine and serotonin response to cardiopulmonary bypass. *Journal of Thoracic and Cardiovascular Surgery* **44**, 638–41.

Riegel, W., Spillner, G., Schlosser, V., Horl, W.H. 1988: Plasma levels of main granulocyte components during cardiopulmonary bypass. *Journal of Thoracic and Cardiovascular Surgery* **95**, 1014–9.

Robicsek, F., Masters, T.N., Niesluchowski, W. 1983: Vasomotor activity during cardiopulmonary bypass. In: J. Utley (ed.), *Pathophysiology and techniques of cardiopulmonary bypass.* Baltimore, MD: Williams & Wilkins, 1–13.

Rocke, D.A., Gaffin, S.L., Wells, M.T. *et al.* 1987: Endotoxemia associated with cardiopulmonary bypass. *Journal of Thoracic and Cardiovascular Surgery* **93**, 832–7.

Romero, E.G., Castillo-Olivares, J.L., O'Connor, F. 1973: The importance of calcium and magnesium ions in serum and cerebrospinal fluid during cardiopulmonary bypass. *Journal of Thoracic and Cardiovascular Surgery* **66**, 668–72.

Rosendorf, L.L., Daicoff, G., Baer, H. 1974: Sources of gram negative infection after open-heart surgery. *Journal of Thoracic and Cardiovascular Surgery* **67**, 195–201.

Rousou, J.A., Engleman, R.A., Amisimowicz, L., Dobbs, W.A. 1985: A comparison of blood and fluosolDA for cardiopulmonary bypass. *Journal of Cardiovascular Surgery* **26**, 447–53.

Royston, D., Fleming, J.S., Desai, J.B. *et al.* 1986: Increased production of peroxidation products associated with cardiac operations. Evidence of free radical generation. *Journal of Thoracic and Cardiovascular Surgery* **91**, 759–66.

Rudy, L.W., Heyman, M.A., Edmunds, L.H. 1970a: Distribution of systemic blood flow during total cardiopulmonary bypass in rhesus monkeys. *Surgical Forum* **21**, 149–51.

Rudy, L.W., Heymann, M.A., Edmunds, L.H. 1970b: Distribution of systemic blood flow during cardiopulmonary bypass. *Journal of Applied Physiology* **34**, 194–96.

Sade, R.M., Stroud, M.R., Crawford, F.A. Jr *et al.* 1985: A prospective randomized study of hydroxyethyl starch, albumin, and lactated Ringer's solution as a priming fluid for cardiopulmonary bypass. *Journal of Thoracic and Cardiovascular Surgery* **89**, 713–22.

Salama, A., Hugo, F., Heinrich, D. *et al.* 1988: Deposition of terminal C5b-9 complement complexes on erythrocytes and leukocytes during cardiopulmonary bypass. *New England Journal of Medicine* **318**, 408–14.

Salzman, E.W., Weinstein, M.J., Weinstraub, R.M. *et al.* 1986: Treatment with desmopressin acetate to reduce blood loss after cardiac surgery. A double-blind randomized trial. *New England Journal of Medicine* **314**, 1402–6.

Saxton, G.A., Andrews, C.B. 1960: An ideal heart pump with hydrodynamic characteristics analogous to the mammalian heart. *Transactions of the American Society for Artificial Organs* **6**, 288–91.

Schaff, H.V., Hauer, J.M., Bell, W.R. *et al.* 1978: Autotransfusion of shed mediastinal blood after cardiac surgery – a prospective study. *Journal of Thoracic and Cardiovascular Surgery* **75**, 632–7.

Schaff, H.V., Mashburn, J.P., McCarthy, P.M. *et al.* 1989: Natriuresis during and after early cardiopulmonary bypass: relationship to atrial natriuretic factor, aldosterone, and antidiuretic hormone. *Journal of Thoracic and Cardiovascular Surgery* **98**, 979–86.

von Segesser, L.K., Turina, M. 1989: Cardiopulmonary bypass without systemic heparinization. *Journal of Thoracic and Cardiovascular Surgery* **98**, 386–96.

Senning, A. 1954: Extracorporeal circulation combined with hypothermia. *Acta Chirugica Scandinavica* **107**, 516–24.

Shah-Mirany, J., Najafi, H., Serry, C. *et al.* 1970: Pathophysiological alterations in perfused and nonperfused lungs during cardiopulmonary bypass. *Annals of Thoracic Surgery* **10**, 402–8.

Shaw, P.A., Bates, D. 1986: Early intellectual dysfunction following coronary bypass surgery. *Quarterly Journal of Medicine* **58**, 59–86.

Shaw, P.J., Bates, D., Cartlidge, N.E. *et al.* 1987: Neurologic and neuropsychological morbidity following major surgery: comparison of coronary artery surgery and peripheral vascular surgery. *Stroke* **18**, 700–7.

Silva, J. Jr, Hoeksema, H., Fekety, F.R. 1974: Transient defects in phagocytic functions during cardiopulmonary bypass. *Journal of Thoracic and Cardiovascular Surgery* **67**, 175–83.

Slogoff, S., Reul, G.J., Keats, A.S. 1990: Role of perfusion pressure and flow in major organ dysfunction after cardiopulmonary bypass. *Annals of Thoracic Surgery* **50**, 911–18.

Smith, P.C.C., Treasure, T. 1986: Cerebral consequences of cardiopulmonary bypass. *Lancet* **1**, 823–5.

Smith, E.E.J., Naftel, D.C., Blackstone, E.H., Kirklin, J.W. 1987: Microvascular permeability after cardiopulmonary bypass. *Journal of Thoracic and Cardiovascular Surgery* **94**, 225–33.

Spaeth, E.E., Roberts, G.W., Yadwadkar, S.R. *et al.* 1973: The influence of fluid shear on the kinetics of blood coagulation reactions. *Transactions of the American Society for Artificial Internal Organs* **19**, 179–87.

Stanley, P., Bertranou, E., Forest, F., Langevin, L. 1971: Toxicity of ethylene oxide sterilization of polyvinyl chloride in open-heart surgery. *Journal of Thoracic and Cardiovascular Surgery* **61**, 309–14.

Stein, J.H., Ferris, T.F. 1973: The physiology of renin. *Archives of Internal Medicine* **131**, 860–72.

Stibbe, J., Kluft, C., Brommer, E.J. *et al.* 1984: Enhanced fibrinolytic activity during cardiopulmonary bypass in open-heart surgery in man is caused by extrinsic (tissuetype) plasminogen activator. *European Journal of Clinical Investigation* **14**, 375–82.

Stone, J.J., Piccione, W., Berrizbeitia, L.D. *et al.* 1986: Hemodynamic, metabolic, and morphological effects of cardiopulmonary bypass with a fluorocarbon primary solution. *Annals of Thoracic Surgery* **41**, 419–24.

Stoney, W.S., Alford, W.C., Burrus, G.R. 1980: Air embolism and other accidents using pump oxygenators. *Annals of Thoracic Surgery* **29**, 336–40

Subramanian, V., Lowman, J., Gans, H. 1968: Effect of extracorporeal circulation on retoculoendothelial function. *Archives of Surgery* **97**, 330–5.

Swan, H.J.C., Paton, B. 1960: The combined use of hypothermia and extracorporeal circulation in cardiac surgery. *Journal of Cardiovascular Surgery* **1**, 169–75.

Taggart, D.P., Reece, I.J., Wheatley, D.J. 1987: Cerebral deficit after elective cardiac surgery. *Lancet* **1**, 47.

Tamari, Y., Aledort, L., Puszkin, E. *et al.* 1975: Functional changes in platelets during extracorporeal circulation. *Annals of Thoracic Surgery* **19**, 639–47.

Tan, C-K., Glisson, S.N., El-Etr, A.A., Ramakrishnaiah, K.B. 1976: Levels of circulating norepinephrine and epinephrine before, during, and after cardiopulmonary bypass in man. *Journal of Thoracic and Cardiovascular Surgery* **71**, 928–31.

Tarhan, S., Moffitt, E.A. 1971: Anaesthesia and supportive care during and after cardiac surgery. *Annals of Thoracic Surgery* **11**, 64–89.

Taylor, K.M. 1995: Pulsatile and non-pulsatile perfusion in cardiac surgery: the continuing controversy. In: T.R. Graham, C.T. Lewis (eds), *Mechanical circulatory support*. London: Eward Arnold, 106–17.

Taylor, K.M., Bremner, W.F., Gray, C.E. 1976: Anterior pituitary fuunction during cardiopulmonary bypass. *British Journal of Surgery* **63**, 161–2.

Taylor, K.M., Bain, W.H., Maxted, K.J. Hutton, M.M., McNab, W.Y., Caves, P.K. 1978a: Comparative studies of pulsatile and nonpulsatile flow during cardiopulmonary bypass. I. Pulsatile system employed and its hematologic effects. *Journal of Thoracic and Cardiovascular Surgery* **75**, 569–73.

Taylor, K.M., Wright, G.S., Reid, J.M. *et al.* 1978b: Comparative studies of pulsatile and nonpulsatile flow during cardiopulmonary bypass. II. The effects on adrenal secretion of cortisol. *Journal of Thoracic and Cardiovascular Surgery* **75**, 574–8.

Taylor, K.M., Wright, G.S., Bain, W.H., Caves, P.K., Beastall, G.S. 1978c: Comparative studies of pulsatile and nonpulsatile flow during cardiopulmonary bypass. III. Response of anterior pituitary gland to thyrotropin-releasing hormone. *Journal of Thoracic and Cardiovascular Surgery* **75**, 579–84.

Taylor, K.M., Bain, W.H., Russell, M., Brannan, J.J., Morton, J.J. 1979a: Peripheral vascular resistance and angiotensin II levels during pulsatile and non-pulsatile cardiopumonary bypass. *Thorax* **34**, 594–8.

Taylor, K.M., Brannan, J.J., Bain, W.H., Caves, P.K., Morton, J.J. 1979b: Role of angiotensin II in the development of peripheral vasoconstriction during cardiopulmonary bypass. *Cardiovascular Research* **13**, 269–73.

Taylor, K.M., Bain, W.H., Morton, J.J. 1980: The role of angiotensin II in the development of peripheral vasoconstriction during open heart surgery. *American Heart Journal* **100**, 935–7.

Taylor, K.M., Bain, W.H., Davidson, K.G., Turner, M.A. 1982: Comparative clinical study of pulsatile and non-pulsatile perfusion in 350 consecutive patients. *Thorax* **37**, 324–30.

Tennenberg, S.D., Bailey, W.W., Cotter, L.A. *et al.* 1985: The effects of methylprednisolone on complement mediated neutrophil activation during cardiopulmonary bypass. *Surgery* **100**, 134–42.

Teoh, K.H., Christakis, G.T., Weisel, R.D. *et al.* 1988: Dipyridamole preserved platelets and reduced blood loss after cardiopulmonary bypass. *Journal of Thoracic and Cardiovascular Surgery* **96**, 332–41.

Tollefsen, D.M., Blinder, M.A. 1995: Heparin. In: L.E. Hoffman (ed.), *Haematology: basic principles and practice*. Edinburgh: Churchill Livingstone.

Trocchio, C.R., Sketel, J.O. 1995: Mechanical pumps for extracorporeal circulation. In: C.T. Mora (ed.), *Cardiopulmonary bypass: principles and techniques of extracorporeal circulation*. New York, NY: Springer-Verlag, 220–37.

Tufo, H.M., Ostfeld, A.M., Shekelle, R. 1970: Central nervous system dysfunction following open-heart surgery. *Journal of the Americal Medical Association* **212**, 1333–40.

Turnier, E., Osborn, J.J., Gerbode, F., Popper, R.W. 1972: Magnesium and open-heart surgery. *Journal of Thoracic and Cardiovascular Surgery* **64**, 694–705.

Uretzky, G., Landsburg, G., Cohn, D., Wax, Y., Borman, J.B. 1987: Analysis of microembolic particles originating in extracorporeal circuits. *Perfusion* **2**, 9–17.

Utley, J.R., Todd, E.P., Wachtel, C.C. *et al.* 1976: Effect of hypothermia, hemodilution, and pump oxygenation on organ water content and blood flow. *Surgical Forum* **27**, 217–9.

Utley, J.R., Wachtel, C., Cain, R.B. *et al.* 1981: Effects of hypothermia, hemodilution, and pump oxygenation on organ water content, blood flow and oxygen delivery, and renal function. *Annals of Thoracic Surgery* **31**, 121–33.

Utoh, J., Yamamoto, T., Kambara, T. *et al.* 1988: Complement conversion and leukocyte kinetics in open heart surgery. *Japanese Journal of Surgery* **18**, 259–67.

Uozumi, T., Manabe, H., Kawashima, Y., Hamanaka, Y., Monden, Y., Matsumo, K. 1972: Plasma cortisol, corticosterone and non-protein bound cortisol in extra-corporeal circulation. *Acta Endocrinologica* **69**, 517–35.

Viinamaki, O., Nuutinen, L., Hanhela, R. *et al.* 1986: Plasma vasopressin levels during and after cardiopulmonary bypass in man. *Medical Biology* **64**, 289–92.

Wachtfogel, Y.T., Kucich, U., Greenplate, J. *et al.* 1987: Human neutrophil degranulation during extracorporeal circulation. *Blood* **69**, 324–30.

Wallwork, J., Davidson, K.G. 1980: The acute abdomen following cardiopulmonary bypass surgery. *American Journal of Surgery* **146**, 133–7.

Ware, J.A., Reaves, W.H., Horak, J.K., Solis, R.T. 1983: Detective platelet aggregation in patients undergoing surgical repair of anoxic congenital heart disease. *Annals of Thoracic Surgery* **36**, 289–94.

Weedn, R.J., Coalson, J.J., Greenfield, L.J. 1970: Effects of oxygen and ventilation on pulmonary mechanics and ultrastructure during cardiopulmonary bypass. *American Journal of Surgery* **120**, 584–90.

Welling, R.E., Rath, R., Albers, J.E. 1986: Gastrointestinal complications after cardiac surgery. *Archives of Surgery* **121**, 1178–80.

Wellons, H.A. Jr., Nolan, S.P. 1973. Prevention of air embolism due to trapped air in filters used in extracorporeal circuits. *Journal of Thoracic and Cardiovascular Surgery* **65**, 476–8.

Wenger, R.K., Lukasiewicz, H., Mikuta, B.S. *et al.* 1989: Loss of platelet fibrinogen receptors during clinical cardiopulmonary bypass. *Journal of Thoracic and Cardiovascular Surgery* **97**, 235–9.

Wheeldon, D.R., Bethune, D.W., Gill, R.D. 1990: Vortex pumping for routine cardiac surgery: a comparative study. *Perfusion* **5**, 135–43.

Whittlesey, G.C., Kundu, S.K., Salley, S.O. *et al.* 1988: Is heparin necessary for extracorporeal circulation? *Transactions of the American Society for Artificial Internal Organs* **34**, 823–6.

Wilson, I.C., Gardner, T.J., DiNatale J.M., Gillinov, A.M., Curtis, W.E., Camerspon, D.E. 1993: Temporary leukocyte depletion reduces ventricular dysfunction during prolonged postischaemic reperfusion. *Journal of Thoracic and Cardiovascular Surgery* **228**, 123–32.

Witoszka, M.M., Tamura, H., Indeglia, R. *et al.* 1973: Electroencephalographic changes and cerebral complications in open-heart surgery. *Journal of Thoracic and Cardiovascular Surgery* **66**, 855–64.

Wolk, L.A., Wilson, R.F., Burdick, M. *et al.* 1985: Changes in antithrombin, antiplasmin, and plasminogen during and after cardiopulmonary bypass. *American Surgeon* **51**, 309–13.

Wright, G. 1986: Blood cell trauma. In: K.M. Taylor (ed.), *Cardiopulmonary bypass: principles and management.* Cambridge: Cambridge University Press, 249–65.

Yeboah, E.D., Petrie, A., Pead, J.L. 1972: Acute renal failure and open heart surgery. *British Medical Journal* **1**, 415–18.

Zwischenberger, J.B., Cilley, R.E., Kirsh, M.M. *et al.* 1986: Does continuous monitoring of mixed venous oxygen saturation (SvO_2) accurately reflect oxygen delivery ($13O_2$) and oxygen consumption (vO_2) following coronary artery bypass grafting (CABG)? *Surgical Forum* **37**, 66–72.

Zwischenberger, J.B., Kirsch, M.M., Deehert, R.E. 1987: Suppression of shivering decreases oxygen consumption and improves hemodynamic stability/during post-operative rewarming. *Annals of Thoracic Surgery* **43**, 428–31.

4

Anaesthesia for cardiopulmonary bypass

LINDA NEL AND JOHN WW GOTHARD

KEY POINTS

- The requirements of the ideal cardiac anaesthetic are haemodynamic stability, appropriate analgesia and lack of patient awareness, and where relevant, the ability to awaken rapidly and smoothly.
- Knowledge of relevant pathophysiology and pharmacology is more important than the employment of a standard 'cardiac anaesthetic'.
- The effects of cardiopulmonary bypass on drug concentrations are variable and complex.
- Transoesophageal echocardiography (TOE) is becoming an increasingly valuable tool in intra-operative monitoring of haemodynamics and morphology.
- The evolution of 'fast track' management, with early post-surgery extubation requires modification of both cardiopulmonary bypass and anaesthetic techniques.
- In off-pump cardiac surgery, tissue stabilization devices optimize the surgical environment more effectively than pharmacological manipulation, and little modification of anaesthetic technique is required.

INTRODUCTION

There are a number of accepted techniques applicable to cardiac surgery and cardiopulmonary bypass. New drugs continue to be developed and introduced into clinical practice so there are bound to be differences of opinion as to the optimal anaesthetic for a particular cardiac procedure. There is substantial evidence, however, that it is not the initial choice of a particular anaesthetic technique or group of drugs that is crucial to outcome, but rather the manner in which these techniques and drugs are applied in different clinical circumstances.

Reves *et al.* (1995) stated in an editorial:

> the point is that drugs with very different sites and mechanisms of action can be given to achieve the same hemodynamic and other efficacy end-points during cardiac anesthesia.

These authors concluded that there is no such entity as a 'cardiac anaesthetic', and what is required to anaesthetize patients with ischaemic heart disease is knowledge of the pathophysiology of the disease and the clinical pharmacology of any number of anaesthetic vaso-active drugs at the clinician's disposal. The outcome of surgery for ischaemic heart disease may be influenced by the manner in which anaesthesia is conducted, but of paramount importance is that the surgeon achieves adequate revascularization without significantly impairing myocardial function. Similarly, the success of valvular heart surgery depends on the efficient replacement or functional repair of valves with minimal myocardial depression.

Standard approaches to anaesthesia for cardiopulmonary bypass are well described in numerous textbooks (Kaplan, 1993; Gothard and Kelleher, 1999). In this chapter we describe aspects of cardiac anaesthesia that have changed over the last few years. We will, therefore, be discussing recent advances and controversial aspects of anaesthetic and peri-operative management for cardiopulmonary bypass. In addition, we include a short section on the anaesthetic management of off-pump cardiac surgery. A basic knowledge of the conduct of anaesthesia for cardiac surgery will be assumed. This chapter will, additionally, be confined to subject matter directly pertinent to the practice of cardiac anaesthesia and the role of anaesthesia in cardiopulmonary bypass.

PRE-OPERATIVE DRUG THERAPY

Anaesthetic evaluation of patients for cardiac surgery includes consideration of the effects of pre-operative drugs that the patient has been taking. Cardiac drugs are, with few exceptions, usually continued up to the time of surgery. This is particularly important in patients who have unstable angina, where stopping medications (including aspirin) might precipitate persistent ischaemia. Some adjustment of anaesthetic and cardiopulmonary bypass techniques may then be necessary where particular drugs have been used. Non-cardiac medications are not considered here.

Aspirin is usually discontinued for a week before surgery in coronary patients with stable disease. The prolonged anti-platelet action of aspirin compounds the platelet dysfunction caused by cardiopulmonary bypass, and predisposes to excessive peri-operative bleeding. If it has not been possible to withdraw aspirin because of unstable angina, or even scheduling problems, it may be necessary to take measures to protect native platelets (such as aprotinin therapy) and platelet infusions will be required to treat any excess post-operative bleeding. Pre-operative heparin infusion, in unstable angina for example, is associated with heparin resistance, and infusion of fresh frozen plasma (a source of anti-thrombin III) may be necessary to correct the deficit (Ranucci et al., 1999). Patients anticoagulated with warfarin should be managed individually depending upon the reason for the anticoagulation and the urgency of the surgery. In patients with atrial fibrillation, for example, withdrawing anticoagulation for short periods is less crucial than in subjects who have a prosthetic mitral valve in situ. Fresh frozen plasma may be necessary to acutely correct coagulation in subjects taking warfarin facing urgent surgery. Vitamin K should be avoided because this will make anticoagulation very difficult post-operatively.

Beta-adrenergic blocking agents are usually continued up to the time of surgery, although some anaesthetists choose to withhold them in the immediate pre-operative period if the patient is markedly bradycardic. It may be necessary to increase heart rate intra-operatively with drugs such as atropine or even with epicardial pacing. Some clinicians use isoprenaline to increase heart rate, but this drug should be used with extreme caution in patients with ischaemic heart disease because it can cause an excessive tachycardia. Isoprenaline also lowers diastolic pressure (β_2 effect) and this can further compromise coronary flow. Calcium channel-blocking agents are also continued up to the time of surgery. A recent retrospective study suggests that pre-operative use of calcium channel blockers might increase blood product use after cardiopulmonary bypass (Mychaskiw et al., 2000). On the other hand, withholding calcium channel-blockers or beta-adrenergic blocking agents for an appreciable time can precipitate tachycardia in the case of beta-blocking agents or a worsening of angina on withdrawal of both classes of drugs. This is obviously undesirable and should be avoided.

Angiotensin converting enzyme inhibitors (ACE inhibitors) have been found to predispose to an unacceptable degree of vasodilatation during and after cardiopulmonary bypass in some patients (Tuman et al., 1995). Some anaesthetists, therefore, choose to omit ACE inhibitors on the day of surgery, although we prefer to continue these drugs up to and including the morning of surgery, and to treat hypotension on cardiopulmonary bypass with vasoconstrictors. Nicorandil, a potassium channel-opening drug that is being used increasingly in the treatment of angina, may also be associated with excessive vasodilatation on cardiopulmonary bypass (Falase et al., 1999). We have not, however, found it necessary to withdraw this drug before cardiopulmonary bypass.

Anti-arrhythmic agents are not discontinued pre-operatively. In the case of digoxin, if there is evidence of toxicity, elective surgery should be deferred to allow correction. Individual anaesthetists may choose to withhold the dose immediately preceding surgery but this method is no longer widely practised. Attention must be paid to correcting hypokalaemia and hypomagnesaemia as these can precipitate signs of digoxin toxicity (Heerdt and Heerdt, 1992).

ANAESTHETIC DRUGS

Modern anaesthetic agents and techniques have led to increased safety and stability of general anaesthesia. It is probably true to say that specific choice of anaesthetic agents has become less important in cardiac anaesthesia than the care with which the anaesthetic is administered in order to maintain haemodynamic stability. Propofol has evolved as an extremely useful drug both intra-operatively and in the post-operative period. It is commonly used in conjunction with medium- to high-dose intravenous opioids, such as fentanyl, and more recently interest has been shown in its combination with the short acting opioid remifentanil. Total intravenous anaesthesia can therefore be used as a sole technique for cardiac anaesthesia, but in the main the majority of clinicians also administer inhalational agents in a combined technique.

Propofol

Propofol is now a well-established intravenous anaesthetic agent that can be used both for induction (as a bolus) and for the maintenance of general anaesthesia (as an infusion, using a nomogram based on the subject's weight or with a specific programmable infusion pump). It is non-cumulative and allows rapid smooth awakening on discontinuation of an infusion. After a bolus intravenous dose of propofol the plasma concentration falls rapidly because of the immediate distribution of the lipid-soluble drug from plasma to tissue. The drug is later metabolized in the liver and excreted renally. Significant accumulation of propofol does not occur after short-term infusion of the drug, but the half-life can be considerably prolonged after chronic infusion in the intensive care unit and therefore it should be used with caution in this context.

Propofol can cause significant systemic hypotension, particularly following a bolus injection for induction. This effect is principally caused by a decrease in systemic vascular resistance, but there may also be an element of direct myocardial depression. Propofol should therefore only be used for induction in fit patients with good ventricular function. It should probably not be used in patients with significant outflow tract obstruction, for example, or in those with aortic stenosis and hypertrophic cardiomyopathy. Elderly people are also susceptible to the cardiovascular effects of the drug and it may be preferable to use an alternative drug, for example etomidate, for induction in this group of patients. Propofol is better tolerated as an infusion and the cardiovascular effects can be minimized if the drug is administered slowly. Partly for this reason, propofol is mainly used as an infusion during cardiac surgery either as part of a total intravenous technique or to provide anaesthesia during cardiopulmonary bypass, when patient 'awareness' can occur.

Propofol also has an important role to play in the immediate post-operative period, when ventilated patients can be sedated for a few hours with a non-cumulative intravenous technique. This allows relatively rapid awakening of many patients when they have been rewarmed and stabilized in the first few hours after surgery. At this point patients can be adequately sedated with low doses of propofol while systemic opioids are infused to establish analgesia. In this way patients readily tolerate the presence of an oro-tracheal tube and rarely remember these early hours in the intensive care unit, or indeed the process of weaning from ventilation and extubation.

Propofol has proved to be an extremely useful drug in the management of patients undergoing cardiac surgery, as discussed above. It has also established a role in the management of severe head injuries, where its ability to reduce cerebral oxygen consumption while preserving the 'coupling' of perfusion to metabolism limits intracranial pressure surges and leads to better neurological outcome. Inhalational agents, such as isoflurane, also reduce cerebral oxygen consumption, but because they 'uncouple' perfusion from metabolism, relative overperfusion results in higher intracranial pressure in patients with reduced intracranial compliance, such as those with severe head injury or large intracranial tumours. It was hoped that the beneficial effects of propofol shown in this group of patients could be extrapolated to improved neuroprotection in patients undergoing cardiac surgery and cardiopulmonary bypass. Disappointingly, no study to date has shown that propofol infusion before, during or after cardiopulmonary bypass confers consistently better neurological outcomes. A large prospective trial by Roach et al. (1999) recently found no difference in neurological outcome between two groups randomized to receive either isoflurane via the oxygenator or an infusion of propofol while on cardiopulmonary bypass, to maintain anaesthesia. Of concern, however, was the finding that propofol was associated with an increased need for vasoconstrictor drugs in order to maintain perfusion pressure and also with increased cerebral lactate production (and hence anaerobic metabolism) during rewarming (Souter et al., 1998). Hindman and Todd (1999) commented, in an editorial, that although propofol is associated with better outcomes with ischaemic cerebral insults (such as large cerebral bleeds and massive head injury), it seems ineffective at limiting neuronal damage from microemboli, which are a known aetiological factor in bypass-associated neuronal injury. Although it may be expected that the reduction in cerebral blood flow produced by propofol anaesthesia might be effective in reducing the number of microemboli that enter the cerebral circulation, this does not appear to translate into improved neurological outcome.

Remifentanil

Remifentanil is a potent opioid with an ultra-short duration of action. It is a fentanyl derivative with an ester linkage and is rapidly broken down by non-specific plasma esterases, producing essentially inactive metabolites. Its duration of action appears unaffected by abnormal butyryl cholinesterases (that is, its metabolism proceeds normally in patients with suxamethonium apnoea), or abnormal renal or hepatic function.

Remifentanil is administered as a continuous infusion as part of a 'balanced' anaesthetic technique. Unlike any other currently available opioid, its clearance from plasma is not prolonged by a preceding steady-state infusion. It is a pure μ-agonist with a terminal half-life of 10–20 minutes (Thompson and Rowbotham, 1996). Rosow (1999) reported that in an initial dose-finding trial, discontinuation of a wide range of infusions (0.025 μg/kg/min to 2 μg/kg/min, the latter being a very large dose) produced a spontaneously breathing subject, ready for extubation within three to seven minutes. In another study, Kapila *et al.* (1995) reported that following a three-hour infusion, full recovery of spontaneous respiration had occurred within 15 minutes for remifentanil, compared with over 45 minutes for an equipotent infusion of alfentanil. The obvious caveat here is that if remifentanil is used in major surgery, adequate alternative analgesia (for example, other opioids or epidural analgesia) must be established before the remifentanil infusion is discontinued.

These novel properties of remifentanil may find a role in the management of the increasing numbers of patients who undergo coronary artery bypass grafting (CABG) and are extubated within hours of surgery in 'fast-track' programmes (*see below*). Intra-operatively, remifentanil is used to provide stable opioid-based anaesthesia without the prolonged recovery period and delay in extubation that an equipotent dose of fentanyl or alfentanil would produce. Remifentanil can thus be used in doses sufficient to produce sympatholysis and suppression of the stress response to major surgery intra-operatively.

Initial enthusiasm for remifentanil in the mid-1990s has been tempered by a number of clinical observations in its use. It has proved difficult to overlap the termination of a remifentanil infusion with the commencement of alternative post-operative analgesia without either under- or overdosing the longer-acting opioid, thus mitigating the benefit of the remifentanil infusion in the first place. If adequate analgesia is not established immediately, it appears that the resultant pain is more resistant to treatment than if a longer-acting drug had been used throughout (Albrecht *et al.*, 1999). There have also been concerns raised about the propensity of a remifentanil bolus, given at induction of anaesthesia, to cause severe hypotension and bradycardia in subjects with coronary artery disease and this practice can no longer be recommended in this group of patients (Wang *et al.*, 1999; Elliott *et al.*, 2000).

The effects of cardiopulmonary bypass on remifentanil levels in a steady-state infusion have yet to be extensively studied.

Inhalational agents

Modern inhalational agents, such as isoflurane, desflurane and sevoflurane, have far fewer undesirable side-effects than older agents, such as halothane. On its introduction to clinical practice isoflurane was heralded as the ideal inhalational agent for cardiac anaesthesia because it preserved cardiac output with reduced peripheral resistance and did not significantly depress myocardial contractility. Subsequently, a number of studies in animals and man suggested that isoflurane could cause a deleterious redistribution of coronary blood flow increasing flow to healthy areas of myocardium by diverting it from potentially ischaemic areas supplied by diseased coronary arteries – the so-called 'coronary steal effect'. These early concerns regarding the coronary steal effect of isoflurane have largely subsided and it is considered to be a safe drug when used in moderate concentrations as part of a balanced anaesthetic technique. Caution should be exercised, however, if ischaemic ECG changes are noted or when high concentrations of isoflurane are used. There is a lack of recent large studies demonstrating any major advantages between these commonly used inhalational agents in cardiac patients.

Factors influencing choice between these agents probably rest more with issues of cost and local practice than with any discernible clinical differences. In practice most units in the UK currently use isoflurane in adults and reserve sevoflurane for inhalational induction in children. Inhalational agents are easy to use intra-operatively and, aside from the coronary steal effect ascribed to isoflurane, they may provide particular benefits to the ischaemic myocardium.

During coronary artery surgery, myocardial ischaemia with subsequent reperfusion can lead to so-called 'ischaemia-reperfusion injury' with variable manifestations ranging from myocardial infarction and myocardial 'stunning' to reperfusion arrhythmias. Reviewing available data, Ross and Foex (1999) concluded that potent inhalational agents, such as isoflurane, halothane and sevoflurane, given before an ischaemic insult, confer significant protection against myocardial ischaemic-reperfusion injury. The mechanisms for this effect include preservation of ATP levels, reduction of calcium overload and free radical scavenging in ischaemic myocardium, thus preserving myocyte integrity. The protection appears to be comparable between available agents (Ross and Foex, 1999; Coetzee *et al.*, 2000). The effect is not seen with intravenous agents such as propofol.

Inhalational agents can also be administered via the oxygenator during cardiopulmonary bypass. Intra-operative awareness appears to be more common in cardiac anaesthesia than in general anaesthesia for other procedures (Phillips *et al.*, 1993) and inhalational agents continued during cardiopulmonary bypass are likely to minimize the possibility of awareness occuring, particularly during the rewarming phase. The use of adjuvant agents such as opioids and benzodiazepines reduce the minimal alveolar concentration of inhalational agents, but there is a 'ceiling effect' and these cannot be relied on to produce satisfactory anaesthesia–amnesia on their own (Hilgenburg, 1981). On the other hand inhalational agents will only prevent awareness if given continuously, and it is important to prevent vaporizers from being turned down (or off) when vasodilatation occurs on bypass. For this reason it may be preferable to rely on an infusion of propofol to prevent awareness during cardiopulmonary bypass.

If inhalational agents are used during cardiopulmonary bypass the question of dosage arises. Hypothermia has long been known to reduce the minimal alveolar concentration requirements in animal models for inhalational agents (Eger et al., 1965; Vitez et al., 1974). This reduction is of the order of about five per cent per degree Celsius (Mets, 2000) and at 20°C the need for inhalational agents is removed (Antognini, 1993). How this translates into how much inhalational agent is actually given on cardiopulmonary bypass is variable.

Lastly, occupational exposure of theatre staff to inhalational agents should be reduced by the use of scavenging devices fitted to the oxygenator outlet (Hoerauf, 1997).

ANAESTHETIC DRUGS AND CARDIOPULMONARY BYPASS

The commencement, running and termination of cardiopulmonary bypass all affect the established concentrations of anaesthetic agents and adjuvants (Table 4.1). The effects are complex, and often unpredicted by theoretical models, thus detailed studies of each anaesthetic drug are necessary. Gedney and Ghosh (1995) and Mets (2000) have written excellent reviews that cover the topic extensively. In general, the factors that influence alterations in drug concentration are as follows:

1 The volume and nature (colloid or crystalloid) of the pump priming fluid.
2 *Effects of dilution*: all plasma drug levels decrease acutely as cardiopulmonary bypass is commenced due to dilution by the pump priming fluid.
3 *Protein binding of the drug*: some drugs are extensively protein bound, however, it must be borne in mind that the active portion of the drug (that is, that which is free to bind to receptors) is the unbound fraction.
4 *Alterations in acid-base balance during cardiopulmonary bypass*: this also affects protein binding of drugs.

Table 4.1 *Effects of cardiopulmonary bypass on plasma concentrations of various anaesthetic drugs**

Drug and mode of administration	Commencement of CPB	During CPB	After CPB
Fentanyl: bolus at induction of anaesthesia	↓ (Haemodilution in circuit prime, sequestration to circuit components)	Stable, after initial change	Early rise on reventilating lungs, from drug sequestered in lungs
Fentanyl: infusion before, during and after CPB	↓ (Haemodilution in circuit prime, sequestration to circuit components)	↑ (Slow rise as CPB continues)	Early rise as above, then ↑↑ levels, as elimination half-life is prolonged post-CPB
Propofol: infusion	↓ (Haemodilution in circuit prime, sequestration to circuit components) Increased free fraction due to reduced protein binding	↑ (Reduced clearance)	Normal clearance
Midazolam: bolus at induction	↓ (Haemodilution in circuit prime, sequestration to circuit components) Increased free fraction due to reduced protein binding	–	↑ (Drug concentrated in plasma as pump prime is excreted)
Midazolam: infusion	↓ (Haemodilution in circuit prime, sequestration to circuit components) Increased free fraction due to reduced protein binding	↑ (Slow rise as CPB continues)	↑ (Drug concentrated in plasma as pump prime is excreted, also prolongation of elimination half-life)
Alfentanil: bolus	↓ (Haemodilution)	Stable – clearance unchanged during CPB	Clearance not altered by CPB
Alfentanil: continuous infusion	↓ (Haemodilution)	Stable – clearance unchanged during CPB	Clearance not altered by CPB

CPB = cardiopulmonary bypass.
*From Gedney and Ghosh (1995) and Mets (2000).

5 *Alterations in tissue perfusion while on cardiopulmonary bypass*: the lungs are isolated from the circulation for the majority of cardiopulmonary bypass, and hepatic and renal blood flow are reduced, altering metabolism of various drugs. Hepatic blood flow may be improved by the use of pulsatile cardiopulmonary bypass, but this technique is not widely used.

6 *Hypothermic techniques*: a reduction in body temperature has a measurable effect on the kinetics of enzyme systems and generally reduces the rate of drug metabolism. As noted above, hypothermia also reduces the minimal alveolar concentration for anaesthetic vapours.

7 *Materials used to construct the bypass circuit and oxygenator*: some drugs, such as propofol, fentanyl and isoflurane, bind avidly to various components of the cardiopulmonary bypass circuit, thus reducing their concentrations.

8 *Mode of drug administration*: in general a drug given as a bolus before cardiopulmonary bypass will exhibit more unstable levels during cardiopulmonary bypass than the same drug given by infusion while on cardiopulmonary bypass.

9 *Volume of distribution of the drug*: if a drug has a large volume of distribution and substantial tissue reserves have built up then back-diffusion from tissues tends to stabilize the plasma concentration during bypass (for example, digoxin).

10 *Effects of cardiopulmonary bypass on the ability of liver and kidneys to clear the drug post-operatively*: agents such as fentanyl and diazepam show prolongation of elimination half-life after cardiopulmonary bypass.

11 *Effects of haemoconcentration*: highly protein-bound drugs, such as midazolam, show an increase in plasma concentration when the excess crystalloid volume from the prime is excreted post-operatively.

INTRA-OPERATIVE DRUG THERAPY

Several non-anaesthetic agents are administered intra-operatively by anaesthetists and perfusionists, including various electrolytes and inotropes. Calcium (Ca^{++}), magnesium (Mg^{++}) and bicarbonate are physiologically ubiquitous, have important functions and are each subject to fluctuations in the setting of cardiac disease and cardiopulmonary bypass. Inotropic agents, such as beta-agonists and phosphodiesterase inhibitors, have an important role in the management of low-output states and in aiding separation from cardiopulmonary bypass. Agents involved in anticoagulation, haemostasis and antifibrinolysis are not included in this discussion.

Calcium

Calcium (Ca^{++}) has wide-ranging physiologic functions. Detailed descriptions of Ca^{++} physiology can be found in a reference text (Guyton and Hall, 1996). Briefly, its most important roles in the cardiovascular system include:

- *Action potential (electrical) generation and propagation*: conduction through the AV node occurs as a slower inward Ca^{++} current, rather than a sodium current, thus being important in normal atrio-ventricular delay.
- *Electromechanical coupling*: the arrival of an action potential at the cell membrane of a myocardial cell prompts the opening of voltage-gated calcium channels in the cell membrane and then the sarcoplasmic reticulum (an intracellular Ca^{++} store). Ca^{++} floods into the cytosol and binds to troponin C, causing myocardial contraction. Myocardial relaxation occurs as the Ca^{++} levels fall due to active extrusion from the cytosol into the sarcoplasmic reticulum and the extracellular fluid. In the heart (but not in skeletal muscle), the initial calcium current from the T-tubules in the cell membrane is important in triggering the subsequent, much larger influx from the sarcoplasmic reticulum, thus myocardial but not skeletal muscle contractility is dependent on extracellular Ca^{++} concentration.
- *Control of peripheral vasomotor tone*: actin–myosin interaction in vascular smooth-muscle cells.
- *Central role in platelet function and blood coagulation*: actin–myosin interaction causes structural changes in activated platelets. Ca^{++} binds specifically to activated clotting factors.

Intact cells actively maintain a calcium concentration in the cytosol about 1000 times lower than that in the extracellular fluid. Ca^{++} moves between intra- and extracellular compartments via ion channels, specific or non-specific, voltage or ligand-gated. Its intracellular actions are mediated by a complex set of calcium-binding proteins and enzymes.

Calcium has been found to play a central role in so-called ischaemia-reperfusion injury of the myocardium (Ross and Foex, 1999). Cytosol Ca^{++} overload occurs when ischaemic or hypoxic myocardial cells are reperfused. This is associated with ATP depletion and the generation of destructive oxygen free radicals. A characteristic spectrum of injury, ranging from temporary myocardial stunning and reperfusion arrhythmias to myocardial necrosis, results. Inhalational anaesthetic agents (*as discussed above*) and magnesium (*see below*) have both been found to protect the myocardium against ischaemia-reperfusion injury when given before the ischaemic-reperfusion insult. As both of these substances are known to have actions that physiologically antagonize those of Ca^{++} this is thought to be the mechanism of the protective effect.

The total concentration of Ca^{++} in plasma is about 2.25–2.55 mmol/L, of which about half is ionized (actively maintained within the narrow range 1.0–1.25 mmol/L) and the rest is bound to various anions and proteins. The ionized fraction is the most important physiologically. This is the Ca^{++} level that should be monitored and corrected intra-operatively, particularly before attempting to wean the patient from cardiopulmonary bypass (Aguilera and Vaughan, 2000). Changes in plasma pH alter the proportion of ionized to un-ionized calcium acutely by altering the solubility of Ca^{++} in plasma: acidosis increases the proportion of ionized calcium and alkalosis (for example, hyperventilation) reduces it. Rapid infusion of citrated blood products also leads to an acute reduction in ionized calcium. These effects are important in the context of cardiac surgery and cardiopulmonary bypass: alterations in plasma pH and blood product transfusion lead to fluctuations in ionized calcium levels, which have a direct effect on myocardial contractility.

Until the potential adverse effects of inappropriate calcium administration became known, it was common practice for anaesthetists to give intravenous boluses (5–10 mg/kg of 10 per cent calcium chloride) of calcium during separation from cardiopulmonary bypass, taking advantage of the transient (10–20 minutes) positive inotropic effects produced. DeHert et al. (1997) demonstrated, however, that this technique also increases diastolic ventricular stiffness, producing a short-lived diastolic dysfunction lasting up to 10 minutes after a bolus of calcium chloride in patients just weaned from cardiopulmonary bypass. In addition, Janelle et al. (2000) showed that intravenous boluses of calcium chloride reduce blood flow through grafted internal mammary artery conduits transiently after cardiopulmonary bypass. However, the latter study failed to show any new wall motion abnormalities (that is, no evidence of ischaemia) during this time. In an accompanying editorial Koski (2000) cautioned that this evidence should not be used to justify withholding calcium when its use is warranted, that is, when ionized calcium levels are low. In summary, present evidence supports the practice of appropriately treating low ionized calcium levels intra-operatively, but that inappropriate use of calcium can contribute to the problems of ischaemia-reperfusion injury, diastolic dysfunction and arterial conduit spasm, particularly in the period immediately after separation from cardiopulmonary bypass.

Magnesium

Magnesium (Mg^{++}) is the second most common intracellular cation. Its physiological functions are legion, and its physiology and pharmacology have been the subject of several recent reviews (Fawcett et al., 1999; Boyd and Thomas, 2000). Measurement of total serum magnesium levels (normally 0.76–0.96 mmol/L) is potentially misleading when used to diagnose deficiency. Ionized levels are more useful but more difficult to measure. Subjects with cardiac disease are more likely to have a magnesium deficiency, as drugs such as diuretics and ACE inhibitors cause increased renal losses.

The actions of magnesium can be conveniently, although somewhat artificially, thought of as falling into two categories:

1 *Its essential 'physiological' functions*: magnesium *is* central to normal aerobic metabolism, being a co-factor in a large number of enzyme reactions. This makes it important in maintaining cellular integrity.
2 *Its 'pharmacological' actions*: including calcium antagonism both intracellularly and at calcium ion channels. It has membrane stabilizing effects and, importantly, inhibits the release of catecholamines. These effects tend to be seen following an intravenous bolus or when plasma levels are higher than normal.

It is important to appreciate that most of the clinical uses of magnesium extend to this second category, rather than purely being aimed at treating a state of deficit.

Magnesium has been found to limit myocardial ischaemia-reperfusion injury when given before reperfusion or immediately within the first two minutes after reperfusion in animal models (du Toit and Opie, 1992). The timing of this dose appears to be critical. Magnesium given during the time frame stated above appears to prevent cytosolic calcium overload and preserves cellular integrity. This protective effect is not seen if it is given later. This protection appears to translate into improved post-ischaemic left ventricular function in human studies both in the surgical and non-surgical setting (thrombolytic therapy leading to reperfusion in acute myocardial infarction). The failure of magnesium to improve outcome in the magnesium arm of the ISIS-4 (Fourth International Study of Infarct Survival Collaborative Group) trial is argued to have been due to its late administration, falling outside the two-minute 'window' thus failing to protect against ischaemia-reperfusion injury.

Magnesium is also used for myocardial protection in cardioplegic solutions. Magnesium is used to treat and prevent both atrial and ventricular arrhythmias in cardiac surgical patients. Plasma magnesium levels are reduced during cardiopulmonary bypass, and plasma ionized magnesium levels remain low post-operatively (Brookes and Fry, 1993). There is thus a state of relative deficit which is pro-arrhythmic. This, together with the 'pharmacological' effects of magnesium (excitable membrane stabilization and suppression of catecholamine release), makes it a logical agent for arrhythmia prophylaxis and treatment in the cardiac surgical patient. There is no general agreement about the optimal regimen for this purpose: Boyd and Thomas (2000) cite several studies with widely varying magnesium doses before cardiopulmonary bypass (range 0.01 g/kg to 0.057 g/kg) and after cardiopulmonary bypass (range 0.01 g/kg to 0.17 g/kg), some as boluses, others as infusions. (Note: 1 g = 4.2 mmol = 8 mEq.) Higher dose regimens are more often associated with adverse effects of magnesium administration, that is, short-lived bradycardia and hypotension (responsive to volume) have been reported.

Magnesium has several potential side-effects, particularly when used in higher dose ranges for its 'pharmacological' actions. These include:

- muscle weakness (synergistic with non-depolarizing neuromuscular blocking drugs)
- bradycardia (managed with temporary pacing)
- hypotension (often responsive to volume)
- platelet inhibition measured in patients within 24 hours of cardiopulmonary bypass, probably compounding any underlying platelet dysfunction already present, but of unknown significance on its own (Gries *et al.*, 1999).

Care should be exercised when giving magnesium to subjects with renal impairment, as there is diminished magnesium excretion in this group, with increased risk of side-effects.

In summary, prophylactic magnesium has been shown to reduce ischaemia-reperfusion injury and the incidence of post-operative arrythmias in cardiac surgical patients. The peri-operative use of magnesium in this way is not universally accepted, however (Grigore and Mathew, 2000). Although there are concerns about the adverse effects, in practice these do not appear to contribute significantly to morbidity. There remains uncertainty about the optimal dosage regimen.

Bicarbonate

The bicarbonate buffering system is the single most important extracellular pH buffer. The reaction involved is described by the following equation:

$$H^+ + HCO_3 - H_2CO_3^- \leftrightarrow H_2O + CO_2$$

so that buffering of protons by bicarbonate (HCO_3^-) produces water and carbon dioxide, which is eliminated by the lungs, forming a so-called 'open system'. A detailed description of bicarbonate physiology can be found in reference texts and will not be discussed in detail here. Bicarbonate is administered intravenously as its sodium salt, sodium bicarbonate, in states of metabolic acidosis. This is only a holding measure, however, raising pH and

temporarily ameliorating the physiological effects of the acidosis. Once this has been achieved other measures must be instituted to treat the primary cause of the acidosis, for example reduced cardiac output or hypoperfusion on cardiopulmonary bypass. There are potential problems associated with the use of sodium bicarbonate. It is formulated as a sodium salt (usually 8.4 per cent [1 mmol/L/mL]) and can cause hypernatraemia and hyperosmolality. There are also concerns that the carbon dioxide generated by proton buffering may back-diffuse into myocardial cells, causing intracellular acidosis, with further impairment of myocardial contractility. Landow and Visner (1993), however, note that available evidence shows that this phase is short-lived and is followed by improved contractility and responsiveness to inotropes (that is impaired by acidosis) and conclude that bicarbonate should not be withheld where it is appropriate. The increase in pH produced by bicarbonate affects the solubility of other ionic species in plasma, as noted above, ionized calcium and magnesium levels fall, as does potassium (K^+). These secondary changes can have significant effects of their own (for example, reduced ionized calcium can reduce myocardial contractility, as discussed above) and may even be used therapeutically (for example, in hyperkalaemia). Other agents that may be used to correct metabolic acidosis include carbicarb (Leung *et al.*, 1994) and tris–(hydroxymethyl)–aminomethane (THAM).

INOTROPIC AGENTS AND VASOCONSTRICTORS

Peri-operative inotrope administration is an integral part of anaesthesia for cardiac surgery. Patients with poor ventricular function may be commenced on inotropes before surgery, or else they may be used to aid separation from cardiopulmonary bypass. Increasingly, the role of these agents is extending beyond purely cardiac support to include renal and mesenteric protection, and possibly modulation of the inflammatory response produced by surgery and cardiopulmonary bypass. Inotropic agents all act to increase cardiac contractility and improve systolic function at a given pre-load. Some also improve diastolic function producing better ventricular filling at a given pre-load. Inotropes may affect both pulmonary and systemic vascular tone. Inotropic drugs which also cause vasodilatation (so-called 'inodilators') reduce ventricular stroke-work, but may induce hypotension and reduce aortic root pressure, thus compromising coronary perfusion. Drugs mainly producing vasoconstriction may maintain perfusion pressure at the expense of increased ventricular stroke work and may also cause constriction in arterial coronary conduits.

Unwanted effects of inotropes include tachycardia and arrhythmias, and increased myocardial oxygen consumption, possibly precipitating ischaemia. Each drug has its own effect and side-effect profile, affecting its suitability in different clinical situations. These drugs are usually short-acting and given as titratable infusions. Inotropic agents used in established clinical practice at present fall into two broad groups: the catecholamines and the phosphodiesterase type III inhibitors. Other drugs, such as aminophylline and digoxin, exhibit inotropic effects that are largely incidental to their primary purpose. Thyroxine has also been used to maintain responsiveness to adrenergic agents in cardiac surgical patients.

The catecholamine, or adrenergic, group of drugs include adrenaline, noradrenaline, dopamine, isoprenaline, dobutamine and dopexamine. The former three are naturally occurring, and the latter three are synthetic. These all act directly at adrenergic receptors, which fit into three groups: alpha (α), beta (β) and dopaminergic (DA). Alpha receptor stimulation increases cell-membrane permeability to calcium. Beta-receptor stimulation activates adenyl cyclase, increasing cytosolic cyclic adenosine monophosphate (cAMP) levels. There are subtypes of each. Their most important cardiovascular functions are:

- α_1: vasoconstriction of most systemic vascular beds
- α_2: pre-synaptic inhibition of noradrenaline release
- β_1: increased sinus rate, A-V conduction and myocardial contractility
- β_2: peripheral vasodilation of some peripheral vascular beds, for example skeletal muscle.

(β_2 receptors also occur on myocardium, in lesser numbers than β_1, but are not down-regulated to the same extent in cardiac failure, thus becoming relatively more important in this setting.)

Each of the drugs mentioned above has a different profile of activity at these receptors: Adrenaline is predominantly a β_1 and β_2 agonist, with dose-dependent α_1 effects. Dobutamine is a β_1 agonist, whereas isoprenaline stimulates β_1 and β_2 receptors, and is useful in treating bradycardia. Noradrenaline given intravenously is an α-agonist, causing vasoconstriction. Dopamine has been used in low 'renal' doses (3 μg/kg/min) for 'renal support' in critically ill patients, but evidence of definite benefit in this regard has been controversial. One recent study (Schneider et al., 1999) suggests that a combination of low-dose dopamine and a low bypass flow rate is particularly deleterious to splanchnic perfusion, reflected as a low gastric mucosal pH, and the authors suggest that this may increase the incidence of post-cardiopulmonary bypass vasodilatory shock. Dopexamine is a relatively new agent. It stimulates dopaminergic and β_2 receptors, improving splanchnic and renal perfusion. It has been shown (Wilson et al., 1999) to improve outcome when used prophylactically to 'pre-optimize' high risk

non-cardiac surgical patients. Phelan et al. (1991), in an earlier study, demonstrated that routine CABG patients who received dopexamine peri-operatively showed improved lactate clearance post-operatively. Honkonen et al. (1998) also demonstrated that dopexamine efficiently offloads the right ventricle by reducing pulmonary vascular resistance after cardiac surgery. It is a relatively weak inotrope in its own right, however, and its place in cardiac surgery remains to be determined.

Phosphodiesterase (Type III) inhibitors (PDE3 inhibitors) increase cytosolic cyclic AMP levels, improving myocardial systolic and diastolic function. Increased levels of cyclic GMP in the peripheral vasculature also leads to vasodilatation, thus reducing after-load, with the possible additional benefit of relieving internal mammary artery spasm. These drugs are thus inodilators, and exert their action at a post-receptor level, hence their efficacy is not dependent upon receptor characteristics and density, in contrast to the adrenergic agents. They act synergistically with adrenergic agents, however, and tachyphylaxis is not a feature of their use. Amrinone, enoximone and milrinone are examples of these drugs. As a group, they have a longer half-life than the adrenergic agents, and are given as a loading dose which is usually then followed by an infusion. Milrinone is a particularly useful drug as it has a shorter half-life than enoximone and does not have to be given via a dedicated intravenous line.

Caution should be exercised in the use of PDE3 inhibitors, however, because of the potential hypotensive effect discussed above. Some authors (Lewis et al., 2000) fail to comment on significant vasodilatation following their use in weaning patients from cardiopulmonary bypass. Many clinicians find that the degree of dilatation produced requires the concurrent use of constrictors, such as noradrenaline or vasopressin, in order to maintain an acceptable perfusion pressure. Fogg and Royston (1998) comment in an editorial, however, that the use of a single prophylactic loading dose of milrinone (50 μg/kg/min) after aortic clamp removal but before weaning from cardiopulmonary bypass allows the vasodilation to be dealt with relatively easily whilst still on cardiopulmonary bypass. The positive inotropic effects persist into the post-cardiopulmonary bypass period, often eliminating the need for a further milrinone infusion. These authors advocate that this approach is sufficiently safe to consider using prophylactically in all high-risk subjects before weaning from cardiopulmonary bypass.

Maintenance of perfusion pressure while on cardiopulmonary bypass can be achieved by manipulation of either bypass flow-rate or systemic vascular resistance. Vasoconstrictors, such as phenylephrine and methoxamine, are direct-acting sympathomimetic amines that can be given as boluses to maintain perfusion pressure during cardiopulmonary bypass. Many cardiac anaesthetists use metaraminol as a vasoconstrictor peri-operatively. This drug is a synthetic amine with both direct and indirect sympatho-mimetic actions. It acts mainly via α-adrenoreceptors but also retains β activity. This latter property is useful therapeutically as it will increase heart rate slightly in addition to increasing vascular resistance. Noradrenaline is an α-adrenergic agonist usually given as an infusion where systemic vascular resistance is persistently low. It is often used in combination with PDE3 inhibitors.

Vasodilatory hypotension, or post-perfusion syndrome, is seen in some patients after cardiac surgery and cardiopulmonary bypass. This is a complex entity and is associated with endothelial injury and the release of cytokines and other inflammatory mediators, with subsequent massive vasodilatation and hypotension requiring the use of pressor agents. Argenziano et al. (1998) found, in a prospective study, that a low ejection fraction (<0.35) and ACE-inhibitor use pre-operatively were independent predictors of this syndrome. They also found that affected subjects had inappropriately low serum arginine vasopressin (a naturally occuring non-adrenergic vasoactive substance) levels and responded well to low-dose arginine vasopressin infusion, with reduced need for noradrenaline with its attendant side-effects when used in high dosage. Tuman et al. (1995), in a very large prospective study, confirmed the association of chronic ACE-inhibitor use and poor ventricular function with post-perfusion syndrome. They also identified duration of cardiopulmonary bypass, re-operative surgery, increasing age and opioid anaesthesia as predisposing factors.

MONITORING

Technology is always advancing, and in some respects has become cheaper, so that facilities for monitoring patients during cardiopulmonary bypass are constantly improving. There is also growing awareness that providing a good outcome for patients is not only of paramount importance but can be cost-effective. At a relatively simple level, there is increasing interest in the use of ultrasound monitoring to aid the placement of central venous lines. As far as more complex monitoring is concerned, there is much debate as to the present and future role of the pulmonary artery catheter (Stocking and Lake, 2000), in particular in comparison with the less invasive monitoring modality of transoesophageal echocardiography.

ULTRASOUND GUIDANCE FOR CENTRAL VENOUS CANNULATION

Percutaneous internal jugular vein cannulation is usually the preferred route for central venous access before cardiac surgery. First described by English et al. (1969) this procedure can be carried out safely in the majority of patients by use of a variety of approaches. In a small number of attempts at cannulation complications can occur. These include failure of cannulation, misplaced cannulae, carotid or arterial puncture, bleeding and pneumothorax. Carotid puncture (or even laceration) is a particularly serious complication prior to cardiac surgery as the patient will require full heparinization before cardiopulmonary bypass, which may exacerbate bleeding and cause haematoma formation. Laceration of arterial structures within the thorax by attempting to cannulate the internal jugular vein via a 'low approach' may cause intra- and post-operative bleeding that is difficult to detect and treat. In addition, damage to the carotid artery must further increase the risk of patients sustaining cerebral damage during cardiopulmonary bypass.

Hatfield and Bodenham (1999) recently demonstrated that a simple two-dimensional ultrasound device can be used successfully to aid central venous access when difficulties or complications have been encountered initially. Scott (1999), in an accompanying editorial, also advocated the use of an ultrasound scanner to delineate the anatomy of the internal jugular vein before cannulation, particularly in the difficult case. The presence (or absence) and size of the internal jugular vein can be ascertained on the selected side of cannulation. Abnormal anatomy can be delineated and, importantly, the position of the internal jugular vein in relation to the carotid artery can be imaged. In this way many of the pitfalls of 'blind' cannulation may be avoided. Portable ultrasound devices are relatively inexpensive and should be available to cardiac anaesthetists to help them to deal with difficult central venous access and as an aid to teaching.

THE ROLE OF THE PULMONARY ARTERY CATHETER

The balloon flotation pulmonary artery catheter was introduced over 30 years ago and the reader of a book of this nature will be familiar with the direct and indirect variables that can be measured via the catheter. Of particular value in the management of cardiac surgery patients is the measurement of pulmonary capillary wedge pressure (PCWP), which is an indirect measure of left atrial pressure.

In addition, several specialized versions of the pulmonary artery catheter have been developed to provide (as required) a pacing facility, the measurement of thermodilution cardiac output, fibre-optically measured mixed–venous oxygen saturation, right ventricular ejection fraction and continuous cardiac output. The information obtained from a thermodilution cardiac output pulmonary artery catheter, combined with arterial and central venous pressures, can be used to calculate a number of derived variables. These include systemic vascular resistance, pulmonary vascular resistance and stroke volume. This information can be invaluable in haemodynamic management of the cardiac patient undergoing surgery, particularly if inotropic or mechanical support is required for myocardial failure. Pulmonary artery catheter placement is certainly a particularly invasive form of monitoring and can lead to a significant number of complications, despite the sophisticated design and manufacture of modern catheters (Table 4.2). There is also concern that the information derived from pulmonary artery catheters does not affect outcome, particularly in the general critical care setting (Dalen and Bone, 1996).

Prospective studies are now underway to investigate the effect of pulmonary artery catheters on outcome in patients admitted to general critical care units (Angus and Black, 2001), but no such study has been initiated in patients undergoing routine cardiac surgery. A recent report (Ramsey *et al.*, 2000) looked retrospectively at the clinical and economic effects of pulmonary artery catheters in more than 13,000 patients who underwent routine coronary artery surgery in community-based medical centres in the USA. The use of pulmonary artery catheters differed widely from institution to institution, some centres recording little or no use in over 200 patients. Overall, however, more than 50 per cent of the hospitals recorded at least 65 per cent usage of pulmonary artery catheters, and 40 per cent of institutions had a greater than 85 per cent usage. In-hospital mortality was significantly higher in the patients who were managed with a pulmonary artery catheter. This is perhaps not surprising considering that the likelihood of receiving a pulmonary artery catheter increased with increasing age, severity of illness and when the initial hospital admission was urgent. Patients with Medicare or private insurance were also more likely to receive a pulmonary artery catheter, reflecting the difference in method of renumeration of clinicians in the USA compared with the UK. The most interesting finding of the study was that mortality in the pulmonary artery catheter groups was highest in those institutions with a low overall pulmonary artery catheter usage. This suggests that 'experience with pulmonary artery catheter use (or lack thereof) may influence outcome'.

Table 4.2 *Complications of pulmonary artery catheter placement*

Infection
Thrombosis and embolism
Rhythm disturbances
Pulmonary haemorrhage
Pneumothorax or vascular damage during insertion
Knotting of catheter

In essence, clinicians need to be trained in the use of pulmonary artery catheters, particularly in interpretation of the data obtained, in order to provide optimal care of the patient. Despite the controversies discussed it is likely that the pulmonary artery catheter will remain an important part of cardiac anaesthetists' armamentarium for the foreseeable future (Stocking and Lake, 2000). The increasing use and refinement of TOE, combined with the development of other technologies to measure cardiac output, such as transpulmonary aortic thermodilution and intravascular pulse contour analysis (Sakka *et al.*, 2000; Zollner *et al.*, 2000), may eventually provide much of the information derived from a pulmonary artery catheter, but in a less invasive manner. This is particularly relevant in the operating theatre where patients are anaesthetized and intubated, and therefore the additional information available from TOE can be obtained easily. In the later stages of intensive care, patients are less likely to tolerate the presence of a TOE probe, however.

TRANSOESOPHAGEAL ECHOCARDIOGRAPHY (TOE)

TOE is now a well-established technique that provides an enormous amount of haemodynamic and morphological information. The technology is constantly improving and is now in routine use intra-operatively in most large cardiac surgery centres. Table 4.3 lists the advantages,

Table 4.3 *Intra-operative transoesophageal echocardiography (TOE)*

Advantages
- Non-invasive, low-risk procedure
- Good image quality
- Does not interfere with surgery
- Continuous monitoring of myocardial function

Uses
- Assessment of global or regional myocardial function
- Monitoring myocardial ischaemia (regional wall motion abnormalities)
- Assessment of ventricular filling
- Evaluating surgical repair of congenital defects
- Assessment of valvular function (also following repair)
- Measurement of intra-cardiac gradients and flow
- Visualization:
  - intra-cardiac air
  - atheroma (especially at the aortic cannulation site)
  - thrombi
  - myxomata
  - aortic dissection

Complications
- Dental injury
- Damage to airway or oesophagus
- Bacteraemia
- Distraction from patient care

uses and potential complications of TOE. This list is not exhaustive, however, and the reader is referred to a recent text for a full description of TOE in anaesthesia (Poelaert and Skarvan, 2000).

TOE is a well-tolerated and relatively non-invasive technique. The evidence regarding the effectiveness of TOE in the peri-operative period has been reviewed by the American Society of Anesthesiologists and the Society of Cardiovascular Anesthesiologists (Practice Guidelines for Perioperative Transesophageal Echocardiography, 1996) and evaluation of the literature, combined with expert opinion from the task force, produced guidelines for the use of TOE in the peri-operative period. The task force divided the indications for TOE into three categories based on published evidence and expert opinion.

Category I indications are those supported by the strongest evidence or expert opinion that TOE improves outcome. Category I indications relevant to cardiac surgery are listed in Table 4.4. Category II and Category III indications are supported by less convincing evidence that TOE improves outcome, but it is likely that some of these indications will move into Category I as technology

Table 4.4 *Indications for transoesophageal echocardiography (TOE) during cardiac surgery*

Haemodynamic instability
Evaluation of left and right ventricular function:
- global and regional
- systolic and diastolic
- valvular function
Assessment of haemodynamic function
Detection of hypovolaemia
Cardiac tamponade
Acute pulmonary embolism
Dynamic left ventricular outflow tract obstruction
Cardiac surgery
Cardiac valve reconstruction
Cardiac valve replacement
Myocardial revascularization in patients with poor function
Surgical correction of congenital heart disease
Aortic dissection
Minimally invasive heart surgery
Minimal access heart surgery
Pulmonary embolectomy
Resection of intra-cardiac tumours and thrombi
Aneurysmectomy
Myotomy for hypertrophic cardiomyopathy
Heart transplantation
Battista's operation
Myocardial laser revascularization
Localization of intra-cardiac foreign bodies, electrodes, catheters, etc.

(Category I indications from Practice Guidelines for Perioperative Transesophageal Echocardiography. 1996: *Anesthesiology* **84**, 986–1006.)

and expertise improve. TOE is now well established for monitoring the cardiac surgical patient. There remain two major problems preventing its use from being more widespread in the UK. These are the cost of the equipment (and staff to run it) and the training of the relevant clinicians and technical staff involved. Images and flow information are relatively easy to obtain with TOE, but the accurate interpretation of this data requires a trained operator, whether an anaesthetist, cardiologist or technician. Surgeons are unlikely to make major intra-operative decisions on the basis of TOE data provided by an inexpert, inadequately trained operator.

THORACIC EPIDURAL ANALGESIA

Over the last decade, there has been a revival in interest in the use of thoracic epidural anaesthesia during cardiac surgery to supplement the general anaesthetic techniques described above. The epidural space is the space surrounding the spinal cord and its nerves and membranes, within the vertebral canal. The space is approached posteriorly, between two vertebrae, and a narrow gauge catheter threaded into the space to a variable distance. Local anaesthetic agents, such as bupivicaine and other drugs (most usually opioids such as fentanyl or diamorphine), are then injected or infused into the epidural space. Local anaesthetics act predominantly on nerve roots as they leave the vertebral canal laterally at the intervertebral foraminae, but opioids have a more central action. A specific volume of agent will spread in a roughly predictable fashion, so that a given number of segments will be anaesthetized. The nerves affected are both somatic (that is, sensory or motor) and autonomic (sympathetic: parasympathetic elements are found only in the sacral segments of the cord and so are not relevant to a discussion about thoracic epidural analgesia) (Armitage, 1990).

Thoracic epidurals for use in cardiac surgery are usually placed in the high thoracic region. Here, the dense somatic anaesthesia is useful intra-operatively, enabling both lower doses of opioids to be used and blunting the stress response to surgery (Loick *et al.*, 1999). Post-operatively, the excellent analgesia has been shown to improve respiratory function by removing the inhibitory influences of pain on chest wall and diaphragm movement. Indeed, Meisner *et al.* (1997) concluded in a recent publication that thoracic epidural analgesia does reduce the incidence of post-operative pulmonary complications in patients with heart disease. This is relevant in patients with underlying lung disease and has also been found to be useful in fast-track programmes (*see below*).

The regional sympatholysis produced by thoracic epidural analgesia has been used in some centres to treat angina refractory to other measures in the non-surgical setting (Blomberg *et al.*, 1989). Interestingly, this has been shown not only to relieve the pain of angina (transmitted along afferent autonomic pathways) but also to reduce ST changes, thus specifically treating the ischaemia. Blomberg *et al.* (1990) also showed that thoracic epidural analgesia produced selective dilatation of stenotic epicardial segments of the coronary bed, thus improving oxygen delivery preferentially to ischaemic myocardium. In addition, by blunting output from the sympathetic cardio-accelerator nerves, heart rate, wall tension and consequently myocardial oxygen demand are reduced. These effects translate into a more favourable myocardial oxygen balance. Advocates of the use of thoracic epidural analgesia for coronary artery surgery feel that these beneficial effects outweigh the additional risks of this analgesic technique. Indeed, thoracic epidural analgesia has been shown to reduce the release of Troponin T, a marker of myocardial cell damage, in patients undergoing CABG (Loick *et al.*, 1999).

Although remarkably safe statistically, there are several potential complications of thoracic epidural placement. The most catastrophic of these is paraplegia produced by compression caused by a haematoma in the confined space of the vertebral canal. This may be heralded by a so-called 'bloody tap' at the time of insertion of the epidural. Haematoma formation is more common in patients with coagulopathies. In patients about to undergo cardiac surgery and cardiopulmonary bypass (with full heparinization), there is obviously a danger that haematoma formation will proceed unrestricted and even a tiny bleed could become significant. Furthermore, because of lower mean perfusion pressures on cardiopulmonary bypass compared with normal physiological pressures, a small haematoma may, in theory, induce a greater area of cord ischaemia while on cardiopulmonary bypass than may otherwise have been expected. Centres regularly placing thoracic eipdural catheters for cardiac surgery advocate placing them one to eight hours preoperatively to allow any minor bleeding to settle and clot to stabilize before heparinization. Patients in whom a bloody tap (and thus a more significant bleed) is noted will have surgery delayed. A comprehensive review of the subject by Riedel and Wright (1997) stated that 'to date, no complications related to spinal haemorrhage before, during or after CABG have been reported after the use of thoracic epidural analgesia', however, the potential for this disastrous complication means that precautions to prevent it should remain rigorous. It is also likely, we believe, that this complication is under-reported.

There is a significant incidence of failure of thoracic epidural analgesia where an incomplete block, or no block at all, is achieved (McCleod *et al.*, 2001). Other adverse events associated with the use of epidurals include inappropriately high blocks (causing respiratory embarrassment in the unventilated patient) and unwanted cardiovascular effects (such as resistant bradycardia and hypotension) mean that patients should be closely observed by appropriately trained staff whilst thoracic epidural analgesia is in use. Effective and regular use of thoracic epidural analgesia requires a significant service commitment from anaesthesia and related personnel in departments that are often overstretched to begin with. Thoracic epidural analgesia is safest, and probably used most effectively in centres where it is common practice to do so, rather than sporadically as isolated cases. It appears unlikely that the technique will be widely used for routine surgery.

An alternative approach to the spinal cord and its nerve roots is direct injection of local anaesthetics and/ or opioids into the cerebrospinal fluid that surrounds these structures within the spinal meninges, a so-called 'intrathecal injection'. Djaiani *et al.* (2000) and Zarate *et al.* (2000) reported, in separate studies, that injection of morphine a water-soluble opioid (which thus disperses widely through the spinal intrathecal space) into the lumbar intrathecal space after induction of anaesthesia, achieves an improvement in respiratory function after cardiac surgery that is comparable with that achieved by thoracic epidural analgesia. The needle used in this procedure is much smaller than the large gauges used for thoracic epidural analgesia. In addition, a catheter is not placed, therefore the risk of bleeding into the vertebral canal is much smaller, making this procedure theoretically safer when performed so soon before heparinization. Further studies are needed regarding this approach, although a number of units have been using intrathecal opioids since the use of this technique underwent a renaissance in the 1980s (Fitzpatrick and Moriaty, 1988).

CEREBRAL INJURY AND CARDIOPULMONARY BYPASS

Neurological injury continues to be a major problem in patients after cardiopulmonary bypass. Cerebral injury manifests itself in several ways. Four neurological and cognitive abnormalities have been observed after coronary artery surgery on cardiopulmonary bypass: stroke; post-operative delerium; short-term cognitive changes; and possible long-term cognitive changes (Selnes and McKhann, 2001). Of these complications, overt stroke is the most serious and is variously reported at an incidence of 1.5–5.2 per cent. Equally worrying in many ways is a recent report (Newman *et al.*, 2001) that has identified long-term cognitive changes, despite initial improvement, in patients after cardiopulmonary bypass. This group studied 261 patients who had undergone CABG on cardiopulmonary bypass. There was a 53 per cent incidence in cognitive decline at initial discharge from hospital,

36 per cent at six weeks post-discharge, 24 per cent at six months and 42 per cent at five years. The cognitive function at discharge was a significant predictor of long term function. Cerebral injury after cardiac surgery is a complex subject that has been reviewed extensively in a recent text (Newman and Harrison, 2000). It is worthwhile summarizing here the main practical consequences of recent work in this field.

It is now considered that, during cardiopulmonary bypass, cerebral emboli constitute the major cause of neurological injury (Hindman and Todd, 1999). Cerebral microemboli occurring during cardiac surgery consist of atheromatous debris, microbubbles, fat and small fibrin or platelet complexes. Little is known about how these different microemboli affect the brain, but it seems that atheromatous thrombi play a major role in the causation of cerebral injury. Cerebral injury after cardiopulmonary bypass rises dramatically in patients over the age of 70 years (Murkin, 1999). This mirrors the incidence of atheroma found in the ascending aorta in relation to age. Thus, cannulation and cross-clamping of the aorta, plus partial clamping for the placement of the proximal end of coronary artery grafts, is implicated in the aetiology of cerebral injury after cardiopulmonary bypass. Atheromatous material is broken away during these manouevres and, as some of these are undertaken during off-pump cardiac surgery, avoiding cardiopulmonary bypass is unlikely to eliminate neurological injury in cardiac surgery. Other sources of emboli include microemboli from bubble oxygenators, fat from cardiotomy suction, and cellular aggregates and particulate matter from the bypass pump circuit. In addition, emboli can occur directly from manipulation of the aorta, as discussed above, and may be generated during the cardiac surgery itself. This latter category includes air embolism from an inadequately de-aired heart and particulate matter after intra-cardiac surgery, such as replacement of a calcified aortic valve. The subject of embolic phenomena during cardiac surgery has recently been reviewed by Rorie and Stump (2000).

To reduce the extent and incidence of cerebral injury during cardiopulmonary bypass it appears logical to minimize the potential 'cerebral load' of emboli. The microembolic load to the brain has been measured or estimated by use of transcranial doppler techniques. This remains a research tool, however, so the majority of effort clinically has been in trying to minimize embolic phenomena.

Aortic atheroma can be estimated at surgery by digital palpation. Cannulation and clamping sites can then be chosen to avoid major areas of plaque. TOE is more sensitive than palpation in assessing the ascending aorta for plaque. It is difficult to visualize the transverse and descending aorta with TOE, however, and some groups advocate hand-held epi-aortic ultrasound scanning in this context. TOE has the advantage in that it can also be used to assess de-airing of the heart after intra-cardiac procedures.

Minimizing cardiotomy suction has been shown to decrease cerebral emboli, and a filter placed in the arterial line also cuts down the cerbral embolic count with improved neuropsychological outcome. Other relatively simple strategies that can be undertaken to either cut down the cerebral 'embolic load' or to minimize the effects created include an alpha-stat blood gas strategy, the use of moderate hypothermia and the avoidance of excessive rewarming.

An alpha-stat blood gas management strategy during cardiopulmonary bypass is associated with a lesser incidence of neurological dysfunction when compared with pH-stat management (Stephan et al., 1992). This seems particularly relevant when bypass times exceed 90 minutes (Murkin, 1999). A pH strategy creates a luxury and excessive perfusion of the brain on bypass and therefore is likely to increase the number of emboli reaching the organ.

Hypothermia decreases the size of gas bubbles and increases the solubility of gases. In addition, it provides cerebral protection against anoxia. Moderate hypothermia also modifies cerebral metabolism to mitigate the effects of ischaemia. Release of glutamine and dopamine mediate histopathological cellular injury in ischaemic models and a temperature decrease from 36°C to 33°C prevents this (Rorie and Stump, 2000). Whether hypothermia is of benefit in the majority of cardiac surgical patients remains a matter for debate. It may be that avoiding hyperthermia is of more importance.

Hyperthermia during rewarming is likely to exacerbate cerebral injury caused by excess perfusion and metabolic changes. Hyperthermia worsens the outcome after cerebral ischaemia in a non-cardiac setting, and most workers in the field now warn against overheating patients after cardiopulmonary bypass. In this respect it is important to keep water temperatures down in the heat exchanger, particularly in high-risk patients such as the elderly. Cook et al. (1996) found that despite efforts to avoid large temperature gradients during rewarming, jugular bulb temperatures were invariably greater than 38°C and higher than the simultaneously measured nasopharyngeal temperature.

Lastly, there has been considerable interest in the use of drug therapy as a cerebral protectant during cardiac surgery and cardiopulmonary bypass (Hindman and Todd, 1999). As discussed earlier in this chapter, burst suppression with propofol has not been shown to reduce the incidence of peri-operative cerebrovascular dysfunction (Roach et al., 1999). Other drugs that have been investigated in this respect include barbiturates, calcium-channel blocking agents and adenosine-regulating agents. Of these drugs acadesine, an adenosine-regulating agent, has perhaps shown the most promise in providing neuroprotection (Multicenter Study of Perioperative

Ischaemia, 1995), but has not been introduced into clinical practice. At present considerable interest is being shown in the role of aprotinin, a serine protease inhibitor, as an anti-inflammatory agent for patients undergoing cardiopulmonary bypass. Aprotinin inhibits plasmin and also inhibits many other enzymatic processes involved in the inflammatory response to cardiopulmonary bypass. Levy *et al.* (1995) found that aprotinin reduced the incidence of stroke at two different dose levels after cardiopulmonary bypass. A meta-analysis (Smith and Muhibaer, 1996) also indicated that aprotinin may reduce neurological damage after cardiopulmonary bypass. Further controlled studies are required, however, to confirm that this effect is real and devoid of significant complications.

POST–OPERATIVE FAST TRACKING

The need to perform ever increasing numbers of cardiac operations, coupled with financial constraints and the limited availability of post-operative intensive care facilities, has led to the evolution of so-called 'fast-track' management of selected cardiac surgical patients over the past two decades (Aps, 1995). Various interpretations exist, but essentially this means appropriate peri-operative management to enable safe 'early' extubation, usually within 10 hours, after completion of surgery (Cheng, 1998). The level of nursing care can then be stepped down after extubation, enabling a cost-reduction of approximately 50 per cent per patient for immediate post-operative care, and higher patient turnover. In order to justify this approach, it has to be shown to be at least as safe as conventional post-operative care in an intensive care setting. Fast-track management protocols have now been successfully instituted in many cardiac centres.

Several factors need to be considered in predicting the likelihood that a given patient will meet the criteria for safe extubation within hours of the completion of surgery. Accepted criteria for extubation are that the patient is:

1 Haemodynamically stable, on little or no inotropic therapy.
2 Not bleeding significantly.
3 Awake, neurologically intact and co-operative.
4 Normothermic.
5 Breathing satisfactorily, with adequate gas exchange.

Pre-operative selection criteria for fast-track candidates are variable between centres and have evolved as the practice has become more widely spread. Criteria such as age, body mass index, anticipated complexity of surgery, pre-existing organ failure (including cardiac), recent myocardial infarction or stroke have been used to exclude patients deemed to have unacceptably high risk for fast-track management. London *et al.* (1998), in a retrospective

study of 304 male veterans, showed that age and pre-operative intra-aortic balloon pump use were the only consistent pre-operative variables associated with delayed extubation after cardiac surgery. In fact, the study demonstrated that intra-operative events and practices were more strongly associated with time to extubation than pre-operative factors. Cheng (1998) argued that in view of this, all patients should be potential candidates for fast-tracking and that only adverse intra- and post-operative events should modify this intention. Intra-operative events associated with prolonged time to extubation include narcotic dose, major inotrope use, use of an arterial graft, platelet transfusion and delay between termination of surgery and transfer to the intensive care unit.

Anaesthetic factors that affect the ability to fast-track patients include:

1 *Narcotic dose*: high-dose fentanyl regimes lead to delayed return of adequate ventilatory drive and awakening. Remifentanil may have a place, although as noted above, the need to establish adequate post-operative analgesia may obviate its benefits.
2 *Good post-operative analgesia*: thoracic epidural analgesia has benefits in this regard (*see above*).
3 *Post-operative normothermia*: achieved with the use of patient warming devices after adequate rewarming on cardiopulmonary bypass. Some centres also advocate the use of generous doses of GTN during the rewarming phase of cardiopulmonary bypass in order to rewarm the periphery.

Cardiopulmonary bypass factors that affect the ability to fast-track patients include:

1 *Use of hypothermia*: Leslie and Sessler (1998) note that hypothermia 'does have potential benefits to the patient, including protection from cerebral ischaemia' and conclude that 'mild core hypothermia (approximately 34°C) may represent the optimal balance between risks and benefits for fast-track patients'.
2 *Duration of cardiopulmonary bypass*: this correlates with pulmonary dysfunction, electrolyte derangement, poor post-operative cardiac function and coagulopathy (requiring the transfusion of platelets), which delay post-operative extubation (London *et al.*, 1998).

Patients who have undergone successful off-pump CABG (*see below*) are, in general, good candidates for post-operative fast-tracking.

ANAESTHETIC ASPECTS OF OFF–PUMP CABG

Before the advent of effective and safe cardiopulmonary bypass, coronary artery surgery could only be performed on the beating heart and only certain coronary arteries could be accessed this way. This limited revascularization was nonetheless performed during the 1960s (Olearchyk, 1988), but was subsequently superseded by more effective surgery on a motionless heart with full cardiopulmonary bypass.

Despite the increasing safety of cardiopulmonary bypass, its cost and the physiological derangements it induces remain substantial (for example, diffuse neurological dysfunction, systemic inflammatory reaction, pulmonary dysfunction), and since the mid-1990s there has been a resurgence of interest in off-pump bypass surgery. Surgical and anaesthetic techniques (Maslow et al., 1999) have evolved that minimize the haemodynamic derangements produced by tilting and manipulating the heart for access to the posterior and lateral aspects of the heart. Specialized retractors and epicardial tissue stabilizers have enabled access to posterior and distal vessels, increasing the safety and efficacy of this technique. The surgical learning curve is steep for these procedures and a perfusionist should be available on stand-by during off-pump CABG for urgent initiation of cardiopulmonary bypass should this become necessary. Details of the procedures are beyond the scope of this chapter.

Several surgical approaches for off-pump CABG have been used. One such approach, minimally invasive direct CABG, avoids median sternotomy, making use instead of a lateral anterior thoracotomy (or similar approach) for access to the heart and internal mammary artery (Acuff et al., 1996). The use of a double-lumen endobronchial tube for one-lung ventilation to facilitate take-down of the internal mammary artery may be necessary. This approach is best suited to patients with single lesions of proximal coronary arteries as the surgical access to the myocardium is restricted to a small area.

Surgical techniques are presently returning to the traditional median sternotomy, however, with its excellent access to the heart. Co-operation between surgeon and anaesthetist has to be close, particularly during the performance of the distal anastomosis when application of tissue stabilizers and surgical manipulation of the native vessel induce variable amounts of ischaemia distally. The tilting and manipulation of the heart necessary for access to posterior vessels may also be poorly tolerated by certain patients.

The aims of anaesthesia for off-pump CABG remain broadly similar to those for conventional CABG. As the distal anastomoses are performed, patients are fluid-loaded and placed in the Trendelenberg (head-down) position in order to preserve venous return to the heart and reduce distortion of the right ventricle, thus minimizing haemodynamic changes induced by tilting or torsion of the heart. Blood pressure is often increased pharmacologically during this stage of the procedure in order to maintain coronary perfusion, and the use of inotropes to maintain cardiac output may be necessary.

If the patient does not tolerate these manoeuvres (for example, developing severe ischaemia, arrhythmias or acute severe output failure) it is sometimes necessary to resort to conventional cardiopulmonary bypass at this stage. When the proximal anastomoses are performed, blood pressure is often decreased pharmacologically in order to reduce shear stresses on aortic plaque while the aortic side-clamp is in place.

Most centres make routine use of intra-operative TOE (see above) and/or pulmonary artery catheterization in order to monitor haemodynamic changes induced by tilting the heart. TOE is also useful for monitoring the presence and extent of ischaemia demonstrable by the development of new wall motion abnormalities. Ischaemia is induced by application of tissue stabilization systems and performance of the distal anastomoses, but TOE is somewhat limited because the tilting and rotation of the heart needed for access to the posterior descending and circumflex vessels distorts the images. TOE is also used to guide the placement of the aortic side-clamp to avoid displacement and embolization of athero-sclerotic plaque.

Before the development of tissue stabilization systems such as the 'Octopus' (Medtronic), pharmacological manipulation by the anaesthetist was commonly used to slow the heart and render the surgical field 'quiet' to enable the surgeon to perform the distal ends of the coronary bypass grafts. Drugs used include calcium channel blockers, beta-adrenergic blockers (such as Esmolol) and various cholinergic drugs, with or without the use of intermittent pacing facilities to 'rescue' any bradyarrhythmias or asystole induced (Lampa and Ramsay, 1999; McCue et al., 2000). These manoeuvres are not without risk and are not necessary where tissue stablization devices are used. The use of microaxial pumps, such as the Hemopump (Medtronic) to maintain cardiac output during lifting or kinking of the heart may be useful in extending the use of off-pump CABG to higher-risk patients (Meyns et al., 1999; Peterzen et al., 1999). The myocardial ischaemia caused during fashioning of the distal anastomoses is 'warm', transient and restricted to the region supplied by the native coronary artery, rather than 'cold', global and for longer periods, such as that during many types of cardiopulmonary bypass. Cardioplegia is not used. Other measures may be taken during off-pump CABG to protect the myocardium. These include ischaemic pre-conditioning, intravenous magnesium and the use of potent inhalational agents (see above) before the ischaemic insult.

SUMMARY

In this chapter we have attempted to summarize some of the recent advances in the anaesthetic management of patients undergoing cardiac surgery and cardiopulmonary bypass. No doubt as perfusion and surgical techniques improve cardiac anaesthesia will continue to develop. Areas where therapeutic progress is likely to be made include the treatment of the inflammatory response, cerebral protection, myocardial protection (including management of ischaemia-reperfusion injury) and the introduction of newer inotropes. It is too early to predict where the most significant advances will be made.

REFERENCES

Acuff, T.L., Landreneau, R.J., Griffith, B.P., Mack, M.J. 1996: Minimally invasive coronary artery bypass grafting. *Annals of Thoracic Surgery* **61**, 135–7.

Aguilera, I.M., Vaughan, R.S. 2000: Calcium and the anaesthetist. *Anaesthesia* **55**, 779–90.

Albrecht, S., Schittler, J., Yarmush, J. 1999: Post-operative pain management after intra-operative remifentanil. *Anesthesia and Analgesia* **89**, S40–5.

Angus, A., Black, N. 2001: Wider lessons of the pulmonary artery catheter trial (editorial). *British Medical Journal* **322**, 446.

Antognini, J. 1993: Hypothermia eliminates isoflurane requirements at 20°C. *Anesthesiology* **78**, 1152–6.

Aps, C. 1995: Fast-tracking in cardiac surgery. *British Journal of Hospital Medicine* **54**, 139–42.

Argenziano, M., Chen, J.M., Choudhri, A.F. *et al.* 1998: Management of vasodilatory shock after cardiac surgery: identification of predisposing factors and use of a novel pressor agent. *Journal of Thoracic and Cardiovascular Surgery* **116**, 973–80.

Armitage, E.N. 1990: Lumbar and thoracic epidural anaesthesia. In: J.A.W. Wildsmith, E.N. Armitage (eds), *Principles and practice of regional anaesthesia*. Edinburgh: Churchill Livingstone, 87–98.

Blomberg, S., Curelau, I., Emanuelsson, H. *et al.* 1989: Thoracic epidural anaesthesia in patients with unstable angina pectoris. *European Heart Journal* **10**, 437–44.

Blomberg, S., Emmanuelsson, H., Kvist, H. *et al.* 1990: Effects of thoracic epidural anesthesia on coronary arteries and arterioles in patients with coronary artery disease. *Anesthesiology* **73**, 840–7.

Boyd, W.C., Thomas, S.J. 2000: Pro: magnesium should be administered to all coronary artery bypass graft surgery patients undergoing cardiopulmonary bypass. *Journal of Cardiothoracic and Vascular Anesthesia* **14**, 339–43.

Brookes, C., Fry, C. 1993. Ionised magnesium and calcium in plasma from healthy volunteers and patients undergoing cardiopulmonary bypass. *British Heart Journal* **69**, 404–8.

Cheng, D.C.H. 1998: Fast track cardiac surgery pathways: early extubation, process of care, and cost containment (editorial). *Anesthesiology* **88**, 1429–33.

Coetzee, J.F., le Roux, P.J., Genade, S., Lochner, A. 2000: Reduction of postischaemic contractile dysfunction of the isolated rat heart by sevoflurane: comparison with halothane. *Anesthesia and Analgesia* **90**, 1089–97.

Cook, D., Orzulak, T., Daly, R., Burda, D. 1996: Cerebral hyperthermia during cardiopulmonary bypass in adults. *Journal of Thoracic and Cardiovascular Surgery* **111**, 268–9.

Dalen, J.E., Bone, R.C. 1996: Is it time to pull the pulmonary artery catheter? *Journal of the American Medical Assocation* **276**, 916–18.

DeHert, S., Ten Broecke, P., DeMulder, P.A. *et al.* 1997: Effects of calcium on left ventricular function after cardiopulmonary bypass. *Journal of Cardiothoracic and Vascular Anesthesia* **11**, 864–9.

Djaiani, G., Bowler, I., Hall, J. *et al.* 2000: A combination of remifentanil and intrathecal morphine improves pulmonary function following CABG. *Anesthesia and Analgesia* **90**, SCA64.

du Toit, E.F., Opie, L.H. 1992: Modulation of severity of reperfusion stunning in the isolated rat heart by agents altering calcium flux at onset of reperfusion. *Circulation Research* **70**, 960–7.

Eger, E. II, Saidman, L.J., Brandstater, B. 1965: Temperature dependence of halothane and cyclopropane anesthesia in dogs: correlation with some theories of anesthetic action. *Anesthesiology* **26**, 764–70.

Elliott, P., O'Hare, R., Bill, K.M. *et al.* 2000: Severe cardiovascular depression with remifentanil. *Anesthesia and Analgesia* **91**, 58–61.

English, I.C.W., Frew, R.M., Pigott, J.F., Zaki, M. 1969: Percutaneous catheterisation of the internal jugular vein. *Anaesthesia* **24**, 521–6.

Falase, B., Bajal, B.S., Wall, T.J. *et al.* 1999: Nicorandil-induced peripheral vasodilatation during cardiopulmonary bypass. *Annals of Thoracic Surgery* **67**, 1158–9.

Fawcett, W.J., Haxby, E.J., Male, D.A. 1999: Magnesium: physiology and pharmacology. *British Journal of Anaesthesia* **83**, 302–20.

Fitzpatrick, G.J., Moriaty, D.C. 1988: Intrathecal morphine in the management of pain following cardiac surgery. A comparison with IV morphine. *British Journal of Anaesthesia* **60**, 639–44.

Fogg, K.J., Royston, D. 1998: Improved performance with single dose phosphodiesterase inhibitor? (editorial). *British Journal of Anaesthesia* **81**, 663–5.

Gedney, J.A., Ghosh, S. 1995: Pharmacokinetics of analgesics, sedatives and anaesthetic agents during cardiopulmonary bypass. *British Journal of Anaesthesia* **75**, 344–51.

Gothard, J.W.W., Kelleher, A. 1999: *Essentials of cardiac and thoracic anaesthesia*. Oxford: Butterworth-Heinemann.

Gries, A., Bode, C., Gross, S. *et al.* 1999: The effect of intravenously administered magnesium on platelet function in patients after cardiac surgery. *Anesthesia and Analgesia* **88**, 1213–19.

Grigore, A.M., Mathew, J.P. 2000: Con: magnesium should not be administered to all coronary artery bypass graft surgery patients undergoing cardiopulmonary bypass. *Journal of Cardiothoracic and Vascular Anesthesia* **14**, 344–6.

Guyton, A.C., Hall, T.E. (eds). 1996: *Textbook of medical physiology* (ninth edition). Philadelphia, PA: WB Saunders.

Hatfield, A., Bodenham, A. 1999: Portable ultrasound for difficult central venous access. *British Journal of Anaesthesia* **82**, 822–6.

Heerdt, P.M., Heerdt, M.B. 1992: The rational pharmacology of digoxin. *Journal of Clinical Anesthesia* **4**, 419–35.

Hilgenberg, J.C. 1981: Intraoperative awareness during high-dose fentanyl–oxygen anesthesia. *Anesthesiology* **54**, 341–3.

Hindman, B.J., Todd, M.M. 1999: Improving neurologic outcome after cardiac surgery (editorial). *Anesthesiology* **90**, 1243–7.

Hoerauf, K., Harth, M., Wild, K., Hobbhaun, J. 1997: Occupational exposure to desflurane and isoflurane during cardiopulmonary bypass: is the gas outlet of the membrane oxygenator an operating theatre pollution hazard? *British Journal of Anaesthesia* **78**, 378–80.

Honkonen, E.L., Kaukinen, L., Kaukinen, S. *et al.* 1998: Dopexamine unloads the impaired right ventricle better than Iloprost, a prostacyclin analog after coronary artery surgery. *Journal of Cardiothoracic and Vascular Anesthesia* **12**, 647–53.

Janelle, J.M., Urdaneta, F., Martin, T.D., Lobato, E.B. 2000: Effects of calcium chloride on grafted internal mammary flow after cardiopulmonary bypass. *Journal of Cardiothoracic and Vascular Anesthesia* **14**, 4–8.

Kapila, A., Glass, P.S.A., Jacobs, J.R. *et al.* 1995: Measured context-sensitive half-times of remifentanil and alfentanil. *Anesthesiology* **83**, 968–75.

Kaplan, J.A. 1993: *Cardiac anesthesia.* Philadelphia, PA: WB Saunders.

Koski, G. 2000: Internal mammary artery spasm: is calcium the culprit? (editorial). *Journal of Cardiothoracic and Vascular Anesthesia* **14**, 1–3.

Lampa, M., Ramsay, J. 1999: Anesthetic implications of new surgical approaches to myocardial revascularization. *Current Opinion in Anesthesiology* **12**, 3–8.

Landow, L., Visner, M.S. 1993: Does $NaHCO_3$ exacerbate myocardial acidosis? *Journal of Cardiothoracic and Vascular Anesthesia* **17**, 340–51.

Leslie, K., Sessler, D.I. 1998: The implications of hypothermia for early tracheal extubation following cardiac surgery. *Journal of Cardiothoracic and Vascular Anaesthesia* **12** (Suppl. 2), 30–4.

Leung, J.M., Landow, L., Franks, M. *et al.* 1994: Safety and efficacy of intravenous carbicarb in patients undergoing surgery: comparison with sodium bicarbonate in the treatment of mild metabolic acidosis. *Critical Care Medicine* **22**, 1540–9.

Levy, J.H., Pifarre, R., Schaff, H.V. *et al.* 1995: A multicenter, double-blind, placebo-controlled trial of aprotinin for reducing blood loss and the requirement for donor-blood transfusion in patients undergoing repeat coronary artery bypass grafting. *Circulation* **92**, 2236–44.

Lewis, K.P., Appadurai, I.R., Pierce, E.T. *et al.* 2000: Prophylactic amrinone for weaning from cardiopulmonary bypass. *Anaesthesia* **55**, 627–33.

Loick, H.M., Schmidt, C., Van Aken, H. *et al.* 1999: High thoracic epidural anesthesia but not clonidine, attenuates the perioperative stress response via sympatholysis and reduces the release of Troponin T in patients undergoing coronary artery bypass grafting. *Anesthesia and Analgesia* **88**, 701–9.

London, M.J., Shroyer, A.L., Coll, J.R. *et al.* 1998: Early extubation following cardiac surgery in a veterans population. *Anesthesiologia* **88**, 1447–58.

Maslow, A., Aronson, S., Jacobsohn, E. *et al.* 1999: Case conference: off-pump coronary artery bypass graft surgery. *Journal of Cardiothoracic and Vascular Anaesthesia* **13**, 764–81.

McCleod, G.A., Davies, H.T.O., Munnoch, N. *et al.* 2001: Postoperative pain relief using thoracic epidural analgesia: outstanding success and disappointing failures. *Anaesthesia* **56**, 75–81.

McCue, M.G., Sakwa, M., Ohanian, N.S. *et al.* 2000: Pharmacological electrical arrest with intermittent pacing facilitates off-pump bypass surgery. *Anesthesia and Analgesia* **90**, SCA48.

Meisner, A., Rolf, N., Van Aken, H. 1997: Thoracic epidural anesthesia and the patient with heart disease: benefits, risks and controversies. *Anesthesia and Analgesia* **85**, 517–28.

Mets, B. 2000: The pharmacokinetics of anesthetic drugs and adjuvants during cardiopulmonary bypass. *Acta Anaesthesiologica Scandinavica* **44**, 261–73.

Meyns, B., Sergeant, P., Siess, T. *et al.* 1999: Coronary artery bypass graft with biventricular microaxial pumps. *Perfusion* **14**, 287–90.

Multicenter Study of Perioperative Ischaemia (McSPI) Research Group. 1995: Effects of acadesine on morbidity and mortality following coronary artery bypass graft surgery. *Anesthesiology* **83**, 658–73.

Murkin, J.M. 1999: Etiology and incidence of brain dysfunction after cardiac surgery. *Journal of Cardiothoracic Anesthesia* **13**, 12–17.

Mychaskiw, G., Hoehner, P.J., Aziz, A.A., Heath, B.J., Eichhorn, J.H. 2000: Pre-operative exposure to calcium channel blockers suggests increased blood product use following cardiac surgery. *Anesthesia and Analgesia* **90**, SCA15.

Newman, M.F., Kirchner, J.L., Phillips-Bute, B. *et al.* 2001: Longitudinal assessment of neurocognitive function after coronary-artery bypass surgery. *New England Journal of Medicine* **344**, 395–402.

Newman, S.P., Harrison, M.J.G. 2000: *The brain and cardiac surgery.* The Netherlands: Harwood Academic Publishers.

Olearchyk, A.S., 1988: Vasilii I Kolesov: a pioneer of coronary revascularization by internal mammary coronary artery grafting. *Journal of Thoracic and Cardiovascular Surgery* **96**, 13–18.

Peterzen, B., Lonn, U., Babi'c, A. *et al.* 1999: Anesthetic management of patients undergoing coronary artery bypass grafting with the use of an axial flow pump and a short-acting β-blocker. *Journal of Cardiothoracic and Vascular Anesthesia* **13**, 431–6.

Phelan, D., White, M., McDonagh, P.D., McGovern, E., Luke, D. 1991: Prophylactic peri-operative dopexamine hydrochloride: a controlled study of tissue oxygenation. *Clinical Intensive Care* **2** (Suppl to 3), 37–40.

Phillips, A.A., McLean, R.F., Devitt, J.H., Harrington, E.M. 1993: Recall of intra-operative events after general anaesthesia and cardiopulmonary bypass. *Canadian Journal of Anaesthesia* **40**, 922–6.

Poelaert, J., Skarvan, K. 2000: *Transoesophageal echocardiography in anaesthesia.* London: BMJ Books.

Practice Guidelines for Perioperative Transesophageal Echocardiography. 1996: *Anesthesiology* **84**, 986–1006.

Ramsey, S.D., Saint, S., Sullivan, S.D. *et al.* 2000: Clinical and economic effects of pulmonary artery catheterization in nonemergent coronary artery bypass graft surgery. *Journal of Cardiothoracic and Vascular Anesthesia* **14**, 113–18.

Ranucci, M., Isgro, G., Cazzaniga, A., Soro, G. *et al.* 1999: Predictors for heparin resistance in patients undergoing coronary artery bypass grafting. *Perfusion* **14**, 437–42.

Reves, J.G., Sladen, R.N., Newman, M.F. 1995: Cardiac anesthetic: is it unique? *Anesthesia and Analgesia* **81**, 895–6.

Riedel, B.J.C., Wright, G. 1997: Epidural anesthesia in coronary artery bypass grafting surgery. *Current Opinion in Cardiology* **12**, 515–21.

Roach, G.W., Newman, M.F., Murkin, J.M. *et al.* 1999: Ineffectiveness of burst suppression therapy in mitigating peri-operative cerebrovascular dysfunction (The Multicenter Study of Perioperative Ischaemia Research Group). *Anesthesiology* **90**, 1255–64.

Rorie, K.D., Stump, D.A. 2000: Techniques and limitations of embolus detection. In: S.P. Newman, M.J.G. Harrison (eds),

The brain and cardiac surgery. The Netherlands: Harwood Academic Publishers, 185–98.

Rosow, C.E. 1999: An overview of remifentanil. *Anesthesia and Analgesia* **89**, S1–3.

Ross, S., Foex, P. 1999: Protective effects of anaesthetics in reversible and irreversible ischaemia-reperfusion injury. *British Journal of Anaesthesia* **82**, 622–32.

Sakka, S.G., Reinhart, K., Wegscheider, K. *et al.* 2000: Is the placement of a pulmonary artery catheter still justified solely for the measurement of cardiac output? *Journal of Cardiothoracic and Vascular Anaesthesia* **14**, 119–24.

Schneider, M., Valentine, S., Fledge, R.M. *et al.* 1999: The effect of different bypass flow rates and low-dose dopamine on gut mucosal perfusion and outcome in cardiac surgical patients. *Anaesthesia and Intensive Care* **27**, 13–19.

Scott, D.H.T. 1999: 'In the country of the blind, the one-eyed man is King' (editorial). *British Journal of Anaesthesia* **82**, 820–1.

Selnes, O.A., McKhann, G.M. 2001: Coronary-artery bypass surgery and the brain (editorial). *New England Journal of Medicine* **344**, 451–2.

Smith, P.K., Muhibaier, L.H. 1996: Aprotinin safe and effective only with the full-dose regimen. *Annals of Thoracic Surgery* **62**, 1575–7.

Souter, M.J., Andrews, P.J.D., Alston, R.P. 1998: Propofol does not ameliorate cerebral venous oxyhemoglobin desaturation during hypothermic cardiopulmonary bypass. *Anesthesia and Analgesia* **86**, 926–31.

Stephan, H., Weyland, A., Kazmaier, S. *et al.* 1992: Acid-base management during hypothermic cardiopulmonary bypass does not affect cerebral metabolism but does affect blood flow and neurological outcome. *British Journal of Anaesthesia* **69**, 51–7.

Stocking, J.E., Lake, C.L. 2000: The role of the pulmonary artery catheter in the year 2000 and beyond (editorial). *Journal of Cardiothoracic and Vascular Anesthesia* **14**, 111–12.

Thompson, J.P., Rowbotham, D.J. 1996: Remifentanil – an opioid for the 21st century. *British Journal of Anaesthesia* **76**, 341–3.

Tuman, K.J., McCarthy, O'Connor, C.J. *et al.* 1995: Angiotensin-converting enzyme inhibitors increase vasoconstrictor requirements after cardiopulmonary bypass. *Anesthesia and Analgesia* **80**, 473–9.

Vitez, T., White, P., Eger, E. 1974: Effects of hypothermia on halothane MAC and isoflurane MAC in the rat. *Anesthesiology* **41**, 80–1.

Wilson, J., Woods, I., Fawcett, I. *et al.* 1999: Reducing the risk of major elective surgery: randomized-controlled trial of preoperative optimisation of oxygen delivery. *British Medical Journal* **318**, 1099–103.

Wang, J.Y.Y., Winship, S.M., Thomas, D.S. *et al.* 1999: Induction of anaesthesia in patients with coronary artery disease: a comparison between sevoflurane–remifentanil and fentanyl–etomidate. *Anaesthesia and Intensive Care* **27**, 363–8.

Zarate, E., Latham, P., White, P.F. *et al.* 2000: Fast track cardiac anesthesia: use of remifentanil combined with intrathecal morphine as an alternative to sufentanil during desflurane anesthesia. *Anesthesia and Analgesia* **91**, 283–7.

Zollner, C., Haller, M., Weis, M. *et al.* 2000: Beat to beat measurement of cardiac output by intravascular pulse contour analysis: a prospective criterion study in patients after cardiac surgery. *Journal of Cardiothoracic and Vascular Anesthesia* **14**, 125–9.

5

Monitoring and safety in cardiopulmonary bypass

JONATHAN M JOHNSON, STEPHEN ROBINS AND JONATHAN AJ HYDE

KEY POINTS

- Cardiopulmonary bypass is an artificial environment with its own potential for severe morbidity and mortality.
- Monitoring of cardiopulmonary bypass is the responsibility of the perfusionist, and begins with pre-operative assessment and anticipation of potential procedures.
- Although the perfusionist is ultimately responsible, the safety of cardiopulmonary bypass is dependent on a team approach, and communication with the surgeon and anaesthetist is critical.
- The current generation of heart lung machines and cardiopulmonary bypass-related equipment are technologically advanced and contain automatic alarm and safety features in all appropriate places.
- Cardiopulmonary bypass is a dynamic situation and problems may occur very suddenly.
  Meticulous attention to detail will ensure that the majority of these can be identified and rectified expeditiously.
- Continuous audit and data collection systems, national guidelines and standardized protocols are all available and are fundamental requirements for safe and effective cardiopulmonary bypass.

INTRODUCTION

Despite the numerous developments optimizing its conduct, cardiopulmonary bypass is an artificial environment and confers a shock-like state on the body. Extensive research over the last 50 years has endeavoured to reduce the pathophysiological effects of cardiopulmonary bypass to a minimum, as detailed elsewhere in this book. Nonetheless, there will always be morbidity and mortality associated with its use, and there is continuing scope for improvement. It is, therefore, crucially important that this complication rate is not added to by circuit-related and equipment-related issues. This chapter deals with the monitoring and control aspects of all component parts of the delivery of cardiopulmonary bypass.

Since cardiopulmonary bypass is a dynamic medium, adverse events may happen surprisingly quickly, and may become compounded if problems are not identified and addressed expeditiously. The potential for harm to the patient is enormous, therefore a constant state of awareness is paramount. In addition, it is important to realize that although the different components are physically independent, they are all interlinked and co-dependent from a functional point of view. Therefore, an unidentified problem in one parameter may well affect another, leading to a potentially lethal spiral of events. Conversely, correction of the error in one parameter does not necessarily mean that the other areas will all 'auto-correct', so everything should be scrupulously re-checked.

Cardiac surgery is a multidisciplinary event involving a large number of people from a variety of different fields and specialities. The actual operation involving the use of cardiopulmonary bypass (as in the majority of cases) necessitates constant communication between several key personnel in the operating theatre. This communication is, in effect, the most important part of the whole monitoring process. A factor that is frequently overlooked is that the monitoring of cardiopulmonary bypass, although largely the responsibility of the perfusionist, also requires detailed input from both the anaesthetist and the surgeon. All three of these personnel can effect large changes on the conduct of cardiopulmonary bypass and must work synergistically, providing each other with details of important changes and information.

Each isolated component of cardiopulmonary bypass (such as oxygenation, fluid balance or anticoagulation) needs careful regulation and a system of alarms or 'fail-safes' to prevent potential accidents from occurring. To monitor, by definition, means to check, record, track, supervise or control something on a regular basis. All of these definitions are particularly pertinent to the conduct of perfusion.

Monitoring by the perfusionist does not necessarily begin with the initiation of cardiopulmonary bypass and end when cardiopulmonary bypass is terminated. Monitoring in cardiopulmonary bypass begins with knowledge and planning of the intended procedure, anticipation of unplanned extra procedures, setting up of the circuit and close attention to patient-related details. The perfusionist's pre-operative checklist addresses some of these details and in a way is analogous to a pilot's pre-flight checklist. Monitoring does not necessarily end with discontinuation of bypass either. There is occasionally the need to re-establish cardiopulmonary bypass quickly, in which case circuit-readiness and re-anticoagulation (amongst other things) need rapid and careful attention.

Although the bulk of this chapter will deal with equipment and device-related monitoring and their requisite alarms, the individual patient and operative factors must never be underestimated. In addition, clinical perfusionists are usually responsible for the regulation of a number of adjuncts to cardiac surgery, such as extracorporeal membrane oxygenation, ventricular assist devices and intra-aortic balloon pumps. It is not within the remit of this chapter to deal with these latter devices, therefore attention will focus upon cardiopulmonary bypass alone. Equally, the anaesthetic equipment includes many components that are responsible for 'monitoring' the patient, such as the ventilator, central venous lines, pulmonary artery flotation catheter, urinary catheter and arterial line. These are not within the scope of this chapter either.

Lastly, in order to maintain a centralized regulatory control over the conduct of perfusion, a set of formal guidelines have been drawn up by the Society of Clinical Perfusion Scientists in conjunction with the Society of Cardiothoracic Surgeons of Great Britain and Ireland and the Association of Cardiothoracic Anaesthetists. These may be downloaded from the internet (www.scps.org.uk/Resources/Bypassrecommendations.doc) or can be found in the Appendix at the end of this chapter.

FLOW REGULATION

Gas flow

The gas flow or 'sweep rate' is the term used for the quantity of ventilatory gas delivered to the gas inlet of the oxygenator. The almost universal use of membrane oxygenators (as opposed to the older bubble devices) allows independent control of oxygenation and removal of carbon dioxide (CO_2) by varying not just the actual flow of gas but also the ratio between the gas constituents. In most cases, the ventilating gas is a mixture of medical air and oxygen, although there may be times when the addition of other gases such as CO_2 may be appropriate. Control of the ventilating gas is usually brought about by the use of a gas blender (Fig. 5.1).

The gas flow path is composed of, and will therefore pass through, various components. These include:

- gas source (or multiple sources for different gases)
- gas hoses
- gas blender
- vaporizer
- oxygen analyser
- oxygenator
- scavenging facility
- capnograph.

The total gas flow and fraction of inspired oxygen (FiO_2) required for a particular patient is dependent on several factors: patient size, efficiency and size of the oxygenator and temperature. In general, a larger patient requires a greater gas flow and FiO_2 at any given temperature. However, a decrease in temperature reduces overall oxygen demand and allows a decrease in the FiO_2. Control of the removal of CO_2 is achieved by varying the total gas flow. A higher total gas flow will increase the removal of CO_2 and therefore lead to a compensatory lower arterial pCO_2. A lower gas flow will obviously bring about the opposite effect.

The monitoring of gas flow must start before initiating cardiopulmonary bypass. Patient size determines the initial settings for gas flow and FiO_2. Most oxygenator manufacturers recommend a 1:1 starting ratio of blood:gas flow rate. However, in practice a gas flow such as this will be too high in the majority of cases, and would almost always require adjustment after blood gas analysis.

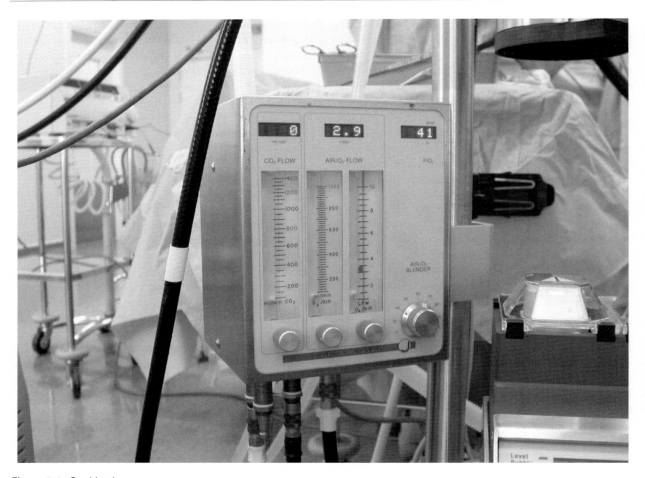

Figure 5.1 *Gas blender.*

During cardiopulmonary bypass, perfusionists must monitor the adequacy of gas flow and FiO_2 continuously. They need to check that gas not only *appears* to flow from the gas blender to the oxygenator (a simple visual check) but also that gas flow is bringing about the desired effect in terms of oxygenation and removal of CO_2. This can be achieved both by blood gas analysis and by visual observation of the relative difference in colour between the arterial and venous blood.

GAS LEAKAGES

All the component parts listed above need to be connected together and therefore have the potential for leaks at any of the joints. Such a leak, if undetected by the perfusionist, could lead to inadequate oxygenation. The use of an oxygen analyser is a recommended standard and provides useful information, although somewhat limited. It only confirms to the perfusionist that what is set on the gas blender is actually being delivered as far as the analyser. It does not, however, imply that the ventilating gas actually reaches the oxygenator further downstream in the gas path. The use of a capnograph attached to the exhaust port

of the oxygenator may arguably be a better way of determining whether or not the gas has actually reached the oxygenator. Providing the capnograph has the facility to set off an alarm when it fails to detect a pre-set gas flow, it increases the chances of identifying a leak in the gas path. The use of a capnograph in this part of the circuit offers the additional benefit of providing valuable information about concentrations of volatile anaesthetic agents delivered from the vaporizer. It will also assist with the management of arterial pCO_2 and should, in the authors' view, be an integral circuit component at this point (McClosky *et al.*, 1994).

Arterial flow

The delivery of oxygen (O_2) to the tissues is dependent on two independent factors: blood flow and O_2 content of the blood. Adequate patient oxygenation must, therefore, depend to a large extent on the accurate measurement of arterial blood flow and the constant monitoring of that flow throughout the duration of cardiopulmonary bypass. This regulation of flow is entirely the domain of the perfusionist and may be adjusted to meet the requirements of the surgeon and anaesthetist if required.

Flow for an individual patient is calculated before cardiopulmonary bypass as part of the pre-operative perfusion assessment, and is based on their size. The height and weight of a patient are used to derive the body surface area (usually from a standardized nomogram). This is then usually multiplied by a cardiac index of 2.4 L/min/m² resulting in an 'ideal' arterial blood flow rate expressed as litres per minute, which is regulated by the perfusionist at the arterial pump. This calculated flow serves as a minimum flow rate during periods of normothermia, but obviously the flow rate can be reduced transiently to improve operating conditions for the surgeon.

DIFFERENCES IN FLOW GENERATION

Laminar arterial blood flow is generated by either a roller or a centrifugal pump in most cases, although pulsatile flow may be added to either type (Fig. 5.2 and Fig. 5.3). Although both types of pump produce easily controlled forward movement of blood, they do so in very different ways. This has important implications for the way flow is monitored and controlled by the perfusionist.

Roller flow

The roller pump is a partially occlusive positive displacement pump, the roller heads repeatedly compressing the circuit tubing onto a solid backing plate or 'raceway'. Output from a roller pump is determined by both the revolutions per minute (RPM) and the stroke volume of the tubing in contact with the rollers, which in turn is determined by tubing diameter. Assuming the stroke volume remains constant, pump output is controlled by varying the RPM. Regular calibration of the roller pump is necessary to ensure that the flow displayed on the pump module is accurate, as it may fluctuate during repeated pump cycles. Under these regulated conditions, flow from a roller pump will remain constant for any given RPM. The pressure generated by this flow will vary according to the resistance to that flow in the form of the circuit (fixed resistance) and the patient (variable resistance). When monitoring blood flow, perfusionists must be aware that in the presence of an obstruction to flow on either the input or the output of the pump, the roller pump will continue to deliver the pre-set flow. In this way, the roller pump is said to be 'pressure insensitive'. Inadvertent clamping of the arterial line, for example, would, therefore, lead to overpressurization of the bypass circuit, and the potential for circuit disruption. The almost 100 per cent occlusion of the tubing in a roller pump ensures that if the pump stops, there is no significant retrograde flow of blood from the aorta back past the rollers of the pump. This is important since there is always the possibility of entraining air into the aorta around the arterial cannula. Appropriate adjustment of

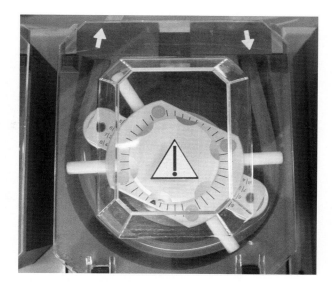

Figure 5.2 *Roller pump.*

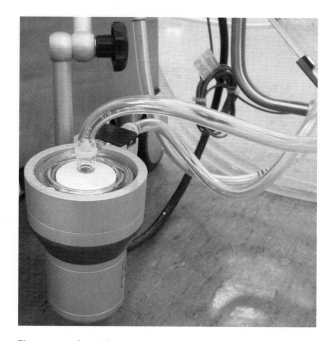

Figure 5.3 *Centrifugal pump.*

the occlusion of the rollers by the perfusionist during the pre-operative setting up of the bypass machine is, therefore, important in preventing both retrograde flow and damage to blood components.

Centrifugal flow

The centrifugal pump is a non-occlusive kinetic pump. It produces flow by imparting energy to blood within a rotating pump head. Various designs of centrifugal pump are in clinical use, but the two most common basic designs are the vaned impeller and the constrained vortex. Output from a centrifugal pump is determined by pre-load (the volume of blood in the venous reservoir on cardiopulmonary bypass), the RPM, and the after-load (a combination of the fixed resistance of the bypass circuit and the variable systemic vascular resistance of the patient). The centrifugal pump is, therefore, in contrast to the roller pump a 'pressure sensitive' device. This means that at a constant RPM, any change in either pressure or resistance will bring about a change in flow. Perfusionists, therefore, must constantly be aware of the need to adjust blood flow (using RPM) if changes in the arterial pressure of the patient cause significant changes to flow. In a centrifugal pump, if the arterial line is inadvertently clamped or occluded, pressure within the bypass circuit will briefly continue to increase (to a low maximal level) and then flow will simply stop. When using a centrifugal pump, perfusionists must also be aware that the console delivery of RPM does not, in itself, imply forward flow of blood. Since there is no occlusive device between the inflow and outflow ports of the centrifugal pump head, flow through the head is possible in either direction. Perfusionists must be aware that if forward flow ceases for any reason, retrograde flow may ensue.

Flow from a centrifugal pump is measured by a flow probe within the bypass circuit. In some designs of centrifugal pump the flow probe is separate from the pump head and may be situated anywhere within the circuit. It is important that this flow probe is placed in the correct orientation (otherwise forward flow will be displayed as negative or retrograde flow). The flow probe must always be zeroed to ensure accurate flow measurements.

Suction and venting

CARDIOTOMY SUCTION

Cardiotomy suction is fairly universal in its application to cardiac surgery utilizing cardiopulmonary bypass. The only real variables are the number of suckers used and the rate of suction. Some surgeons prefer to keep suction limited or low as there is some evidence of blood cellular destruction at higher levels (De Jong *et al.*, 1980). It is rare to avoid suction altogether, however, as it helps to provide the surgeon the best possible view of the operating field and to ensure that spilt blood is returned to the patient's circulation.

Suction is usually run as a separate circuit at the cardiopulmonary bypass machine, using a roller pump head to apply the requisite negative pressure. The surgeon will use the suction as required and direct it to clear the operative field of blood.

VENTING

A similar circuit (or even the same one) can be used for the different purpose of intra-cardiac venting. In this case, the 'patient' end of the suction tubing is attached to a special-tipped cannula that can be placed inside one of the heart chambers (usually the left ventricle) or great vessels (most commonly the pulmonary artery, pulmonary vein or aorta). This technique enables perfusionists to decompress the heart in order to prevent overdistension, which may damage future myocardial function. Since the venting circuit is connected to the inside of the heart or great vessels, it is important to monitor the RPM and flow through the vent continually. This usually operates at lower RPMs than normal cardiotomy suction, often simply being left 'open' (to gravity) rather than employing active negative pressure. Another option, used less frequently, is to employ a 'gravity-only' vent circuit that reduces the amount of time the blood is in contact with the rollers of the pump.

COMPLICATIONS

There are several problems associated with the use of cardiotomy suction, all of which are avoidable. The main factor seems to be that suction is a major source of haemolysis during cardiopulmonary bypass (Osborn *et al.*, 1962), as mentioned above. Haemolysis is a multifactorial event, part of which is compounded by the co-aspiration of air from the surgical field. The air–blood interface causes turbulence and shear stresses (Malinauskas *et al.*, 1988), which can damage blood components. These effects may be exacerbated when high suction flow rates are used, but it should not be forgotten that high negative pressures are also generated by occlusion of the suction catheter tip. This should be noted well by many surgeons who regard the perfusionist's constant call of 'sucker blocked' as an irritation! In order to alleviate these problems the perfusionist and surgeon should ensure that the suction catheter is placed below the blood level, thus minimizing the aspiration of air, and that the tip is always free of debris and potential blockage. It is also advised that the lowest possible flow is used on the roller pump governing the suction circuit, even to the point of leaving it in the 'off' position when not in use. This will greatly aid the reduction of air intake and blood cellular damage (De Jong *et al.*, 1977).

If an active vent is attached to an aortic root cardioplegia cannula, perfusionists must always be aware of the possibility of introducing a negative pressure into the cardioplegia line. This negative pressure has the potential to draw gases out of solution, which could potentially be introduced into the coronary circulation when cardioplegia is next administered.

Other methods of reducing red cell damage include the use of a cell salvage machine in place of cardiotomy suction. This, however, is of limited use and presents perfusionists with a problem when major blood loss occurs. The other important point, of course, is that the cell saver cannot be connected to the vent circuit.

One particularly important point that needs stressing is that the roller pumps that are used for cardiotomy suction and intra-cardiac venting should have their occlusion settings checked before each procedure, to help reduce blood cell damage. Perfusionists should also meticulously check the direction of the roller pump, particularly that of the vent. This ensures that the vent flow is not accidentally reversed with the potentially disastrous complication of pumping air into the heart, causing major distal air embolism (Lewis and Czaplicka, 1990).

Another major safety concern is the accidental suction of blood after the reversal of anticoagulation by the systemic administration of protamine. Protocols vary as to the timing of cessation of suction related to protamine administration, but the safest position to adopt is no further suction after administration has started. On the occasions that it is required, the emergency reinstitution of cardiopulmonary bypass may be delayed if it has received sufficient protamine to cause any clotting within the cardiopulmonary bypass circuit. This potential delay whilst a new circuit is set up and primed could obviously have serious consequences. It is, therefore, important that perfusionists receive notification from the anaesthetist when protamine is about to be administered to ensure suction is terminated (despite pleas from the surgeon) and that the above situation does not arise.

Cardioplegia delivery

Cardioplegia may be administered independently from a 'bag', or may be delivered from the heart–lung machine. Delivery from the pump is becoming more and more popular, particularly with advocates of warm or tepid blood cardioplegia. Its delivery from the pump utilizes a separate roller pump (or pumps) and is therefore dependent on all the standard features pertaining to the circuit as mentioned elsewhere.

During the delivery of cardioplegia factors such as flow rate, pressure, temperature, concentration, dilution and time all interact with each other. Although there are many different techniques of delivering blood cardioplegia from the pump, broadly speaking all methods fall into one of two categories: fixed delivery volume or fixed delivery time. Some techniques require delivery of a fixed volume at a particular pressure, which means that flow rate, and therefore duration, will depend upon the resistance to that flow. The resistance is also multifactorial and depends upon:

- circuit tubing
- cannula
- site of delivery (antegrade or retrograde)
- dilution (and, therefore, viscosity)
- anatomy of the coronary vessels.

Other techniques require constant flow rate for a predetermined time at variable pressures, and resistance encountered is less of an issue. During cardioplegia delivery perfusionists are monitoring all the above parameters, and strive to maintain them within agreed standardized limits. A higher than expected pressure is likely to be an indication of obstruction to flow caused by inadvertent clamping of the cardioplegia line, malpositioning of the cardioplegia cannula or anatomical variations. A lower than expected pressure for a given flow may indicate the presence of significant aortic regurgitation if cardioplegia is being delivered into the aortic root. It is important that perfusionists are not tempted to exceed high pressure limits, which could result in damage to structures such as coronary ostia and the coronary sinus. Electrical activity should be closely monitored after cardioplegia delivery to ensure complete arrest, and the time since the last delivery should be noted and regularly communicated to the surgeon.

TEMPERATURE CONTROL

One of the fundamental requirements of an extracorporeal circulation is the facility to control, manipulate and monitor the body temperature of the patient. The use of profound hypothermic techniques also increases the need for meticulous temperature monitoring. A heat exchanger within the bypass circuit allows blood to be warmed or cooled. In turn, the temperature modification may be reversed as required, thereby warming or cooling the body tissues as blood re-enters the circulation. In general terms, temperature is measured in two specific places: the bypass circuit and the patient.

The temperature of the blood within the circuit will vary as it passes through the various components, including the heat exchanger itself, so it is important to measure temperature at specific sites within the circuit. This system of monitoring will allow optimal temperature management.

Water temperature

The basis of the ability to adjust the temperature of the blood is dependent upon the temperature setting of a water reservoir within the heater–cooler. Water temperature is usually measured directly within the heater–cooler itself. However, loss of heat as the water passes through the heater–cooler tubing to the heat exchanger (dependent upon room temperature and tubing length) will mean that the temperature measured is almost always an overestimate.

Some oxygenators have a water temperature port within the heat exchanger providing a more accurate

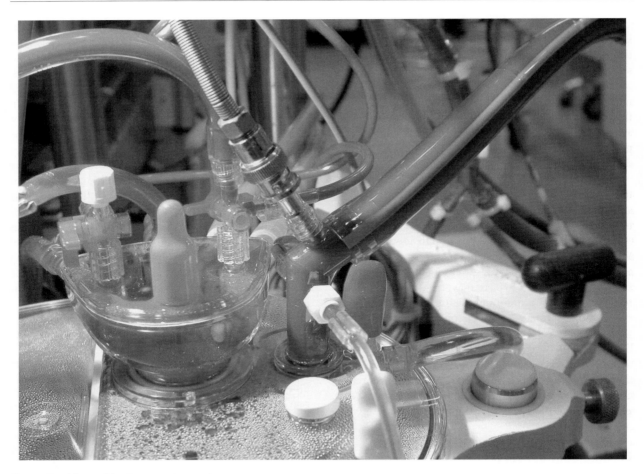

Figure 5.4 *Venous blood temperature probe.*

value. Water temperature is important, not just in terms of heat exchange under normal conditions, but it gives perfusionists an early warning of heater–cooler malfunction, which could potentially lead to dangerous overheating of the blood.

Venous blood

The venous blood temperature provides a crude indication of whole body temperature, in much the same way as mixed venous oxygen saturation provides information about whole-body oxygen consumption (Fig. 5.4). It is usually measured in close proximity to the venous reservoir. Therefore, depending on the variable length of the venous line, it probably underestimates the true venous blood temperature due to heat loss from the circuit between the patient and the reservoir. The actual value is not one that perfusionists will ever attempt to manipulate, but depends upon manipulation of other factors. However, the gradient between the venous blood temperature and the temperature of water in the heat exchanger is important and will be discussed later.

Arterial blood

In terms of patient safety, the arterial blood temperature is probably the most important temperature monitored by perfusionists. It is usually measured at the point of exit of blood from the oxygenator. If the blood temperature is excessively deranged in either direction, there is a likelihood that the blood and its components could be damaged, but also that infusion of such blood could result in damage to vulnerable tissues. In particular, there is always the potential for cerebral hyperthermia if the temperature of the delivered blood is allowed to be too high. In practical terms it is easy to heat blood to 39°C or more during rewarming, given the maximum water temperature of the heater–cooler. Blood re-enters the circulation by way of the ascending aorta and quickly reaches the brain, so excessive heating must be avoided. Even under normal circumstances an increase in brain temperature would lead to an increase in oxygen demand and consequent blood flow, which may be undesirable. During the rewarming phase of cardiopulmonary bypass, cerebral hyperthermia may be disastrous as the increased temperature and oxygen demand coincides with a phase of the bypass when there may already be a mismatch in cerebral oxygen supply or demand (Enomoto *et al.*, 1996). This is because this is the stage of the operation when flow is often lowered for short periods of time to allow application or removal of side-biting clamps to the aorta. These manoeuvres already carry the threat of relative hypoperfusion and the increased possibility of embolic activity, added to which is the increased embolic activity due to rewarming (Donald and Fellows, 1960).

The site of measurement of arterial blood temperature at the oxygenator is probably the most practical and useful. It might be assumed that a more appropriate site would be at the point of re-entry of blood into the circulation. However, it could be argued that knowledge of blood temperature at the oxygenator is important in terms of reduction of damage of blood elements therein. This is coupled with the knowledge that the temperature of the blood can only decrease *en route* to the aortic cannula and that it therefore represents a 'maximum' blood temperature.

TEMPERATURE GRADIENTS

During both cooling and rewarming, the perfusionist will set a target arterial blood temperature. This produces a temperature 'gradient', or difference between the *actual* temperature and the *target* temperature. Too steep a gradient in either direction carries the danger of too rapid a rise or fall in temperature with its attendant risks, therefore there are pre-set standards of gradients that should not normally be exceeded. Temperature gradients are discussed more fully in a later section of this chapter.

Patient monitoring

In general terms, patient temperature monitoring is performed for two reasons. The first is to satisfy the need to know actual 'body temperature' (and therefore, confirm the adequacy of cooling or rewarming). The second is to derive an indirect measurement of brain temperature. Historically, investigators and clinicians attempted to measure accurate 'core' temperature. However, knowledge of core temperature on its own does not give perfusionists enough information relating to whole-body temperature. Ideally, temperature should be measured at a number of different sites to provide a better overall appreciation of whole-body temperature. For this reason, temperature is sometimes measured at more than one of several specified sites, each with its own inherent advantages and disadvantages. In practice, however, many centres use only one or two measurement sites, the most common of which is the nasopharynx.

NASOPHARYNGEAL TEMPERATURE

A probe in this position has long been thought of as a true indication of core temperature, and a reliable surrogate cerebral temperature measurement site. A nasopharyngeal temperature of 37°C is often the target for 'full' rewarming of the patient. The common post-bypass temperature afterdrop (Ramsey *et al.*, 1985) is sometimes cited as a reason in some centres to rewarm the patient to a higher target nasopharyngeal temperature of 38°C. The potential disadvantages of this approach are that it requires arterial blood temperature to be increased to above 38°C for extended periods of time, and that inaccuracy and potential underestimation of true brain temperature may lead to dangerously high values. Accurate placement of the nasopharyngeal probe is essential to provide reliable and consistent results. It is not uncommon for small adjustments to the position of the probe during rewarming to produce apparently large changes in the displayed temperature.

OTHER MEASUREMENT SITES

Other common sites of temperature monitoring include the following:

- oesophageal
- rectal
- bladder
- tympanic membrane
- skin.

The position of an oesophageal probe is important to prevent inadvertent measurement of myocardial temperature – particularly important when the heart is selectively cooled with cold cardioplegia and/or topical cooling (Cooper and Kenyon, 1957). Rectal temperature was originally perceived to be a core temperature; however, it has been largely abandoned now. This is because of problems with accuracy caused by the presence of faeces, and in general, temperature measured at this site tends to underestimate the true core temperature (Severinghaus, 1962). Rectal temperature changes more slowly than nasopharyngeal temperature. A target rectal temperature of 35°C during rewarming can only be achieved by prolonging the rewarming period if an excessively high arterial blood temperature is to be avoided. Bladder temperature has been shown to depend on urine flow (Imrie and Hall, 1990), which may vary considerably during cardiopulmonary bypass. Tympanic membrane temperature has been shown to underestimate brain temperature (Wallace *et al.*, 1974), with the added disadvantage of potential perforation of the membrane as a complication.

Cooling and rewarming

The relative efficiency of modern heat exchangers and heater–coolers allows rapid changes in patient temperature to be achieved. However, there are several disadvantages to bringing about changes in temperature too quickly.

Rewarming too quickly to a core temperature of 37°C, rapidly followed by immediate discontinuation of bypass, is likely not only to require a higher than desirable arterial blood temperature, but is very unlikely to have achieved adequate whole body rewarming, and will almost certainly result in a rapid post-bypass afterdrop. Similarly, attempting to cool a patient too quickly is unlikely to result in a homogenous reduction in temperature for all organs of the body, which may be particularly important when, for example, there is a need for more profound hypothermia coupled with circulatory arrest. In addition to this, there is a high possibility of the production of gaseous microemboli when the temperature of blood is increased too quickly. This eventuality can happen within the heat exchanger during the rewarming period if the gradient between the circulating water and venous blood temperatures exceeds 10–12°C. Perfusionists will therefore prevent this gradient being exceeded during the rewarming phase.

Perhaps more dangerously, the infusion of a perfusate that is much cooler than body tissues during a period of rapid cooling can lead to the production of gaseous microemboli, this time within the patient's circulation (Butler, 1990). Again, unless there is a need to cool rapidly that outweighs the potential disadvantage of the production of microemboli, perfusionists will use a similar maximal gradient that, in turn, produces slower, but probably more uniform cooling.

ANTICOAGULATION AND CLOTTING

The use of extracorporeal circulation during cardiac surgery inevitably means that blood comes into contact with non-endothelial or artificial surfaces. The thrombogenic nature of this surface necessitates full systemic anticoagulation in order to prevent clotting within the circuit. Heparin has traditionally been used to achieve anticoagulation during cardiac surgery, and its reversal is achieved with protamine sulphate. This has been the accepted standard since early animal experiments and the first human cardiopulmonary bypass procedures in the early 1950s. Although heparin may be considered to exhibit many advantageous properties, such as speed of onset and relatively easy reversal, one of its disadvantages is undoubtedly the fact that there is huge inter-patient variation in response to a fixed-dose bolus (Esposito et al., 1983). This highly variable response means that in order to administer heparin safely and effectively, its activity needs to be measured accurately. From a perfusionist's point of view, over-heparinization is not considered to be a problem during cardiopulmonary bypass. However, the use of too large a dose of heparin during bypass may lead to problems with reversal of anticoagulation or bleeding, which may be attributable to heparin rebound (Martin et al., 1992). A much greater problem for perfusionists is the situation where anticoagulation is insufficient. This will prevent the commencement of cardiopulmonary bypass due to the risks of clotting within the circuit. There are three potential consequences of under-heparinization:

1 The formation of major clot within part of the circuit could produce a potential blockage. This may lead to the requirement for removal or replacement of that part, necessitating the temporary interruption of bypass and its consequences.
2 Small amounts of *undetected* clot within the circuit could potentially embolize to a position further upstream in the circuit itself, or, much more dangerously, be transmitted into the patient's circulation.
3 Formation of any clot within the circuit will deplete clotting factors and therefore delay the return to a normal clotting status once cardiopulmonary bypass is discontinued.

In most cardiac surgical centres, anticoagulation is monitored by devices which measure activated clotting time (ACT). Basically, these devices work by mixing whole blood with an activating substance (usually celite, kaolin or a mixture of both) that triggers contact activation. The device has an inbuilt means of detecting the presence of clot. It also displays the time taken from the start of the test (when blood was first introduced) until clot is detected. There are several different devices currently available on the market for measuring ACT, as follows.

• *Hemochron analyser* (International Technidyne Corporation): this consists of a pre-aligned magnet within a test tube and a magnet detector within the test well (Fig. 5.5) (Zucker et al., 1999). A 2 mL sample of whole blood is first added to the test tube containing the activator (either celite or kaolin), the tube is then agitated and placed into the test well. The tube is warmed and rotated within the test well. Formation of a clot causes the magnet to move within the tube in such a way that the detector senses a change in the magnetic field and stops the timer. The instrument gives an audible beep and displays the coagulation time in seconds.
• *HemoTec analyser* (Medtronic Inc.): this device consists of two plastic cartridges that are pre-warmed immediately before the test is performed. A sample of 0.4 mL of whole blood is injected into each of the cartridges, which are then placed back into the heat block of the analyser. Each cartridge contains a plunger, at the top of which is a flag, that is engaged by a lifting device within the analyser when the test is started. Movement of the plunger mixes the blood with the activator (kaolin). Continued active rising and passive falling of the plunger back through the blood agitates the sample until a clot starts to form.

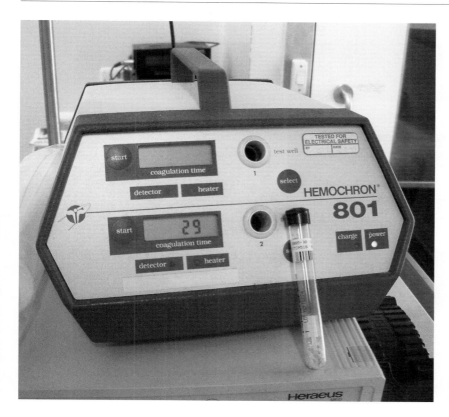

Figure 5.5 *Hemochron 801 analyser and test tube.*

Clot formation itself affects the rate at which the plunger can fall. A photo-optic detector stops the timer when the slowing or stopping of the plunger occurs, and the ACT is displayed in seconds for each of the two cartridges, displaying a mean result.

- *Actalyke Mini ACT Test System* (Helena Laboratories Inc.): this system is similar to the Hemochron device, but differs in two important ways. First, there are two magnetic detectors within the test well, instead of just one. Second, the activator contained in the MAX-ACT test tubes is described by the manufacturers as a 'cocktail' of celite, kaolin and glass particles. This so-called maximum activation, combined with the presence of two detectors instead of one leads, in most cases, to the detection of clot at an earlier point in time, and therefore, to shorter ACTs.

- *Hemochron Jr Microcoagulation system* (International Technidyne Corporation): this is a cartridge-based system using a sample of 15 microlitres of whole blood (Fig. 5.6). The sample is automatically drawn into the test channel of the machine (excess blood being drawn into a waste channel, thereby improving the consistency of results which may be affected by varying sample size in other devices). After mixing with the activator (silica, kaolin and phospholipid mixture), the blood moves within the test channel between two LED optical detectors. The speed at which the blood moves between the detectors is

measured. As clot begins to form, blood flow is impeded and the movement slows. The instrument recognizes that a clot endpoint has been reached when the flow falls to a predetermined rate. Detection of this point causes the instrument's digital timer to display the celite-equivalent ACT value in seconds. A useful advantage of this device is that the result is obtained more quickly in real time than the value in seconds of the celite equivalent result that it displays. This is particularly useful when bypass needs to be initiated quickly.

Since each device may give a different result for the same given blood sample (Salmenperä *et al.*, 1995), it is important that perfusionists are aware which is being used. It is also necessary that perfusionists ensure that results are standardized by adhering to strict protocols relating to the test procedure and specific use of equipment.

ACTIVATED CLOTTING TIME

The normal pre-heparin value expected for an ACT is in the range of 90–130 seconds. The target minimum value of the ACT during cardiopulmonary bypass varies from one institution to the next. However, most centres use a target in the range of 400–480 seconds. The optimal minimal value has still not been clearly defined. A value of 400 seconds was used for many years, based on the work of Young *et al.* (1978), who detected fibrin monomers

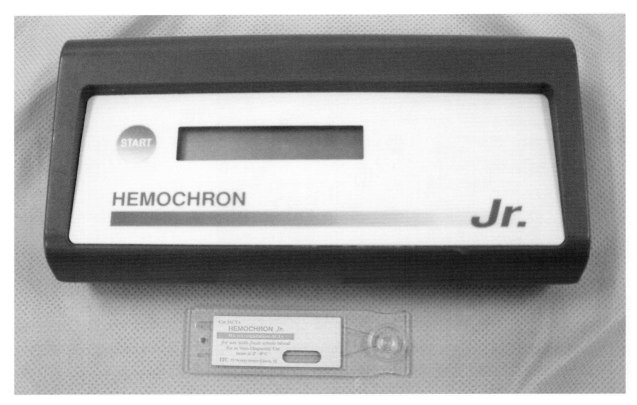

Figure 5.6 *Hemochron Jr. and cartridge.*

in six out of nine monkeys after 30 minutes of bypass. Of the six monkeys, five had an ACT that was below 400 seconds. Bull *et al.* (1975) showed that clots do not form in the circuit with an ACT above 300 seconds, but went on to suggest that an ACT value of at least 480 seconds would add a reasonable margin of safety in preventing sub-clinical coagulation activity, given the potential inaccuracy of the test which may have a coefficient of variation approaching 10 per cent.

It is important that perfusionists adhere to the agreed protocol for the particular institution, and maintain strict consistency when performing ACTs in order to allow maximum accuracy and safety. The ACT is measured pre-heparinization to provide a baseline value that can be used as a reference point for the reversal of heparin later in the operation. Following a bolus of 3–4 mg (300–400 units) per kg bodyweight of heparin, the ACT is repeated at approximately five minutes after administration. The result of this ACT determines whether initiation of cardiopulmonary bypass or even the introduction of blood to the circuit via the cardiotomy suckers is possible.

There are a number of patient-specific conditions that may affect the ACT. Heparin resistance may be caused by:

- antithrombin III (ATIII) deficiency
- pre-operative heparin therapy
- endocarditis

- systemic inflammatory conditions
- pre-operative infusions of glyceryl trinitrate (GTN) (debatable).

Heparin sensitivity may be seen in obese patients where lean body mass is much lower that actual body weight and where there is a deficiency of platelets or other clotting factors (factor VIII and fibrinogen). Hypothermia and haemodilution also bring about an artificial increase in the ACT.

Once bypass has been established, the perfusionist will repeat the ACT at regular appropriate intervals. Usually this is likely to be approximately every 20–30 minutes. However, there are situations which merit more frequent ACT measurement. These include the situation where an unexpected result has been obtained, a period where the ACT may be expected to change more quickly, and after the administration of additional heparin on bypass. Following termination of bypass and administration of protamine, another ACT is performed to assess the adequacy of heparin reversal; ideally, the value returning to close to the original baseline level.

Aprotinin and ACT

Perfusionists must take extra care when monitoring ACTs in patients who have received aprotinin (Trasylol). Ideally,

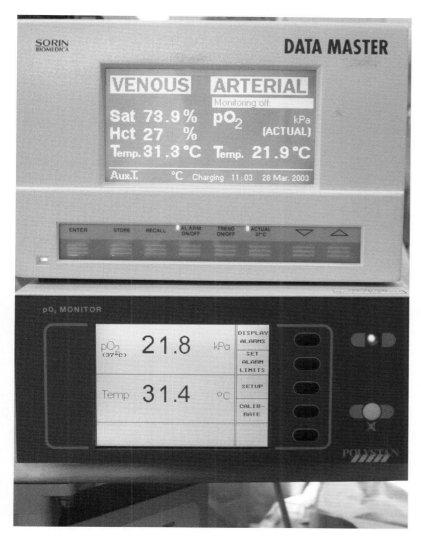

Figure 5.7 *In-line monitors.*

the ACT should be measured using a kaolin-based system as this is not affected by aprotinin. Celite-based systems may give a false reading mimicking heparin sensitivity and are extended in the presence of aprotinin. This is potentially dangerous as it could lead to underheparinization due to a falsely high ACT result. If celite ACTs are used in the presence of aprotinin, a target value of 750 seconds has been put forward as a safe minimum value to allow for the false reading (Hunt *et al.*, 1992).

BLOOD GAS ANALYSIS

The changes in many of the physiological parameters brought about by cardiopulmonary bypass are often rapid and without warning. It follows that the means to monitor or measure those changes must allow the results of any analyses to be readily available within a reasonable time. Typically, these parameters may be measured by any one or combination of the following:

- bench top blood gas analysers
- extracorporeal circuit-based in-line monitors
- hand-held cartridge-based analysers.

In most centres, a bench top blood gas analyser is available within, or in close proximity to, the operating theatre. It is essential that this analyser is maintained strictly according to the manufacturer's guidelines and that a programme of daily quality control is used to validate all results obtained from it. In-line monitors consist of sensors (usually one arterial and one venous) placed within the extracorporeal circuit and connected to a monitor that displays a continuously changing value for a number of parameters measured in real time. In the more basic monitors, these parameters may be arterial pO_2, arterial blood temperature, venous saturation of O_2, haematocrit and venous blood temperature (Fig. 5.7). In the more complex monitors, such as the CDI 500 (Terumo Cardiovascular Systems), other parameters are displayed.

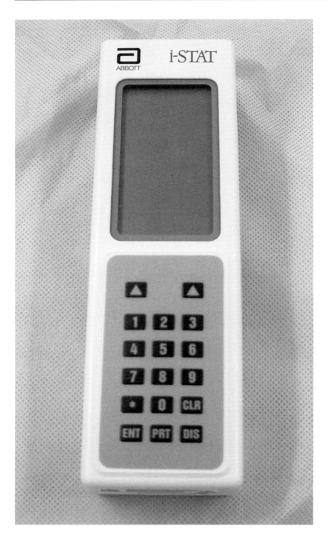

Figure 5.8 *i-Stat blood gas analyser.*

It is often the case that where in-line monitoring is used, the bench top blood gas analyser serves as the 'gold standard' against which the in-line monitor is compared and, in some cases, calibrated. An alternative to the bench top analyser is the hand-held device, such as the i-Stat (Fig. 5.8), which allows perfusionists to measure various parameters by use of a wide choice of different cartridges. The parameters that are necessary to measure or derive for the safe conduct of cardiopulmonary bypass are:

- pO_2
- pCO_2
- oxygen saturation
- pH
- base excess
- bicarbonate
- potassium
- glucose
- lactate
- haemoglobin or haematocrit.

In addition to the above, it may be desirable in some situations to measure sodium, calcium and magnesium. Perfusionists will also attempt to maintain each of these parameters within agreed limits.

INDICATIONS FOR ARTERIAL BLOOD GASES ANALYSIS

In basic terms, blood gas analysis is performed during cardiopulmonary bypass for the following reasons.

- *To assess oxygenator function*: the blood gas result will confirm what the perfusionist has very likely already observed, both by the difference in colour of the arterial and venous blood, and by the display of arterial pO_2 on the in-line monitor. A pO_2 in excess of 100 mmHg or 13 Kpa implies that the haemoglobin is fully saturated with oxygen and that the oxygenator is, therefore, functioning satisfactorily. However, this has to be evaluated in the context of each individual situation. For example, if the pO_2 is only 100 mmHg but requires an FiO_2 of 100 per cent at a temperature of 28°C, then clearly the oxygenator is struggling to achieve sufficient gas exchange.
- *Adequacy of perfusion*: assessment of the adequacy of perfusion is multifactorial. However, the results of arterial blood gases analysis can assist with this assessment. Perfusionists strive to conduct the bypass in such a way that the results of blood gas analysis reflect relatively normal acid-base and electrolyte status. An arterial blood gas gives perfusionists certain information relating to oxygenator function and the delivery of oxygen to the patient. In addition to this, an abnormal pH and/or an increasing metabolic acidosis will alert them to the possibility of inadequate perfusion. The use of venous blood gas measurement (to confirm results which may already be displayed on the in-line monitor) will also allow perfusionists to assess oxygen consumption. This, in turn, will add to their overall ability to assess the adequacy of perfusion.

In addition to these two main monitoring indications arterial blood gases measurement has a number of other applications. Perhaps the most important of these are alpha-stat and pH-stat regulation when utilizing hypothermic bypass, and they are dealt with in detail elsewhere in this book.

FLUID BALANCE

General regulation

The importance of monitoring the level of blood in the venous reservoir will be discussed later in this chapter. However, changes in this level are not only caused by mechanical obstructions to venous return or arterial flow, but are also dependent upon a change in circulating volume. Perfusionists must be aware of a number of important factors that will affect both the volume status of the patient during cardiopulmonary bypass, and also the choice of volume replacement fluid where necessary. Pre-operatively, the presence of anaemia, low body weight, renal dysfunction, heart failure and valve disease are likely to have a bearing on fluid balance and requirements during bypass. Patients may frequently present for cardiac surgery in either a volume-depleted or a volume-overloaded state.

The priming of the bypass circuit is, therefore, a fundamental part of the pre-operative set-up and may have profound implications on fluid balance both during and after the case. Many adult cardiac surgical centres use a standard priming volume of approximately 2 L (Lilley, 2002), which is usually a mixture of crystalloid and colloid solutions. More recently, however, there has been a trend towards reduced priming volumes in the adult population. Even in departments where this is not the standard regime, specific patient conditions will, on occasion, prompt perfusionists to alter the prime in content and/or volume. Perfusionists should also be aware of, and make allowances for, the potential change in the pre-operative haemoglobin during the pre-bypass period as a result of fluid infusions and/or autologous donation of blood.

RESERVOIR LEVELS

The venous reservoir is situated in advance of the main arterial pump and contains an integral cardiotomy filter. It allows temporary storage of a variable volume of blood in order to buffer the fluctuations in balance between venous return and arterial flow. In addition to this it performs a filtering function of blood from both venous return and cardiotomy suction. The level of blood within the reservoir may vary to large extents throughout the whole of the bypass procedure. Broadly speaking, there are two main types of reservoir in current clinical practice.

Probably the most common is the 'hard shell' variety, which is essentially a hard plastic graduated cylinder. It has the advantages of more accurate and easier volume measurement, better venous air handling, a large capacity of 3.5–4 L, it is more straightforward to prime and allows much easier connection to a level sensing device (see below). Its disadvantages are that it contains a blood:gas interface since the reservoir is open to atmosphere. This means that it is much easier to entrain air into the arterial pump under certain circumstances, with the potential to lead to a massive arterial air embolism.

The alternative type is the 'soft shell' variety, which is basically a soft, collapsible plastic bag. This type of reservoir has little or no blood:gas interface since it is closed to the atmosphere, but usually has a smaller capacity, may be seen to have more difficulty handling venous air, and does not easily allow the use of level detection devices.

Perfusionists must constantly monitor the level in the reservoir throughout the course of bypass, both in terms of the actual volume present at any one time and also the rate of change of volume. A relatively rapid change (usually a drop in level) requires immediate diagnosis of the cause. This may be caused by any of a number of different factors, such as a change in the position of the heart, a problem with or occlusion of venous cannulation, and occult loss of circulating volume (e.g. within the pleural cavity).

Monitoring of the level in the reservoir is performed in conjunction with central venous pressure (CVP) monitoring and observation of the position of the heart to give the perfusionist a clearer idea of the potential causes of change. Perfusionists should be aware that a prolonged increase in the CVP, if accompanied by a low mean arterial pressure (MAP), results in a reduced cerebral perfusion pressure. This may be exacerbated by a reduction in arterial blood flow if the high CVP has also caused a significant drop in reservoir level. Not only can the level in the reservoir suddenly decrease, but it may also rise unexpectedly, if, for example, flow of the arterial pump is significantly reduced or even interrupted completely for some reason.

Maintenance of appropriate reservoir levels is a fine balancing act that may alter without warning, and inattention to it can have devastating consequences. The minimal level at which a reservoir should be operated is to some extent dependent on the individual device and its design. Perfusionists should be aware of the manufacturer's recommended minimum operating level. At lower levels, there is an increase in the chances of entrainment of air caused by vortexing of the blood at the reservoir outlet. In addition to this, gaseous microemboli not removed by the filter in the reservoir have less time to 'settle out' at lower operating levels. The use of level and air emboli alarms is paramount and will be discussed in a later section.

Volume losses and gains

During bypass, there are several factors that perfusionists need to attend to constantly in order to monitor the loss of and addition to the circulating volume.

VOLUME LOSSES

As cardiopulmonary bypass progresses, fluid can be lost via several routes.

- *Loss into the interstitial space*: this is associated with the use of haemodiluting priming fluids that lower the plasma oncotic pressure. There is no direct means of measurement of interstitial fluid, but accumulation of excess interstitial fluid and development of oedema (with the potential consequence of reduced tissue perfusion) should be prevented by limiting the addition of fluid during bypass.

- *The production of urine*: monitoring urine production during bypass is important not just in terms of maintenance of renal function but also in the wider context of fluid balance. Excessive urine production will have a knock-on effect on the overall fluid balance of the patient and adjustments can be made by the perfusionist and anaesthetist working together.

- *Blood loss*: this may simply be the overt loss of blood temporarily into the pericardial cavity during bypass, for which the cardiotomy suckers are used to return the blood to the bypass circuit. However, blood loss may also be concealed in the form of loss into the pleural space if open, or even loss from the conduit harvesting site. More ominously, but fortunately rarely, loss into another body cavity may occur, such as into the abdomen as a result of abdominal aortic rupture.

- *Use of a haemofilter*: the use of a haemofilter during bypass to remove excessive volume is sometimes necessary, but will obviously reduce the circulating volume. The perfusionist will monitor the volume of haemofiltrate to ensure excessive volume is not removed.

- *Use of a cell-saver*: on occasions where a cell-saver is used during bypass, volume may be temporarily lost from the circuit and returned having been processed and concentrated. The concentration, by definition, results in a large loss of circulating volume.

- *Circuit leakage*: although rare, this cause of volume loss must be diagnosed and addressed expeditiously to avoid potential disaster. It may take the form of a very small slow leak from one of the components in the circuit and may be tolerated if the perceived risk of changing the component outweighs the benefit. Alternatively, it may take the form of a much more major leak or circuit disruption requiring immediate cessation of bypass in order to rectify the source of the problem.

VOLUME GAINS

Similarly, an increase in circulating volume during bypass can occur for several reasons.

- *The addition of fluid into the venous reservoir by the perfusionist*: as mentioned earlier, this should be kept to a minimum, but is unavoidable if the level in the reservoir reaches a critical level and it is inappropriate to further reduce arterial blood flow.

The fluid added under such circumstances depends upon local protocols, with which perfusionists should be fully conversant. In particular, the use of allogeneic blood transfusion, where indicated, should be carried out with strict adherence to the relevant safety checks for such transfusions.

- *Cardioplegia*: delivery of blood cardioplegia from the cardiopulmonary bypass machine usually involves mixing a crystalloid component with oxygenated blood in an agreed ratio to allow for a predetermined dilution and final concentration of potassium. Perfusionists must constantly be aware of how much volume has been added in the form of the crystalloid component. Similarly, if crystalloid cardioplegia is used (delivered by the anaesthetist from the head of the table), an awareness of delivery volumes is required, with careful monitoring of the resultant haematocrit and potassium.

- *Topical cooling and slush*: in addition to cardioplegia, some surgeons use topical cooling or ice 'slush' which may or may not be removed from the operative field by a separate sucker to prevent excessive haemodilution. If it is carelessly drawn into the cardiotomy suckers it will clearly have the effect of increasing overall fluid volume in the circuit.

ALARMS AND SAFETY

Perfusionists are the first line of defence in preventing critical incidents relating to cardiopulmonary bypass from occurring. As a fundamental adjunct, modern extracorporeal circuits employ a wide array of alarms that assist perfusionists with the safe monitoring of cardiopulmonary bypass. It is important to note that any alarm is operator-dependent and is only of any use when it is set, calibrated, switched on and fully functioning. Perfusionists must ensure that all alarms are in good working order, and that the override function of an alarm is only used when absolutely necessary.

Alarms involved in cardiopulmonary bypass circuits may serve one or both of two main functions. The first is to alert the perfusionist by way of an audible and/or visual alarm to a problem. The second is to slow or stop the main arterial pump, thereby limiting the possibility of further problems and potential patient harm.

The main alarms involved in the bypass circuit are as follows.

Reservoir level

This alarm requires an electronic probe to be attached to the reservoir at a predetermined minimum level (Fig. 5.9).

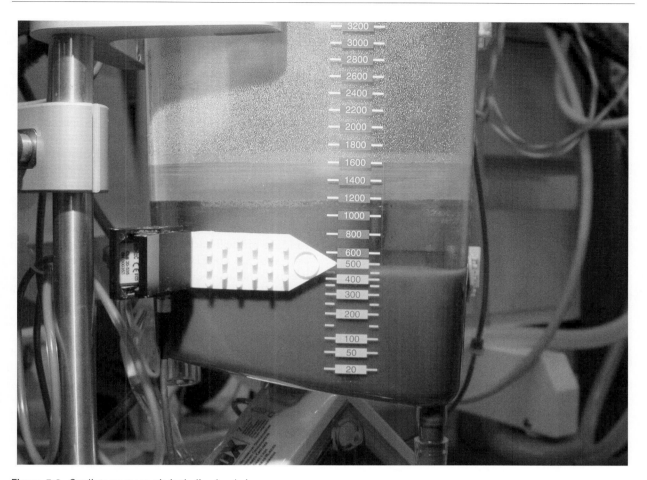

Figure 5.9 *Cardiotomy reservoir, including level alarm sensor.*

The probe is usually attached by connection to a self-adhesive sticker placed by the graduations of the reservoir. The older level sensors worked by ultrasonics and consequently needed a transmission layer of ultrasonic gel. They did not always work effectively on some hard shell venous reservoirs, and on some occasions the gel 'dried out' leading to multiple false alarms.

Most modern detectors use a metal self-adhesive strip that utilizes the principle of capacitance. Basically, the level detector works by sensing the presence of fluid (blood or clear fluid) through the plastic of the cardiotomy reservoir. The heart–lung machine will give an audible and/or visual alarm when the level of fluid falls close to the pre-set limit, alerting the perfusionist to a potential problem, and slowing the arterial pump. At this stage, perfusionists should endeavour to ascertain the reason for a fall in the level of blood in the reservoir and rectify this appropriately. If the problem persists, and the level in the reservoir actually drops below the pre-set limit the arterial pump will stop so that the reservoir does not empty completely and air is not entrained into the arterial pump, and ultimately the patient's circulation. The audible alarm alerting perfusionists to the fact that the pump has been stopped is usually different in tone to the alarm that signifies slowing of the pump.

Air bubble detection

The main function of the bubble detector in an extracorporeal circuit is to prevent massive arterial air embolism, which carries an extremely high mortality. The principle behind modern bubble detectors is ultra-sound. A high frequency transmitter or receiver is clamped around tubing within the circuit, usually requiring the use of an ultrasonic gel to aid contact (Fig. 5.10). If a bubble is detected, the arterial pump (connected to the bubble detector electronically) will respond in different ways, depending on the size of the bubble detected. Smaller bubbles (approximately 0.3–3 mm) are registered by the sensor and displayed to the perfusionist as microbubble activity. Bubbles in this range do not stop the arterial pump. An attempt should be made by the perfusionist to ascertain the cause of microbubble activity, and appropriate action taken to

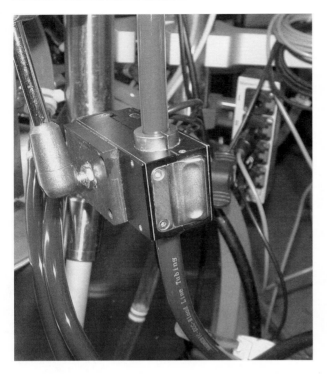

Figure 5.10 *Air bubble detector on bypass circuit tubing.*

reduce this activity. Larger bubbles (greater than 3 mm) will produce an audible and visual alarm condition, and immediately stop the arterial pump. This effectively terminates cardiopulmonary bypass, and the perfusionist must identify and remove the bubble from the circuit before reinstituting bypass.

The *ideal* position for the bubble detector within the circuit is unclear. If the detector is placed close to the patient as a last line of defence after all the components of the circuit, it will be able to detect air bubbles arising from any point. However, orientation of the tubing, height of the operating table, distance between the detector and the aortic cannula, speed of the pump and the potential for continued flow of blood by inertia even after the pump has stopped means that there is still a chance that the bubble will enter the patient's circulation. A bubble detector placed much further back within the circuit between the venous reservoir and the oxygenator, effectively acts as a second level detector. In this position, it would fail to detect any air exiting from the oxygenator itself, either due to a fault arising with the oxygenator or inadequate priming.

Considering the above, the ideal position of the detector is arguably close to the outlet of the oxygenator, maximizing the distance to the patient. An additional benefit of this position is the presence of the arterial line filter downstream of the detector, which will assist perfusionists with the removal of any bubbles detected.

Circuit pressures

Pressure is measured at various points within the extracorporeal circuit, including pre- and post-oxygenator and in the cardioplegia line. Post-oxygenator pressure is commonly referred to as 'arterial line pressure'. This is essential for perfusionists to monitor resistance to arterial pump flow. Additional information can be gained by the use of a pre-oxygenator pressure that is measured at a point between the arterial pump and the oxygenator. The difference between the pre- and post-oxygenator pressure gives perfusionists information about the resistance to flow through the oxygenator. Under normal circumstances, the difference in pressure, or ΔP, stays relatively constant but will vary to some extent with changes in arterial pump flow. However, in rare circumstances the pre-oxygenator pressure can increase significantly as a result of 'oxygenator thrombosis', which could lead to the need for an oxygenator change-out (Fisher, 1999).

Historically, pressure was measured and displayed using a 'Tycos' pressure gauge. The disadvantage of these devices is that they cannot be connected to any kind of alarm system and linked in any way to the arterial or cardioplegia pump to cause automatic slowing or stopping. They do, of course, provide not only a very visual analogue display of the value of a particular pressure, but also information relating to the pulsatility of that given pressure. This is particularly useful immediately following aortic cannulation, to confirm the accurate positioning of the cannula within the aortic lumen.

The use of electronic pressure displays in most cardiopulmonary bypass machines allows various parameters to be alarmed and linked to the arterial pump. For each of the pressures being measured, perfusionists will set alarms to give an alert of any abnormality. This may be an excessively high positive pressure, or an excessive negative pressure. A detected pressure that is approaching the pre-set high limit will slow the pump initially, and alert the perfusionist with an audible or visual alarm. The pump will be stopped automatically if the high-pressure condition persists and the high-pressure limit is reached. The function of the high-pressure limit is to prevent major overpressurization, with the potential for causing damage to the cardiopulmonary bypass components and even circuit rupture. It follows that the limits for pressure alarms should be set at a realistic and appropriate level. Perfusionists must treat an overpressurization alarm seriously, and respond accordingly.

Patient systemic pressures

Although not strictly extracorporeal circuit monitoring, perfusionists must constantly monitor the patient's MAP. In many centres, perfusionists directly control the MAP

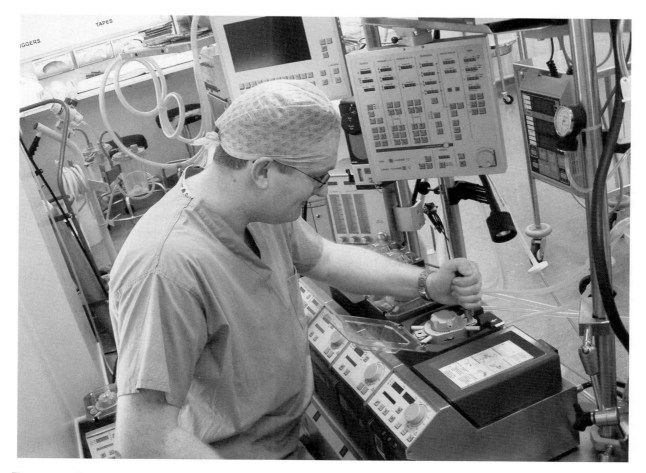

Figure 5.11 *Hand-cranking a roller pump.*

with the use of vasoconstrictor and vasodilator drugs, and as a consequence have an effect on arterial blood flow. The MAP will generally be maintained according to an agreed protocol. Commonly, a target range for MAP is 50–60 mmHg, but this can vary and be increased if there is a perceived higher risk of low pressure-related complications, such as stroke and renal dysfunction. The CVP is also closely monitored throughout bypass by the perfusionist, and its relevance has already been discussed in previous sections.

Other alarms

Historically, heart–lung machines relied solely on mains electricity. If mains power was interrupted for any reason, the heart–lung machine would cease to function. In this situation, perfusionists would be faced with having to manually drive or 'hand crank' the arterial pump to maintain perfusion (Fig. 5.11). Modern heart–lung machines have a built-in battery back-up unit that allows continuation of bypass in the presence of a complete mains failure. Perfusionists must be aware of the alarm on the heart–lung machine that will alert them to a mains failure.

They must also be aware of the display of the available voltage or time and the need to conserve battery power if the mains failure persists.

Failure of the piped gas supply to an operating theatre could have potentially disastrous consequences for the patient on bypass. The gas blender connected to the piped gas supply has an alarm to alert the perfusionist in the event of a gas failure. An alternative source of gas should be readily available for use with the minimum of delay. The importance of the gas failure alarm cannot be stressed too strongly, and its function must be tested on a regular basis.

Centrifugal pumps allow retrograde flow under certain conditions, as previously discussed. This type of pump has an alarm to indicate negative flow, and perfusionists can set alarms to indicate zero or low flow.

In cases where blood cardioplegia is delivered from the heart–lung machine, one or more separate pumps are involved to mix oxygenated blood from the oxygenator with a crystalloid component containing the cardioplegic agent. This system relies upon constant flow through the oxygenator at a rate which exceeds the speed of the cardioplegia pump. If for any reason flow through the oxygenator falls or even stops, the cardioplegia pump continuing to rotate will effectively be attempting to draw blood from a closed system. Under these circumstances, it is possible that air may be drawn across the membrane of the oxygenator as the cardioplegia pump creates an excessively negative pressure on the blood side of the membrane. Once air is present in the blood of the cardioplegia system, it is also a possibility that this could be inadvertently infused into the patient's aorta. To avoid this potentially catastrophic event, modern heart–lung machines link the cardioplegia delivery system to the arterial pump in such a way that if the arterial pump stops, the cardioplegia pump also stops. An alarm on the cardioplegia pump will alert the perfusionist as to the cause of cessation of the cardioplegia pump.

Since temperature and other parameters such as the on-line pO_2, SVO_2 and Hct are electronically recorded, they can all have alarms set to notify perfusionists of abnormal values.

DATA AND AUDIT

Traditionally, perfusionists have manually recorded the parameters during cardiopulmonary bypass in the form of a perfusion record or chart. Data recorded in this way allow perfusionists to be selective in terms of what and when to record. Other obvious disadvantages of perfusion charts are the need for storage and the difficulty in preventing loss of data in certain circumstances, such as fire. A physical record, such as a paper chart, may not have the required longevity if there is a need to keep records over a long period of time.

A more recent development is that heart–lung machines are supplied with integral data acquisition or management systems. These automatically record data relating to any parameter monitored by the heart–lung machine, and can even receive data from external devices. In addition, perfusionists can input the relevant details of consumable items used, members of staff involved, procedure performed and details of the patient's pre-operative status. Data are usually recorded on a memory card integral to the heart–lung machine, which can be downloaded to a computer after the procedure, or directly to a laptop computer situated close to the heart–lung machine. This eliminates any subjectivity attached to manual recording of data.

Once recorded and stored, data can be secured and analysed. There are various uses for this data.

- Easy audit of variables, such as consumable items, procedures performed, staff involved, and patient-related variables, such as age, sex and body mass index.
- Easy audit of intraoperative variables, such as methods of myocardial protection, cardioplegia volumes and

times, perfusion times, cross-clamp times, circulatory arrest time, and various pressures and flows.
- Easy graphical representation of intraoperative variables, such as flows and pressures. If required, these graphs can form part of a printout at the end of each case, and may be attached to the patient's notes.
- Assist with investigation of critical incidents. This can prove invaluable where the stress of a situation in the operating theatre may have made it difficult to record the sequence and timing of events accurately. The ability of the automatic data recording system to record values at, for example, 15-second intervals, may even later expose events that inadvertently went unnoticed at the time by the perfusionist or surgeon. The possibility of being able to learn from such data in a way that it helps to prevent any repetition of incidents that may be harmful to patients cannot be overstressed. It is entirely likely that this type of data recording will become a legal requirement in the future.
- Assists with research projects related to retrospective and prospective analysis of variables.
- Allows the safe and easy evaluation of new products.

Overall, the use of both manually recorded charts and automatic data management systems should help to raise perfusionists' awareness of various trends relating to their patient care, and should help to improve the quality and safety of the bypass procedure.

PROTOCOLS

We have referred to the use of protocols several times during this chapter and believe that the formulation of up to date protocols or guidelines is an essential part of providing safe cardiopulmonary bypass to patients.

In order to formulate such protocols perfusionists must consider both surgical and anaesthetic techniques as well as perfusion practices.

Protocols allow perfusionists to deliver consistent, standardized perfusion based on agreed safe practice.

Broadly speaking, protocols can be divided into two groups:

1 Protocols relating to the provision of cardio-pulmonary bypass under normal circumstances. These may detail specific requirements for different surgeons, anaesthetists and procedures.
2 Protocols relating to the procedures that may become necessary in abnormal or emergency situations (e.g. oxygenator failure).

Such protocols ensure that each member of the team understands their role in the event of an emergency situation (e.g. massive air embolism). They are also useful as an adjunct to the training of student perfusionists and for the induction of new members of the perfusion team. Well-written protocols not only ensure safe practice but allow perfusionists autonomy to make independent decisions without having to constantly refer to the anaesthetist or surgeon. This in no way overrides the fact that surgeons maintain overall responsibility for patients, but allows them to delegate responsibility for the safe conduct of bypass to perfusionists within previously agreed limits, allowing them to operate without the distraction of monitoring adequate perfusion.

Emergency procedure protocols should also be used regularly to practise such procedures in a wet-lab environment to allow these important manoeuvres to be performed more quickly, safely and efficiently when such situations arise in the more stressful environment of a surgical procedure.

SUMMARY

The issue of monitoring during cardiopulmonary bypass is not optional but mandatory. The conduct of cardiopulmonary bypass is constantly improving in terms of safety and reduction of adverse effects. This is largely attributable to meticulous monitoring and alarm systems throughout all aspects of the provision of extracorporeal circulation. Cardiopulmonary bypass begins with careful planning of the procedure, assessment of the patient, and a standardized and thorough set-up protocol. Monitoring should not end until the patient has left theatre, and in some instances even later.

Fortunately, the current generation of cardiopulmonary bypass machines (and all other equipment associated with the conduct of cardiopulmonary bypass) are 'state of the art' and have inbuilt alarms and autoregulatory systems that are able to address most eventualities. Unfortunately, any machine is only as good as its operator, therefore obsessive attention to detail is required by perfusionists in order to avoid mishaps of human error.

Finally, it is important to realize that although perfusionists have responsibilty for the heart–lung circuit and its management, optimum patient care is a multidisciplinary event. This means that good lines of communication with the anaesthetist, the surgeon and other members of theatre staff are paramount at all times.

REFERENCES

Bull, M.H., Huse, W.M., Bull, B.S. 1975: Evaluation of tests used to monitor heparin therapy during extracorporeal circulation. *Anesthesiology* **43**, 346–53.

Butler, B. 1990: Gaseous microemboli: a review. *Perfusion* **5**, 81–99.

Cooper, K.E., Kenyon, J.R. 1957: A comparison of temperatures measured in the rectum, oesophagus and on the surface of the aorta during hypothermia in man. *British Journal of Surgery* **44**, 616–19.

De Jong, J.C.F., Ten Duis, H.J., Smit Sibinga, C.T. *et al.* 1977: Hematological damage by blood/air interfaces in open heart surgery. *Proceedings of the European Society for Artifical Organs* **4**, 532–43.

De Jong, J.C.F., Ten Duis, H.J., Smit Sibinga, C.T. *et al.* 1980: Haematological aspects of cardiotomy suction in cardiac operations. *Journal of Thoracic and Cardiovascular Surgery* **79**, 227–36.

Donald, D.E., Fellows, J.L. 1960: Relation of temperature, gas tension and hydrostatic pressure to the formation of gas bubbles in extracorporeally oxygenated blood. *Surg Forum* **10**, 589–92.

Enomoto, S., Hindman, B.J., Dexter, F. *et al.* 1996: Rapid rewarming causes an increase in the cerebral metaboli rate for oxygen that is temporarily unmatched by cerebral blood flow. A study during cardiopulmonary bypass in rabbits. *Anaesthesiology* **84**, 1392–400.

Esposito, R.A., Culliford, A.T., Colvin, S.B. *et al.* 1983: The role of the activated clotting time in heparin administration and neutralization for cardiopulmonary bypass. *Journal of Thoracic and Cardiovascular Surgery* **85**, 174–85.

Fisher, A.R. 1999: The incidence and cause of emergency oxygenator changeovers. *Perfusion* **14**, 207–12.

Hunt, B.J., Segal, H., Yacoub, M. 1992: Aprotinin and heparin monitoring during cardiopulmonary bypass. *Circulation* **86**, 410–12.

Imrie, M.M., Hall, G.M. 1990: Body temperature and anaesthesia. *British Journal of Anaesthesia* **64**, 346–54.

Lewis, G.S., Czaplicka, B.S. 1990: *In vitro* comparison of three vent valves. *Journal of Extra Corporeal Technology* **22**, 125–30.

Lilley, A. 2002: The selection of priming fluids for cardiopulmonary bypass in the UK and Ireland. *Perfusion* **17**, 315–19.

Malinauskas, R., Sade, R.M., Dearing, J.P. *et al.* 1988: Blood damaging effects in cardiotomy suction return. *Journal of Extra Corporeal Technology* **20**, 41–6.

Martin, P., Horkay, F., Gupta, N.K. *et al.* 1992: Heparin rebound phenomenon – much ado about nothing? *Blood Coagulation & Fibrinolysis* **3**, 187–91.

McClosky, D.B., Strickler, R.F., Reusch, G.W. 1994: Alpha-stat capnography for the Sorin Monolyth oxygenator. *J Extra Corporeal Technology* **26**, 64–7.

Osborn, J.J., Cohn, K., Hait, M. *et al.* 1962: Hemolysis during perfusion: sources and means of reduction. *Journal of Thoracic and Cardiovascular Surgery* **43**, 459–64.

Ramsey, J.G., Ralley, F.E., Whalley, D.G. *et al.* 1985: Site of temperature monitoring and prediction of afterdrop after open-heart surgery. *Canadian Anaesthetists Society Journal* **32**, 607–12.

Salmenperä, M.T., Levy, J.H., Harker, L.A. 1995: Hemostasis and cardiopulmonary bypass. In: C.T. Mora, R.A. Guyton, D.C. Finlayson, R.L. Rigatti (eds) *Cardiopulmonary bypass – Principles and Techniques of Extracorporeal Circulation.* New York: Springer-Verlag Inc., 88–113.

Severinghaus, J.W. 1962: Temperature gradients during hypothermia. *Acad Sci USA* **15**, 515–21.

Wallace, C.T., Marks, W.E., Adkins, W.Y. *et al.* 1974: Perforation of the tympanic membrane, a complication of tympanic thermometry during anaesthesia. *Anaesthesiology* **41**, 290–1.

Young, J.A., Kisker, C.T., Doty, D.B. 1978: Adequate anticoagulation during cardiopulmonary bypass determined by activated clotting time and the appearance of fibrin monomer. *Annals of Thoracic Surgery* **26**, 231–40.

Zucker, M., Jobes, C., Siegel, M. *et al.* 1999: Activated clotting time (ACT) testing: analysis of reproducibility. *Journal of Extra Corporeal Technology* **31**, 130–4.

APPENDIX

Recommendations for standards of monitoring and alarms during cardiopulmonary bypass

Published by the Society of Clinical Perfusion Scientists of Great Britain & Ireland, the Association of Cardiothoracic Anaesthetists and the Society of Cardiothoracic Surgeons of Great Britain & Ireland, February 2001.

MEMBERSHIP OF THE WORKING PARTY

Brian Glenville	Society of Cardiothoracic Surgeons of Great Britain & Ireland
Tim Graham	Society of Cardiothoracic Surgeons of Great Britain & Ireland
John Kneeshaw	Association of Cardiothoracic Anaesthetists
Richard Reeves	Society of Clinical Perfusion Scientists of Great Britain & Ireland
Kathy Sherry	Association of Cardiothoracic Anaesthetists
Ken Taylor	Society of Cardiothoracic Surgeons of of Great Britain & Ireland
Mike Weatherall	Society of Clinical Perfusion Scientists of Great Britain & Ireland
Gerry Webb	Society of Clinical Perfusion Scientists of Great Britain & Ireland
David Whitaker	Association of Cardiothoracic Anaesthetists
Julian Williams	Society of Clinical Perfusion Scientists of Great Britain & Ireland

This document is available on the following websites:

- Society of Clinical Perfusion Scientists of Great Britain & Ireland (www.scps.org.uk)
- Association of Cardiothoracic Anaesthetists (www.acta.org.uk)
- Society of Cardiothoracic Surgeons of Great Britain & Ireland (www.scts.org).

INTRODUCTION

It is accepted that monitoring during the operative period reduces risks for patients. In 1988 the Association of Anaesthetists of Great Britain and Ireland first published Recommendations for Standards of Monitoring during Anaesthesia and Recovery. Within these recommendations it was recognized that additional monitoring may be required during cardiopulmonary bypass.

The aim of this document is to determine standards for monitoring and alarms during cardiopulmonary bypass. This includes monitoring for the onset of and weaning from cardiopulmonary bypass, for example confirmation of anticoagulation and ventilation of the lungs. These standards are for use in conjunction with the Society of Clinical Perfusion Scientists of Great Britain and Ireland Standards of Practice document[1] and local protocols.

Sources of reference include publications from the Society of Clinical Perfusion Scientists of Great Britain and Ireland,[1] the Association of Anaesthetists of Great Britain and Ireland[2] and the American Society of Extra-Corporeal Technology[3] as well as two UK surveys.[4,5]

Within these Recommendations for Standards of Monitoring and Alarms during Cardiopulmonary Bypass 'on site facility' is defined as on the hospital site and 'near patient facility' is defined as within or in close proximity to the cardiac theatre.

The recommended monitors and alarms that should be used during cardiopulmonary bypass are considered by the Society of Clinical Perfusion Scientists of Great Britain and Ireland, the Association of Cardiothoracic Anaesthetists and the Society of Cardiothoracic Surgeons of Great Britain and Ireland to be the minimal monitoring requirements during cardiopulmonary bypass. All centres undertaking cardiac surgery involving cardiopulmonary bypass should plan to institute these standards of monitoring and alarms by 1 January 2004.

It is accepted that special clinical circumstances, for example emergency surgery or failure to insert a urinary catheter, may on some occasions preclude complete monitoring. There may be additional monitoring requirements during cardiopulmonary bypass for paediatric patients.

Only an accredited clinical perfusion scientist registered with the college of Clinical Perfusion Scientists of Great Britain and Ireland can undertake or supervise the conduct of cardiopulmonary bypass.[1,6,7] A named and accredited clinical perfusion scientist not distracted by other clinical commitments, in close proximity and freely available, must supervise a trainee undertaking a cardiopulmonary bypass.[1]

The safe conduct of cardiopulmonary bypass is a joint responsibility of surgeons, anaesthetists and clinical perfusionists and requires a high level of communication between the team members. At all times during the conduct of cardiopulmonary bypass a surgeon, an anaesthetist and a clinical perfusion scientist *must* be present in the operating room.

The Recommendations for Standards of Monitoring and Alarms during Cardiopulmonary Bypass will be reviewed in the year 2005.

GENERAL RECOMMENDATIONS

All monitors and alarms used should be *calibrated and maintained regularly* according to the manufacturer's instruction and the recommended service schedule.

During cardiopulmonary bypass the electrocardiograph (ECG), intravascular pressures and core body temperature should be *continuously displayed and visible to the clinical perfusion scientist, surgeon and anaesthetist*. This will normally entail the use of a main monitor with at least one additional slave screen monitor.

MONITORING OF CLINICAL PARAMETERS ACQUIRED DIRECTLY FROM THE PATIENT

The following should be monitored continuously:

- electrocardiograph (ECG)
- systemic arterial pressure
- central venous pressure
- core body temperature.

Urine output should be monitored using a freely draining urinary catheter. Local protocols should dictate the frequency of measurement.

Pulse oximetry should be continuously displayed when there is a spontaneous pulsatile circulation.

Expired carbon dioxide tension/concentration should be continuously displayed while the lungs are being ventilated.

MONITORING ASSOCIATED WITH THE CARDIOPULMONARY BYPASS CIRCUIT

The following should be monitored continuously:

- *Venous oxygen saturation* of the blood in the venous return line of the cardiopulmonary bypass circuit.
- *Arterial oxygen tension or saturation* of the blood in the arterial line of the cardiopulmonary bypass circuit.
- *Continuity of the fresh gas flow to the oxygenator* using an in-line flow meter or rotameter.[2]
- *Oxygen concentration of the fresh gas flow to the oxygenator* using an oxygen analyser with alarms and sited after the oxygen blender and vaporiser if used.[2]
- *Blood flow rate* generated by the arterial pump of the cardiopulmonary bypass circuit.
- *Arterial line pressure* of the cardiopulmonary bypass circuit.
- *Cardioplegia delivery line pressure* when cardioplegia is delivered using the heart–lung machine.
- *Temperature of the blood* in the cardiopulmonary bypass circuit.
- *Temperature of water* in the heater–cooler system.

Activated clotting time (ACT) to confirm anticoagulation should be measured after heparinization and before cardiopulmonary bypass. Confirmation of anticoagulation within 20 minutes before the start of cardiopulmonary bypass should be considered if the time between initial heparinization and the start of cardiopulmonary bypass is greater than one hour. During cardiopulmonary bypass the ACT should be measured at intervals. Local protocols should dictate the frequency of measurement.

Filtrate volume should be measured when a haemofilter or concentrator is being used.

The following measurements should be available at a near patient facility. Local protocols should dictate the frequency of measurements:

- *Blood gases.*
- *Red cell concentration* (haemoglobin or haematocrit).
- *Serum potassium.*
- *Blood sugar.*

The following measurements should be available at an on-site facility:

- clotting studies
- serum calcium
- serum lactate
- serum magnesium.

SAFETY DEVICES

Local protocols for the conduct of cardiopulmonary bypass should be formulated by all hospitals undertaking cardiac surgery using cardiopulmonary bypass. Examples of UK protocols can be seen on the Society of Clinical Perfusion Scientists of Great Britain and Ireland website (www.scps.org.uk).

The following should be used:

- *Power failure alarm* with a *battery-powered back-up unit* for the cardiopulmonary bypass machine.
- *Bubble detector* on the arterial line of a roller pump cardiopulmonary bypass circuit with an *alarmed automatic pump cut out facility*.
- *Level sensor* on a hard shell venous reservoir system in the cardiopulmonary bypass circuit with an *alarmed automatic pump cut out facility*.
- *Anaesthetic gas-scavenging apparatus* whenever volatile agents are used in the cardiopulmonary bypass circuit.[8]
- *Out of range temperature alarm* on the heater–cooler unit.

REFERENCES

1 Society of Clinical Perfusion Scientists of Great Britain and Ireland. *Standards of practice.* London, 1999. (www.scps.org.uk)
2 Association of Anaesthetists of Great Britain and Ireland. *Recommendations for standards of monitoring during anaesthesia and recovery.* Association of Anaesthetists of Great Britain and Ireland, London, 2000. (www.aagbi.org)

3   American Society of Extra-Corporeal Technology. *AmSECT guidelines for perfusion practice.* American Society of Extra-Corporeal Technology, 1998. (www.amsect.org)

4   Cockroft S. Use of monitoring devices during anaesthesia for cardiac surgery: a survey of practices at public hospitals within the United Kingdom and Ireland. *Journal of Cardiothoracic and Vascular Anaesthesia* 1994, **8**(4): 382–5.

5   Weatherall M, Sherry KM. Monitors and alarms used by perfusionists during cardiopulmonary bypass. *The Perfusionist* 2000; **24**(3),10.

6   Royal College of Anaesthetists. *Guidelines for the provision of anaesthetic services.* Royal College of Anaesthetists, London, 1999. (www.rcoa.ac.uk)

7   Department of Health. *The employment of clinical perfusionists in the NHS, the Department of Health's guidance on best practice for the employment of clinical perfusionists in the NHS.* December, 1999.

8   Health Services Advisory Committee. *Anaesthetic agents: controlling exposure under COSHH.* London, HMSO, 1995.

6

Priming fluids for cardiopulmonary bypass

PIET W BOONSTRA AND Y JOHN GU

KEY POINTS

- Although it is established practice to prime the bypass circuit with a clear priming fluid, there is no clear consensus as to which fluid or combination of fluids is best.
- The use of clear fluid prime results in significant haemodilution, which improves blood rheology and tissue oxygenation, especially during hypothermia.
- The use of colloid in the priming fluid may help to maintain colloid oncotic pressure and reduce tissue oedema. However, there is some impairment of haemostasic mechanisms and a low but measurable incidence of anaphylactic reaction.
- Factors such as expense and ease of handling may help determine choice of priming fluid.

INTRODUCTION

Priming the extracorporeal circuit with an appropriate volume of an appropriate fluid is a prerequisite for the initiation of cardiopulmonary bypass. During the early years of open-heart surgery, the whole extracorporeal circuit was primed with fresh heparinized homologous blood (Zuhdi *et al.*, 1960). Shortly afterwards, the disadvantages and complications associated with blood priming demanded a search for alternative priming fluids

(Gadboys *et al.*, 1962). Nowadays, blood as priming fluid is rarely used for routine adult cardiopulmonary bypass, and instead a variety of artificial fluids are used to prime the extracorporeal circuit (Shah, 1992). This chapter reviews the classification and characteristics of priming fluids, the relationship between priming fluids and haemodilution, and the body's reactions to the priming fluids, such as the allergic reactions and influences in blood coagulation and haemostasis. Some general principles for choosing the right priming fluid are discussed.

CLASSIFICATION OF PRIMING FLUIDS

Crystalloid solutions

Crystalloid solutions are fluids that mimic normal plasma electrolyte concentrations but do not contain any colloid substances. They are usually equivalent to plasma in osmolarity but have no oncotic activity (Table 6.1). In general, crystalloids are considered to be more effective than colloids in expanding the extracellular compartment and are eliminated very rapidly by the kidneys. However, crystalloids reduce body colloid oncotic pressure and may result in increased fluid shifts from the intravascular space to the extravascular space (Beattie *et al.*, 1974), and this may in turn predispose the patient to pulmonary and peripheral oedema. Nonetheless, crystalloid fluids are cheap and are associated with a lower risk of anaphylactoid reactions than colloid fluid, and are used in most cardiac centres worldwide.

Table 6.1 *Physicochemical characteristics of priming fluids for cardiopulmonary bypass (crystalloids)*

	Dextrose 5%	Saline 9%	Lacteted Ringer's solution	Balanced solution	Mannitol 10%
Osmolarity (mOsm/kg)	292	290	278	294	620
COP (mmHg)	0	0	0	0	0
Na$^+$ (mmol/L)	0	154	131	140	0
K$^+$ (mmol/L)	0	0	5	5	0
Ca^{++} (mmol/L)	0	0	2	0	0
Cl$^-$ (mmol/L)	0	154	111	98	0
Mg^{++} (mmol/L)	0	0	0	1.5	0
Lactate (mmol/L)	0	0	29	0	0
Acetate (mmol/L)	0	0	0	27	0
Gluconate (mmol/L)	0	0	0	23	0

COP = colloid osmotic pressure. (Adapted partly from Tobias and Fryer, 1981.)

Dextrose

Five per cent dextrose was one of the first crystalloids to be used as priming fluid in the heart–lung machine following the abandonment of blood priming (Zuhdi *et al.*, 1961). Five per cent dextrose is slightly hyptonic and acidotic and becomes more so as dextrose is metabolized *in vivo* (Tobias and Fryer, 1981). In the early years of cardiopulmonary bypass, when compared with banked blood as priming fluid, five per cent dextrose reduced the mechanical damage to erythrocytes (Zuhdi *et al.*, 1961) and had a positive effect on intra-operative and post-operative diuresis (Cooley *et al.*, 1962). Crystalloid prime containing dextrose has also been found to lead to decreased perioperative fluid requirement and reduced post-operative fluid retention (Mets and Keats, 1991). However, there are also a number of disadvantages of using dextrose as a priming fluid. As the dextrose is metabolized the dilutional effect on plasma bicarbonate may cause systemic metabolic acidosis (Ing *et al.*, 1977). Furthermore, as serum glucose and insulin concentrations are elevated because of the effects of cardiopulmonary bypass (Hewitt *et al.*, 1972) adding dextrose to the prime may further increase the level of blood glucose, which may be of concern in diabetic patients (Mills *et al.*, 1973). More recently, experimental evidence has suggested that glucose-containing priming solution might increase the risk of cardiopulmonary bypass-related neurological complications, although clinical evidence is lacking (Hindman, 1995; Metz, 1995). Possibly this lack of clinical effect is caused by the protective effect of hypothermia in clinical cardiopulmonary bypass (Martin *et al.*, 1994).

BALANCED CRYSTALLOID FLUIDS

Balanced crystalloids are fluids formulated to have a neutral pH and concentrations of electrolyte ions similar to human plasma. Ringer's lactate fluid, or Hartmann's solution, is a typical example of a balanced crystalloid, and contains lactate as a source of bicarbonate (Tobias and Fryer, 1981). However, a large volume of fluid containing lactate should be used with caution in diabetic patients, as lactate may be converted into glucose *in vivo* through the gluconeogenic pathway (Thomas and Alberti, 1978). A further example of a balanced crystalloid is Plasmolyte solution, which contains acetate and gluconate for bicarbonate production. It also contains magnesium, which is an important intracellular cation involved in cellular process of energy transfer (Khan *et al.*, 1973) and in myocardial adenosine triphosphate metabolism (Storm and Zimmerman, 1997).

MANNITOL

Mannitol is a hypertonic, low molecular weight crystalloid widely used in clinical practice as a diuretic (Lant, 1985). As a volume expander, mannitol draws fluid initially across the capillary into plasma. It then rapidly diffuses into interstitial fluid and increases the volume of the whole extracellular phase by withdrawing water from body cells. A particular advantage of mannitol is its protective effect on renal function. In adult cardiopulmonary bypass, priming fluid containing 10 g of mannitol provided only an transient diuresis during the bypass period, compared with control patients who did not receive mannitol (Fisher *et al.*, 1998). However, an increased dose of 20 g of mannitol resulted in a significantly greater diuresis than both the control group and the 10-g group, and this diuretic effect continued for three hours during the post-bypass period. Furthermore, patients receiving 30 g of mannitol had an even greater diuresis, which lasted four hours. The diuretic effect of mannitol lasted for up to 12 hours after patients' arrival in the intensive care unit despite indications that the crystalloid had already been cleared from the body.

Table 6.2 *Physicochemical characteristics of solutions for cardiopulmonary bypass (colloids)*

	Albumin 5%	Dextran-40 10%	Dextran-70 6%	Gelatin-U 3.5%	Gelatin-S 3%	HES 6%	HES 10%
Mw (daltons)	69,000	40,000	70,000	35,000	35,000	450,000	264,000
Mn (daltons)	69,000	25,000	39,000	15,000	14,000	71,000	63,000
Osmolarity (mOsm/kg)	300	308	308	302	–	310	354
COP (mmHg)	19–20	160	78	–	–	25–30	55–60
T½ conc (hours)	–	2.5	25.5	2.5	–	25.5	2.5
Duration of PVE (hours)	2–8	2–12	6–48	2–4	–	6–24	2–12
Elimination	17 days	12–45 hours	–	168 hours	168 hours	24–67 days	1.9 days

Mw = Average molecular weight; Mn = number average molecular weight; COP = colloid osmotic pressure; T½ conc = half-life of concentration; PVE = plasma volume expansion; Gelatin-U = urea-linked gelatin; Gelatin-S = succinyl-linked gelatin; HES = hydroxyethyl starch.
(Adapted partly from Tobias and Fryer (1981) and Mishler (1984).)

Colloid solutions

In an attempt to maintain a higher level of colloid osmotic pressure during cardiopulmonary bypass, a number of colloid solutions have been used as priming fluids. Decades ago, human serum albumin as pump prime was an attractive alternative in achieving blood-free priming for open-heart surgery. However, potential problems, such as the transmission of viral diseases as well as cost issues, prompted the use of other, artificial, colloids as priming fluids, such as dextrans, gelatins, and more recently, hydroxyethyl starch. The physical and chemical characteristics of these substances are summarized in Table 6.2.

ALBUMIN

Albumin is a naturally occurring colloid product that has a molecular weight of about 69,000 daltons (Brown *et al.*, 1979). Under physiological circumstances, albumin accounts for 75–80 per cent of the plasma oncotic pressure responsible for the maintenance of body plasma volume. When used as priming fluid, albumin is usually in combination with crystalloid fluid. The amount of albumin used in pump prime is usually based on the calculation that it should be able to compensate for the drop of intravascular colloid osmotic pressure caused by the infusion of crystalloid fluid. However, despite its theoretical advantages in preserving the colloid oncotic pressure, a randomized study showed that the addition of 200 mL of 25 per cent albumin in the bypass circuit had no beneficial effect on peri-operative fluid balance, cardiopulmonary function and renal function (Marelli *et al.*, 1989).

In addition to its putative favourable effect in maintaining the body fluid balance, albumin was also reported to prevent protein denaturation, caused by blood–material interaction in the extracorporeal circuit (Kurusz *et al.*, 1982). In addition, a recent study showed that adding a low concentration of albumin to the pump prime (3 mL of 25 per cent albumin solution in 2000 mL of priming fluid), reduced platelet loss during bypass (Palanzo *et al.*,

1999a). This protective effect on platelets by albumin is even more marked than the use of a heparin-coated extra-corporeal circuit (Palanzo *et al.*, 1999b).

As a human blood product, albumin may induce ana-phylactic or anaphylactoid reactions, and may also carry the risk of transmission of viral disease (McClelland, 1998). For these reasons, and because albumin is rather expensive, a number of synthetic colloid fluids are used more frequently as priming fluids.

DEXTRANS

Dextrans are also naturally occurring colloids with an average molecular weight of either 40,000 daltons (Dextran 40) or 70,000 daltons (Dextran 70) (Gruber, 1975). The dextran molecule is a polysaccharide, produced from sucrose by the bacterium *Leuconostoc mesenteroides*. Dextran 40 has a colloid osmotic pressure twice as high as that of plasma, and so has a strong effect in mobilizing water from the extravascular into the intravascular space. Dextran 40 prepared in 10 per cent solution is a more effective volume expander than Dextran 70, as it contains almost twice as much colloid per litre. However, the action of the Dextran 40 is much less sustained, as the small molecules allow it to be rapidly eliminated by the kidneys. As a priming fluid for cardiopulmonary bypass, dextrans reduce blood viscosity and prevent the adhesion of leukocytes in the microcirculation (McGrath *et al.*, 1989). It is recommended that the total dose of dextran infusion does not exceed 1.5 g/kg per day as dextrans may impair haemostasis. This dose should be further limited in patients undergoing cardiopulmonary bypass because heparin is used in these patients. Anaphylactoid reactions to dextrans may occur, but the incidence of reaction is much lower than that caused by gelatin (Ring and Messmer, 1977).

GELATINS

Gelatins are manufactured from bovine collagen and have an average molecular weight of 30,000 to 35,000 dalton.

Two types of gelatins are used as priming fluid for cardiopulmonary bypass: urea-linked gelatin and succinyl-linked gelatin. The former is the result of cross-linking polypeptides with hexamathyl di-isocyanate, whereas the latter is modified by the addition of succinic acid anhydride to become succinylated or modified fluid gelatin. This modification results in a lower isoelectric point with a corresponding increase in the net negative charge, so that the retention time within the circulation is significantly prolonged (Van der Lindon and Schmartz, 1992). An important difference between these two solutions is that the urea-linked gelatin contains calcium, and because of clot formation should not be mixed with citrated blood. In addition, plasma calcium concentration may increase as a result of using urea-linked gelatin as priming solution (Himpe et al., 1991), and high concentrations of calcium at the end of cardiopulmonary bypass may lead to coronary vasoconstriction (Engleman et al., 1984). Although gelatins were originally considered free of adverse effects on haemostasis (Himpe et al., 1991), more recent studies have indicated that there is a negative effect on blood coagulation both in healthy volunteers (De Jonge et al., 1998) and in patients undergoing cardiopulmonary bypass (Tigchelaar et al., 1997). This is particularly true when patients receive a total dose of more than 3.5 L of gelatin peri-operatively (Tabuchi et al., 1995). A further disadvantage of gelatin is its relatively high incidence of anaphylactoid reactions compared with other artificial colloids (Laxenaire et al., 1994).

HYDROXYETHYL STARCH

Hydroxyethyl starch is a synthetic colloid that consists of hydroxyethylated polymers of glucose, derived from amylopectin. The physical and chemical characteristics of hydroxyethyl starch can be defined by both their average molecular weight and their molar substitution ratio, that is, the ratio of replacement of glucose group by hydroxyethyl group during production. For instance, hetastarch has an average molecular weight of 450,000 daltons with a molar substitution of 0.7, so that it is labelled as 450/0.7. Similarly, pentastarch is labelled as 200/0.5, which means that it has a relatively low molecular weight of 250,000 daltons with a low molar substitution ratio of 0.5. In principle, the average molecular weight of hydroxyethyl starch determines its colloidal effect, whereas the molar substitution ratio determines its half-life and pharmacokinetics in vivo. Therefore, hydroxyethyl starch with a relatively lower average molecular weight and lower ratio of molar substitution has a greater oncotic pressure and a shorter plasma half-life than the starch with a higher molecular weight and molar substitution ratio.

Hydroxyethyl starch (450/0.7) was first used as priming fluid for cardiopulmonary bypass in 1975 and found to be as effective and safe as crystalloid priming fluids (Lee et al.,

1975). Compared with albumin as a colloid priming fluid, hydroxyethyl starch appeared to achieve the similar clinical effects of volume expansion in cardiac surgical patients (Kirklin et al., 1984; Sade et al., 1985) with low incidence of anaphylactoid reactions (Palanzo et al., 1982). However, it is retained in the reticulo-endothelial system and it may cause impairment of haemostasis (Stump et al., 1985; Treib et al., 1996a). The medium molecular weight hydroxyethyl starch (200/0.5, pentastarch) was introduced as priming solution for cardiopulmonary bypass during the late 1980s (London et al., 1989) and has become popular in recent years, especially in Europe (Treib et al., 1999). However, the adverse effects of the 200/0.5 starch solution on haemostasis have also been reported (Mortelmans et al., 1995). More recently, a new 130/0.4 hydroxyethyl starch solution was developed with an improved metabolic elimination profile (Waitzinger et al., 1998). Preliminary evaluation using this solution as priming fluid in patients undergoing cardiopulmonary bypass revealed that this new medium molecular weight starch was associated with an improved haemostasis, largely as a consequence of increased concentration of von Willebrand Factor (Van Oeveren et al., 1999). Further observation has indicated that it was safe to be used in cardiac surgical patients in volumes up to 3 L during the whole peri-operative period (Gallandat Huet, unpublished observation).

PRIMING FLUIDS AND HAEMODILUTION

Adding non-blood priming fluids to the extracorporeal circuit produces haemodilution. As a consequence, body oxygen transport may be influenced because of reduced concentration of red blood cells, whilst the colloid osmotic pressure may drop as a result of diluted plasma proteins.

Maintenance of body oxygenation

Adequate body oxygenation depends upon oxygen delivery by haemoglobin to various organs and tissues. In normal volunteers, oxygen delivery can be sustained when the haemoglobin level is reduced to 10 g/dL by increased cardiac output (Woodson et al., 1978). In patients undergoing cardiopulmonary bypass, oxygen transport is not only influenced by the haemoglobin level, but also by the pump flow of the heart–lung machine and by the degree of hypothermia. Body oxygen consumption reduces considerably under hypothermia, so that the total requirement for oxygen is also reduced. In addition, oxygen solubility in plasma increases as temperature decreases. It has been estimated that body oxygen requirement declines progressively to 50 per cent of normal as temperature falls to 30°C, and to 20 per cent of normal at a temperature of 20°C

(Gott *et al.*, 1962). However, blood viscosity rises as body temperature falls, which in turn may increase the systemic vascular resistance, and reduce tissue oxygen delivery. This effect is compensated for by haemodilution with improved rheological characteristics and better flow.

Maintenance of intravascular colloid osmotic pressure

Colloid osmotic pressure is the pressure that prevents free movement of water and salt across the semi-permeable capillary membrane. Under physiological circumstances, the colloid osmotic pressure is greater in the intravascular compartment than in the interstitial compartment because the capillary membrane does not allow plasma proteins to move from the intravascular side to the inter-stitial side. This imbalance of colloid osmotic pressure across the capillary counteracts the imbalance in hydro-static pressure, which is modulated by the Starling force (Starling, 1896).

Theoretically, an ideal artificial colloid used as priming fluid should exert an effect on colloid osmotic pressure and viscosity similar to that of plasma. In reality, however, there are considerable differences between colloids with regard to their weight average molecular weight (Mw) and their number average molecular weight (Mn) (*see* Table 6.2). Usually, Mw is greater than Mn because the large molecules contribute more to the measured effect than the smaller ones (Van der Linden and Schmartz, 1992). Albumin solution contains an equal size of mol-ecules, so that their Mw and Mn are the same. In contrast, artificial colloids almost always differ in Mw and Mn because of differing particle size and shape during chem-ical preparation. The theoretical advantage of this is that the smaller molecules may reduce blood viscosity and promote blood flow distribution, whereas the larger ones may serve to prolong the effect of plasma expansion.

During cardiopulmonary bypass, the colloid osmotic pressure may drop as a result of haemodilution. This is particularly the case when large proportions of crystal-loids are used in the priming solution. A low intravascular colloid osmotic pressure may result in the shift of water from the intravascular compartment to the interstitial compartment, leading to tissue oedema. The normal ref-erence range of colloid osmotic pressure is 25–30 mmHg (Weil *et al.*, 1974). However, in patients undergoing car-diopulmonary bypass, a lower limit of 15–16 mmHg can be tolerated without leading to tissue oedema and organ dysfunction (Schupback *et al.*, 1978). A recent study com-pared the effect of three colloids on colloid oncotic pres-sure (Tigchelaar *et al.*, 1998). In patients receiving gelatin prime the colloid osmotic pressure was maintained throughout the operation. However in patients receiving either hydroxyethyl starch or human albumin, colloid oncotic pressure fell after infusion of crystalloid cardio-plegic solution. The lowest level of colloid osmotic pres-sure detected during operation was 12.8 mmHg but it returned to the baseline of around 20 mmHg in all three groups six hours after bypass in the intensive care unit. A colloid osmotic pressure of as low as 9 mmHg has been observed in patients undergoing cardiopulmonary bypass without any post-operative problems (Hoeft *et al.*, 1991). However, such a low level is probably best avoided in patients who have already have risk factors for post-operative pulmonary dysfunction.

Advantages of haemodilution

The most obvious advantage of haemodilution for patients undergoing cardiopulmonary bypass is that directly associated with the avoidance of homologous blood as pump priming. In comparison with blood prime, haemo-dilution with the use of clear priming fluids has reduced post-operative renal failure, pulmonary insufficiency, thrombo-embolic events, as well as complications associ-ated with homologous blood transfusion. As haemodilu-tion increasingly is accepted as a safe and effective means for cardiac surgical patients, the need for donor blood as pump priming is also dramatically reduced. Furthermore, haemodilution is associated with a reduction of blood viscosity and increased tissue perfusion as a result of reduced systemic vascular resistance. As a consequence, body metabolism is improved with a notable absence of metabolic acidosis (Messmer, 1975).

BODY REACTIONS TO PRIMING FLUIDS

Anaphylactoid reactions to priming fluids

Anaphylactoid reactions to various sorts of synthetic col-loids were well documented when colloids were first introduced into clinical practice as volume expanders. The typical clinical symptoms of anaphylactoid reaction include skin flush, urticaria, tachycardia and hypoten-sion. Very occasionally, life-threatening events, such as shock and cardiorespiratory arrest, may occur.

In general, the occurrence of anaphylactoid reaction to these synthetic colloid substitutes is very low, at around 0.033 per cent. In a large-scale German study, including 200,906 infusion of colloid volume substitutes in 31 hos-pitals (Ring and Messmer, 1977), the incidence of severe reaction was found to be 0.008 per cent for dextran, 0.038 per cent for gelatin and 0.006 per cent for hydroxyethyl starch. A somewhat higher incidence was observed recently in a French multicentre study, showing an overall frequency of severe form of reaction of 0.219 per cent in

19,593 patients (Laxenaire *et al.*, 1994). The various synthetic colloids did differ in their incidence for anaphylactoid reactions, being 0.273 per cent for dextrans, 0.345 per cent for gelatins and 0.058 per cent for hydroxyethyl starch. Anaphylactoid reaction to the natural product albumin was found to be 0.099 per cent.

According to its definition, anaphylactoid reaction is similar to anaphylactic reaction in its clinical manifestation, but is not mediated immunologically by an antigen–antibody reaction. However, involvement of specific antibodies against these synthetic colloids was repeatedly reported (Hedin *et al.*, 1976; Hedin *et al.*, 1979; Kreimeier *et al.*, 1995). Antibodies against dextrans were found in approximately 70 per cent of healthy volunteers or surgical patients who received dextran infusion (Hedin *et al.*, 1976). These dextran-reactive antibodies predominantly belong to the IgG class (Kraft *et al.*, 1982), and may induce an immune-complex anaphylaxis clinically resembling as a type III allergic reaction (Laubenthal and Messmer, 1992). Dextran-induced anaphylactoid reaction can be successfully prevented by the use of a substance called haptan, which binds to the antibody to form a haptan–dextran complex (Ljungström *et al.*, 1988). With haptan inhibition, the incidence of dextran-induced anaphylactoid reaction is greatly reduced (Ljungström, 1993). Antibodies against either urea-linked gelatin or the succinyl-linked gelatin were not thoroughly documented in the literature, although antibodies to raw unmodified gelatin were found both in animals and man (Mishler, 1984). Anaphylactoid reaction to hydroxyethyl starch is usually not considered to be associated with antibodies (Kraft *et al.*, 1992) until a recent report that high titres of hydroxyethyl-starch-reactive antibodies were found in serum of an aortic surgical patient at the time of reaction (Kreimeier *et al.*, 1995).

Blood coagulation and haemostasis

Priming fluids, either crystalloids or colloids, may influence the normal blood coagulation system and haemostasis. These effects are more marked when a large volume of priming is applied. Because of a decreased concentration of clotting factors, it may be anticipated that there should be some degree of coagulopathy and impairment of haemostasis as a result of haemodilution. However, during the early years of haemodilution, it was observed that haemodilution with crystalloid solution actually enhanced blood coagulation (Tocantins *et al.*, 1959). This hypercoagulable state induced by haemodilution was independent of the nature of the crystalloid diluent, and all crystalloid solutions produced similar effects. The mechanism of enhanced blood coagulation by haemodilution is most likely to be caused by the imbalance of plasma thrombin and anti-thrombin

concentration resulting in a relative decrease in the antithrombin capacity (Ruttmann *et al.*, 1996). A recent *in vivo* study on healthy volunteers has further demonstrated that infusion of 1000 mL saline solution over a period of 30 minutes resulted in a significant increase of platelet aggregation. This increased platelet aggregation was accompanied by a drop in circulating antithrombin III that was far more marked than could be explained by haemodilution itself (Ruttmann *et al.*, 1998).

Of perhaps more clinical significance are those colloid fluids that may impair post-operative haemostasis. Dextrans are known to affect both the antihaemophilic factor (Factor VIII) and platelet function, and thus have been used as an antithrombotic agent for deep venous thrombosis prophylaxis (Åberg *et al.*, 1979; Fredin *et al.*, 1989). Because of these inhibitory effects on blood coagulation system, a dose limitation of 1.0–1.5 g/body weight of dextrans is usually recommended (Mishler, 1984). Although gelatins were considered to have no adverse effects on haemostasis in early years (Himpe *et al.*, 1991), they may diminish the efficacy of aprotinin on haemostasis in cardiac surgical patients (Tabuchi *et al.*, 1995). When albumin was used as priming solution, aprotinin significantly decreased post-operative blood loss. However, this haemostatic effect by aprotinin disappeared in patients who received gelatin prime. The inhibitory effect of gelatin on haemostasis is largely caused by its inhibition on platelet ristocetin agglutination during the bypass period. Platelet aggregation capacity induced by ADP showed no difference between gelatin and albumin (Tigchelaar *et al.*, 1997). This negative effect of gelatin on ristocetin-induced platelet aggregation has recently been demonstrated in healthy volunteers who received 1 L of gelatin-based plasma substitute (De Jonge *et al.*, 1998). Also, the circulating levels of both von Willebrand factor and the ristocetin co-factor dropped significantly after gelatin infusion, suggesting that gelatin impairs the primary haemostasis mediated by von Willebrand factor.

The effect of hydroxyethyl starch on blood coagulation and haemostasis was well recognized during early years of observation as reflected by reduced platelet function and prolonged bleeding time (Thompson and Gadsden, 1965; Lewis *et al.*, 1966). These negative effects on haemostasis are likely to be attributed to the chemical characteristics of hydroxyethyl starch, which is quite similar to dextran. A remarkable inhibitory effect of hydroxyethyl starch was noticed on factor VIII (Strauss, 1981; Stump *et al.*, 1985). According to some reports, hydroxyethyl starch may induce a type I von Willebrand-like syndrome recognized by a marked reduction in Factor VIII coagulant activity, von Willebrand's factor antigen and Factor VIII-related riscocetin cofactor (Sanfelippo *et al.*, 1987; Treib *et al.*, 1996a). High molecular weight starch (450/0.7) has been reported to be associated with a greater impairment on haemostasis than the starch solution with a relatively low molecular weight (200/0.5) (Strauss *et al.*, 1988; Boldt *et al.*, 1993; Treib *et al.*, 1996b). The adverse effects of hydroxyethyl starch on haemostasis (represented by high blood loss) have also been reported in patients receiving the 200/0.5 starch as priming solution (Mortelmans *et al.*, 1995). In contrast there are other observations indicating that the 200/0.5 starch solution did not increase post-operative bleeding as compared with albumin priming (London *et al.*, 1992; Tigchelaar *et al.*, 1997). The inhibitory effects of hydroxyethyl starch on haemostasis and von Willebrand factor seem to be not only associated with its *in vitro* molecular weight, but also associated with the so-called '*in vivo* molecular weight', a description depending on its degree of substitution (Treib *et al.*, 1997, 1999). This is supported by our recent observation that the new 130/0.4 hydroxyethyl starch solution, which has a relatively lower degree of substitution, causes less reduction in von Willebrand factor than the 200/0.5 starch when compared as priming fluids for bypass (Van Oeveren *et al.*, 1999).

CHOICE OF PRIMING FLUIDS FOR CARDIOPULMONARY BYPASS

Although numerous studies have been performed over the past three decades to compare different types of pump prime, there is still no simple consensus with regard to the best choice of priming fluids for cardiopulmonary bypass. Crystalloid solutions are easy to handle during priming and de-airing of the extracorporeal circuit. They are considerably cheaper than colloids and are free of anaphylactoid reactions. Improved post-operative pulmonary and renal function have been observed by the use of crystalloid priming alone (Sade *et al.*, 1985; Marelli *et al.*, 1989; Scott *et al.*, 1995). However, a major drawback of a crystalloid is its inability to maintain the colloid pressure. For this reason, many institutions choose to add albumin into the priming solution to compensate for this effect. Colloid solutions are inexpensive alternatives that have similar efficacy to albumin in maintaining the colloid pressure for cardiopulmonary bypass patients (Himpe *et al.*, 1991; Tigchelaar *et al.*, 1998). However, adverse effects on blood coagulation and the occasional occurrence of allergic reactions have raised some questions about the suitability of these synthetic colloids when used as priming fluids (Mortelmans *et al.*, 1995; Bothner *et al.*, 1998).

Overall, the choice of priming fluids for cardiopulmonary bypass varies from institution to institution. A recent British survey containing 38 cardiac surgical teams working in 32 centres revealed that almost all the teams used crystalloids as priming fluids (Hett and Smith, 1994). Among them, 54 per cent used crystalloids alone and 44 per cent used synthetic colloids mixed with

Table 6.3 *A British survey of different priming fluids used for cardiopulmonary bypass*

Priming solutions	Frequency of use (%)
Hartmann's alone	42
Hartmann's + synthetic colloid	26
Ringer's alone	5
Ringer's + synthetic colloid	7
Plasmalyte alone	5
Plasmalyte + synthetic colloid	2
Hartmann's + dextrose saline	2
Dextrose saline + synthetic colloid	7
Normal saline + synthetic colloid	2

(Adapted from Hett and Smith (1994).)

crystalloids (Table 6.3). In the future, more options can be anticipated for composing a specific priming solution for individual patients as more advanced synthetic products with improved efficacy and safety become available.

REFERENCES

Åberg, M., Hedner, U., Bergentz, S.E. 1979: Effect of dextran on factor VIII (antihemophilic factor) and platelet function. *Annals of Surgery* **189**, 243–7.

Beattie, H.W., Evens, G., Garnett, E.S., Regoezci, E., Webber, C.E., Wong, K.L. 1974: Albumin and water fluxes during cardiopulmonary bypass. *Journal of Thoracic and Cardiovascular Surgery* **67**, 926–31.

Boldt, J., Knothe, C., Zickmann, B., Andres, P.U., Hempelmann, G. 1993: Influence of different intravascular volume therapies on platelet function in patients undergoing cardiopulmonary bypass. *Anesthesia and Analgesia* **76**, 1185–90.

Bothner, U., Georgieff, M., Vogt, N.H. (1998) Assessment of the safety and tolerance of 6% hydroxyethyl starch (200/0.5) solution: a randomized, controlled epidemiology study. *Anesth Analg* **86**, 850–55.

Brown, J.R., Shockley, P., Behrens, P.Q. 1979: Albumin: sequence, evolution and structural models. In: D.H. Bing, ed. *The chemistry and physiology of the human plasma proteins.* New York, NY: Pergamon Press: 23–40.

Cooley, D.A., Beall, A.C. Jr., Grondin, P. 1962: Open-heart operations with disposable oxygenators, 5% dextrose prime and normothermia. *Surgery* **52**, 713–19.

De Jonge, E., Levi, M., Berends, F., van der Ende, A.E., ten Cate, J.W., Stoutenbeek, C.P. 1998: Impaired haemostasis by intravenous administration of a gelatin-based plasma expander in human subjects. *Thrombosis and Haemostasis* **79**, 286–90.

Engleman, R.M., Hadij-Rousou, J.M., Breyer, R.H. *et al.* 1984: Rebound vasospasm after coronary revascularization in association with calcium antagonist withdrawal. *Annals of Thoracic Surgery* **37**, 469–72.

Fisher, A.R., Jones, P., Barlow, P., Kennington, S., Saville, S., Farrimond, J. *et al.* 1998: Influence of mannitol on renal function during and after open-heart surgery. *Perfusion* **13**, 181–6.

Fredin, H., Bergqvist, D., Cederholm, C., Lindblad, B., Nyman, U. 1989: Thromboprophylaxis in hip arthroplasty. Dextran with graded compression or pre-operative dextran compared in 150 patients. *Acta Orthopedica Scandinavica* **60**, 678–81.

Gadboys, H.L., Slonim, R., Litwak, R.S. 1962: Homologous blood syndrome: 1. Preliminary observations on its relationship to clinical cardiopulmonary bypass. *Annals of Surgery* **156**, 793–804.

Gott, V.L., Bartlett, M., Long, D.M., Lillehei, C.W., Johnson, J.A. 1962: Myocardial energy substrates in the dog heart during potassium and hypothermic arrest. *Journal of Applied Physiology* **17**, 815–19.

Gruber, U.F. 1975: Dextran and the prevention of post-operative thromboembolic complications. *Surgical Clinics of North America* **55**, 679–96.

Hedin, H., Richter, W., Ring, J. 1976: Dextran-induced anaphylactoid reactions in man. Role of dextran-reactive antibodies. *International Archieves of Allergy and Applied Immunology* **52**, 145–59.

Hedin, H., Kraft,D., Richter, W., Scheiner O., Devey, M. 1979: Dextran-reactive antibodies in patients with anaphylactoid reactions to dextran. *Immunobiology* **156**, 289–90.

Hett, D.A., Smith, D.C. 1994: A survey of priming solutions used for cardiopulmonary bypass. *Perfusion* **9**, 19–22.

Hewitt, R.L., Woo, R.D., Ryen, J.R., Drapanas, T. 1972: Plasma insulin and glucose relationships during cardiopulmonary bypass. *Surgery* **71**, 905–12.

Himpe, D., Van Cauwelaert, P., Neels, H. *et al.* 1991: Priming solutions for cardiopulmonary bypass: comparison of three colloids. *Journal of Cardiothoracic and Vascular Anesthesia* **5**, 457–66.

Hindman, B. 1995: Con: glucose priming solutions should not be used for cardiopulmonary bypass. *Journal of Cardiothoracic and Vascular Anesthesia* **9**, 605–7.

Hoeft, A., Korb, H., Mehlhorn, U., *et al.* 1991 Priming of cardiopulmonary bypass with human albumin or Ringer lactate: Effect on colloid pressure and extravascular lung water. *British Jouranal of Anaesthesia* **66**, 73–80.

Ing, T.S., Wu, C., Rosenberg, J.C., Ng, P.S.Y., Su, W.S., Bernard, A.A., Wilson, R.F. 1977: Cerebrospinal fluid changes in experimental cardiopulmonary bypass during hemodilution with glucose water. *Neurology* **27**, 85–9.

Khan, R.M.S., Hodge, J.S., Bassett, H.F.M. 1973: Magnesium in open-heart surgery. *Journal of Thoracic and Cardiovascular Surgery* **66**, 185–91.

Kirklin, J.K., Lell, W.A., Kouchoukos, N.T. 1984: Hydroxyethyl starch versus albumin for colloid infusion following cardiopulmonary bypass in patients undergoing myocardial revascularization. *Annals of Thoracic Surgery* **37**, 40–6.

Kraft, D., Hedin, H., Richter, W. *et al.* 1982: Immunoglobulin class and subclass distribution of dextran-reactive antibodies in human reactors and non reactors to clinical dextran. *Allergy* **37**, 481–9.

Kraft, D., Sirtl, C., Laubenthal, H. *et al.* 1992: No evidence for the existence of preformed antibodies against hydroxyethyl starch in man. *Euroupean Surgical Research* **24**, 138–42.

Kreimeier, U., Christ, F., Kraft, D., Lauterjung, L., Niklas, M., Peter, K. *et al.* 1995: Anaphylaxis due to hydroxyethyl-starch-reactive antibodies. *Lancet* **346**, 49–50.

Kurusz, M, Schneider, B., Conti, V. 1982: Albumin pretreatment of autotransfusion apparatus. *Journal of Extra Corporeal Technology* **14**, 467–9.

Lant, A. 1985: Diuretics: clinical pharmacology and therapeutic use. *Drugs* **29**, 57–87.

Laubenthal, H., Messmer, K. 1992: Allergic reactions to dextrans. In: J.F. Baron, ed. *Plasma volume expansion.* Paris: Arnette Blackwell: 86–96.

Laxanaire, M.C., Charpentier, C., Feldmann, L. *et al.* 1994: Anaphylactoid reactions to colloid plasma substitutes: incidence, risk factors, mechanisms. A French prospective multicentre study. *Annales Francaises D anesthesic ETDE Reanimation* **13**, 301–10.

Lee, W.H., Rubin, J.W., Huggins, M.P. 1975: Clinical evaluation of priming solutions for pump oxygenator perfusion. *Annals of Thoracic Surgery* **19**, 529–36.

Lewis, J.H., Szeto, I.L.F., Bayer, W.L., Takaori, M., Safar, P. 1966: Severe hemodilution with hydroxyethyl starch and dextrans. Effects on plasma protein, coagulation factors and platelet adhesiveness. *Archives of Surgery* **93**, 941–50.

Ljungström, K.G. 1993: Safety of dextran compared to other colloids. Ten years of experience with hapten inhibition. *Infusionsther Transfusionsmed* **20**, 206–10.

Ljungström, K.G., Renck, H., Hedin, H., Richter, W., Wiholm, B.E. 1988: Hapten inhibition and detrans anaphylaxis. *Anaesthesia* **43**, 729–32.

London, M.J., Ho, J.S., Triedman, J.K., Verrier, E.D., Levin, J., Merrick S.H. *et al.* 1989: A randomised clinical trial of 10% pentastarch (low molecular weight hydroxyethyl starch) versus 5% albumin for plasma volume expansion after cardiac operations. *Journal of Thoracic and Cardiovascular Surgery* **97**, 785–97.

London, M.J., Franks, M., Verrier, E.D., Merrick, S.H., Levin, J., Mangano, D.T. 1992: The safety and efficacy of ten percent pentastarch as a cardiopulmonary bypass priming solution. *Journal of Thoracic and Cardiovascular Surgery* **104**, 284–96.

Marelli, D., Paul, A., Samson, R. *et al.* 1989: Does the addition of albumin to the priming solution in cardiopulmonary bypass affect clinical outcome? A prospective randomized study. *Journal of Thoracic and Cardiovascular Surgery* **98**, 751–6.

Martin, T.D., Craver, J.M., Gott, J.P. *et al.* 1994: Prospective, randomized trial of retrograde warm cardioplegia: myocardial benefit and neurologic threat. *Annals of Thoracic Surgery* **57**, 298–304.

McClelland, D.B. 1998: Safety of human albumin as a constituent of biologic therapeutic products. *Transfusion* **38**, 690–99.

McGrath, L.B., Gonzalez-Lavin, L., Neary, M.J. 1989: Comparison of dextran 40 with albumin and Ringer's lactate as components of perfusion prime for cardiopulmonary bypass in patients undergoing myocardial revascularization. *Perfusion* **4**, 41–9.

Messmer, K. 1975: Hemodilution. *Surg Clin North Am* **55**, 659–78.

Metz, S. 1995: Pro: Glucose priming solutions should be used for cardiopulmonary bypass. *J Cardiothorac Vasc Anesth* **9**, 603–604.

Metz, S., Keats, A.S. 1991: Benefits of a glucose-containing priming solution for cardiopulmonary bypass. *Anesthesia and Analgesia* **72**, 428–34.

Mills, N.L., Baudet, R.L., Isom, D.W., Spencer, F.C. 1973: Hyperglycemia during cardiopulmonary bypass. *Annals of Surgery* **177**, 203–5.

Mishler, J.M. 1984: Synthetic plasma volume expanders – their pharmacology, safety and clinical efficacy. *Clinics in Haematology* **13**, 75–92.

Mortelmans, Y.J., Vermaut, G., Verbruggen, A.M., Arnout, J.M., Vermylen, J., van Aken, H. *et al.* 1995: Effects of 6% hydroxyethyl starch and 3% modified fluid gelatin on intravascular volume and coagulation during intraoperative hemodilution. *Anesthesia and Analgesia* **81**, 1235–42.

Palanzo, D.A., Parr, G.V.S., Bull, A.P., Williams, D.R., O'Neill, M.J., Waldhausen, J.A. 1982: Hetastarch as a prime for cardiopulmonary bypass. *Annals of Thoracic Surgery* **34**, 680–3.

Palanzo, D.A., Zarro, D.L., Montesano, R.M., Manley, N.J. 1999a: Albumin in the cardiopulmonary bypass prime: how little is enough? *Perfusion* **14**, 167–72.

Palanzo, D.A., Zarro, D.L., Manley, N.J., Montesano, R.M., Quinn, M., Gustafson, P.A. 1999b: Effect of surface coating on platelet count drop during cardiopulmonary bypass. *Perfusion* **14**, 195–200.

Ring, J., Messmer, K. 1977: Incidence and severity of anaphylactoid reactions to colloid volume substitutes. *Lancet* **1**, 466–9.

Ruttmann, T.G., James, M.F.M., Viljoen, J.F. 1996: Haemodilution induces a hypercoagulable state. *British Journal of Anaesthesia* **76**, 412–14.

Ruttmann, T.G., James, M.F.M., Aronson, I. 1998: *In vivo* investigation into the effects of haemodilution with hydroxyethyl starch (200/0.5) and normal saline on coagulation. *British Journal of Anaesthesia* **80**, 612–16.

Sade, R.M., Stroud, M.R., Crawford Jr, F.A., Kratz, J.M., Dearing, J.P., Bartles, D.M. 1985: A prospective randomized study of hydroxyethyl starch, albumin, and lactated Ringer's solution as priming fluid for cardiopulmonary bypass. *Journal of Thoracic and Cardiovascular Surgery* **89**, 713–22.

Sanfelippo, M.J., Suberviola, P.D., Geimer, N.F. 1987: Development of a von Willebrand-like syndrome after prolonged use of hydro-xyethyl starch. *American Journal of Clinical Pathology* **88**, 653–5.

Schupback, P., Pappova, E., Schilt, W. *et al.* 1978: Perfusate oncotic pressure during cardiopulmonary bypass: optimum level as determined by metabolic acidosis, tissue edema, and renal function. *Vox Sanguinis* **35**, 332–44.

Scott, D., Cannata, J., Mason, K. *et al.* 1995: A comparison of albumin, polygeline and crystalloid priming solutions for cardiopulmonary bypass in patients having coronary artery bypass graft surgery. *Perfusion* **10**, 415–24.

Shah, M.V. 1992: Priming fluids for cardiopulmonary bypass. In: P.H. Kay, ed. *Techniques in extracorporeal circulation* (third edition). Oxford: Butterworth-Heinemann: 72–7.

Starling, E.H. 1896: On the absorption of fluids from the connective tissue spaces. *Journal of Physiology* (London) **19**, 312–26.

Storm, W., Zimmerman, J.J. 1997: Magnesium deficiency and cardiogenic shock after cardiopulmonary bypass. *Annals of Thoracic Surgery* **64**, 572–7.

Strauss, R.G. 1981: Review of the effects of hydroxyethyl starch on the blood coagulation system. *Transfusion* **21**, 299–302.

Strauss, R.G., Stansfield, C., Henriksen, R.A., Villhauer, P.J. 1988: Pentastarch may cause fewer effects on coagulation than hetastarch. *Transfusion* **28**, 257–60.

Stump, D.C., Strauss, R.G., Henriksen, R.A., Petersen, R.E., Saunders, R. 1985: Effects of hydroxyethyl starch on blood coagulation, particularly factor VIII. *Transfusion* **25**, 349–54.

Tabuchi, N., de Haan, J., Gallandat Huet, R.C.G., Boonstra, P.W., van Oeveren, W. 1995: Gelatin use impairs platelet adhesion during cardiac surgery. *Thrombosis and Haemostasis* **74**, 1447–51.

Thomas, D.J., Alberti, K.G. 1978: Hyperglycaemic effects of Hartmann's solution during surgery in patients with maturity onset diabetes. *Br J Anaesth*, **50**, 185–8.

Thompson, W.L., Gadsden, R.H. 1965: Prolonged bleeding times and hypofibrinogenemia in dogs after infusion of hydroxyethyl starch and dextran. *Transfusion* **5**, 440–6.

Tigchelaar, I., Gallandat Huet, R.C.G., Korsten, J., Boonstra, P.W., van Oeveren, W. 1997: Hemostatic effects of three colloids plasma substitutes for priming solution in cardiopulmonary bypass. *Euroupean Jouranal of Cardiothoracic Surgery* **11**, 626–32.

Tigchelaar, I., Gallandat Huet, R.C.G., Boonstra, P.W., van Oeveren, W. 1998: Comparison of three plasma expanders used as priming fluid in cardiopulmonary bypass. *Perfusion* **13**, 297–303.

Tobias, M.A., Fryer, J.M. 1981: Which priming fluids? In: Longmore, D. ed. *Towards safer cardiac surgery*. Lancaster: MTP Press: 401–26.

Tocantins, L.M., Carroll, R.T., Holburn, R.N. 1959: The clot accelerating effect of dilution of blood and plasma. Relation to the mechanism of coagulation of nornal and hemophiliac blood. *Blood* **6**, 720–39.

Treib, J., Haass, A., Pindur, G. *et al.* 1996a: Highly substituted hydroxyethyl starch (HES200/0.62) leads to Type-I von Willebrand syndrome after repeated administration. *Haemostasis* **26**, 210–13.

Treib, J., Haass, A., Pindur, G. *et al.* 1996b: All medium starches are not the same: influence on the degree of hydroxyethyl substitution of hydroxyethyl starch on plasma volume, hemorrheologic conditions and coagulation. *Transfusion* **36**, 450–5.

Treib, J., Haass, A., Pindur, G. 1997: Coagulation disorders caused by hydroxyethyl starch. *Thromb Haemost* **78**, 974–83.

Treib, J., Baron, J.F., Grauer, M.T., Strauss, R.G. 1999: An international view of hydroxyethyl starches. *Intensive Care Medecine* **25**, 258–68.

Van der Linden, P., Schmartz, D. 1992: Pharmacology of gelatins. In: J.F. Baron, ed. *Plasma volume expansion*. Paris: Arnette Blackwell: 67–74.

Van Oeveren, W., Siemons, W., Huet, R.C.G. 1999: Preserved endothelial and formed blood element function after use of medium molecular weight hydroxyethyl starches in cardiac surgery. *British Journal of Anaesthesia* **82** (Suppl. 1), 75.

Waitzinger, J., Bepperling, F., Pabst, G. *et al.* 1998: Pharmacokinetics and tolerability of a new hydroxyethyl starch (HES) specification (HES 130/0.4) after single dose infusion of 6% or 10% solutions in healthy volunteers. *Clinical Drug Investigation* **16**, 151–60.

Weil, M.H., Morissette, M., Michaels, S. *et al.* 1974: Routine plasma colloid osmotic pressure measurements. *Crit Care Med* **2**, 234–79.

Woodson, R.D., Wills, R.E., Lenfant, C. 1978: Effect of acute and established anemia on O_2 transport at rest, submaximal and maximal work. *Journal of Applied Physiology* **44**, 36–43.

Zuhdi, N., McCollough, B., Carey, J., Greer, A. 1960: The use of citrated banked blood for open heart surgery. *Anesthesiology* **21**, 496–501.

Zuhdi, N., McCollough, B., Carey, J., Krieger, C., Greer, A. 1961: Hypothermic perfusion for open-heart surgical procedures: report on the use of a heart–lung machine primed with 5% dextrose in water inducing hemodilution. *J Int Coll Surg* **35**, 319–26.

7

Filters in cardiopulmonary bypass

FARAH NK BHATTI AND TIMOTHY L HOOPER

KEY POINTS

- Emboli in the extracorporeal circuit may arise from a variety of sources and be either particulate or gaseous in nature.
- Microemboli originating from the extracorporeal circuit have been strongly implicated in the development of neurological injury following cardiac surgery, and also in post-operative dysfunction of other organs.
- Filters of varying designs and pore size may be incorporated in appropriate parts of the extracorporeal circuit to minimize embolic load.
- Pre-bypass filters are of benefit in reducing emboli caused by spallation during priming.
- The benefits of arterial filters in reducing embolic load and improving outcome have been well established and their use is now routine.
- The use of leucodepleting filters is less well established, but they may be of particular benefit during reperfusion of the post-ischaemic myocardium.

INTRODUCTION

Filters are used in the extracorporeal circuit to prevent potentially harmful matter (both particulate and gaseous) entering a patient's systemic circulation whilst on cardiopulmonary bypass. This chapter begins by reviewing potential sources of emboli in cardiac surgery and their association with neurological impairment. Filter design and physical characteristics are covered, together with their clinical applications, including arterial line filtration. The chapter then focuses on more recent work on the role of leucocyte-depleting filters, which, in addition to removing emboli, may further improve outcomes by preventing potential damage caused by the activation of leucocytes during cardiopulmonary bypass.

HISTORICAL NOTE

It was work performed concurrently by Swank and Patterson in the 1960s that led to the production of the first commercially available filters for use in the extracorporeal circuit (Berman and Marin, 1986). Swank described the presence of microaggregates in stored blood, which led to him to develop a dacron wool depth filter to remove them (Swank, 1961). This was then used to filter blood in the cardiotomy reservoir in patients undergoing open heart surgery (non-randomized study) and found to lead to a subjective improvement in general patient well-being and to less mental confusion (Osborn et al., 1970). Post-mortem studies also revealed that patients in the filtered group had fewer emboli in their brains compared to the non-filtered group (13 per cent versus 33 per cent).

Meanwhile, Patterson had developed a prototype polyester screen filter that was shown in animal studies to decrease microemboli and to improve neurological status

(Patterson and Twitchell, 1971). The first filters available on the market were a dacron wool depth filter by Pioneer–Swank for use in the cardiotomy line and a polyester mesh screen filter by Pall Medical for use in both the cardiotomy and arterial lines.

SOURCES OF EMBOLI

Emboli present in the extracorporeal circuit can be either gaseous or particulate and can be from a variety of sources, including the equipment and the surgical site, as well as being generated when blood contacts the foreign surfaces in the circuit (Pearson, 1986). If they reach the patient, they have a direct route into the systemic circulation with resultant damage to end organs, in particular the brain.

Particulate emboli

The main sources of particulate emboli are the surgical site, the extracorporeal circuit and any drugs or solutions added to the circuit.

Debris from the surgical site can include atheroma, calcium, fat, bone fragments, denatured proteins, hair or suture material, as well as platelet and leucocyte aggregates. These can all be returned to the circuit via the cardiotomy suction lines. Surgical techniques can be adjusted to minimize the risk from certain embolic phenomena; for example, in an extensively atheromatous aorta a single cross-clamp technique with the use of pedicled arterial grafts would minimize the trauma to the aorta during coronary artery surgery (Barbut and Gold, 1996). Intracardiac procedures are associated with higher rates of neurological complications than extracardiac procedures because of air as well as calcium and atheromatous debris directly entering the aorta; thus, meticulous surgical debridement and venting are necessary (Nussmeir, 1996; Utley, 1996).

The extracorporeal circuit itself may be the source of embolic particles. Evidence of spallation and shredding of the luminal surface of polyvinyl chloride (PVC) and silicone circuit tubing has been observed by scanning electron microscopy opposite the site of pump roller heads, although this is more common with silicone rubber tubing (Orenstein et al., 1982; Pearson, 1986). In addition, Orenstein et al. (1982) found evidence of silicone in areas of micro-infarcts in kidneys from patients who died after cardiopulmonary bypass, presumably caused by silicone emboli from the antifoaming agent used.

All intravenous solutions contain a permissible number of contaminant particles ranging from 0.2 μm to 20 μm. This particle load increases as the solutions are handled and mixed. Of particular relevance is the administration of crystalloid cardioplegia solution as it enters the coronary circulation directly. Studies have shown that a number of cardioplegic solutions (commercially available as intravenous solutions to which specific sterile agents are added) can cause a reduction in coronary blood flow that is partially reversed if a 0.8 μm filter is used (Robinson et al., 1984; Hearse et al., 1985). This reversibility implies that the contaminants in the solutions cause coronary vasoconstriction rather than vessel occlusion. Another study described the presence of particles of varying sizes plugging the coronary capillaries in biopsies taken from pigs and humans who underwent cardiac arrest with Bretschnieider's solution (Hellinger et al., 1997). The same study observed that a terminal 0.2 μm filter significantly reduced the number of particles in the solution.

Gaseous emboli

Sources of gaseous emboli include the oxygenator, the heat exchanger, the roller pump and the surgical site (Pearson, 1986).

The bubble oxygenator is inherently more likely to generate gaseous microemboli than a membrane oxygenator. This risk can be minimized by the use of defoaming agents, maintaining an adequate reservoir in the oxygenator to allow any microbubbles to settle, and by maintaining low gas to blood flows. The introduction and acceptance of membrane oxygenators has led to a reduction of gaseous emboli from this source.

Increases in temperature decrease the solubility of gases in blood. A temperature gradient greater than 10°C between the water inflow and blood entering a heat exchanger has been shown to significantly increase the number of gaseous microemboli generated (Clark et al., 1975). It is therefore important to try and use as low a gradient as is practical whilst rewarming the patient.

A further potential source of gaseous emboli is the roller pump, as cavitation can occur because of the negative pressures generated behind the pump (Bass and Longmore, 1969). Other causes include gaseous microemboli in drugs and solutions added into the circuit, air from the cardiotomy suction and agitation of the oxygenator.

The surgical site can be the source of gross amounts of air entering either the extracorporeal circuit or the aorta directly. Air can be entrained at the venous cannulation site if the snares are inadequate, and this may enter the systemic circulation if there is a patent foramen ovale; air can also enter during aortic cannulation. Removal of the aortic cross-clamp and the start of cardiac ejection are also periods when air can enter the circulation if the left heart has been opened. Transcranial Doppler studies have shown that there are an increased number of emboli detected at these times (Nussmeir, 1996).

EMBOLI AND NEUROLOGICAL COMPLICATIONS

Neurological injury (both stroke, as well as more subtle cognitive changes) after a period of extracorporeal circulation may be caused by a number of factors, including cerebral hypoperfusion and loss of cerebral autoregulation, but microemboli undoubtedly play a role (Utley, 1996). A number of studies have implicated the involvement of microemboli in neurological deficits following cardiac surgery. Pugsley and colleagues employed transcranial Doppler ultrasonography to detect microemboli in the middle cerebral artery in patients undergoing elective coronary artery bypass graft (CABG) surgery (Pugsley et al. 1994). Patients were randomized to either having a 40 µm arterial line filter or not having a filter. Neuropsychological testing was performed at 8 days and 8 weeks post-operatively, and patients in the non-filtered group were significantly more likely to have a deficit. The patients in the non-filtered group had more high-intensity transcranial signals detected. Furthermore, there was a relationship between the number of high-intensity signals detected and the likelihood of having a neuropsychological deficit at 8 weeks post-surgery. A similar finding relating embolic load to neuropsychological deficits was made by Stump and colleagues (Stump et al., 1993). These authors found that of 167 patients undergoing elective coronary artery surgery, those with neuropsychological deficits at 5–7 days post-operatively had almost twice as many emboli detected in their left common carotid arteries as those without deficits. Barbut and colleagues showed that the number of emboli detected by transcranial Doppler ultrasonography in patients undergoing CABG surgery was significantly related to a number of adverse outcomes, including strokes and major cardiac complications as well as prolonged hospital stay (Barbut et al., 1997).

Further evidence for microembolic events being related to neurological injury has been found from post-mortem studies carried out by Moody and colleagues in patients who had recently undergone extracorporeal circulation (Moody et al., 1990; Moody et al., 1995; Stump et al., 1996). These workers found small capillary and arteriolar dilatations (SCADs) in all the brains when stained with alkaline phosphatase and these were felt to represent the 'footprints' of microemboli that have been removed by the reagents used in the staining process. These SCADs have not been seen in the brains of patients undergoing non-cardiac surgery and are thought to be formed by silicone or fat emboli from the circuit and suction lines.

USES OF FILTERS

Filters can be incorporated into a number of places in the extracorporeal circuit in order to minimize the embolic load presented to the patient (Marshall, 1988, 1992). The different types of filters available are listed in Table 7.1. Clear fluid filters include those for filtering crystalloid cardioplegia as well pre-bypass filters to clear the pump prime of any circulating debris. These are made from extremely fine membranes and range in size from 0.2 microns to 0.8 microns. All blood and blood products, as well as autologous blood that has been pre-donated or salvaged during the operation, are recommended to be filtered before infusion using 20–40 micron screen or depth filters (see below) to remove any cellular aggregates and other contaminants from the operative site. Incidentally, all transfusion products are depleted of leucocytes (and microaggregates) before being dispensed by blood banks in a number of countries to avoid transmission of infections such as new variant CJD and cytomegalovirus (CMV), and also to reduce other white cell-associated transfusion complications. Lastly, screen or depth filters are used in the arterial and cardiotomy lines to filter both particulate and gaseous microemboli from the circulating blood.

Table 7.1 *Summary of filter types*

Filter position	Pore size	Function
Pre-bypass filter	0.2–5.0 µ	Reduction of particulate contamination from circuit prime (Bacterial and endotoxin – 0.02 µ only)
Cardiotomy (integral)	20–200 µ	Reduction of gross particle and air emboli contamination from suction lines
Arterial line	20–200 µ	Reduction of particle and air embolic load in arterial line
Crystalloid cardioplegia	0.2–0.8 µ	Reduction of particulate contamination from cardioplegia (Bacterial and endotoxin – 0.2 µ only)
Gas line	0.02 µm	Reduction of particulate and microbial contamination from gas lines
Blood transfusions and salvaged blood	20–40 µ	Reduction of micro-aggregates and debris from stored or salvaged blood
Intra-aortic deployable	120–200 µ	Reduction of atherosclerotic plaque debris upon clamp removal

FILTER DESIGN

Safety of the patient is a prime consideration when using filters. They must be biocompatible and be of a pore size and configuration that does not cause trauma to blood components, both cells and proteins. Thus, ideally, haemolysis and thrombocytopenia should be minimal and inflammatory mediators should not be activated.

Filters used for retaining microemboli in the cardiotomy reservoir and the arterial filter are either of a screen or a depth design (but usually screen filters). Depth filters consist of a packed medium, such as Dacron wool or porous plastic foam, that creates multiple tortuous channels for the blood to traverse. Large particles are stopped at the surface of the filter and smaller ones continue through the channels (which present a large surface area to the blood) where they may impact and then adhere to the fibres, particularly at places where the blood flow changes directions (the emboli having greater inertia and thus tending to continue in the same direction). This type of filter becomes more efficient the deeper and narrower it is. The efficiency of filtration is also a function of the type of material used, the diameter of the fibres and how densely they are packed together (Swank and Seaman, 2000). Screen filters consist of a meshwork of woven polymer threads that have a specific pore size of 20–40 μm (most commonly 40 μm). All particles greater than the specified pore size will be stopped at the surface by direct interception. Their efficacy is improved by increasing their surface area and this is usually achieved by pleating.

Microbubbles larger than the pore size of the device will be prevented from crossing the filter until a certain pressure differential is reached across the filter medium, after which point they will be forced through. This is because adhesive forces hold a layer of water on the filter medium while cohesive forces hold water within the pores of the filter and these have to be displaced if the gas is to pass through the filter. The pressure required to do this is termed the bubble pressure point (BPP) and is determined by the pore diameter (d), the surface tension of the liquid (γ, a measure of cohesion) and the wetting angle of the liquid or solid (θ, a measure of adhesion), and is defined by the following formula:

$$BPP = \frac{4\gamma \cos\theta}{d}$$

The BPP for a 40-micron polyester screen filter is of the order of 37 mmHg, although the typical pressure across the filter is only a few mmHg (since there is such a large surface area present). As more gas bubbles are trapped at the filter surface, the available area open for filtration decreases and thus the pressure across the filter rises. Even if half the membrane surface was to be occluded, the pressure would double and still only be about 6 mmHg, well below the BPP. When gas is retained in the filter, it rises to a vent port and is led away by a vent line at the top of the filter to a low-pressure area, such as the oxygenator or cardiotomy reservoir. Reduction of micro-gas emboli prior to them challenging the screen filter can be enhanced further by careful design. By creating a tangential flow in a circular filter, a centrifuge effect can be induced in the blood flow that will 'squeeze' and separate the low-density gas bubbles towards the centre of the induced centrifugal flow. The natural buoyancy of gas emboli, with this centrifuge effect, will divert considerable amounts of air emboli to a central vent for removal. An additional coalescing ring downstream of the centrifuge may trap any micro-air emboli that escape the centrifuge effect. Other filters have an integral self-venting hydrophobic membrane that facilitates escape of collected gas out to the atmosphere and this also means there is no loss of flow because these filters do not require an open vent-line back to the venous reservoir to remove air emboli. Filter design, in terms of flow direction, also has a bearing on the efficiency of gas elimination, with top entry, circular flow designs being more effective than bottom blood entry filters (Spielberg and Matkovich, 1986).

ARTERIAL LINE FILTERS

Evidence of benefits

Many studies have been directed at evaluating the efficacy of arterial line filters. Guidon and colleagues compared three different filters (Dacron wool, polyester screen and polyurethane foam) in dogs and found that when clotted blood was infused into the circulation, all three filters were successful in trapping the debris and preventing emboli lodging in the pulmonary vasculature (Guidon *et al.*, 1976). Gourlay evaluated 13 different arterial line filters for their ability to handle both microbubbles and gross air. All the filters varied in their characteristics, with the Swank depth filter being most efficient (Gourlay and Taylor, 1988). The results did not, however, relate to filter pore size and all the filters were better than if none were present in the circuit. Turning to clinical studies, Pugsley used a transcranial Doppler system to demonstrate that inclusion of an arterial line filter in patients undergoing open heart surgery (with a bubble oxygenator) led to fewer microembolic events detected in the middle cerebral artery (Pugsley, 1989). Sellman and colleagues employed a pulsed Doppler ultrasound system to analyse both size and intensity of microbubbles in the arterial line of patients undergoing coronary artery surgery with a bubble oxygenator and found that use of an arterial line filter was associated with both a decrease in size and number of microbubbles detected (Sellman *et al.*, 1990). Other clinical studies have related adverse neurological outcome to arterial line filters not being included in the circuit, as described previously (Pugsley *et al.*, 1994; Barbut *et al.*, 1997). Taggart and co-workers recently showed that levels of S-100 protein (a specific astroglial cell protein whose level is thought to correlate with cerebral injury) were significantly reduced when they used an arterial line filter during elective coronary surgery (with a membrane oyxgenator) (Taggart *et al.*, 1997). Thus, there is good evidence that arterial line filters are effective in decreasing microembolic load to the patient as well as improving outcome.

Current status

The use of arterial line filters has increased over the last 20 years, although there was an initial drop after the introduction of membrane oxygenators. Silvay and co-workers questioned a range of people, including surgeons, perfusionists and anesthesiologists, at a meeting in 1993 and found that 92 per cent routinely used arterial line filters, in contrast with only 64 per cent in 1982 (Silvay *et al.*, 1995). A more recent review of perfusion practice between 1996 and 1998 in the USA revealed that 98.5 per cent of respondents used an arterial line filter (Mejak *et al.*, 2000).

LEUCOCYTE–DEPLETING FILTERS

Theoretical benefits of leucodepletion

Cardiopulmonary bypass results in the activation of a number of inflammatory and immune responses after the exposure of cellular and humoral components of blood to the foreign surfaces of the extracorporeal circuit. Further activation of the inflammatory system is stimulated by localized ischaemia followed by reperfusion, as well as by endotoxin released from the hypoperfused gastrointestinal tract (Kirklin, 1991; Asimakopoulos, 1999). This inflammatory response can lead to the clinical sequelae defined by the systemic inflammatory response syndrome (SIRS) and ranging from mild changes to multi-organ failure.

Neutrophils play a central role in this inflammatory process as well as in ischaemia–reperfusion injury. They are activated both directly and because of stimulation by a range of proinflammatory cytokines, including C3a and C5a, IL-1 and TNFα. The neutrophils, in turn, secrete a range of inflammatory mediators that further amplify the process by activating complement and recruiting more leucocytes. In addition to plugging capillaries, activated neutrophils express adhesion molecules on their surface, which allow them to bind to endothelial cells leading to the generation of oxygen-derived free radicals and the release of proteolytic enzymes, both of which lead to endothelial cell damage.

A number of strategies have been proposed to try and minimize this inflammatory response, and thus the clinical complications and cost that can ensue. One strategy is that of leucodepletion using specially designed filters (Ortalano, 1995). This can take the form of having a leucocyte-depleting filter in the arterial line, or else targeting the leucodepletion to the heart alone – either when cardioplegia is administered or during the period of coronary reperfusion. Additionally, salvaged blood or residual circuit blood can also be leuco-reduced by the use of specific filters before being reinfused. The role of leucocyte depletion in cardiac surgery has been the subject of two recent reviews (Matheis *et al.*, 2001; Morris, 2001). Although *in vitro* studies have shown the efficacy of leucodepleting filters in removing white cells, the results from clinical studies looking for improvements in clinical outcome have been more mixed.

In vitro studies

A number of *in vitro* studies have been conducted to ascertain whether leucocyte-depleting filters are efficient at decreasing circulating white cells. Thurlow and colleagues perfused an extracorporeal circuit, containing either a leucocyte-depleting filter or a standard arterial line filter, with human blood for 60 minutes. Among the variables studied, total white cell counts were monitored as well as the number of leucocytes expressing antigens associated with activation by the use of monoclonal antibodies. A 40 per cent reduction in leucocytes was seen in the leucocyte-depleting filter group, with neutrophils decreasing by 70 per cent, whereas the standard filter group had a minimal reduction in these two parameters (Thurlow *et al.*, 1995). The fall was steepest in the first 15 minutes of perfusion, after which a steady state was reached. The leucocyte-depleting filter group also showed a fall in leucocytes positive for CD67, CD11b, CD45Ro and L selectin (markers of activated leucocytes) while no consistent trend was seen in the other group, suggesting that activated leucocytes were possibly being removed by the leucocyte-depleting filters.

Similarly, another laboratory study found that leucodepletion of human blood was more effective during the first 30 minutes of perfusion through a leucocyte-depleting filter (Baksaas *et al.*, 1997). Here, white cell counts together with markers of complement and leucocyte activation were studied in both leucocyte-depleting filter and standard arterial filter groups over 2 hours of perfusion. Although the initial reduction of total white cells was more marked in the leucocyte-depleting filter group, overall leucocyte counts were not significantly different between the two groups. In contrast to the previous study, however, both groups had raised levels of myeloperoxidase (a marker of leucocyte degranulation), C3bc and TCC (complement activation products) and CD11b (an adhesion molecule present on activated neutrophils), with no significant intergroup differences. Again it was concluded that the levelling off of white cells might reflect a steady state in which the filter either released and trapped a similar number of cells or else became saturated. In this study, however, there was some evidence that perhaps neutrophils trapped on the filter were being activated preferentially.

Clinical studies of efficacy

What is clear from the *in vitro* studies is that the efficacy of leucocyte-depleting filters appears to decrease with time. This has been borne out by further clinical studies. Whilst evaluating a leucocyte-depleting filter for blood cardioplegia during routine cardiac surgery, the Heggie group found that the percentage of leucocyte reduction decreased with increasing volume of cardioplegia (Heggie *et al.*, 1998). Although overall leucocyte reduction in the cardioplegia was 70 per cent, that in the first 400 mL was 98.4 per cent as opposed to only 25 per cent for aliquots delivered above 4 L. Whilst the efficacy of the leucocyte-depleting filter decreased with increasing volume, it was shown to be safe to use, with low resistance, no haemolysis and a degree of platelet reduction comparable to standard arterial line filters. Similarly, Roth and colleagues found that the efficiency of their leucocyte-depleting filter decreased with each dose of blood cardioplegia delivered, leading these authors to conclude that the filter was only effective for the first 800 mL of cardioplegia (Roth *et al.*, 1997). The leucocyte depletion rates were improved when two leucocyte-depleting filters were used in series.

Leucocyte depletion throughout cardiopulmonary bypass

One approach to decrease white cell numbers has been to incorporate leucocyte-depleting filters in the arterial line for the whole period of extracorporeal circulation during open heart surgery. Studies have come to varied conclusions as to the clinical benefits gained by employing such a strategy.

In one study, 36 patients undergoing routine coronary artery or aortic valve surgery were randomized to either a leucocyte-depleting filter or standard arterial line filtration throughout cardiopulmonary bypass (Palanzo *et al.*, 1993). Post-operatively the patients in the leucocyte-depleting filter group had better arterial oxygenation and spent less time ventilated (both statistically significant). In addition, use of leucocyte-depleting filters was deemed to be cost effective, with an average saving of just under $3000 per patient.

A recent trial compared four different anti-inflammatory strategies (standard/aprotonin/leucocyte-depleting filter or heparin-bonded circuit) in 400 patients undergoing both coronary and valve surgery (Gott *et al.*, 1998). In the low risk patient group, use of a leucocyte-depleting filter led to average length of stay decreasing by 1 day and the average per patient cost falling by approximately $2000. Further evidence of biochemical and clinical benefit from use of a leucocyte-depleting arterial line filter came from a study by DiSalvo and colleagues who studied patients undergoing emergency coronary artery surgery. Both Troponin T and creatinine phosphokinase-MB (CKMB) levels were lower in the group with a leucocyte-depleting filter (DiSalvo *et al.*, 1996). Levels of total glutathione were higher in the leucocyte-depleting filter group, demonstrating that this group had been subjected to less oxidative stress, and there was also a lower incidence of arrhythmias and a greater tendency to return to sinus rhythm.

Although the above studies had a number of positive findings, there are other studies showing little if any benefit gained by the use of leucocyte-depleting filters over standard arterial line filters. A study of 32 patients undergoing CABG surgery found that the leucocyte-depleting filter group had significantly higher levels of elastase, again leading to the suggestion that the filter may be responsible for activating neutrophils (Mihaljevik *et al.*, 1995). The same study found no improvement in a number of respiratory parameters, including intubation time, oxygenation index and pulmonary vascular resistance. Similarly, Johnson and colleagues found that use of a leucocyte-depleting filter in CABG surgery did not benefit the patients. Other than an improved blood pressure and lower pulmonary shunt at a single time point (4 hours), there was no benefit to patients in terms of shorter hospital stay, improved cardiorespiratory status or lower levels of inflammatory markers such as IL6, TNFα and malondialdehyde (Johnson *et al.*, 1995).

Further evidence against the routine incorporation of a leucocyte-depleting arterial line filter came from a study which showed there was no significant difference in arterial oxygenation, time on a ventilator or hospital stay when compared with the use of a standard arterial filter (Lust *et al.*, 1996). Mair and colleagues found no beneficial changes in arterial oxygenation, inotrope requirement or levels of CKMB and Troponin I post-operatively in patients undergoing coronary surgery when a leucocyte-depleting filter was used compared with a conventional filter (Mair *et al.*, 1999). As in the study by Mihaljevik and co-workers, levels of plasma elastase were elevated in the leucocyte-depleting arterial filter group, although this did not lead to any adverse effects (Mihaljevik *et al.*, 1995). Thus, while there is some evidence that the use of leucocyte-depleting arterial line filters is cost effective and leads to some improvement in cardiac and respiratory function, much of the data point to little evidence of clinical benefit.

Leucodepletion after cross–clamp removal

Another strategy with leucocyte-depleting filters has been to incorporate them in the arterial line after removal of the aortic cross-clamp, so that leucocytes are depleted at the time that reperfusion of the myocardium and lungs takes place. This approach, also known as 'strategic leucocyte depletion', has been shown to be effective in decreasing white cell counts both during reperfusion and post-operatively in patients undergoing coronary surgery (Baksaas et al., 1999). The same study, failed however, to demonstrate any significant attenuation in the levels of a number of inflammatory markers, including myeloperoxidase, C3bc, TCC, IL-6 and IL-8. A fall in systemic leucocyte count when using a leucocyte-depleting arterial line filter during the period of reperfusion was also noted by a group that demonstrated a decrease in inotropic requirement, with a lower CKMB after coronary artery surgery (Hachida et al., 1995).

Leucodepletion of blood cardioplegia

Yet another way of employing leucocyte-depleting filters is to use them during delivery of blood cardioplegia to the myocardium. This strategy aims to decrease the number of leucocytes present in the capillaries of the myocardium during the period of ischaemia and thus to limit subsequent damage during the period of reperfusion. When this approach was applied to coronary artery surgery Browning and colleagues demonstrated effective leucocyte depletion in the cardioplegia delivered as demonstrated by previous authors (Browning et al., 1999; Heggie, 1998). No attenuation in the rise of oxidized glutathione gradient across the myocardium or reduction in post-operative CKMB or Troponin-T was observed in this study, however, suggesting that no additional protection was offered to the myocardium by this manoeuvre. De Vecchi and colleagues (1997) demonstrated that the use of leucocyte-depleted blood cardioplegia was clinically beneficial in patients with impaired left ventricular function undergoing coronary artery surgery (De Vecchi et al., 1997). They found that these patients had less evidence of lipid peroxidation and a trend to faster improvements in cardiac index. This finding was not mirrored in patients with normal ventricular function and may suggest that the compromised ventricle is more likely to benefit from strategies to improve myocardial function.

Leucodepletion of coronary reperfusate

Lastly, depleting leucocyte from blood reperfusing the coronary arteries after aortic cross-clamp removal has been investigated. An early study by Pearl and colleagues evaluated the effects of using leucodepleted blood to reperfuse transplanted human hearts. In a double-blind randomized trial in 20 patients undergoing orthotopic heart transplants, these authors perfused one group of 9 patients with warm whole blood and a second group with warm leucocyte-depleted blood for 10 minutes (with cardioplegia solution added for the first 3 minutes). They found significantly less coronary sinus release of CKMB and thromboxane B2 (a marker of leucocyte activation) in the leucodepletion group (Pearl et al., 1992). As well as biochemical evidence of decreased myocardial injury, there was also a trend towards a shorter duration of inotropic support in the leucodepleted group; however, there was no difference in clinical outcomes between the two groups.

The Sawa group looked at leucocyte-depleted blood reperfusion of the heart following both elective and emergency CABG surgery. Reperfusion of the heart with whole blood, terminal cardioplegia solution or leucocyte-depleted terminal cardioplegia solution was compared for both groups. In the emergency cases, the leucocyte-depleted group had significantly lower peaks of CKMB and less dopamine requirement at time of weaning from bypass compared with the other two groups, whereas no differences were noted in the elective CABG group (Sawa et al., 1994). This finding led these authors to conclude that leucodepletion of the coronary reperfusate may have a role in attenuating reperfusion injury when the myocardium is in a critical state, in this case ischaemic. The same group followed up this work by undertaking a similar protocol of reperfusion in patients with left ventricular hypertrophy (>300 mg) undergoing aortic valve replacements (Sawa et al., 1996). In addition to looking at biochemical markers of myocardial damage and leucocyte activation, biopsies were taken from the apex of the heart and scored for damage to myocardial and endothelial cells as well as the number of adherent neutrophils present. At 20 minutes after reperfusion, the leucocyte-depleted group had well preserved myocardium and less damage to both myocytes and endothelial cells than the other two groups, as well as less neutrophil adhesion. There was also a lower CKMB rise and less malondialdehyde in the coronary effluent in the leucodepletion group and a trend towards better cardiac indices. Thus, reperfusion of hearts with leucodepleted blood in these studies appears to lead to biochemical, structural and functional benefits.

Summary of leucodepletion

In summary, leucocyte-depleting filters attenuate the leucocytosis seen during and after cardiopulmonary bypass. The reason why the total leucocyte count does not fall per se may either be saturation of the filters or else the mobilization of white cells from the body's reserves.

The use of leucodepleting filters in certain circumstances appears to have some beneficial clinical effects. Certainly, they appear to be most effective in maintaining cardiac function both biochemically and functionally when used while reperfusing the aortic root after ischaemia or during a dose of terminal cardioplegia (hot shot). In addition, compromised left ventricles (e.g. hypertrophied or ischaemic) appear to benefit more than normal hearts.

SUMMARY

In conclusion, it is both desirable and standard practice to employ both cardiotomy and arterial line filters (Treasure, 1989; Mejak et al., 2000). Pre-bypass filters are also employed by the majority of people in the USA (Mejak et al., 2000). Evidence for the use of leucocyte-depleting arterial line filters is still mixed and this area requires further evaluation (Whitaker et al., 2001). Other novel uses for filters are also under review, such as an intra-aortic filter to prevent atheromatous debris from the aorta directly entering the systemic circulation (Reichenspurner et al., 2000). The area of filter use in cardiac surgery therefore remains an area of active research.

REFERENCES

Asimakopoulos, G. 1999: Mechanisms of the systemic inflammatory response. *Perfusion* **14**, 269–77.

Baksaas, S.T., Videm, V., Mollnes, T.E., Pedersen, T., Karlsen, H., Svennevig, J.L. 1997: Effects on complement, granulocytes and platelets of a leukocyte-depletion filter during *in vitro* extracorporeal circulation. *Scandinavian Cardiovascular Journal* **31**, 73–8.

Baksaas, S.T., Flom-Halvorsen, H.I., Øvrum, E., Videm, V., Mollnes, T.E., Brosstad, F. *et al.* 1999: Leucocyte filtration during cardiopulmonary reperfusion in coronary artery bypass surgery. *Perfusion* **14**, 107–17.

Bass, R.M., Longmore, D.B. 1969: Cerebral damage during open heart surgery. *Nature* **222**, 30.

Barbut, D., Gold, J.P. 1996: Aortic atheromatosis and risk of cerebral embolization. *Journal of Cardiothoracic and Vascular Anesthesia* **10**, 24–30.

Barbut, D., Lo, Y., Gold, J.P., Trifiletti, R.T., Yao, F.S., Hager, D.N. *et al.* 1997: Impact of embolisation during coronary artery bypass grafting on outcome and length of stay. *Annals of Thoracic Surgery* **63**, 998–1002.

Berman, L., Marin, F. 1986: Micropore filtration during cardio-pulmoanary bypass. In: Taylor KM, ed. *Cardiopulmonary Bypass. Principles and Management.* London: Chapman & Hall: 355–74.

Browning, P.G., Pullan, M., Jackson, M., Rashid, A. 1999: Leukocyte-depleted cardioplegia does not reduce reperfusion injury in hypothermic coronary artery bypass surgery. *Perfusion* **14**, 371–7.

Clark, R.E., Dietz, D.R., Miller, J.G. 1975: Continuous detection of microemboli during cardiopulmonary bypass in animals and man. *Circulation* **54**, 74–8.

De Vecchi, E., Paroni, R., Pala, M.G., Di Credico, G., Agape, V., Gobbi, C. *et al.* 1997: Role of leucocytes in free radical production during myocardial revascularisation. *Heart* **77**, 449–55.

DiSalvo, C., Louca, L.L., Pattichis, K., Hooper, J., Walesby, R.K. 1996: Does activated neutrophil depletion on bypass by leukocyte filtration reduce myocardial damage? *Journal of Cardiovascular Surgery* **37** (Suppl. 1, no 6), 93–100.

Gott, J.P., Cooper, W.A., Schmidt, F.E., Morris Brown, W., Wright, C.E., Merlino, J.D. *et al.* 1998: Modifying risk for extracorporeal circulation: trial of four antiinflammatory strategies. *Annals of Thoracic Surgery* **66**, 747–54.

Gourlay, T., Taylor, K.M. 1988: Evaluation of a range of arterial line filters: Part II. *Perfusion* **3**, 29–35.

Guidon, R., Laperche, Y., Martin, L., Awad, J. 1976: Disposable filters for microaggregate removal from extracorporeal circulation. *Journal of Thoracic and Cardiovascular Surgery* **71**, 502–16.

Hachida, M., Hanayama, N., Okamura, T., Akasawa, T., Maeda, T., Bonkohara, Y. *et al.* 1995: The role of leukocyte depletion in reducing injury to myocardium and lung injury during cardiopulmonary bypass. *ASAIO Journal* **41**, M291–M294.

Hearse, D.J., Erol, C., Robinson, L.A., Maxwell, M.P., Braimbridge, M.V. 1985: Particle-induced coronary vasoconstriction during cardioplegic infusion. *Journal of Thoracic and Cardiovascular Surgery* **89**, 428–38.

Heggie, A.J., Corder, J.S., Crichton, P.R., Hesford, J.W., Bingham, H., Jeffries, S. *et al.* 1998: Clinical evaulation of the new Pall leucocyte-depleting blood cardioplegia filter. *Perfusion* **13**, 17–25.

Hellinger, A., Piotrowski, J., Konerding, M.A., Burchard, W.G., Doetsch, N., Peitgen, K. *et al.* 1997: Impact of particulate contamination in crystalloid cardioplegic solutions: studies by scanning and transmission electron microscopy. *Thoracic and Cardiovascular Surgeon* **45**, 20–6.

Johnson, D., Thompson, D., Mycyk, T., Burnbridge, B., Mayers, I. 1995: Depletion of neutrophils by filter during aortocoronary bypass surgery transiently improves postoperative cardiorespiratory status. *Chest* **107**, 1253–9.

Kirklin, J.K. 1991: Prospects for understanding and eliminating the deleterious effects of cardiopulmonary bypass. *Annals of Thoracic Surgery* **51**, 529–31.

Lust, R.M., Bode, A.P., Yang, L., Hodges, W., Chitwood, W.R. 1996: In-line leukocyte filtration during bypass clinical results from a randomised prospective trial. *ASAIO Journal* **42**, M819–822.

Mair, P., Hoermann, C., Mair, J., Puschendorf, B., Balogh, D. 1999: Effects of a leucocyte depleting arterial line filter on perioperative proteolytic enzyme and oxygen free radical release in patients undergoing aortocoronary bypass surgery. *Acta Anaesthesiology Scandinavica* **43**, 452–7.

Marshall, L. 1988: Filtration in cardiopulmonary bypass: past, present and future. *Perfusion* **3**, 135–47.

Marshall, L. 1992: Filtration in cardiopulmonary bypass. In: Kay, P.H., ed. *Techniques in Extracorporeal Circulation.* Oxford: Butterworth-Heinemann: 56–71.

Matheis, G., Scholz, M., Simon, A., Dzemali, O., Moritz, A. 2001: Leukocyte filtration in cardiac surgery: a review. *Perfusion* **16**, 361–70.

Mejak, B.J., Stammers, A., Rauch, E., Vang, S., Viessman, T. 2000: A retrospective study on perfusion incidents and safety devices. *Perfusion* **15**, 51–61.

Mihaljevik, T., Tonz, M., von Segesser, L.K., Pasic, M., Grob, P., Fehr, J. et al. 1995: The influence of leukocyte filtration during cardiopulmonary bypass on postoperative lung function. *Journal of Thoracic and Cardiovascular Surgery* **109**, 1138–45.

Moody, D.M., Bell, M.A., Challa, V.R., Johnston, W.E., Prough, D.S. 1990: Brain microemboli during cardiac surgery or aortography. *Annals of Neurology* **28**, 477–86.

Moody, D.M., Brown, W.R., Challa, V.R., Stump, D.A., Reboussin, D.M., Legault, C. 1995: Brain microemboli associated with cardiopulmonary bypass: a histologic and magnetic resonance imaging study. *Annals of Thoracic Surgery* **59**, 1304–7.

Morris, S.J. 2001: Leukocyte reduction in cardiovascular surgery. *Perfusion* **16**, 371–80.

Nussmeier, N.A. 1996: Adverse neurological events: risks of intracardiac versus extracardiac surgery. *Journal of Cardiothoracic and Vascular Anesthesia* **10**, 31–7.

Orenstein, J.M., Sato, N., Aaron, B., Buchoholz, B., Bloom, S. 1982: Microemboli observed in deaths following cardiopulmonary bypass surgery: silicone antifoam agents and polyvinyl chloride tubing as sources of emboli. *Human Pathology* **13**, 1082–90.

Ortolano, G.A. 1995: Potential for reduction in morbidity and cost with total leucocyte control for cardiac surgery. *Perfusion* **10**, 283–90.

Osborn, J.J., Swank, R.L., Hill, J.D., Aguilar, M.J., Gerbode, F. 1970: Clinical use of a Dacron wool filter during perfusion for open-heart surgery. *Journal of Thoracic and Cardiovascular Surgery* **60**, 575–81.

Palanzo, D.A., Manley, N.J., Montesano, R.M., Yeisley, G.L., Gordon, D. 1993: Clinical evaluation of the Leukogard (LG-6) arterial line filter for routine open heart surgery. *Perfusion* **8**, 489–96.

Patterson, R.H., Twitchell, J.B. 1971: Disposable filter for microemboli, use in cardiopulmonary bypass and massive transfusions. *JAMA* **215**, 76–8.

Pearl, J.M., Drinkwater, D.C., Laks, H., Capouya, E.R., Gates, R.N. 1992: Leukocyte-depleted reperfusion of transplanted human hearts: a randomized, double-blind clinical trial. *Journal of Heart and Lung Transplantation* **11**, 1082–92.

Pearson, D.T. 1986: Microemboli: gaseous and particulate. In: Taylor, K.M., ed. *Cardiopulmonary Bypass. Principles and Management*. London: Chapman & Hall: 313–53.

Pugsley, W. 1989: The use of Doppler ultrasound in the assessment of microemboli during cardiac surgery. *Perfusion* **4**, 115–22.

Pugsley, W., Klinger, L., Paschalis, C., Treasure, T., Harrison, M., Newman, S. 1994: The impact of microemboli during cardiopulmonary bypass on neuropsychological functioning. *Stroke* **25**, 1393–9.

Reichenspurner, H., Navia, J.A., Berry, G., Robbins, R.C., Barbut, D., Gold, J.P. et al. 2000: Particulate emboli capture by an intra-aortic filter device during cardiac surgery. *Journal of Thoracic and Cardiovascular Surgery* **119**, 233.

Robinson, L.A., Braimbridge, M.V., Hearse, D.J. 1984: The potential hazard of particulate contamination of cardioplegic solutions. *Journal of Thoracic and Cardiovascular Surgery* **87**, 48–58.

Roth, M., Bauer, E.P., Reuthebuch, O., Klovekorn, W.P. 1997: Single leukocyte filter (Pall BC1B) fails in multidose cold blood cardioplegia. *Journal of Thoracic and Cardiovascular Surgery* **113**, 1116–17.

Sawa, Y., Matsuda, H., Shimazaki, Y., Kaneko, M., Nishimura, M., Amemiya, A. et al. 1994: Evaluation of leukocyte-depleted terminal blood cardioplegic solution in patients undergoing elective and emergency coronary artery bypass grafting. *Journal of Thoracic and Cardiovascular Surgery* **108**, 1125–31.

Sawa, Y., Taniguchi, K., Kadoba, K., Nishimura, M., Ichikawa, H., Amemiya, A. et al. 1996: Leukocyte depletion attenuates reperfusion injury in patients with left ventricular hypertrophy. *Circulation* **93**, 1640–6.

Sellman, M., Ivert, T., Stensved, P., Hogberg, M., Semb, B.K.H. 1990: Doppler ultrasound estimation of microbubbles in the arterial line during extracorporeal circulation. *Perfusion* **5**, 23–32.

Silvay, G., Ammar, T., Reich, D.L., Vela-Cantos, F., Joffe, D., Ergin, A.M.J. 1995: Cardiopulmonary bypass for adult patients: a survey of equipment and techniques. *Cardiothoracic and Vascular Anesthesia* **9**, 420–4.

Spielberg, R., Matkovich, V.I. 1986: Gas microemboli – detection, quantitation and elimination. *Chemical Engineering Communication* **47**, 175–83.

Stump, D.A., Tegeler, C.H., Rogers, A.T. 1993: Neuropsychological deficits are associated with the number of emboli detected during cardiac surgery. *Stroke* **24**, 509.

Stump, D.A., Rogers, A.T., Hammon, J.W., Newman, S.T. 1996: Cerebral emboli and cognitive outcome after cardiac surgery. *Journal of Cardiothoracic and Vascular Anaesthesia* **10**, 113–19.

Swank, R.L. 1961: Alteration of blood on storage: measurement of adhesiveness of ageing platelets and leukocytes and their removal by flitration. *New England Journal of Medicine* **265**, 728–33.

Swank, R.L., Seaman, G.V.F. 2000: Microfiltration and micoemboli: a history. *Transfusion* **40**, 114–19.

Taggart, D.P., Bhattacharya, K., Meston, N., Standing, S., Kay, J.D.S., Pillai, R. et al. 1997: Serum S-100 protein concentration after cardiac surgery: a randomized trial of arterial line filtration. *European Journal of Cardiothoracic Surgery* **11**, 645–9.

Thurlow, P.J., Doolan, L., Sharp, R., Sullivan, M., Smith, B. 1995: Studies of the effect of Pall leucocyte filters LG6 and AV6 in an *in vitro* simulated extracorporeal circulatory system. *Perfusion* **10**, 291–300.

Treasure, T. 1989: Interventions to reduce cerebral injury during cardiac surgery – the effect of arterial line filtration. *Perfusion* **4**, 147–52.

Utley, J.R. 1996: Techniques for avoiding neurological injury during cardiac surgery. *Journal of Cardiothoracic and Vascular Anaesthesia* **10**, 38–44.

Whitaker, D.C., Stygall, J.A., Newman, S.P., Harrison, M.J. 2001: The use of leucocyte-depleting and conventional arterial line filters in cardiac surgery: a systematic review of clinical studies. *Perfusion* **16**, 433–6.

8

The inflammatory response to cardiopulmonary bypass

SAEED ASHRAF

KEY POINTS

- Cardiopulmonary bypass produces a whole-body inflammatory response, characterized by disturbances in vascular tone, fluid shifts, capillary permeability, and blood and organ dysfunction.
- This inflammatory response is initiated by contact of blood with the extracorporeal circuit and is mediated by a number of complex biochemical pathways.
- Although complex, an understanding of these pathways may help in devising strategies to attenuate the inflammatory response.
- A number of therapeutic modalities have been shown to reduce the inflammatory response 'in the test tube', but have not found widespread clinical application.
- Improving biocompatibilty by the use of heparin-bonded circuits has major potential for reducing the inflammatory response in the clinical setting.
- Development of severe systemic inflammatory response syndrome (SIRS), whilst rare, requires active supportive medical management.

INTRODUCTION

The cornerstone of the astonishing progress in cardiac surgery has been the development of cardiopulmonary bypass involving extracorporeal circulation. Whilst modern cardiopulmonary bypass makes open heart surgery possible, it also induces a physiological challenge to body systems. In most patients, the functional reserves of injured organs are sufficient to overcome this trauma, but in severely ill patients and those at the extremes of age, the morbidity of cardiopulmonary bypass may influence operative outcome. Cardiopulmonary bypass damages specific blood elements, introduces emboli and, more importantly, initiates a series of complex reactions that attempt to defend the body against bleeding, thrombosis and invasion by foreign organisms and substances. These defence reactions during and after cardiopulmonary bypass create disturbances in vascular tone, fluid balance, capillary permeability, blood and organ function that are collectively described as the 'whole-body inflammatory response' (Chenoweth et al., 1981; Kirklin et al., 1983; Kirklin, 1991). This whole-body inflammatory response (or 'post-pump' syndrome) is caused by the interaction of blood with non-endothelial surface, as well as turbulence, cavitation, osmotic forces and shear stresses. These factors not only activate but also injure blood elements (Kirklin *et al.*, 1983; Kirklin and Barratt-Boyes, 1986). Clinically, this syndrome is characterized by hypotension and coagulopathy, and has been linked to post-operative organ dysfunction (Casey, 1993). This 'post-pump' syndrome tends to be more common in infants than older children (Kirklin *et al.*, 1983; Kirklin *et al.*, 1986) and is thus being seen more frequently with the trend towards definitive corrective operations in the neonatal period (Sethia, 1992; Ashraf *et al.*, 1998b).

MEDIATORS OF THE INFLAMMATORY RESPONSE

Blood is a complex fluid made up of both formed and unformed elements. The formed elements include erythrocytes, leucocytes and platelets. Among the unformed elements, the plasma proteins may be particularly vulnerable to cardiopulmonary bypass. Activation of these blood elements initiates a number of biological pathways, including the coagulation, fibrinolytic, kallikrein and complement cascades and cytokines.

The coagulation, fibrinolytic and kallikrein systems

Immediately after the onset of bypass, Hageman factor (Factor XII) is activated because of massive contact of

blood with non-endothelial surfaces (Verska, 1977). Factor XII then activates not only the coagulation cascade but also other cascades. Even with appropriate heparinization during bypass, there is evidence of ongoing micro-coagulation, with consumption of clotting factors. The onset of cardiopulmonary bypass also activates the fibrinolytic cascades, and increased levels of the active fibrinolytic agent, plasmin, have been detected shortly after the initiation of cardiopulmonary bypass (Backmann *et al.*, 1975). Plasmin may further activate pre-kallikrein, the complement system and Hageman factor. The kallikrein cascade is activated by Hageman factor and by other events, and results in the production of bradykinin, which in turn increases vascular permeability, dilates arterioles, initiates smooth muscle contraction and generates pain (Ellison *et al.*, 1980). Kallikrein itself can activate Hageman factor and can also activate plasminogen to form plasmin, which illustrates the complex interaction between these systems (Figure 8.1).

Complement activation

Complement is a group of circulating glycoproteins that become activated in response to immunological, traumatic, infectious or foreign-body stimulus. Two pathways exist for complement activation: the classic pathway, which is usually initiated via interaction with antigen–antibody complexes, and the alternative or properdin pathway, activated by exposure of blood to foreign surfaces.

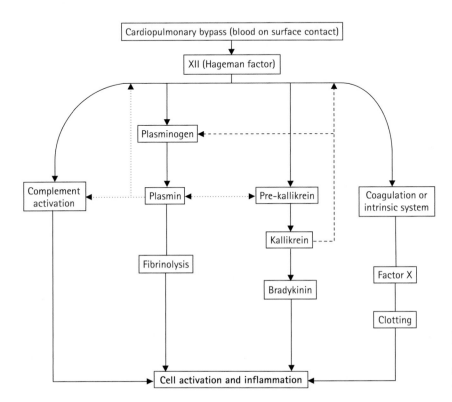

Figure 8.1 *Induction of coagulation, fibrinolytic, kallikrein and complement systems after contact of blood with the cardiopulmonary bypass circuit.*

Complement activation during cardiopulmonary bypass leads to the formation of anaphylatoxin C3a and C5a mainly via the alternative pathway (Chenoweth *et al.*, 1981; Kirklin *et al.*, 1983). Activation of the classic pathway, which is generally recognized by C4a formation, occurs at blood or air interfaces (Chenoweth *et al.*, 1981) and through the formation of heparin–protamine complexes (Fehr and Rohr, 1983; Kirklin *et al.*, 1986). The anaphylatoxins C3a and C5a have similar physiological effects in many patients after cardiopulmonary bypass, including vasoconstriction and increased capillary permeability (Bjork *et al.*, 1985). Complement activation has been demonstrated during operative procedures without cardiopulmonary bypass, but the magnitude of activation is relatively small compared with that during cardiopulmonary bypass. Furthermore, the level of the C3a remains normal throughout cardiac operations not involving cardiopulmonary bypass (Kirklin *et al.*, 1983).

The level of C3a rises dramatically with commencement of cardiopulmonary bypass and peaks at the end of bypass. Its level is related to the duration of cardiopulmonary bypass and returns to pre-cardiopulmonary bypass values after 48 hours (Kirklin *et al.*, 1983). Less substantial generation of C3a can be induced by plasmin and kallikrein (Ward *et al.*, 1983). An overall index of morbidity was also determined, which related significantly to higher levels of C3a, longer duration of cardiopulmonary bypass, and younger age at operation (Kirklin *et al.*, 1983). C5a receptor sites have been demonstrated on human neutrophils by Chenoweth and Hugli (1978). Activation of the alternative pathway produces C5a, which then rapidly binds to neutrophils (limiting its detection in plasma during bypass), resulting in adherence of neutrophils to vascular endothelium (Charo *et al.*, 1986) and is a potentially important event at the time of organ reperfusion. Fosse and colleagues (Fosse *et al.*, 1987, 1994, 1997) also demonstrated increased levels of the terminal complement complex (TCC[C5b-9]) shortly after initiation of cardiopulmonary bypass. The TCC represents the end product of complement activation and requires splitting of C5 into C5a and C5b (Figure 8.2). Patients undergoing thoracotomy without cardiopulmonary bypass show no increase in TCC (Fosse *et al.*, 1987). During cardiopulmonary bypass, deposition of the terminal C5b-9 complement complex on erythrocytes and neutrophils has been demonstrated, which results in intravascular haemolysis and neutrophil activation, respectively (Salama *et al.*, 1988). Since, unlike the anaphylatoxins, this complex is neither rapidly degraded nor bound to specific cell surface receptors, it remains in the plasma as a useful marker of recent complement activation.

Although the widespread inflammatory reaction to cardiopulmonary bypass affects whole body systems, the lung appears particularly susceptible to this challenge, and thus has been studied as a model for the specific organ sequelae of cardiopulmonary bypass (Tennenberg *et al.*, 1990). The causes of post-bypass pulmonary damage are multifactorial, but the neutrophil has generated the greatest current interest as a mediator of this damage. It is hypothesized that a portion of the pulmonary dysfunction after cardiopulmonary bypass results from complement activation via the alternative pathway leading to the generation of the anaphylatoxins C3a and C5a. The C5a is rapidly bound through its receptors to circulating neutrophils, which are then activated and undergo deposition and sequestration in the lung and other organs. The activated neutrophils release superoxide and lysosomal enzymes, which induce direct endothelial damage, alterations in capillary permeability, and accumulation of extravascular water. By using models of complement activation, it has been possible to demonstrate leucopenia, rises in pulmonary artery pressure and impaired oxygenation. These changes are accompanied by histological evidence of sequestration of leucocytes in the capillary bed with endothelial cell damage (Craddock *et al.*, 1977).

Hypothermic cardiopulmonary bypass in neonates and children is often associated with 'capillary leak syndrome', defined as the development of non-cardiogenic generalized oedema, including pleural effusions and/or ascites and blood pressure instability, necessitating volume substitution. There is widespread tissue oedema and an increase in total body water (Maehara *et al.*, 1991; George, 1993), and the syndrome is more marked in small babies of low body weight, undergoing long periods of bypass, with haemodilution. The consequences of capillary leak may be serious, as tissue oedema may lead ultimately

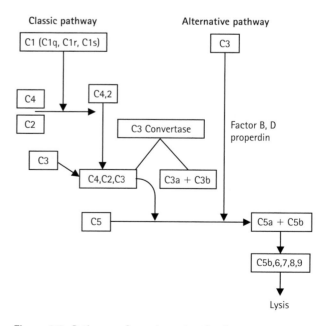

Figure 8.2 *Pathways of complement activation.*

to organ dysfunction, and in particular pulmonary- and cardiac-related morbidity (Elliott *et al.*, 1990). A number of mechanisms may contribute to this process, ranging from the direct physical consequences of haemodilution to fluid overload and the systemic inflammation (Elliott, 1993). Neonates and young children have not yet been fully characterized with respect to their induced inflammatory response. Neonates are reported to have subnormal activity of both the alternative and classical pathway of the complement system compared with adults (Strunk *et al.*, 1979) and immaturity of complement receptors on neutrophils (Melvin, 1990), although Seghaye *et al.* (1993) reported significant complement activation and leucocyte stimulation in neonates and young children undergoing cardiopulmonary bypass. Despite the relatively high prevalence of post-operative 'capillary leak syndrome', in neonates, data on the influence of risk factors, including cardiopulmonary bypass-related inflammatory reaction, are lacking.

Neutrophil activation

Neutrophils are activated during cardiopulmonary bypass by activated complement system (Salama *et al.*, 1988) and also by kallikrein that is cleaved from pre-kallikrein after reaction of Factor XII with the foreign surface. Kallikrein also directly activates neutrophils (Wachtfogel *et al.*, 1983, 1987). Activated neutrophils release powerful proteolytic enzymes, including elastase, collagenase, acid hydrolases, and cathapsin G and D (Wachtfogel *et al.*, 1987; Hind *et al.*, 1988; Butler *et al.*, 1993a). Other active components released by neutrophils include superoxides, hydrogen peroxide, myeloperoxidase, lactoferrin and thromboxane A (Royston *et al.*, 1986; Wachtfogel *et al.*, 1987; Riegel *et al.*, 1988).

An immediate fall in leukocyte numbers with loss of mature granulocytes occurs at the onset of cardiopulmonary bypass, due to a combination of haemodilution, adhesion of neutrophils to the absorbed protein layer in the bypass circuit and pulmonary vascular leucosequestration (Martin *et al.*, 1982; Stahl *et al.*, 1991; Finn *et al.*, 1993). At the end of cardiopulmonary bypass, this transient leucopenia is followed by leucocytosis, especially during rewarming and after the release of the aortic cross-clamp (Finn *et al.*, 1993; Butler *et al.*, 1993b). This rebound leucocytosis is related to the increase in body temperature that is thought to increase blood flow to the bone marrow and induce the mobilization of marginated cells with release of immature neutrophils. Post-operatively, this leucocytosis persists for several days (Ryhanen *et al.*, 1979). There is a positive correlation between the extent of pulmonary vascular leucosequestration, the length of aortic cross-clamp time and total duration of cardiopulmonary bypass (Chenoweth *et al.*, 1981). It has

been claimed that bubble oxygenators cause significantly more leukocyte sequestration than silicone membrane oxygenators (Cavarocchi *et al.*, 1986). Leucocyte activation has been assessed by the release of myeloperoxidase, lactoferrin and plasma leucocyte elastase (Butler *et al.*, 1993b; Fosse *et al.*, 1994, 1997; Menasche *et al.*, 1994, 1995; Ashraf *et al.*, 1997a,b,c, 1998a). The role of plasma lactoferrin remains uncertain, but it has been shown that levels peak before cardiopulmonary bypass (Wachtfogel *et al.*, 1987), with potential increase in production of oxygen-derived free radicals (Ambruso and Johnston, 1981). Lactoferrin and myeloperoxidase, synthesized in early myeloid cells and stored in the granules of the neutrophils, are the mediators of the inflammatory response. Increased levels of myeloperoxidase have been demonstrated during cardiopulmonary bypass both *in vitro* (Havermann and Gramse, 1984) and *in vivo* (Venge *et al.*, 1987; Riegel *et al.*, 1988; Fosse *et al.*, 1994, 1997), as well as during haemodialysis (Horl *et al.*, 1987).

Neutrophil elastase is of importance because of its high intracellular concentration and low substrate specificity. It lies within the azurophilic granules of the neutrophil and is released upon degranulation or disintegration. It is a potent enzyme, and changes in coagulation proteases (McGuire *et al.*, 1982), platelet Gp-Ib hydrolysis (Brower *et al.*, 1985) and exposure of fibrinogen receptors on the platelet surface (Kornecki *et al.*, 1986) are just some of its effects that may be of relevance to the haemorrhagic complications of prolonged cardiopulmonary bypass. Endothelial functional integrity can be damaged by adherent neutrophil release of this enzyme by degrading collagen, elastin, proteoglycan and fibronectin, which form much of the endothelial extracellular matrix and basement membrane (Finn *et al.*, 1993; Fosse *et al.*, 1994, 1997). Free circulating elastase is rapidly bound to the protease inhibitor α1-antitrypsin, and elevated levels of this complex, a marker of neutrophil degranulation, have been detected in patients with acute inflammatory states such as sepsis (Speer *et al.*, 1986), the haemolytic uremic syndrome (Fitzpatrick *et al.*, 1992) as well as after cardiopulmonary bypass (Faymonville *et al.*, 1991; Finn *et al.*, 1993; Fosse *et al.*, 1994; Ashraf *et al.*, 1997a,b,c, 1998a,b). The half-life of elastase-α1-antiprotease complex in plasma is about 1–2 hours (Wachtfogel *et al.*, 1987). During cardiopulmonary bypass the level of elastase-α1-antiprotease complex increases progressively and peaks 1–3 hours after operation (Butler *et al.*, 1993b; Finn *et al.*, 1993; Menasche *et al.*, 1994, 1995; Ashraf *et al.*, 1997a,b,c, 1998a,b). Elastase levels are correlated with duration of cardiopulmonary bypass (Hind *et al.*, 1988, Butler *et al.*, 1993b), suggesting neutrophil degranulation or injury during the period of extracorporeal circulation. Despite peripheral neutrophil activation it is probable that intrapulmonary tissue injury is more closely related to intra-alveolar elastase release (Rocker *et al.*, 1989).

Cytokines

The term 'cytokine' was introduced to group together a number of hormone-like proteins, many of which have been known for quite some time under individual names such as interferon, lymphokine, interleukin, lymphotoxin, lymphocyte activating factor, and others. During the last 10 years, the field of cytokine biology has seen enormous expansion.

CHARACTERISTIC FEATURES OF CYTOKINES

Cytokines are endogenous polypeptides or glycoproteins with a molecular weight generally less than 30 kDa (some cytokines may form higher-molecular-weight oligomer) and produced by a variety of cell types. Their production is usually low or absent and regulated by various inducing stimuli at the level of transcription or translation. Cytokine production is transient and the radius of action is usually short (typical action is autocrine or paracrine, not endocrine) and they produce their action by binding to specific high-affinity cell surface receptors. Most cytokine actions can be attributed to an altered pattern of gene expression in the target cells and thus they serve as intercellular signalling molecules and participate in the regulation of cellular growth, function and differentiation (Evans and Whicher, 1993).

One of the most important feature of cytokines is their ability to stimulate or inhibit the production of other cytokines, that is, function as a cascade system. As a result, many cytokine actions are indirect, that is, caused by an increase or decrease in the level of production of other cytokines, which then results in altered biological response. An example of such mechanisms of cytokine action are the stimulatory effect of IL-1 on IL-2 production and role of this interaction in T-cell proliferation (Evans and Whicher, 1993). In addition to its effect on IL-2, IL-1 also stimulates the production of IL-6 (Tosato and Jones, 1990), IL-8 (Matsushima and Oppenheim, 1989) and monocyte chemotactic and activating factor (MCAF) (Larsen et al., 1989). All of these cytokines are also induced by tumour necrosis factor (TNF), in accordance with the many other similarities seen between the action of IL-1 and TNF. In monocytes both TNF and IL-1 are also autostimulatory and, in addition, stimulate each other's production (Dinarello, 1988).

In addition, there is increasing evidence of the inhibitory action of cytokine on cytokine production. Cytokine inhibitors can be divided into three groups: cytokines themselves; cytokine receptor antagonists; and cytokine-binding molecules. Many cytokines can inhibit or antagonize the activity of other cytokines. Two important examples are interleukin-10 (IL-10) and transforming growth factor-β (TGF-β) (Sironi et al., 1993). IL-10

(originally called 'cytokine synthesis inhibitory factor', appears to act chiefly as an inhibitor of cytokine synthesis) suppresses the in vitro production of TNF-α, IL-1, IL-6 and IL-8 (Fiorentino et al., 1991), whereas TGF-β is a potent inhibitor of IL-1 activity and it has been suggested that this effect is mediated by inhibition of IL-1 receptor expression (Dubois et al., 1990). One example of cytokine receptor antagonist is an IL-1 receptor antagonist (IL-1ra), a naturally occurring antagonist of IL-1 activity (Hannum et al., 1990).

Although complement activation has been incriminated for many years in the development of acute lung and organ injury after cardiopulmonary bypass, more recent studies question the role of complement (Tennenberg et al., 1990). Cytokines are now thought to play an essential role in the pathogenesis of shock and multiple organ failure during sepsis (Glauser et al., 1991), and after cardiopulmonary bypass (Casey, 1993). Several studies have now shown that surgical procedures using cardiopulmonary bypass (both adult and paediatric) cause release of systemic pro-inflammatory cytokines, including TNF-α (Jansen et al., 1991, 1992; Menasche et al., 1994; Hennein et al., 1994), IL-1β (Haeffner-Cavaillon et al., 1989; Menasche et al., 1994), IL-6 (Kawamura et al., 1993; Steinberg et al., 1993; Hennein et al., 1994; Menasche et al., 1994; Butler et al., 1996; Ashraf et al., 1997a,b,c, 1998a,b) and IL-8 (Finn et al., 1993; Kalfin et al., 1993; Kawamura et al., 1993; Steinberg et al., 1993; Hennein et al., 1994; Menasche et al., 1994, 1995; Kawahito et al., 1995; Wan et al., 1996b,c; Ashraf et al., 1997a,b,c, 1998a,b) (Figure 8.3). These important pro-inflammatory cytokines, which are potentially involved in 'post-pump syndrome', are discussed in the following section.

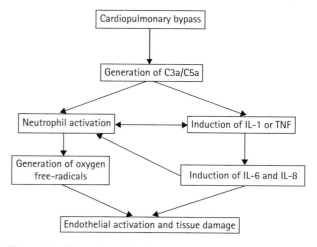

Figure 8.3 Flow chart: induction of cytokines occurring as a consequence of the initial generation of C3a/C5a and neutrophil activation.

INTERLEUKIN-1 (IL-1)

Interleukin-1 was the first leukocyte-derived cytokine to be studied extensively. It represents two biochemically distinct but structurally related molecules, IL-1α and IL-1β (17.5-kDa proteins). These are primarily derived from stimulated mononuclear phagocytes (Haeffner-Cavaillon et al., 1989). Endotoxins (lipopolysaccharide) (Dinarello, 1988, 1989), human complement-derived fragments C5a/C5a desArg (Okusawa et al., 1990) and C3a/C3a desArg (Haeffner-Cavaillon et al., 1987) induce monocytes to produce IL-1 in vitro after a brief exposure period. IL-1α and IL-1β are also produced by several other nucleated cell types, including tissue macrophages, polymorphnuclear leukocytes (PMN), endothelial cells and fibroblasts (Dinarello, 1991). On stimulation of cells, IL-1 genes are transcribed and translated into two precursor polypeptides that are processed by serine proteases into intracellular active forms of IL-1.

Intracellular IL-1, which represents processed IL-1α and IL-1β, has been measured antigenically in cell lysates (Haeffner-Cavaillon et al., 1987, 1989). IL-1 directly mediates multiple aspects of host inflammatory response, including fever, synthesis of hepatic acute phase proteins, release of growth factors and immunoregulatory cytokines, changes in endothelial cell function and permeability, and decreased vascular resistance (Dinarello, 1988, 1989; Butler et al., 1993b). IL-1 has been implicated in the pathogenesis of many different disease states, especially inflammatory and auto-immune disorders. Haeffner-Cavaillon et al. (1989) have shown transiently increased production of IL-1β after cardiopulmonary bypass, maximal at 24 hours, coinciding with a peak in body temperature. In their study, IL-1β production was assessed by measuring functional activity and IL-1 antigen concentration in cell lysates from monocytes of patients during and after cardiopulmonary bypass. By contrast, both plasma IL-1α and IL-1β were not detected in other studies (Finn et al., 1993; Steinberg et al., 1993; Ashraf et al., 1997a,b, 1998a), perhaps reflecting a more important role as a paracrine mediator (Fong et al., 1990) and therefore low circulating concentration. Although there may exist more than one receptor, IL-1α and IL-β seems to cross-react with at least one particular receptor that occur on many different cell types (Moldawer et al., 1987).

TUMOUR NECROSIS FACTOR

Tumour necrosis factor (TNF) was originally described as a leukocyte-derived endotoxin-induced factor, responsible for in vivo and in vitro tumour necrosis, and as cachectin, a molecule that caused the wasting associated with chronic infection (Beutler and Cerami, 1986, 1987). Cachectin/TNF (17-kDa polypeptide) is predominantly macrophage-derived and is termed TNF-α; lymphotoxin TNF is T-cell-derived and is known as TNF-β. Factors triggering TNF synthesis include C5a (Okusawa et al., 1990), IL-1β and Gram-negative endotoxin (Beutler and Cerami, 1987).

In vitro studies have demonstrated that TNF causes induction of the acute phase response by increasing the synthesis of hepatic proteins (Permutter et al., 1986). Its effects on neutrophils include production of oxidative burst, degranulation, increased phagocytic activity and increased expression of leukocyte adhesion molecules (Klebanoff et al., 1986; Tracey et al., 1989). It is detected in the serum of patients experiencing various diseases, including parasitic (Scuderi et al., 1986) and bacterial infections (Waage et al., 1987), different malignant diseases (Balkwill et al., 1987), renal allograft rejection (Maury and Teppo, 1987) and fulminent hepatic failure (Muto et al., 1988). Recently, it has also been implicated in septic lung injury (Marks et al., 1990) and post-ischaemic myocardial depression ('stunning') after cardiopulmonary bypass (Finkel et al., 1992). Some of these effects may be mediated by increased production of nitric oxide with cardiac myocytes (Finkel et al., 1992; Kapadia et al., 1995). Other main targets of TNF-α and IL-1β, are the vessel wall, where these cytokines cause peripheral vasodilatation (Menasche et al., 1994).

However, according to recent literature, the TNF response to cardiopulmonary bypass provides conflicting evidence. No significant detection of plasma TNF has been observed in some studies (Butler et al., 1992; Finn et al., 1993; Steinberg et al., 1993; Seghaye et al., 1996; Ashraf et al., 1997a,b,c, 1998a), whereas Jansen et al. (1991) have shown a significant increase in TNF after the removal of aortic cross-clamp, which was inhibited by dexamethasone administration. Unresolved issues in the measurement of circulating cytokines (mainly IL-1 and TNF following cardiopulmonary bypass) include effects of binding to plasma proteins, assay inhibition by specific plasma proteins, rapid degradation by plasma protease, rapid clearance from the circulation by cell receptors, and transiently elevated levels that are easily missed (Dinarello, 1989).

INTERLEUKIN-6 (IL-6)

IL-6 is a family of at least six differentially modified phosphoglycoproteins. It was isolated independently for its multiple biologic properties and has variously been described as β2-interferon, hepatocyte-stimulating factor, B-cell differentiation factor BSF-2 and hybridoma growth factor (Tosato et al., 1988). IL-6 (26-kDa polypeptide) is a pleiotropic cytokine synthesized by monocytes, endothelial cells and fibroblasts during systemic inflammation and plays a central role in the modulation of the acute phase response (Gieger *et al.*, 1988; Fong *et al.*, 1990). In addition to IL-1 and TNF-α, IL-6 is also the major inducer of the synthesis of acute phase proteins such as C-reactive protein (CRP) by hepatocytes. The 'acute phase response' refers to the large and diverse systemic and metabolic changes that occur in response to events such as trauma and infection. This response is characterized by fever, leucocytosis, thrombocytosis, alteration in the serum concentration of zinc, copper and iron, and release of prostaglandins, leucotrienes, vaso-active amines and increase in acute phase proteins (Nijsten *et al.*, 1987; Heinrich *et al.*, 1990; Butler *et al.*, 1993b). A number of cytokines have been implicated as endogenous pyrogens, including IL-1, TNF-α, interferon-γ, IL-6 and IL-8, but IL-1 and IL-6 are considered the most potent (Nijsten *et al.*, 1987), whereas IL-1, TNF and interferon-β are known to induce the production of IL-6 (Akira *et al.*, 1993).

IL-6 has been detected in serum after burn injury (Nijsten *et al.*, 1987), after elective operation (Butler *et al.*, 1996) and in septic patients (Hack *et al.*, 1989; Billiau and Vandekerckhove, 1991). In response to cardiopulmonary bypass, IL-6 level tends to rise at the time of rewarming reaching its peak 2–4 hours after the completion of cardiopulmonary bypass, before returning to baseline within 48 hours (Steinberg *et al.*, 1993; Butler *et al.*, 1996; Cremer *et al.*, 1996; Seghaye *et al.*, 1996; Ashraf *et al.*, 1997a,b,c, 1998a,b). After cardiopulmonary bypass, fever, leucocytosis, a negative nitrogen balance, increased vascular permeability, and an increase in the synthesis of acute phase response proteins are all compatible with IL-6 release, and the pattern of the IL-6 response (peaking at 4 hours and remaining high at 24 hours post-operation) is consistent with a role as a major mediator of the acute phase response to cardiopulmonary bypass. Salas *et al.* (1990) have shown that, as with several other monocyte-derived cytokines, IL-6 can act on the hypothalamic– pituitary–adrenal axis as well as directly on adrenal cells to release ACTH and corticosteroid into the plasma, respectively, which in turn exert an overall immunosuppressive and anti-inflammatory effect. Moreover, IL-6 may exert anti-inflammatory effects through its ability to inhibit production of other cytokines, such as TNF (Aderka *et al.*, 1989). A counter-regulatory role for systemic IL-6 is also suggested by the observation that in severe infections, peak serum levels of IL-6 follow those of TNF-α and IL-1 (Waage *et al.*, 1989; Lotz, 1993).

INTERLEUKIN-8 (IL-8)

IL-8 is a 10 kDa peptide and was the first known chemoattractant specific for neutrophils. IL-1 and TNF induce the release of IL-8 from fibroblasts (Mielke *et al.*, 1990), endothelial cells (Herbert and Baker, 1993), alveolar macrophages and leucocytes, including neutrophils themselves (Bazzoni *et al.*, 1991). Among cytokines, only IL-1 and TNF have been shown to stimulate IL-8 gene expression at the transcription level. This increase in transcription is rapid, being seen within 1 hour of stimulation and reaching a peak at around 3 hours before falling (Matsushima and Oppenheim, 1989; Finn *et al.*, 1993; Kawahito *et al.*, 1995; Ashraf *et al.*, 1997a,b,c, 1998a,b).

The main activity ascribed to IL-8 is neutrophil chemotaxis, but it may also cause oxygen radical and enzyme release by neutrophils. IL-8 interacts with neutrophils by binding to specific receptors which have been characterized and are distinct from receptors for other cytokines and chemotactic agents such as IL-1, TNF, C5a and platelet activating factor (Samanta *et al.*, 1990). IL-8 appears rapidly to downregulate expression of its receptors on the surface of neutrophils, a process which appears to be accompanied by proteolytic degradation of IL-8 and recycling of receptor to the cell surface. In common with other chemotactic factors, IL-8 appears to cause rapid rise of in cytosolic free Ca^{2+} concentration in human neutrophils (Finn *et al.*, 1993).

A central role for IL-8 in the regulation of neutrophil transendothelial migration has already been demonstrated (Huber *et al.*, 1991). IL-8 has also been shown to bind to the endothelium in the microvasculature in immuno histochemical studies (Rot, 1992). These findings have led to the proposition that IL-8 may bind to specific sites on endothelial cells and thus regulate neutrophil migration. IL-8, released from endothelial or other cell types, could thus guide the neutrophil into intercellular junctions and thence across the endothelial monolayer by controlling changes in expression and function of neutrophil L-selectin and CD11b/CD18 (Finn *et al.*, 1993). Most reports focus on the potent effects of IL-8 on neutrophils; however, it also has effects on other cell types, including basophils, eosinophils and some mononuclear leucocytes (Leonard *et al.*, 1990). Animal studies have revealed that intravenous administration of IL-8 causes neutrophilia, neutrophil sequestration in the lungs and a histological picture that resembles the adult respiratory distress syndrome (Rot, 1992). Recent studies have shown that IL-8 release is correlated with the length of cardiopulmonary bypass and cross-clamp time (Kawamura *et al.*, 1993; Wan *et al.*, 1996b,c), plasma levels of leucocyte elastase and peripheral neutrophils count after cardiopulmonary bypass (Finn *et al.*, 1993).

Summary of cytokine biology

In summary, during and after cardiopulmonary bypass: (1) the release of cytokines occurs under the combined influence of complement-derived anaphylatoxins and

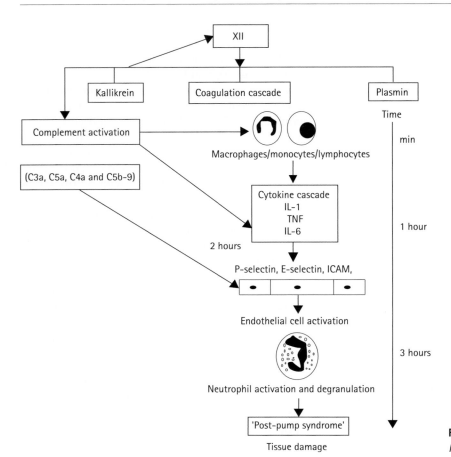

Figure 8.4 *The 'post-pump syndrome'. ICAM = intracellular adhesion molecule.*

endotoxin; (2) the mediating event is then the expression of endothelial adhesion molecules that are upregulated by cytokines and interact with specific receptors concomitantly expressed at the surface of complement-activated polymorphonuclear neutrophils; (3) this interaction finally leads to the firm attachment of neutrophils to endothelial cells and subsequent release of neutrophil-derived cytotoxic proteases and oxygen free radicals. These proteolytic enzymes are responsible for much of the end-organ damage seen after cardiopulmonary bypass (Figure 8.4). A better understanding of the cytokines response to cardiopulmonary bypass may lead in the future to some form of intervention aimed at reducing the incidence and the severity of post-operative complications by modulating the inflammatory reactions associated with cardiopulmonary bypass.

CLINICAL FEATURES OF THE SYSTEMIC INFLAMMATORY RESPONSE SYNDROME (SIRS)

According to the American College of Chest Physicians/ Society of Critical Care Medicine Consensus Conference, the definition of the systemic inflammatory response syndrome (SIRS) is:

> The response to a variety of severe clinical insults (either infectious or non-infectious). The response is manifested by two or more of the following conditions: (1) temperature >38°C; (2) heart rate >90 beats per minute; (3) respiratory rate >20 breaths per minute or PaCO$_2$ <32 mmHg; and (4) white blood count >12,000 cu/mm, or immature (band) form accounting for >10% of neutrophils.

One weakness of this definition is that the clinical features are remarkably non-specific; for example, the presence of pyrexia of more than 38°C and a moderate tachycardia are sufficient to include a patient in the syndrome. SIRS is not a single clinical entity but spectra of responses that may range from the relatively mild through to severe and potentially life-threatening conditions. It is induced in all patients undergoing cardiopulmonary bypass, but the severity of the response syndrome is variable. In a minority of patients (less than 10 per cent) it manifests with severe haemodynamic disturbance. This clinical entity is assumed to be a consequence of nitric oxide synthetase stimulation with high endothelial release of nitric oxide. Nitric oxide stimulates soluble guanylate cyclase, and activates the production of cyclic guanosine 3′,5′ monophasphate, resulting in the relaxation of vascular smooth muscles.

This pathophysiological condition reflects a hyperdynamic circulatory state, including an increased cardiac output in the presence of reduced systemic vascular resistance, requiring treatment by vasoconstrictive agents and fluid replacement. The syndrome is also characterized by generalized increased capillary permeability with consequent transcapillary plasma loss, increased interstitial fluid, leucocytosis, fever, peripheral vasodilatation, haemodynamic instability resulting in low perfusion pressure, and renal dysfunction. The breakdown of red blood cells results in haemoglobinemia, haemoglobinuria and anaemia. Although the widespread inflammatory reaction to cardiopulmonary bypass almost certainly affects all organ systems (coagulation disorders, cerebral and renal dysfunction), the lung appears particularly susceptible to these effects. The occurrence of severe pulmonary oedema without elevated left atrial pressure is a typical feature of SIRS. 'Pump lung' ranges from barely noticeable interstitial oedema to rare but lethal haemorrhagic pulmonary oedema. This results in increased work of breathing, arterial hypoxaemia with increased alveolar arterial oxygen difference and increased fluid in the tracheobronchial tree.

THERAPEUTIC INTERVENTIONS FOR CARDIOPULMONARY BYPASS-RELATED INFLAMMATORY RESPONSE

If systemic inflammatory mediators contribute to the morbidity of cardiopulmonary bypass then limitation of the intensity of the response should be possible with treatment, including among others corticosteroids, oxygen radical scavengers, neutrophilgranule-stabilizers and specific monoclonal antibodies.

Aprotinin is used extensively in cardiac surgery for its ability to reduce post-operative blood loss (Bidstrup et al., 1989), but has also been shown to inhibit kallikrein production and complement and neutrophil activation in vitro (Wachtfogel et al., 1993, 1995). It has also been shown to reduce plasma levels of leucocyte elastase in vivo (van Oeveren et al., 1987). However, Ashraf et al. (1997a) could show no beneficial effect in terms of the release of inflammatory mediators following the use of 'low-dose' aprotinin in adult cardiopulmonary bypass. The use of intravenous corticosteroids to suppress postcardiopulmonary bypass systemic inflammation has had mixed results in the clinical setting. Dexamethasone administration prevents TNF-α, IL-6 and IL-8 production during cardiopulmonary bypass (Jansen et al., 1991; Engelman et al., 1995; Teoh et al., 1995), whereas in another study there was no significant difference in

complement and cytokine production (Andersen et al., 1989). However, recently it has been documented that administration of steroids before heart transplantation and heart– lung transplantation procedures, instead of, as usual, at the end of cardiopulmonary bypass, can significantly inhibit TNF-α and IL-8 production (Wan et al., 1996a, 1997). These results are in agreement with previous studies stressing the crucial importance of the timing of anticytokine interventions (Christman et al., 1995). However, as yet there is no conclusive evidence from in vivo studies that inhibition of pro-inflammatory markers may be achieved after steroid administration and, in fact, higher endotoxin levels have been reported in treated patients (Andersen et al., 1989) and therefore its routine use as prophylaxis during cardiopulmonary bypass is debatable.

Reduction of lung injury may be achieved by inhibiting neutrophil activation. In animal models, neutrophil depletion using filtration technology (Pall filter) protects against cardiopulmonary bypass-induced lung injury (Bando et al., 1990; Hart and Roe, 1993). Such filters remove neutrophils from the circulation, decreasing their availability to promote inflammatory injury (Wilson et al., 1991; Gu et al., 1996). Unfortunately, leucocytes rapidly return to the circulation when the filter is discontinued.

Calcium channel blockers may inhibit neutrophil metabolic pathways involved in the production of injurious substances. The continuous infusion of nifedipine causes significantly lower levels of elastase-α1 antiprotease complex and lactoferrin but not C3a (Riegel et al., 1988). The antioxidants mannitol and allopurinol reduce hydrogen peroxides production during clinical cardiopulmonary bypass (England et al., 1986). Non-enzymatic free radical scavengers, vitamins C and E, have shown a beneficial effect in clinical practice (Ward et al., 1983). Moreover, in a clinical study, haemofiltration (Millar et al., 1993) and modified ultrafiltration (Naik et al., 1991) have shown beneficial effects in children undergoing cardiopulmonary bypass.

There is a variety of additional techniques available to block neutrophil adhesion to the activated endothelium. Specific monoclonal antibodies were developed by cellular biologists as tools to identify adhesion molecules expressed on cytokine-activated endothelium. Today, there is an increasing number of monoclonal antibodies available to block adhesion molecules before neutrophils can adhere. The objective of adhesion therapy after cardiopulmonary bypass should be to prevent neutrophil adherence during the first 24 hours after operation, thereby preventing the neutrophils from mediating widespread organ damage. Monoclonal antibodies blocking selectins (E-selectin, P-selectin), or circulating oligosaccharide antagonists that block the interaction of the neutrophil S-lex ligand with endothelial selectins, prevent the rolling and subsequent adherence of neutrophils. Gillinov et al.

(1993) used the anti-inflammatory agent NPC 15669 to inhibit neutrophil adhesion in a cardiopulmonary bypass model and found a marked decrease in pulmonary injury.

Monoclonal antibodies to endotoxin have been shown to reduce mortality in Gram-negative bacteraemia and septic shock in humans (Ziegler *et al.*, 1991) and, given prophylactically, reduce septic shock and mortality in surgical patients at high risk of Gram-negative infection (Baumgartner *et al.*, 1985). However, concerns have been shown by some investigators that therapeutic interventions that reduce the cytokine related response (by monoclonal antibodies) may result in inhibition of T-cell, B-cell proliferation and lymphokine generation, thus diminishing host defence and making the patient more vulnerable to severe infection (Sharar *et al.*, 1991). There is currently little to justify the proposed use of monoclonal antibodies to endotoxin in routine cardiopulmonary bypass.

EXTRACORPOREAL CIRCUIT MANIPULATION

Reduction of shear-stress

Both roller and centrifugal pumps are commonly used to move blood in extracorporeal circuits. Shear stresses produced by pumps contribute significantly to the pathogenesis of 'post-pump syndrome' (Kirklin *et al.*, 1993). Roller pumps cause blood trauma by surface contact during occlusion, compression of red cells and high shear stresses imparted to the red cells as the pump occludes the tubing (Hessel, 1993). Theoretically, centrifugal pumps are superior to roller pumps, but they still cause blood trauma by surface contact and shear stress on the boundary layer between blood and rotating cones (Hoerr *et al.*, 1987; Berki *et al.*, 1992). Some prospective randomized studies of centrifugal and roller pumps have shown that centrifugal pumps cause greater preservation of platelet number, decreased complement activation, less haemolysis and neutrophil activation (Hoerr *et al.*, 1987; Weeldon *et al.*, 1990; Driessen *et al.*, 1991; Moen *et al.*, 1995), whereas studies carried out by Wahba *et al.* (1995) and the author, in both adult and paediatric groups of patients (Ashraf *et al.*, 1997b, 1998a), have shown no difference between the two pumps in terms of release of the inflammatory markers.

Recently, a prospective randomized study carried out by Richter *et al.* (2000), using patients' own lungs as an oxygenator in a bilateral circuit (Drew–Anderson technique), showed markedly reduced release of postoperative inflammatory mediators and improved clinical outcome after coronary artery bypass graft (CABG) operation. Richter *et al.* (2000) concluded that this technique may be very beneficial in a high-risk group of patients undergoing CABG procedures.

Biocompatibility

Biocompatibility can be defined as the ability of biomaterials to perform without a host response, and is usually expressed as the levels of bioactive substances encountered in the circulation after contact with biomaterials. Because the majority of the inciting events begin as a result of the blood's interaction with the cardiopulmonary bypass circuit, efforts have been focused on altering the components of the extracorporeal circuit. The bubble oxygenator has been shown to result in a greater degree of complement activation and pulmonary leucosequestration, prompting many surgeons to turn to membrane oxygenators (Nilsson *et al.*, 1990). In order to reduce the contact activation of blood components by the exposed surfaces of cardiopulmonary bypass circuit, a number of investigators have investigated heparin-coated bypass circuits. Originally introduced to enable reduction or even elimination of systemic heparinization (Gott *et al.*, 1963; Von Segesser *et al.*, 1992), workers have found decreased activation of systemic inflammatory mediators. Leucocyte activation was diminished, as measured by elastase, lactoferrin and myeloperoxidase release, as were C3a and C5b-9 generation (Videm *et al.*, 1992; Gu *et al.*, 1993; Ovrum *et al.*, 1995; Fosse *et al.*, 1994, 1997). Heparin-coated bypass circuits also resulted in a significant reduction in circulating levels of IL-6 and IL-8 (Steinberg *et al.*, 1995; Weerwind *et al.*, 1995) and improved clinical outcome after cardiopulmonary bypass (Jansen *et al.*, 1991; Ashraf *et al.*, 1997c).

Heparin can be attached to polymers with various ionic preparations or by covalent binding to the surface. At present, two different types of heparinized extracorporeal circuits are available for clinical use: the Duraflo II surface (Baxter Health-care Corp., Bentley Laboratories Division, Irvine, CA, USA) binds heparin partly ionically by means of a proprietary process; the Carmeda BioActive Surface (CBAS, Medtronic, Inc., Minneapolis, MN, USA) covalently binds endpoint-attached degraded heparin. Both these systems have clinically shown improved biocompatibility in terms of reduced complement and granulocyte activation and cytokines release.

PRACTICAL GUIDE TO THE TREATMENT OF SIRS

There are a numbers of ways in which one can modify or minimize the incidence of SIRS after cardiopulmonary bypass. Once SIRS has developed clinically, it should be managed intensively to avoid morbidity and mortality. At present there is no specific treatment for this clinical entity. However, management should be directed towards combating the adverse effects of SIRS on individual organ systems.

Complete haemodynamics should be measured by pulmonary artery catheter (Swan–Ganz). Adequate tissue perfusion pressure is maintained by fluid replacement and vasopressors (noradrenaline, phenylephrine, etc.), guided by haemodynamic measurements (blood pressure, cardiac index and systemic vascular resistance) and urine output (0.5–1.0 mL/kg per hour). The issue of colloid versus crystalloid for fluid replacement is still a matter of debate. Personal preference is for the use of colloids as required and to limit the use of crystalloid to a minimum. Clinical use of steroids in well-established SIRS has so far been disappointing. Recently, there have been a few reports (Andrade et al., 1996; Yiu et al., 1999) of successful use of methylene blue, a guanylate cyclase inhibitor, in treating refractory haemodynamic instability in cases of SIRS following cardiopulmonary bypass. A diuretic dose of dopamine and/or continuous loop diuretic infusion to achieve satisfactory urine output has been routine clinical practice in many centres. However, its efficacy to prevent renal failure remains controversial. In cases of established renal failure, veno–venous haemofiltration has markedly reduced mortality in intensive care units (Jacobson and Webb, 1992). As pulmonary impairment is the most common presentation of SIRS, these patients will invariably require respiratory support. Hospital-acquired infection is a well recognized complication of intensive therapy, and once suspected, every effort should be made to identify the site and the type of organism and appropriate treatment should be started without delay.

SUMMARY

Inflammatory response after cardiopulmonary bypass is considerably more complex than it seemed two decades ago. It is not a single clinical entity but a myriad of responses of the body to a severe insult. A number of inflammatory mediators contribute to it. The commonly accepted roles of cytokines, endotoxin, selectin and nitric oxide in this condition must be defined. Greater awareness of this condition and further research into its pathophysiology and treatment are mandatory for further progress.

REFERENCES

Aderka, A. Le, J., Vilcek, J. 1989: IL-6 inhibits lipopolysaccharide induced TNF production in cultured human monocytes, U937 cells, and in mice. *Journal of Immunology* **143**, 3517–23.

Akira, S., Taga, T., Kishimoto, T. 1993: Interleukin-6 in biology and medicine. *Advances in Immunology* **54**, 1–7.

Ambruso, D.R., Johnston, R.B. 1981: Lactoferrin enhances hydroxyl radical production by human neutrophils, neutrophil particulate fractions, and enzymatic generating system. *Journal of Clinical Investigation* **67**, 352–60.

Andersen, L.W., Baek, L., Thomsen, B.S., Rasmussen, J.P. 1989: Effect of methylprednisolone on endotoxemia and complement activation during cardiac surgery. *Journal of Cardiothoracic Anaesthesia* **3**, 544–9.

Andrade, J.C.S., Batista, M.L., Evora, P.R.B. 1996: Methylene blue administration in SIRS after cardiac operation. *Annals of Thoracic Surgery* **63**, 1209–22.

Ashraf, S., Tian, Y., Cowan, D. et al. 1997a: 'Low-dose' aprotinin modifies hemostasis but not proinflammatory cytokine release. *Annals of Thoracic Surgery* **63**, 68–73.

Ashraf, S., Tian, Y., Cowan, D. et al. 1997b: Proinflammatory cytokine release during paediatric cardiopulmonary bypass: influence of centrifugal and roller pumps. *Journal of Thoracic and Cardiovascular Anaesthesia* **11**, 711–22.

Ashraf, S., Tian, Y., Martin, P. et al. 1997c: Production of proinflammatory cytokine release during paediatric cardiopulmonary bypass: heparin-bonded versus non-bonded oxygenators. *Annals of Thoracic Surgery* **64**, 1790–4.

Ashraf, S., Butler, J., Tian, Y. et al. 1998a: Inflammatory mediators in adults undergoing cardiopulmonary bypass: comparison of centrifugal and roller pumps. *Annals of Thoracic Surgery* **65**, 480–4.

Ashraf, S., Tian, Y., Martin, P. et al. 1998a: Effects of cardiopulmonary bypass on neonatal and paediatric inflammatory profiles. *European Journal of Cardiothoracic Surgery* **12**, 862–8.

Backmann, F., McKenna, R., Cole, E.R., Najafi, H. 1975: The hemostatic mechanism after open-heart surgery. Studies on plasma coagulation factors and fibrinolysis in 512 patients after extracorporeal circulation. *Journal of Thoracic and Cardiovascular Surgery* **70**, 76–85.

Balkwill, F., Osborne, R., Burke, F. 1987: Evidence of tumour necrosis factor/cachectin production in cancer. *Lancet* **1**, 1229–32.

Bando, K., Pillai, R., Cameron, D.E. et al. 1990: Leucocyte depletion ameliorates free radical mediated lung injury after cardiopulmonary bypass. *Journal of Thoracic and Cardiovascular Surgery* **99**, 873–7.

Baumgartner, J.D., McCutchan, J.A., van Melle, G. 1985: Prevention of Gram-negative shock and death in surgical patients by antibody to endotoxin core glycolipid. *Lancet* **2**, 59–63.

Bazzoni, F., Cassatella, M.A., Rossi, F. et al. 1991: Phagocytosing neutrophils produce and release high amounts of the neutrophil-activating peptide1/interleukin-8. *Journal of Experimental Medicine* **173**, 771–4.

Berki, T., Gurbuz, A., Isik, O. et al. 1992: Cardiopulmonary bypass using centrifugal pump. *Vascular Surgery* **26**, 123–34.

Beutler, B., Cerami, A. 1986: Cachectin and tumour necrosis factor as two sides of the same coin. *Nature* **320**, 584–8.

Beutler, B., Cerami, A. 1987: Cachectin: more than a tumour necrosis factor. *New England Journal of Medicine* **316**, 379–85.

Bidstrup, B.P., Royston, D., Sapsford, R.N.J., Taylor, K.M. 1989: Reduction in blood loss and blood use after cardiopulmonary bypass with high dose aprotinin (Trasylol). *Journal of Thoracic and Cardiovascular Surgery* **97**, 364–72.

Billiau, A., Vandekerckhove, F. 1991: Cytokines and their interactions with other inflammatory mediators in the pathogenesis of sepsis and septic shock. *European Journal of Clinical Investigation* **21**, 559–73.

Bjork, J., Hugli, T.E., Smedegard, G. 1985: Microvascular effect on anaphylatoxins C3a and C5a. *Journal of Immunology* **134**, 1115–19.

Brower, M.S., Levin, R.I., Garry, K. 1985: Human neutrophil elastase modulates platelet function by limited proteolysis of membrane glycoproteins. *Journal of Clinical Investigation* **75**, 657–66.

Butler, J., Chang, G.L., Baigrie, R.J., Pillai, R. 1992: Cytokine responses to cardiopulmonary bypass with membrane and bubble oxygenation. *Annals of Thoracic Surgery* **53**, 833–8.

Butler, J., Rocker, G.M., Westaby, S. 1993a: Inflammatory response to cardiopulmonary bypass. *Annals of Thoracic Surgery* **55**: 552–9.

Butler, J., Pillai, R., Rocker, G.M., Westaby, S. 1993b: Effect of cardiopulmonary bypass on systemic release of neutrophil elastase and tumour necrosis factor. *Journal of Thoracic and Cardiovascular Surgery* **105**, 25–30.

Butler, J., Pathi, V.L., Paton, R.D. *et al.* 1996: Acute-phase response to cardiopulmonary bypass in children weighing less than 10 kilograms. *Annals of Thoracic Surgery* **62**, 538–42.

Casey, L.C. 1993: Role of cytokines in the pathogenesis of cardiopulmonary bypass induced multisystem organ failure. *Annals of Thoracic Surgery* **56**, 92–6.

Cavarocchi, N.C., Pluth, J.R., Schaff, H.V. *et al.* 1986: Complement activation during cardiopulmonary bypass: comparison of bubble and membrane oxygenators. *Journal of Thoracic and Cardiovascular Surgery* **91**, 252–8.

Charo, I.F., Yuen, C., Perez, H.D. *et al.* 1986: Chemotactic peptides modulate adherence of human polymorphonuclear leucocytes to monolayers of cultured endothelial cells. *Journal of Immunology* **136**, 3412–19.

Chenoweth, D.E., Hugli, T.E. 1978: Demonstration of specific C5a receptor on intact human polymorphonuclear leukocytes. *Proceedings of the National Academy of Sciences* **75**, 3943–7.

Chenoweth, D.E., Cooper, S.W., Hugli, T.E. *et al.* 1981: Complement activation during cardiopulmonary bypass. Evidence of generation of C3a and C5a anaphylatoxins. *New England Journal of Medicine* **304**, 497–503.

Christman, J., Holden, W.E., Blackwell, T.S. 1995: Strategies for blocking the systemic effects of cytokines in the sepsis syndrome. *Critical Care Medicine* **23**, 995–8.

Craddock, P.R., Fehr, J., Brigham, K.L. *et al.* 1977: Complement and leucocyte-mediated pulmonary dysfunction in hemodialysis. *New England Journal of Medicine* **296**, 769–74.

Cremer, J., Martin, M., Redle, H. *et al.* 1996: Systemic inflammatory response after cardiac operations. *Annals of Thoracic Surgery* **61**, 1714–20.

Dinarello, C.A. 1988: Biology of interleukin-1. *Advances in Immunology* **2**, 108–15.

Dinarello, C.A. 1989: Interleukin-1 and its biologically related cytokines. *Advances in Immunology* **44**, 153–205.

Dinarello, C.E. 1991: Interleukin-1 and interleukin-1 antagonism. *Blood* **77**, 1627–52.

Driessen, J.J., Fransen, G., Rondelez, L. *et al.* 1991: Comparison of the standard roller pump and pulsatile centrifugal pump for extracorporeal circulation during routine coronary artery bypass grafting. *Perfusion* **6**, 303–11.

Dubois, C.M., Ruscetti, F.W., Palaszynski, E.W. *et al.* 1990: Transforming growth factor beta is a potent inhibitor of Interleukin-1 receptor expression: proposed mechanism of inhibition of IL-1 action. *Journal of Experimental Medicine* **172**, 737–44.

Elliott, M.J. 1993: Ultrafiltration and modified ultrafiltration in paediatric open heart operations. *Annals of Thoracic Surgery* **56**, 1518–22.

Elliott, M.J., Hamilton, J.R.L., Clark, I. 1990: Perfusion for paediatric open-heart surgery. *Perfusion* **5**, 1–8.

Ellison, N., Behar, M., MacVaugh, H., Marshall, B.E. 1980: Bradykinin, plasma protein fraction and hypotension. *Annals of Thoracic Surgery* **29**, 15–19.

Engelman, R.M., Rousou, J.A., Flack, J.E. *et al.* 1995: Influence of steroids on complement and cytokine generation after cardiopulmonary bypass. *Annals of Thoracic Surgery* **60**, 801–4.

Evans, S.W., Whicher, J.T. 1993: *The cytokines: physiological and pathophysiological aspects.* New York, NY: Academic Press Inc: 40–3.

England, M.D., Cavarocchi, N.C., O'Brien, J.F. 1986: Influence of antioxidants (manitol and allopurinol) on oxygen free radical generation during and after cardiopulmonary bypass. *Circulation* **74** (Suppl. 3): 134–7.

Faymonville, M.E., Pincemail, J., Duchateau, J. 1991: Myeloperoxidase and elastase as a markers of leucocyte activation during cardiopulmonary bypass in human. *Journal of Thoracic and Cardiovascular Surgery* **102**, 309–17.

Fehr, J., Rohr, H. 1983: *In vivo* complement activation by polyanion–polycation complexes: evidence that C5a is generated intravascularly during heparin–protamine interaction. *Clinical Immunopathology* **29**, 7–14.

Finkel, M.S., Oddis, C.V., Jacob, T.D. *et al.* 1992: Negative inotropic effects of cytokines on the heart mediated by nitric oxide. *Science* **257**, 387–9.

Finn, A., Naik, S., Nigel, K. *et al.* 1993: Interleukin-8 release and neutrophil degranulation after paediatric cardiopulmonary bypass. *Journal of Thoracic and Cardiovascular Surgery* **105**: 234–41.

Fiorentino, D.F., Zlotnik, A., Mosmann, T.R. 1991: IL-10 inhibits cytokine production by activated macrophages. *Journal of Immunology* **147**, 3815–22.

Fitzpatrick, M.M., Shah, V., Filler, G. *et al.* 1992: Neutrophil activation in the haemolytic uraemic syndrome: free and complex elastase in plasma. *Paediatric Nephrology* **6**, 50–3.

Fong, Y., Moldawer, L.L., Shires, G.T., Lowery, S.F. 1990: The biologic characteristics of cytokines and their implication in surgical injury. *Surgery of Gynaecology Obstetrics* **170**, 363–78.

Fosse, E., Mollness, T., Ingvaldsen, B. 1987: Complement activation during major operations with or without cardiopulmonary bypass. *Journal of Thoracic and Cardiovascular Surgery* **93**, 8600–66.

Fosse, E., Moen, O., Johnson, E. *et al.* 1994: Reduced complement and granulocyte activation with heparin-coated cardiopulmonary bypass. *Annals of Thoracic Surgery* **58**, 472–7.

Fosse, E., Thelin, S., Svennevig, J.L. *et al.* 1997: Duraflo 11 coating of cardiopulmonary bypass circuits reduces complement activation, but does not affect the release of granulocyte enzymes in fully heparinized patients: a European multicentre study. *European Journal of Cardiothoracic Surgery* **11**, 320–7.

George, J.F. 1993: Cytokines and mechanisms of capillary leakage after cardiopulmonary bypass. *Journal of Thoracic and Cardiovascular Surgery* 106, 566–7.

Gieger, T., Andus, T., Klapproth, J. *et al.* 1988: Induction of rat acute-phase protein by interleukin-6 *in vivo. European Journal of Immunology* 18, 717–21.

Gillinov, A.M., Redmond, J.M., Zehr, K.J. 1993: Inhibition of neutrophil adhesion during cardiopulmonary bypass: a study in a complement-deficient dog. *Annals of Thoracic Surgery* 57, 345–52.

Glauser, M.P., Zanetti, G., Baumgartner, J.D., Cohen, J. 1991: Septic shock: pathogenesis. *Lancet* 338, 732–6.

Gott, V.L., Whiffen, J.D., Dutton, R.C. 1963: Heparin bonding on colloidal graphite surfaces. *Science* 142, 1297–9.

Gu, Y.J., van Oeveren, W., Akkerman, C. 1993: Heparin-coated circuits reduce the inflammatory response to cardiopulmonary bypass. *Annals of Thoracic Surgery* 55, 917–22.

Gu, Y.J., de Vries, A.J., Boonstra, P.W., van Oeveren, W. 1996: Leucocyte depletion results in improved lung function and reduced inflammatory response after cardiac surgery. *Journal of Thoracic and Cardiovascular Surgery* 112, 494–500.

Hack, C.E., DeGroot, E.R., Felt-Bersma, R.J. 1989: Increased plasma levels of interleukin-6 in sepsis. *Blood* 74, 1704–10.

Haeffner-Cavaillon, N.J.H., Cavaillon, J.M., Laude, M., Kazatchkines, M.D. 1987: C3a(C3a des Arg) induces production and release of interleukin-1 by cultured human monocytes. *Journal of Immunology* 139, 794–9.

Haeffner-Cavaillon, N.J.H., Roussellier, N., Ponzio, O. 1989: Induction of interleukin-1 production in patients undergoing cardiopulmonary bypass. *Journal of Thoracic and Cardiovascular Surgery* 98, 1100–6.

Hannum, C.H., Wilcox, C.J., Arend, W.P. *et al.* 1990: Interleukin-1 receptor antagonist activity of a human interleukin-1 inhibitor. *Nature* 343, 336–40.

Hart, S., Roe, J.A. 1993: Leucocyte depleting filters and cardiothoracic surgery. *Perfusion* 8, 477–82.

Havermann, K., Gramse, M. 1984: Physiology and pathophysiology of neutral proteinases of human granulocytes. In: Horl, W.H., Heidland, A., eds. *Proteinases: potential role in health and disease.* London: Plenum Press: 1–20.

Hennein, H.A., Ebba, H., Rodriguez, J.L. *et al.* 1994: Relationship of the proinflammatory cytokines to myocardial ischemia and dysfunction after uncomplicated coronary revascularization. *Journal of Thoracic and Cardiovascular Surgery* 108, 626–35.

Heinrich, P.C., Castell, J.V., Andus, T. 1990: Interleukin-6 and acute phase response. *Biochemistry Journal* 265, 621–36.

Herbert, C.A., Baker, J.B. 1993: Interleukin-8: a review. *Cancer Investigation* 11, 743–50.

Hessel, E.A. 1993: Cardiopulmonary bypass circuitry and cannulation techniques. In: Gravlee, G.P., Davis, R.F., Utley, J.R., eds. *Cardiopulmonary bypass: principles and practice.* Baltimore, MD: Williams & Wilkins: 233–48.

Hind, C.R.K., Griffin, J.F., Pack, S. 1988: Effect of cardiopulmonary bypass on circulating concentration of leucocyte elastase and free radical activity. *Cardiovascular Surgery* 22, 37–41.

Hoerr, H.R., Kraemer, M.F., Williams, J.L. 1987: *In vitro* comparison of the blood handling by the constrained vortex and twin roller blood pumps. *Journal of Extracorporeal Technology* 19, 316–21.

Horl, W.H., Riegel, W., Schollmeyer, P. 1987: Plasma levels of main granulocyte components in patients dialysed with polycarbonate and cuprophan membranes. *Nephron* 45, 272–6.

Huber, A.R., Kunkel, S.L., Todd, R.F., Weiss, S.J. 1991: Regulation of transendothelial neutrophil migration by endogenous interleukin-8. *Science* 254, 99–102.

Jacobson, D.W., Webb, A.R. 1992: Acute renal support in the ITU. *Current Anaesthesia and Critical Care* 3, 150–5.

Jansen, N.J.G., van Oeveren, W., van der Broek, L. 1991: Inhibition by dexamethasone of the reperfusion phenomena in cardiopulmonary bypass. *Journal of Thoracic and Cardiovascular Surgery* 102, 515–25.

Jansen, N.J.G., van Oeveren, W., Gu, Y.J. *et al.* 1992: Endotoxin release and tumour necrosis factor formation during cardiopulmonary bypass. *Annals of Thoracic Surgery* 54, 744–8.

Jones, D.R., Hill, R.C., Hollingsed, M.J. 1993: Use of heparin-coated cardiopulmonary bypass. *Annals of Thoracic Surgery* 56, 566–8.

Kalfin, R.E., Engelman, R.M., Rousou, J.A. 1993: Induction of interleukin-8 expression during cardiopulmonary bypass. *Circulation* 88, 401–6.

Kapadia, S., Lee, J., Torre-Amione, G. *et al.* 1995: Tumour necrosis factor – a gene and protein expression in adult feline myocardium after endotoxin administration. *Journal of Clinical Investigation* 96, 42–52.

Kawahito, K., Kawakami, M., Fujiwara, T. *et al.* 1995: Interleukin-8 and monocyte chemotactic activating factor responses to cardiopulmonary bypass. *Journal of Thoracic and Cardiovascular Surgery* 110, 99–102.

Kawamura, T., Wakusawa, R., Okada, K., Inada, S. 1993: Elevation of cytokines during open heart surgery with cardiopulmonary bypass: participation of interleukin-8 and 6 in reperfusion injury. *Canadian Journal of Anaesthesia* 40, 1016–21.

Kirklin, J.K. 1991: Prospect for understanding and eliminating the deleterious effects of cardiopulmonary bypass. *Annals of Thoracic Surgery* 51, 529–31.

Kirklin, J.W., Barratt-Boyes, B.G. 1986: The damaging effect of cardiopulmonary bypass. In: Kirklin, J.K., ed. *Cardiac surgery.* Edinburgh: Churchill Livingstone: 51–5.

Kirklin, J.K., Westaby, S., Blackstone, E.H. *et al.* 1983: Complement and damaging effects of cardiopulmonary bypass. *Journal of Thoracic and Cardiovascular Surgery* 86, 845–57.

Kirklin, J.K., Chenoweth, D.E., Naftel, D.C. 1986: Effect of protamine administration after cardiopulmonary bypass on complement, blood elements, and hemodynamic state. *Annals of Thoracic Surgery* 41, 193–9.

Kirklin, J.K., George, J.F., Holman, W. 1993: The inflammatory response to cardiopulmonary bypass. In: Gravlee, G.P., Davis, R.F., Utley, J.R., eds. *Cardiopulmonary bypass: principles and practice.* Baltimore, MD: Williams & Wilkins: 233–48.

Klebanoff, S., Vadas, M.A., Harlan, J.M. 1986: Stimulation of neutrophil by tumour necrosis factor. *Journal of Immunology* 136, 4220–5.

Kornecki, E., Ehrlich, Y.H., De Mars, D.D., Lenox, R.H. 1986: Exposure of fibrinogen receptor on human platelets by surface proteolysis with elastase. *Journal of Clinical Investigation* 77, 750–6.

Larsen, C.G., Anderson, A.O., Oppenheim, J.J., Matsushima, K. 1989: Production of interleukin-8 by human dermal fibroblast and keratinocytes in response to interleukin-1 or tumour necrosis factor. *Immunology* **68**, 31–6.

Leonard, E.J., Skeel, A., Yoshimura, T. *et al.* 1990: Leukocyte specificity and binding of human neutrophil attractant/activating protein 1. *Journal of Immunology* **144**, 1323–30.

Lotz, M. 1993: Interleukin-6: a review. *Cancer Investigation* **11**, 732–42.

Maehara, T., Novak, I., Wyse, R.H., Eliott, M.J. 1991: Perioperative monitoring of total body water by bio-electrical impedance in children undergoing open heart surgery. *European Journal of Cardiothoracic Surgery* **5**, 258–68.

Marks, J.D., Marks, C.B., Luce, J.M. 1990: Plasma necrosis factor in patients with septic shock: mortality rate and incidence of adult respiratory distress syndrome, and effect of methylprednisolone administration. *American Review of Respiratory Disease* **141**, 94–7.

Martin, B.A., Wright, J.L., Thommasen, H., Hogg, J. 1982: Effects of pulmonary blood flow on the exchange between the circulating and marginating pool of polymorphonuclear leukocytes in dog lungs. *Journal of Clinical Investigation* **69**, 1277–85.

Matsushima, K., Oppenheim, J.J. 1989: Interleukin-8 and MCAF: novel inflammatory cytokines induced by IL-1 and TNF. *Cytokine* **1**, 2–13.

McGuire, W.W., Spragg, R.G., Cohen, A.B., Cochrane, C.G. 1982: Studies on the pathogenesis of the adult respiratory syndrome. *Journal of Clinical Investigation* **69**, 543–53.

Maury, C.P., Teppo, A.M. 1987: Raised serum levels of cachectin/tumour necrosis factor alpha in renal allograft rejection. *Journal of Experimental Medicine* **166**, 1132–7.

Melvin, B. 1990: Complement deficiency and neutrophil dysfunction as risk factors for bacterial infection in new-borns and role of granulocyte transfusion in therapy. *Reviews of Infectious Diseases* **12** (Suppl. 4), 401–9.

Menasche, P., Peynet, J., Lariviere, J. *et al.* 1994: Does normothermia during cardiopulmonary bypass increase neutrophil–endothelium interactions? *Circulation* **90**, 275–9.

Menasche, P., Peynet, J., Haeffner-Cavallion, N. *et al.* 1995: Influence of temperature on neutrophil trafficking during clinical cardiopulmonary bypass. *Circulation* **92** (Suppl. 2), 334–40.

Mielke, V., Bauman, J.G., Sticherling, M. 1990: Detection of neutrophil-activating peptide NAP/IL-8 and NAP/IL-8 mRNA in human recombinant IL-1 alpha- and human recombinant tumour necrosis factor-alpha stimulated human dermal fibroblasts. *Journal of Immunology* **144**, 153–61.

Millar, A.B., Armstrong, L., van der Linden, J. 1993: Cytokine production and hemofiltration in children undergoing cardiopulmonary bypass. *Annals of Thoracic Surgery* **56**, 1499–502.

Moen, O., Fosse, E., Brockmeier, V., Andersson, C. 1995: Disparity in blood activation by two different heparin-coated cardiopulmonary bypass system. *Annals of Thoracic Surgery* **60**, 1317–23.

Moldawer, L.L., Gelin, J., Schersten, T., Lundholm, K.G. 1987: Circulating interleukin-1 and tumour necrosis factor during inflammation. *American Journal of Physiology* **253**, 922–8.

Muto, Y., Nouri-Aria, K.T., Meager, A. 1988: Enhanced tumour necrosis factor and interleukin-1 in fulminent hepatic failure. *Lancet* **2**, 72–4.

Naik, S.K., Knight, A., Elliott, M. 1991: A prospective randomized study of a modified technique of ultrafiltration during paediatric open-heart surgery. *Circulation* **84** (Suppl. 3), 422–31.

Nijsten, N.W., DeGroot, E.R., ten Duism, H.J. *et al.* 1987: Serum levels of interleukin-6 and acute-phase responses. *Lancet* **2**, 921.

Nilsson, L., Tyd'en, H., Johansson, O. 1990: Bubble and membrane oxygenators – comparison of post-operative organ dysfunction with special reference to inflammatory activity. *Scandinavian Journal of Thoracic and Cardiovascular Surgery* **24**, 59–64.

van Oeveren, W., Jansen, N.J.C., Bidstrup, B.P. *et al.* 1987: Effect of aprotinin on hemostatic mechanisms during cardiopulmonary bypass. *Annals of Thoracic Surgery* **44**, 640–5.

Okusawa, S., Yancey, K.B., Van der Meer, J.W. 1990: C5a stimulates secretion of tumour necrosis factor from human mononuclear cells *in vitro*. Comparison with secretion of interleukin-1β and interleukin 1-α. *Journal of Experimental Medicine* **171**, 439–48.

Ovrum, E., Mollnes, T.E., Fosse, E. *et al.* 1995: Complement and granulocyte activation in two different types of heparinized extracorporeal circuits. *Journal of Thoracic and Cardiovascular Surgery* **110**, 1623–32.

Permutter, D.H., Dinarello, C.A., Punsal, P.I., Colten, H.R. 1986: Cachectin/tumour necrosis factor regulates hepatic acute phase gene expression. *Journal of Clinical Investigation* **78**, 1349–54.

Richter, S.A., Meisner, H., Tassani, P., Barankay, A., Dietrich, W., Braun, S.L. 2000: Drew–Anderson technique attenuates systemic inflammatory response syndrome and improves respiratory function after coronary bypass grafting. *Annals of Thoracic Surgery* **69**, 77–83.

Riegel, W., Spillner, G., Schlosser, V., Horl, W.H. 1988: Plasma levels of main granulocyte components during cardiopulmonary bypass. *Journal of Thoracic and Cardiovascular Surgery* **95**, 1014–19.

Rocker, G.M., Wiseman, M.S., Pearson, D., Shale, D.J. 1989: Diagnostic criteria for adult respiratory distress syndrome: time for reappraisal. *Lancet* **1**, 120–3.

Rot, A. 1992: Endothelial cell binding of NAP-1/IL-8: role in neutrophil emigration. *Immunology Today* **13**, 291–4.

Royston, D., Fleming, J.S., Desai, J.B. *et al.* 1986: Increased production of peroxidation products associated with cardiac operation: evidence of free radical generation. *Journal of Thoracic and Cardiovascular Surgery* **91**, 759–66.

Ryhanen, P., Herva, E., Hollman, A. *et al.* 1979: Changes in peripheral blood leucocyte counts, lymphocyte subpopulations, and *in vitro* transformation after heart valve replacement. *Journal of Thoracic and Cardiovascular Surgery* **77**, 259–66.

Salama, A., Hugo, F., Heinrich, D. 1988: Deposition of terminal C5b-9 complement complex on erythrocytes and leucocytes during cardiopulmonary bypass. *New England Journal of Medicine* **318**, 408–14.

Salas, M.A., Evans, S.W., Levell, M.J., Whicher, J.T. 1990: Interleukin-6 and ACTH act synergistically to stimulate the release of corticosterone from adrenal gland cells. *Clinical Experimental Immunology* **79**, 470–3.

Samanta, A.K., Oppenheim, J.J., Matsushima, K. 1990: Interleukin-8 (monocyte-derived neutrophil chemotactic factor) dynamically regulates its own receptor expression on human neutrophils. *Journal of Biological Chemistry* **265**, 183–9.

Scuderi, P., Lam, K.S., Ryan, K.J. 1986: Raised levels of tumour necrosis factor in parasitic infections. *Lancet* **2**, 1364–5.

Seghaye, M.C., Duchateau, J., Grabitz, R.G. *et al.* 1993: Complement activation in infant and children: relation to postoperative multiple system organ failure. *Journal of Thoracic and Cardiovascular Surgery* **106**, 978–87.

Seghaye, M.C., Duchateau, J., Grabitz, R.C. *et al.* 1996: Influence of low-dose aprotinin on the inflammatory reaction due to cardiopulmonary bypass in children. *Annals of Thoracic Surgery* **61**, 1205–11.

Sethia, B. 1992: Current status of definitive surgery for congenital heart disease. *Archives of Disease in Childhood* **67**, 981–4.

Sharar, S.R., Winn, R.K., Murry, C.E. 1991: A CD 18 monoclonal antibody increases the incidence and severity of subcutaneous abscess formation after high-dose *Staphylococcus aureus* injection in rabbits. *Surgery* **110**, 213–19.

Sironi, M., Munoz, C., Pollicino, T. 1993: Divergent effect of interleukin-10 on cytokine production by mononuclear phagocytes and endothelial cells. *European Journal of Immunology* **23**, 2692–5.

Speer, C.P., Ninjo, A., Gahr, M. 1986: Elastase-alpha1 proteinase inhibitor in early diagnosis of neonatal septicaemia. *Journal of Paediatrics* **108**, 987–90.

Stahl, R.E., Fisher, C.A., Kucich, U. 1991: Effects of simulated extracorporeal circulation on human leucocyte elastase release, superoxide generation, and procoagulant activity. *Journal of Thoracic and Cardiovascular Surgery* **101**, 230–9.

Steinberg, J.B., Kapelanski, D.P., Olson, J.D., Weiler, J.M. 1993: Cytokine and complement levels in patients undergoing cardiopulmonary bypass. *Journal of Thoracic and Cardiovascular Surgery* **106**, 1008–16.

Steinberg, B.M., Grossi, E., Schwartz, D. *et al.* 1995: Heparin bonding of bypass circuits reduces cytokine release during cardiopulmonary bypass. *Annals of Thoracic Surgery* **60**, 525–9.

Strunk, R.C., Fenton, L.J., Gaines, J.A. 1979: Alternative pathway of complement activation in full term and premature infants. *Paediatric Research* **13**, 641–3.

Tennenberg, S.D., Clardy, C.W., Bailey, W.W., Solomkin, J.S. 1990: Complement activation and lung permeability during cardiopulmonary bypass. *Annals of Thoracic Surgery* **50**, 597–601.

Teoh, K.H., Bradley, C.A., Gauldie, J., Burrows, H. 1995: Steroid inhibition of cytokine-mediated vasodilatation after warm heart surgery. *Circulation* **92** (Suppl. 2), 3447–53.

Tosato, G., Jones, K.D. 1990: Interleukin-1 induces interleukin-6 production in peripheral blood monocytes. *Blood* **75**, 1305–10.

Tosato, G., Seamon, K.B., Goldman, N.D. 1988: Monocyte-derived human B-cell growth factor identified as interferon-b2 (BSF-2, IL-6). *Science* **239**, 502–4.

Tracey, K.J., Valssara, H., Cerami, A. 1989: Cachectin/tumour necrosis factor. *Lancet* **1**, 1122–6.

Venge, P., Nilsson, L., Nystrom, S.O., Aberg, T. 1987: Serum and plasma measurements of neutrophil granule protein during cardiopulmonary bypass; a model; of estimate of human turnover of lactoferrin and myeloperoxidase. *European Journal of Haematology* **39**, 339–45.

Verska, J.J. 1977: Control of heparinization by activated clotting time during bypass with improved post-operative hemostasis. *Annals of Thoracic Surgery* **24**, 170–3.

Videm, V., Mollnes, T.E., Garred, P., Svennevig, J.L. 1991: Biocompatibility of extracorporeal circulation: *in vitro* comparision of heparin-coated and uncoated oxygenator circuits. *Journal of Thoracic and Cardiovascular Surgery* **101**, 654–60.

Videm, V., Svennevig, J.L., Fosse, E. *et al.* 1992: Reduced complement activation with heparin-coated oxygenator and tubings in coronary bypass surgery. *Journal of Thoracic and Cardiovascular Surgery* **103**, 806–13.

Von Segesser, L.K., Weiss, B.M., Garcia, E. *et al.* 1992: Reduction and elimination of systemic heparinization during cardiopulmonary bypass. *Journal of Thoracic and Cardiovascular Surgery* **103**, 790–9.

Waage, A., Halstensen, A., Espevik, T. 1987: Association between tumour necrosis factor in serum and fatal outcome in patients with meningococcal diseases. *Lancet* **1**, 355–7.

Waage, A., Brandtzaeg, P., Halstensen, A. *et al.* 1989: The complex pattern of cytokines in serum from patients with meningococcal septic shock: association between interleukin-6, interleukin-1 and fatal outcome. *Journal of Experimental Medicine* **169**, 333–8.

Wachtfogel, Y.T., Kucich, U., James, H.L. 1983: Human plasma kallikrein releases neutrophil elastase during blood coagulation. *Journal of Clinical Investigation* **72**, 1672–7.

Wachtfogel, Y.T., Kucich, U., Greenplate, J. 1987: Human neutrophil degranulation during extracorporeal circulation. *Blood* **69**, 324–30.

Wachtfogel, Y.T., Hack, C.E., Nuijens, J.H. *et al.* 1995: Selective kallikrein inhibitors alter human neutrophil elastase during extracorporeal circulation. *American Journal of Physiology* **268**, H1352–H1357.

Wahba, A., Philip, A., Bauer, M.F. *et al*, 1995: The blood saving potential of vortex versus roller pump with and without aprotinin. *Perfusion* **10**, 333–41.

Wan, S., DeSmet, J.M., Antoine, M. *et al.* 1996a: Steroid administration in heart and heart-lung transplantation: is the timing adequate? *Annals of Thoracic Surgery* **61**, 674–8.

Wan, S., DeSmet, J.M., Barvais, L. *et al.* 1996b: Myocardium is a major source of proinflammatory cytokines in patients undergoing cardiopulmonary bypass. *Journal of Thoracic and Cardiovascular Surgery* **112**, 806–11.

Wan, S., Marchant, A., DeSmet, J.M. 1996c: Human cytokine response to cardiac transplantation and coronary artery bypass grafting. *Journal of Thoracic and Cardiovascular Surgery* **119**, 76–80.

Wan, S., LeClerc, J., Vincent, J. 1997: Cytokine response to cardiopulmonary bypass: lessons learned from cardiac transplantation. *Annals of Thoracic Surgery* **63**, 269–76.

Ward, P.A., Till, G.O., Beauchamp, C. 1983: Evidence for role of hydroxyl radical in complement and neutrophil-dependent tissue injury. *Journal of Clinical Investigation* **72**, 789–801.

Weeldon, D.R., Bethune, D.W., Gill, R.D. 1990: Vortex pumping for routine cardiac surgery: a comparative study. *Perfusion* **5**, 135–43.

Weerwind, P.W., Maessen, J.G., vanTits, L.J. *et al.* 1995: Influence of Duraflo II heparin treated extracorporeal circuits on the systemic inflammatory response in patients having coronary bypass. *Journal of Thoracic and Cardiovascular Surgery* **110**, 1633–41.

Wilson, I.C., Gardner, T.J., DiNatale, J.M. *et al.* 1993: Temporary leukocyte depletion reduces ventricular dysfunction during prolonged postischemic reperfusion. *Journal of Thoracic and Cardiovascular Surgery* **106**, 805–10.

Yiu, P., Robin, J., Pattison, C.W. 1999: Reversal of refractory hypotension with single-dose methylene blue after coronary artery bypass surgery. *Journal of Thoracic and Cardiovascular Sugery* **118**, 195–6.

Ziegler, E.J., Fisher, C.J., Sprung, C.L. 1991: Treatment of Gram-negative bacteremia and septic shock with HA–1A human monoclonal antibody against endotoxin: a randomized double-blind, placebo-controlled trial. *New England Journal of Medicine* **324**, 429–36.

9

Pulsatile cardiopulmonary bypass

TERRY GOURLAY AND KENNETH M TAYLOR

KEY POINTS

- The importance of pulsatile blood flow to the maintenance of normal physiological function has long been recognized and considerably pre-dates the clinical application of cardiopulmonary bypass.
- The increased energy delivered by pulsatile blood flow maintains capillary patency, and the pulse is responsible for the exchange of fluids at the extracellular level and the maintenance of cell metabolism.
- Roller pumps are commonly used to produce a pulsatile pressure profile, although this rarely resembles a physiological pulse pressure profile.
- There is substantial, but often conflicting, literature on the beneficial effects of pulsatile cardiopulmonary bypass on organ function. None of the literature, however, suggests that pulsatile flow is deleterious.
- It is possible that the optimum maximum benefit of pulsatile flow on renal, gut and brain function may be most apparent in higher risk patients.
- Future improvements in pump and cannula design may allow a truly physiological pulse pressure to be generated with the potential for clear clinical benefit.

technological, pharmacological and surgical developments extending over many years. Fundamental research that led to the evolution of routine cardiopulmonary bypass included the discovery and refinement of heparin (McLean, 1916), which offered effective anticoagulation, without which cardiopulmonary bypass as we know it today would not be possible. Other developments, such as efficient blood oxygenators, the refinement of surgical technique and the development of the pumping technology required to support the circulation during cardiac operations, are all part of the evolution of cardiopulmonary bypass, and pre-date its clinical application by a considerable period. However, despite this long evolutionary period, and considerable achievement leading to the now routine and safe use of cardiopulmonary bypass during cardiac surgery throughout the modern world, a number of controversies have prevailed since the first successful application of this technique in clinical practice. Among the most persistent of these, for example the use of arterial line filtration and hypothermia, is the question of whether it is necessary, or indeed desirable, to employ a pulsatile blood flow regime during the cardiopulmonary bypass phase of the cardiac operation. This has been the focus of continued interest and research throughout the phase of development of cardiopulmonary bypass technology, and continues to attract attention from investigators to the present day.

INTRODUCTION

When Gibbon (1954) carried out the first cardiopulmonary bypass-supported clinical open-heart surgical procedure, it was the culmination of a convergence of

THE EVOLUTION OF PULSATILE PERFUSION

The issue of whether blood flow should be pulsatile or non-pulsatile during cardiopulmonary bypass was raised at a very early stage in its development. However, interest in the importance of pulsatile blood flow to the maintenance of normal physiological function, considerably predates the clinical application of cardiopulmonary bypass. In the latter part of the nineteenth century, physiologists studying the function of isolated organs used a wide variety of novel and innovative technologies in an attempt to replicate normal blood flow and pressure architecture. These perfusion systems, described very eloquently by Bregman *et al.* (1991) in the previous edition of this book, include pendulum, compression plate and cam-driven pumping apparatus, all designed to impart a pulse during artificial maintenance of blood flow. Studies using these perfusion apparatus were very productive in terms of our understanding of the role of the pulsatile nature of blood flow in the maintenance of normal organ function. In the late nineteenth century, Hamel (1889) determined that the presence of pulsatile blood flow is essential to the maintenance of renal function in isolated renal preparations. Early in the last century, Hooker (1910) employed a cam-driven pulsatile pumping system which allowed some control of pulsatile architecture, to study renal blood flow and urinary output in an isolated kidney preparation. He found that increased pulsatile pressure amplitude was associated with enhanced renal blood flow and urine output. Other investigators have attempted to reproduce these results since, with varying degrees of success, but with studies such as these, the interest in the pulsatile nature of blood flow, and the technology that can be employed to produce it, was established.

The advent of clinical cardiopulmonary bypass offered those interested in the field of pulsatile flow a unique research opportunity: the ability to study the effect of pulsatile blood flow in patients under conditions in which the investigators have considerable degree of control over the blood flow environment. With this in mind, a number of pumping systems with a pulsatile flow option were designed for clinical use. However, fears of generating excessive haemolysis, and the technical complexity of the systems, with findings unsupportive of pulsatile flow (Wesolowski *et al.*, 1950), hindered the adoption and development of these technologies, and ensured that non-pulsatile perfusion became the regime of choice for clinical perfusion applications. Research into pulsatile blood flow continued in the ensuing years, using much of the evolving technology of the latter third of the twentieth century. Many investigators used balloon pumps to generate pulsatile flow during cardiopulmonary bypass (Berger and Saini, 1972; Pappas *et al.*, 1975; Biddle *et al.*, 1976). However, once again, technical complexity and fears of generating excessive haemolysis limited widespread use of such systems during routine cardiopulmonary bypass. In the mid-1970s, the Stockert Company from Germany produced a pulsatile roller pump that offered all of the desired characteristics for a clinical device: familiarity, simplicity and safety. This pulsatile roller pump sparked a renewed

interest in pulsatile flow during routine cardiopulmonary bypass, and further research and development of this and alternative pulsatile flow technologies continues to the present day.

PUMPING SYSTEMS FOR PULSATILE PERFUSION

A number of pumping systems have been designed for cardiopulmonary bypass, some of which offer some degree of pulsatility as a clinical option. In the previous edition of this book, Bregman *et al.* (1991) described these pumps as falling broadly into two categories: positive displacement pumps and kinetic pumps. The positive displacement pumps comprise roller and ventricular mechanisms, whereas the kinetic pumps include the centrifugal or forced vortex pumps.

Positive displacement pumps

ROLLER PUMPS

The roller pump is probably the mechanism that is most familiar to clinicians, and is widely used in many pumping applications in other medical specialities, including renal dialysis. The pump works on the very simple principle of milking a constrained piece of tubing of known diameter and length (Fig. 9.1). Typically, the roller pump has two diametrically opposed rollers that ensure the 'positive displacement' of the perfusate, the rollers preventing backflow by performing the function of valves. In 'non-pulsatile' mode, the roller pump rotates at a constant speed, delivering a continuous blood flow, with only a small ripple

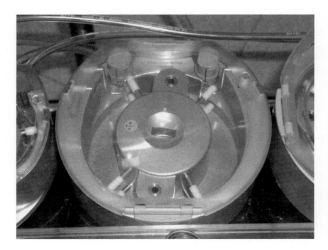

Figure 9.1 *The roller pump head. The roller pump played a significant role in the safe and effective routine application of clinical cardiopulmonary bypass. The pump operates on a simple 'milking' principle and is extremely safe and effective.*

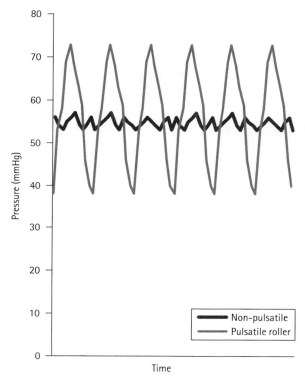

Figure 9.2 *Radial artery pressure profiles taken from patients undergoing pulsatile and non-pulsatile perfusion. The ripple pattern present in the non-pulsatile patient is the result of the pump head rollers making and breaking contact with the tubing in the pump head.*

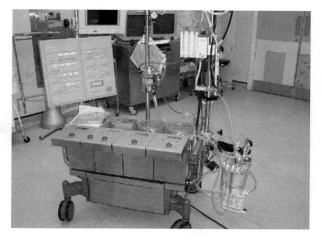

Figure 9.3 *The Stockert pulsatile roller pump, shown here in the operating theatre at Hammersmith Hospital. This pump revolutionized pulsatile flow for routine practice, largely because of its low-inertia pump head and stepping motor technology.*

have formed the basis of much of the ensuing research into pulsatility of blood flow during cardiopulmonary bypass.

The use of the pulsatile roller pump results in a pulsatile pressure profile in the patient that has all the elements of physiological pulsatile pressure: amplitude, frequency and wavelength, but rarely resembles a physiological pulse pressure profile (*see* Fig. 9.2). The principal attraction of pumps of this nature is that they offer a pulsatile flow option, with all of the other benefits of the conventional roller pump mechanism, such as familiarity, a high level of control and safety.

VENTRICULAR PUMPS

Ventricular pumps, or reciprocating pumps, operate in a manner that is very similar to the heart itself. In general terms, during the ejection cycle, these mechanisms operate by compressing a quantity of blood contained within a ventricle or sac. Once the pressure head, against which the pump is operating, is exceeded by the pressure within the ventricle, an outlet one-way valve will open, driven by the pressure differential across it, and blood is ejected through the outlet valve. The fill cycle is driven either passively by the pressure differential at the inlet of the ventricle at the end of the ejection cycle, or actively by generating a negative pressure within the ventricle. The negative pressure required for active drive is generated by withdrawing the compression mechanism, either by mechanical coupling of the compression device to the drive mechanism, or by actively withdrawing the hydraulic drive fluid (Fig. 9.4). The complex nature of this type of pump, along with cost considerations, has limited its use in routine clinical practice. The passive filling system, where the filling cycle is driven solely by the inlet pressure differential, results in a mechanism that is largely incompatible with modern

present in the output flow or pressure pattern (Fig. 9.2) resulting from the action of the rollers making and breaking contact with the tubing. The roller mechanism can be made to deliver a form of pulsatile flow by rapidly accelerating and decelerating the pump head. Early investigators found that by modifying roller pumps in this manner, they could be made to generate some measurable degree of pulsatility (Ogata *et al.*, 1959; Nonoyama, 1960; Nakayama *et al.*, 1963). However, further development of such systems was hampered by fears, principally on the part of clinicians, of generating unacceptably high levels of haemolysis when using these pumps in the pulsatile mode. The introduction of stepping motor technology to clinical pump systems by the Stockert Company from Munich, Germany in the mid-1970s stimulated renewed interest in roller pump generated pulsatile flow. This new pump (Fig. 9.3) had a lightweight, low inertia pump head that was controllable in terms of its position and speed at all times, and offered a new dimension in pulsatile pumps for clinical use, being both controllable and technologically familiar. Early studies demonstrated that fears of excessive haemolysis were unfounded (Taylor *et al.*, 1978). This pump proved to be the model for a number of subsequent mechanisms that

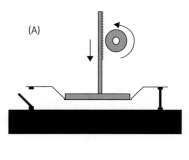

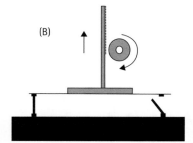

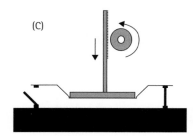

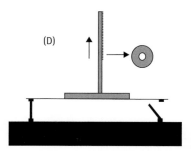

Figure 9.4 *Mode of operation of two common varieties of ventricular pump, active filling system (A and B) and passive filling system (C and D). In both systems the ejection cycles are similar (A and C), driven by the rotating drive wheel coupled to the drive shaft. They differ, however, in the filling cycle (B and D). In the active-fill system the coupling of the drive wheel and shaft remains during filling and the wheel rotates in the opposite direction to that employed during the ejection phase, resulting in the compression plate being actively 'pulled' back to the zero position; the associated negative pressure in the ventricle itself effects ventricular filling. In the passive system, the drive wheel and shaft are de-coupled, and the ventricle fill is powered by the head of pressure in the inlet side of the system.*

clinical cardiopulmonary bypass (Runge *et al.*, 1989). Positioning such a pump within the typical perfusion circuit can be extremely difficult, as it needs to be located significantly below its feeding reservoir to permit passive filling. For this reason, among others, passively filling ventricular pumps are generally employed for ventricular assist where output governance by inflow conditions can be advantageous.

The active filling ventricular systems offer the best option for routine clinical cardiopulmonary bypass application. The action of actively filling the ventricle during the fill cycle by either mechanical coupling of the drive mechanism to the ventricle (Runge *et al.*, 1989), or by hydraulic fluid displacement (Rottenberg *et al.*, 1995), renders the ventricle independent of its position within the perfusion circuit. Systems of this type have been employed for clinical studies with considerable success (Waldenberger *et al.*, 1997; Mutch *et al.*, 1998). However, the introduction of ventricular pumps in routine clinical practice has been hampered by a number of factors, in particular the cost of employing such pumps routinely. The valve mechanism required for the operation of ventricular pumps has always proved prohibitively expensive. Despite the ability of these systems to produce truly pulsatile blood flow (Fig. 9.5), the enthusiasm of clinicians to use them has been tempered by cost consciousness and, to date, experience remains limited.

Kinetic pumps

Kinetic pumps are load-sensitive pumps in which the generation of blood flow is achieved by increasing the

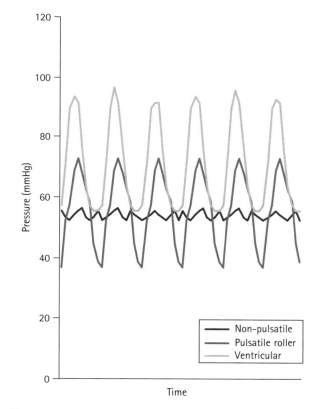

Figure 9.5 *Radial artery pressure profile taken from a patient undergoing perfusion with a ventricular pumping system. The pressure profile has near-physiological architecture.*

velocity of blood at the inlet of the pump head by rotating an impeller (Fig. 9.6). This results in an increase in the kinetic energy of the blood at the outlet, resulting in its

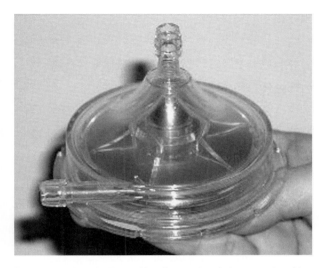

Figure 9.6 *A typical centrifugal pump head, the pump head is shown separated from the drive mechanism. The impeller can be seen in the pump head and the drive magnets are apparent at the base of the mechanism.*

positive displacement. A number of factors influence the blood flow generated by such systems, including input pressure, resistance (or pressure head) against which the pump must operate and the rotational rate of the impeller. Kinetic pumps are, in fact, the only truly non-pulsatile pumps, insofar as the output profile associated with their use has none of the elements normally associated with pulsatility, or the ripple pattern associated with the use of the roller pump mechanism. However, attempts have been made to produce pulsatile flow with such systems with some degree of success. The rapid acceleration of the pump head required to generate flow with any degree of pulsatile content with the kinetic mechanism is mechanically taxing and, it has been suggested, may be associated with the generation of unacceptable degrees of haemolysis. A number of studies have indicated that these fears are unfounded (Takami *et al.*, 1996; Tayama *et al.*, 1997a). However, clinical acceptance of pulsatile centrifugal pumps has been slow to evolve. Many early studies using pulsatile centrifugal systems were not encouraging, with some investigators finding difficulty in generating pulsatile flow that approached physiological proportions (Nishida *et al.*, 1997). Many of these early studies found that these pumps were not associated with many of the perceived advantages of pulsatile perfusion typically seen when using the pulsatile roller pump (Komada *et al.*, 1992). However, recent studies are more encouraging. Orime and co-workers (Orime *et al.*, 1999) found that the new Jostra centrifugal pump, which offers a pulsatile mode of operation, was associated with a similar degree of improved kidney and liver microcirculation normally encountered when using a pulsatile roller pump system. Ongoing study with this device continues to be extremely encouraging (Hata *et al.*, 1999).

Centrifugal or kinetic pumps are truly non-pulsatile instruments under normal operating conditions. However, recent engineering innovations and developments have resulted in kinetic systems that are capable of generating some degree of pulsatile blood flow, and this, coupled with the safety benefits inherent in this mechanism, may spark new interest in clinical studies of pulsatile flow in an area where only combination technologies had previously been considered (Ninomiya *et al.*, 1994).

THE PHYSIOLOGICAL EFFECTS OF PULSATILE PERFUSION

The physiological effects of pulsatile flow used during routine cardiopulmonary bypass have been extensively studied and can be categorized in terms of haemodynamic and metabolic effects. Although the vast majority of evidence is supportive towards the use of pulsatile blood flow during cardiopulmonary bypass, and there is little evidence that is directly contraindicative, the effect of flow modality on the body as a system is extremely complex, not fully understood, and remains controversial.

Haemodynamic effects of pulsatile blood flow

The haemodynamic effects of pulsatile cardiopulmonary bypass are the most immediately apparent to the clinician. One of the most consistently reported clinical findings in this regard relates to the effect of flow modality on systemic vascular resistance, with more physiological levels being maintained in patients undergoing a pulsatile flow regime (Videcoq *et al.*, 1987; Taylor, 1980). Taylor (1980) confirmed this effect (Fig. 9.7) when he demonstrated that patients who undergo non-pulsatile perfusion generally develop a progressive vasoconstriction that, if left unchecked, can seriously compromise the patient in the post-perfusion phase of the cardiac surgical procedure. The vasoconstriction, seen under non-pulsatile flow, often needs to be reversed by pharmacological intervention during the critical post-operative phase. However, Taylor (1980) suggested that pulsatile flow used during cardiopulmonary bypass may represent an alternative strategy to pharmacological intervention in dealing with this unwanted post-operative complication. Although it is clear that pharmacological intervention can successfully moderate the effects of vasoconstriction (Stinson *et al.*, 1977), it is reasonable to argue that prevention by use of pulsatile flow is a more satisfactory and physiological solution than pharmacological cure.

The mechanisms involved in preserving the haemodynamic status under pulsatile flow conditions are complex and, as yet, not fully understood. A number of factors

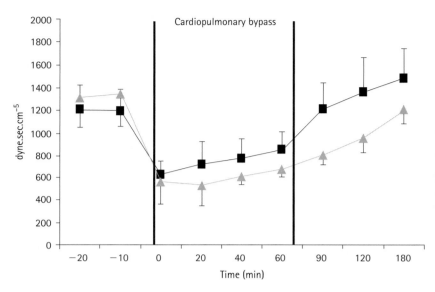

Figure 9.7 *System vascular resistance (SVR) in two groups of patients, one undergoing a pulsatile flow regime (Δ–Δ, n = 50), the other non-pulsatile (■–■, n = 10). There is a rise in SVR in both groups thoughout the perfusion period, which persists into the post-operative period. However, SVR is significantly higher in the non-pulsatile flow group and exceeds the pre-bypass values early in the post-operative phase. The difference between the two groups is significant during the perfusion period, with the pulsatile flow group showing more moderate SVR.*

have been identified as contributing to the vasoconstriction associated with non-pulsatile flow, including activation of the renin-angiotensin (Taylor *et al.*, 1979a; Taylor, 1980; Townsend *et al.*, 1984; Kaul *et al.*, 1990) system, and release of catecholamines, vasopressin and local tissue vasoconstrictors (Hutcheson and Griffith, 1991; Levine *et al.*, 1981; Minami *et al.*, 1990). However, in understanding why these different flow modalities generate different physiological responses in patients undergoing cardiopulmonary bypass, it is necessary to address the fundamental differences between the two regimes in terms of blood flow delivery to the tissues, and to bear in mind that even with regard to this simple mechanism, opinion is divided (Weinstein *et al.*, 1987).

Microcirculatory effects of pulsatile blood flow

Burton (1954) suggested that, as arterial blood pressure begins to decay after systole, blood flow in the microcirculation continues until a specific critical closing pressure in the pre-capillary arterioles is reached, at which point blood flow within the capillaries will cease. He further demonstrated that pulsatility prolongs the period of capillary opening and blood flow. This concept is largely the basis of pulsatile blood flow as a preferred flow modality and may explain many of its perceived benefits. As early as 1938, McMaster and Parsons demonstrated that lymph flow is greatly reduced when blood flow is de-pulsed. Ogata *et al.* (1960) confirmed that capillary blood flow and diameter are affected by the presence of a pulse, irrespective of total blood flow and mean pressure. Concurrently, Takeda (1960) demonstrated that there was a general collapse in capillary structure, coupled to a reduction in blood flow and an increase in capillary shunting

with non-pulsatile blood flow. Once again, in these animal experiments, mean blood flow and arterial pressure were the same in both the pulsatile and non-pulsatile flow arms of the study, indicating that the pulse itself was responsible for the observed benefit. The reduction in capillary diameter and capillary shunting correlates extremely well with the clinical findings of increased peripheral vascular resistance with non-pulsatile flow. It has been suggested, more recently, that it may not be the pulse pressure that is responsible for the maintenance of an open periphery under pulsatile blood flow conditions. Shepard *et al.* (1966) postulated that the critical closing pressure argument is correct, but that it is the energy delivered to the tissues under pulsatile flow conditions which is responsible for the maintenance of an open periphery. They determined, by use of both mathematical and physical modelling, that pulsatile blood flow at the same mean pressure and flow contains up to 2.4 times the energy content of a non-pulsatile blood flow modality. Wilcox *et al.* (1967) confirmed this when he determined that pulsatile blood flow is responsible for the dissipation of significantly more energy through the tissues. Shepard *et al.* (1966) had suggested that the increased energy delivered under pulsatile blood flow conditions is responsible for maintaining capillary patency, and that the pulse itself, which is discernible to the capillary level, is responsible for the exchange of fluids at the extracellular level, thus maintaining cell metabolism. Using a rabbit model Parsons and McMaster (1938) noted that oedema developed in an isolated ear preparation when perfused with non-pulsatile blood flow and that those perfused in a pulsatile manner remained essentially normal. They also found that contrast dye cleared more rapidly from the ear perfused with pulsatile blood flow, suggesting that fluid exchange and clearance is enhanced under pulsatile flow conditions. These findings tend to add weight to those of Shepard *et al.* (1966). Prior *et al.*

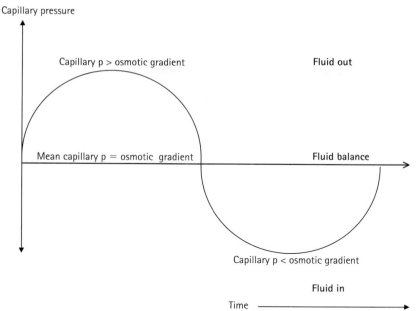

Capillary pressure

Capillary p > osmotic gradient   **Fluid out**

Mean capillary p = osmotic gradient   **Fluid balance**

Capillary p < osmotic gradient

Fluid in

Time

Pulse reverse osmosis suggests that fluid balance is achieved when the mean capillary pressure is equal and opposite to the osmotic gradient. During the systolic phase of the pulse wave the capillary pressure exceeds the osmotic gradient resulting in fluid movement out of the capillary. During diastole the osmotic gradient exceeds the capillary pressure resulting in fluid being drawn back into the capillary.

Figure 9.8 *Pulse reverse osmosis (PRO) as described by Prior* et al. *(1995). (Reproduced with permission of the author.)*

(1995) suggested that the pulse is responsible for the exchange of fluids at the capillary level and that the mean pressure is responsible for the maintenance of fluid balance (Fig. 9.8). This simple relationship, which Prior described as 'pulsed reverse osmosis', suggests that the architecture of the pulse pressure profile at the capillary level, with the mean blood pressure and osmotic pressures in the blood and interstitium, are the factors responsible for the maintenance of fluid balance and the exchange of nutrients at the cellular level. This is largely in keeping with the Starling Principle (Starling, 1896) with the exception that Starling did not recognize the presence or importance of the pulse or differential pore distribution at the capillary level (Prior *et al.*, 1996). This microcirculatory effect may be fundamental to the importance of pulsatile flow in the maintenance of normal physiological function. This theory is gaining support, and is the focus of continued laboratory and clinical research.

Metabolic effects of pulsatile perfusion

The importance of the pulse to metabolic processes has been the focus of research for many decades and the literature on the subject is substantial. Most of the major organ systems have been studied in this regard, and the effects of pulsatile flow on their function and structure have been investigated extensively.

Pulsatile blood flow and the kidney

The effect of pulsatile flow on renal function has been the focus of research for some time, considerably pre-dating

the clinical application of cardiopulmonary bypass. In 1889, using an isolated renal preparation, Hamel (1889) confirmed that the pulse had an important influence on kidney function. These early studies were supported by the work of Gesell (1913), who postulated that the improved kidney function associated with pulsatile flow was the result of improved gas exchange at the capillary level, with enhanced lymph flow. That the pulse itself was associated with the maintenance of renal function was shown by Kohlstaedt and Page (1940), who demonstrated that the absence of pulsatility in blood flow to an isolated kidney preparation was associated with an increase in rennin secretion and a reduction in urine flow. These early findings were the foundation for a substantial body of work in the ensuing years. These results were later supported by a similar study carried out by Many *et al.* (1968), in which the renal arteries of dogs were depulsed. This study confirmed that rennin levels increased in those animals which underwent depulsation and that this was further associated with significant systemic electrolyte and fluid imbalance.

Mavroudis (1978), in his excellent review of the subject, points out that there are those who contest the importance of pulsatile flow. Selkurt (1951), Ritter (1952), Goodyer and Glenn (1951), and Oelert and Eufe (1974) all found that renal function appeared not to be affected by the presence of a pulse in isolated renal preparations, provided the mean blood pressure was maintained at physiological levels. The differences between the modelling methods employed in these studies may, in part, be responsible for the conflicting results. However, the overwhelming bulk of studies carried out using various models of cardiopulmonary bypass tend to support the early findings, which show some degree of renal functional preservation with pulsatile flow in isolated organs.

By using animal cardiopulmonary bypass models, Fintersbuch *et al.* (1961) and Nakayama *et al.* (1963) reported that renal venous return was preserved under pulsatile blood flow conditions, and a loss in normal renal artery configuration was associated with non-pulsatile blood flow. Using a similar model, Barger and Herd (1966) had associated these findings with a shift in intra-renal blood flow, resulting in decreased sodium excretion. The effect of pulsatile flow on renal blood flow was further demonstrated by Boucher *et al.* (1974), who used radioactively labelled microspheres in a bypass model to show that renal blood flow was preserved under pulsatile flow conditions. This effect was further described by Mori *et al.* (1988), who found that, after a period of hypothermic circulatory arrest, renal blood flow was substantially higher and kidneys recovered function more fully and rapidly in dogs exposed to pulsatile blood flow during the reperfusion period, and by Nakamura *et al.* (1989), who reported that renal blood flow, lactate extraction and urine output were higher when pulsatile rather than non-pulsatile cardiopulmonary bypass was employed in a similar canine model. Undar *et al.* (1999), using a piglet model, found once again that organ blood flow, including blood flow to the kidney, was preserved under pulsatile flow conditions. Many of the findings from isolated organ and animal studies has been confirmed in clinical studies. German *et al.* (1972) demonstrated that non-pulsatile blood flow was associated with a more rapid onset of renal hypoxia and acidosis than pulsatile flow, despite apparently adequate total blood flow. Mukherjee *et al.* (1973) subsequently confirmed these findings, reporting decreased tissue PO_2 in the medulla with non-pulsatile blood flow, with increased local lactate levels and decreased oxygen uptake. Taylor *et al.* (1982) described an increase in urine production and a decrease in plasma angiotensin II levels associated with the clinical use of pulsatile blood flow during open-heart surgical procedures. Similarly, Landymore *et al.* (1979) found that urine output was enhanced with pulsatile flow and that plasma rennin levels were higher with non-pulsatile flow. The findings associated with adult cardiac surgery were mirrored in paediatric surgery. Williams *et al.* (1979), in a study of infants, found that urine output in patients undergoing pulsatile flow was twice that of patients who underwent a non-pulsatile flow regime.

In keeping with the findings from animal and *in vitro* studies, not all the clinical findings have been in favour of pulsatile flow. A number of studies tend to indicate that there is no real difference between pulsatile and non-pulsatile flow regimes with regard to renal function. Badner *et al.* (1992) found that the flow regime had little or no effect on renal function, and Louagie *et al.* (1992) concluded that pulsatile blood flow was associated with reduced urine output and reduced creatinine clearance in routine cardiopulmonary bypass patients. The reasons for these results may be associated with a number of variable factors, including the pulse architecture and anaesthetic regime employed, both of which have been shown to have an effect on clinical findings (Mavroudis, 1978; Wright, 1997; Gourlay, 1997; Taylor, 1986). The use of anaesthetic regimes, which have varying haemodynamic effects of their own, with varying pump output profiles may offer some explanation for the conflicting findings relating to the physiological effects of pulsatile flow during cardiopulmonary bypass. Until some degree of consensus can be reached on the ideal blood flow profile and anaesthetic regime, the controversy surrounding pulsatile flow may persist.

The use of pulsatile flow and its effect during routine cardiopulmonary bypass continues to be debated. However, it has been suggested that the optimum benefit from the application of pulsatile flow may be most apparent in high-risk patients. Matsuda *et al.* (1986), suggested that patients who present with pre-operative renal insufficiency may benefit most from the pulsatile flow regime, confirming that renal function is preserved in this patient group only under pulsatile flow conditions.

Pulsatile blood flow and the brain

Despite its inherent, protective, autoregulatory mechanism, the brain is susceptible to injury during cardiopulmonary bypass. A number of factors have been shown to affect the brain during cardiopulmonary bypass (Taylor, 1986), including temperature, blood pressure, blood viscosity, and oxygen and carbon dioxide tension. Early studies by Hill *et al.* (1969) described significant neuropathological manifestations, including histological evidence of focal brain lesions resulting from cardiopulmonary bypass during open heart surgery. Subsequently, a number of studies have confirmed these early findings, and have shown that many of these inappropriate results could be prevented by employing pulsatile flow during the perfusion phase of the operation. Using similar canine models, Sanderson *et al.* (1972) and Taylor (1980) demonstrated that the diffuse brain cell damage associated with non-pulsatile flow was not apparent under pulsatile conditions, and that the level of creatine kinase BB iso-enzyme in cerebrospinal fluid was significantly lower in animals perfused with pulsatile flow, indicating significantly less cerebral injury.

Studies have also confirmed that the flow modality employed has an effect on the physiological response of the brain during cardiac surgery. In a series studies, Taylor *et al.* (1979b) demonstrated that the activity of the hypothalmic–pituitary axis to surgical stress is markedly different in the presence of pulsatile and non-pulsatile blood flow. These workers showed that the anterior pituitary response to thyrotrophin-releasing hormone (TRH) is hampered. The secretion of adrenocorticotrophic hormone (ACTH) and cortisol was also found to be significantly reduced under non-pulsatile flow conditions (Taylor *et al.*, 1980). Philbin *et al.* (1979) had already demonstrated a similar response pattern with vasopressin secretion during non-pulsatile cardiopulmonary bypass. All these findings reflect a major difference in the physiological response of the brain to the perfusion modality, and confirm that pulsatile flow is associated with a more physiological response pattern than non-pulsatile flow.

In addition to maintaining the functional aspect of cerebral activity, pulsatile flow has the effect of preventing the cerebral acidosis normally encountered during the early phase of cardiopulmonary bypass with non-pulsatile flow (Briceno and Runge, 1994). This may be because of the effect of pulsatile flow in maintaining regional cerebral blood flow, which dePaepe *et al.* (1979) and Simpson (1981) suggested may be disrupted during non-pulsatile flow. Kono *et al.* (1990) demonstrated that there was a difference of as much as 25 per cent in the measured cerebral vascular resistance between pulsatile and non-pulsatile groups of patients. This highly significant difference in cerebral vascular resistance, with improved regional blood flow and distribution, may be responsible for the reduced cerebral excess lactate encountered by Mori *et al.* (1981), who suggested that regional blood flow was maintained and anaerobic metabolism was suppressed with the application of pulsatile blood flow, particularly during the critical cooling and rewarming phase of the operative procedure. Other studies, focusing on cerebral oxygen consumption, indicate that pulsatile flow is associated with increased cerebral metabolism under pulsatile flow conditions (Mutch *et al.*, 2000).

These data, suggesting improved cerebral function and metabolism under pulsatile flow conditions, do not go unchallenged. Many investigators suggest that there is no difference between clinically applied pulsatile flow and non-pulsatile flow with regard to cerebral effects. Hindman *et al.* (1995), in a study focusing on cerebral blood flow and cerebral oxygen consumption in a rabbit model, found no difference, in terms of either parameter, between pulsatile and non-pulsatile flow regimes. Similarly, Grubhofer *et al.* (2000) and Kawahara *et al.* (1999) found that there was no change in cerebral oxygenation during cardiopulmonary bypass under pulsatile flow conditions. However, the nature of the pulsatile flow regime applied in these studies, rather than pulsatile flow *per se*, may significantly contribute to these findings.

Pulsatile blood flow and the liver and pancreas

Disruption of the blood flow to the liver and pancreas is a well-documented complication of cardiopulmonary

bypass for cardiac surgery. Interest in the effects of cardiopulmonary bypass on pancreatic function was stimulated by early sporadic and isolated findings which pointed to increased plasma amylase levels associated with non-pulsatile bypass, and by the findings of Feiner (1976), who reported a 16 per cent incidence of ischaemic pancreatitis in patients who had undergone open heart surgery with non-pulsatile blood flow. Baca *et al.* (1979), using a canine model, found that pancreatic function was preserved under pulsatile blood flow conditions and impaired under non-pulsatile conditions. Saggau *et al.* (1980), monitoring insulin levels, with glucose, glucagon and growth hormone, in both human and animal studies, concluded that pulsatile blood flow during the perfusion phase of the operation preserved normal pancreatic function. In a clinical study, Murray *et al.* (1982) were able to demonstrate improved pancreatic function associated with a reduction in the occurance of elevated amylase levels in patients undergoing cardiopulmonary bypass with pulsatile flow. Mori *et al.* (1988) concluded that pancreatic function was preserved in those dogs perfused under both hypothermia and normothermia only in the presence of pulsatile blood flow.

Studies of hepatic function during pulsatile and non-pulsatile cardiopulmonary bypass have generated similar results to that of pancreatic function. Employing serum glutamic-oxayloacetic transaminase (sGOT) as a marker of hepatic injury, Pappas *et al.* (1975) found that pulsatile blood flow was associated with the preservation of hepatic function. Mathie *et al.* (1984) demonstrated that pulsatile cardiopulmonary bypass in dogs preserved both hepatic blood flow and function. This was echoed in the results of a series of clinical studies carried out by Chiu *et al.* (1984), who described normal hepatic function associated with pulsatile blood flow during cardiopulmonary bypass, as reflected in post-operative sGOT levels. Mathie *et al.* (1984) demonstrated that hepatic blood flow showed a typical vasoconstrictive response to non-pulsatile cardiopulmonary bypass, coupled with a reduction in hepatic oxygen consumption. The preservation of more physiological blood flow to the liver and pancreas with pulsatile blood flow when compared to non-pulsatile blood flow, may be the most significant underlying factor in the preservation of normal function and architecture in these tissues.

Pulsatile blood flow and the gut

Abdominal complications associated with cardiopulmonary bypass form a significant part of the reported operative mortality. In one study of 500 open-heart surgical procedures, Gauss *et al.* (1994) reported that 1.8 per cent of the patients exhibited some form of abdominal complication. The mortality rate was high in this group of patients, at 44 per cent, which reflects the seriousness of this complication. In an extremely substantial review of 5924 patients, Baue (1993) confirmed that gastrointestinal problems were responsible for a significant amount of cardiopulmonary bypass-related mortality and morbidity, and suggested that one mechanism leading to these complications was the mesenteric hypoperfusion associated with non-pulsatile blood flow. Many studies have linked this hypoperfusion with gut ischaemia and endotoxaemia (Bowles et al., 1995). Endotoxaemia associated with cardiopulmonary bypass in children has been the focus of study for some time. Anderson and Baek (1992) linked the high levels of endotoxin found in children to increased gut permeability associated with mesenteric ischaemia. Anderson et al. (1987) had earlier demonstrated that the endotoxaemia seen during and after bypass was not associated with pre-operative infection. A number of studies have shown that peak levels of endotoxin occurred after the release of the aortic cross-clamp during the phase of rewarming (Rocke et al., 1987; Jansen et al., 1992). Ohri et al. (1994), using a canine model of bypass, confirmed the importance of the rewarming phase to the pathophysiology of endotoxaemia. These authors further demonstrated that, during this phase of the procedure, there was a disparity between the mesenteric oxygen consumption and oxygen delivery, with an associated increase in gut permeability. Using a porcine model, Tao et al. (1995) demonstrated that the gut mucosa does, indeed, become ischaemic during cardiopulmonary bypass and suggested that this may be caused by two factors: blood flow redistribution and shifting tissue oxygen demand. Riddington et al. (1996) confirmed these findings in the clinical model, demonstrating that patients undergoing cardiopulmonary bypass exhibited increased gut mucosal ischaemia and gut permeability and that endotoxin was detectable in the plasma of 42 per cent of these patients. These workers further found that elevated intestinal pH did not return to normal until the non-pulsatile flow regime was terminated and the heart took over the circulation. Later, Hamulu et al. (1998) described a similar effect.

Fiddian-Green (1990) suggested that pulsatile blood flow may result in improved blood flow to the gut, reducing mucosal ischaemia and increasing oxygen delivery. He further suggested the application of pre-operative gut lavage and parenteral antibiotics as a prophylactic approach to reducing the incidence of endotoxaemia. Reilly and Bulkey (1993) proposed that the vasoactive response in the gut to circulatory shock was mediated by the activation of the rennin-angiotensin system, leading to gut hypoperfusion and ischaemia, which results in increased gut permeability. The maintenance of more physiological circulatory architecture and flow, which Taylor et al. (1979b) associated with a lower level of rennin-angiotensin activation, may explain the lower incidence of gut complications associated with the use of pulsatile flow.

Tissue oxygen consumption

Many investigators and clinicians employ tissue oxygen consumption as an indicator of the adequacy of tissue perfusion during bypass, and pulsatile and non-pulsatile flow are frequently contrasted in this regard. Shepard and Kirklin (1969) described how oxygen consumption declined in calves exposed to non-pulsatile blood flow and that this contrasted with the preservation of tissue oxygen consumption levels in animals undergoing a pulsatile flow regime. In the same study, they described the development of metabolic acidosis in animals undergoing non-pulsatile blood flow. The development of metabolic acidosis, linked to lower oxygen consumption, has been a fairly routine finding with non-pulsatile flow conditions, and many investigators have shown that oxygen consumption is increased and metabolic acidosis is prevented under pulsatile flow conditions (Jacobs et al., 1969; Dunn et al., 1974). That these findings are associated with improved blood flow to the tissues is highlighted in studies that indicate that physiological levels of oxygen consumption are preserved and acidosis prevented when very high blood flow rates are used under non-pulsatile flow conditions (Ogata et al., 1960; Boucher et al., 1974). Boucher et al. (1974) demonstrated that, at flow rates in excess of 200 mL/kg per minute, there was no advantage offered by pulsatile blood flow, but this is in excess of normal clinical blood flow conditions.

Shepard et al. (1966) suggested that there may be three mechanisms which explain the difference between pulsatile and non-pulsatile blood flow conditions with respect to tissue oxygen consumption:

1 The pulse component may break down the boundary layer around cells, enhancing diffusion.
2 The pulse may be responsible for overcoming the capillary critical closing pressure.
3 Interstitial and lymph flow may be enhanced during pulsatile blood flow.

Recent work by Prior et al. (1995) appears to confirm this.

Tissue oxygen consumption is an excellent marker of the adequacy of perfusion. Early recognition of oxygen deficit and the development of tissue acidosis led clinicians to employ core cooling to reduce the metabolic demands of patients undergoing cardiopulmonary bypass. Even when these cooling techniques are employed, pulsatile flow is associated with a higher oxygen demand (Sheperd and Kirklin, 1969), indicating improved tissue perfusion. Modern gas exchange devices can meet the increased oxygen demand associated with pulsatile flow with no difficulty (Gourlay and Taylor, 1994; Gourlay et al., 1997). At the point of maximum demand, when rewarming is taking place, patients being perfused with a non-pulsatile flow regime may already present the regional ischaemic conditions required for the development of reperfusion injury.

Pulsatile flow may offer a simple and effective preventative therapy by maintaining a normal vascular architecture.

FACTORS LIMITING THE EFFICIENT DELIVERY OF PULSATILE BLOOD FLOW

Mechanical pulsatile pumping systems are efficient machines, capable of delivering blood flow with considerable hydraulic power. However, the efficiency of these devices is limited in clinical practice by a number of extrinsic factors. In routine clinical practice, the arterial pump is positioned remotely in terms of the aorta, the vessel into which it generally pumps blood. Ideally, the pump should be positioned close to the aorta, interfacing with it in a similar manner to the aorta with the native heart, but this is, unfortunately, not realistic in conventional clinical perfusion circuits. Between the pump and the aorta one typically finds several large-surface-area, large-volume devices, for example the membrane oxygenator and arterial filter, and a considerable length of flexible tubing. The movement and flexing of the tubing and membrane surfaces all absorb energy, reducing the efficiency of the pulse generator. Many studies have characterized the energy-absorbing properties of these devices when used in typical clinical circuitry (Wright, 1989; Gourlay and Taylor, 1994; Inzoli et al., 1997) (Fig. 9.9). All of these studies show that the in-line devices and the tubing of the perfusion circuit absorb a significant amount of energy. However, the most limiting factor in terms of pulsatile blood flow delivery is the aortic cannula. The diameter of the aortic cannula is often less than 4 or 5 mm, a significant step down from the 8–10 mm of normal arterial tubing. This diametric reduction has a significant effect on the pulse architecture delivered to the aorta. Some investigators have demonstrated that it is possible to generate pulsatile flow of physiological proportions in the aorta through a large cannula (Runge et al., 1992); however, the introduction of large-diameter pipes into the aorta may present an unacceptable additional level of risk to an already complex operative procedure.

THE FUTURE OF PULSATILE PERFUSION

The evolution of pulsatile perfusion has paralleled and embraced the developing technologies of the last century. The level of control offered by the introduction of the 'stepping motor' as part of a pulsatile roller pump had a radical effect on the level of acceptance and clinical use of pulsatile flow systems. Further advances in pump design have resulted in the production of pulsatile pumps that are capable of producing near-physiological pulse pressure or flow profiles, as shown in laboratory studies by Inzoli et al. (1996), Undar et al. (1996), Gourlay (1997) and Wright (1997). However, the limiting factors outlined in the previous section of this chapter still remain at present. Recent developments in clinical cardiopulmonary bypass offer some hope for the future of pulsatile perfusion. Although these recent advances, which include miniaturization of the perfusion circuit (Darling et al., 1998; Suenaga et al., 2000) and moving the entire perfusion apparatus closer to the patient, aided by vacuum-assisted venous drainage (Lau et al., 1999; Munster et al., 1999), suit the requirements for optimising pulsatile cardiopulmonary bypass perfectly, the principal limiting factor, the arterial cannula, remains a serious hurdle to be overcome in terms of pulse transmission. If this cannulation issue can be addressed, it may be possible to reap all the perceived benefits of truly physiological pulsatile flood flow in the near future.

REFERENCES

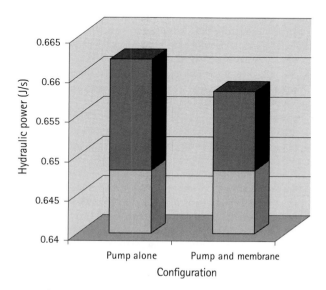

Figure 9.9 *The effect of including a membrane oxygenator in the arterial line of the perfusion circuit on pulsatile hydraulic power. The membrane clearly reduces the energy delivered in the pulsatile domain.*

Anderson, L.W., Baek, L. 1992: Transient endotoxaemia during cardiac surgery. *Perfusion* **7**, 53–8.

Anderson, L.W., Baek, L., Degen, H., Lehd, J., Krasnik, M., Rasmussen, J.P. 1987: Presence of circulating endotoxins during cardiac operations. *Journal of Thoracic and Cardiovascular Surgery* **93**, 115–19.

Baca, I., Beiger, W., Mittmann, U., Saggau, W., Schmidt-Gayk, H., Storch, H.H. 1979: Comparative studies of pulsatile and continuous flow during extracorporeal circulation. Effects on liver function and endocrine pancreas secretion. *Chir Forum Exp Klin Forsch*, 49–53.

Badner, N.H., Murkin, J.M., Lok, P. 1992: Differences in pH management and pulsatile/nonpulsatile perfusion during cardiopulmonary bypass do not influence renal function. *Anesthesia and Analgesia* **75**, 696–701.

Barger, A.C., Herd, J.A. 1966: Study of renal circulation in the un-anaesthetized dog with inert gases (Proceedings of the Third International Congress of Nephrology). *Nephrology* **1**, 174–82.

Baue, A.E. 1993: The role of the gut in the development of multiple organ dysfunction in cardiothoracic patients. *Annals of Thoracic Surgery* **55**, 822–9.

Berger, R.L., Saini, V.K. 1972: Conversion of non-pulsatile cardiopulmonary bypass to pulsatile flow by intra-aortic balloon pumping during myocardial revascularisation for cardiogenic shock. *Circulation* **45** (Suppl. II), 130–7.

Biddle, T.L., Stewart, S., Stuard, I.D. 1976: Dissection of aorta complicating intra-aortic balloon counterpulsation. *American Heart Journal* **92**, 781–4.

Boucher, J.K., Rudy, L.W., Edmunds, L.H. 1974: Organ blood flow during pulsatile cardiopulmonary bypass. *Journal of Applied Physiology* **36**, 86–90.

Bowles, C.T., Ohri, S.K., Nongchana, K., Keogh, B.E., Yacoub, M.H., Taylor, K.M. 1995: Endotoxaemia detected during cardiopulmonary bypass with a modified Limulus amoebocyte lysate asay. *Perfusion* **10**, 219–28.

Bregman, D., Kesselbrenner, M., Sack, J.B. 1991: Pulsatile flow during cardiopulmonary bypass. In: Kay, P., ed. *Techniques in extracorporeal circulation*. London: Butterworth-Heinemann: 211–19.

Briceno, J.C., Runge, T.M. 1994: Monitoring of blood gasses during prolonged cardiopulmonary bypass and their relationship to brain pH, PO_2 and PCO_2. *ASAIO* **40**, M344–50.

Burton, A.C. 1954: Relationship of structure to function of the tissues of the wall of blood vessels. *Physiological Reviews* **34**, 618–42.

Chiu, I.S., Chu, S.H., Hung, C.R. 1984: Pulsatile flow during routine cardiopulmonary bypass. *Journal Cardiovascular Surgery* (Torino) **25**, 530–6.

Darling, E., Kaemmer, D., Lawson, S., Smigla, G., Collins, K., Shearer, I., Jaggers, J. 1998: Experimental use of an ultra-low prime neonatal cardiopulmonary bypass circuit utilizing vacuum-assisted venous drainage. *Journal of Extracorporeal Technology* **30**, 184–9.

dePaepe, J., Pomerantzeff, P.M.A., Nakiri, K., Armelin, E., Verginalli, G., Zerbini, E.J. 1979: Observations of the microcirculation of the cerebral cortex of dogs subjected to pulsatile and non-pulsatile flow during extracorporeal circulation. In: *A propos du debit pulse*. Belgium: Cobe Laboratories Inc.

Dunn, J., Kirsh, M.M., Harness, J., Carroll, M., Straker, J., Sloan, H. 1974: Hemodynamic, metabolic and hematologic effects of pulsatile cardiopulmonary bypass. *Journal of Thoracic and Cardiovascular Surgery* **68**, 138–47.

Feiner, H. 1976: Pancreatitis after cardiac surgery. *American Journal of Surgery* **131**, 684–8.

Fiddian-Green, R.G. 1990: Gut mucosal ischaemia during cardiac surgery. *Seminars in Thoracic and Cardiovascular Surgery* **4**, 389–99.

Fintersbuch, W., Long, D.M., Sellers, R.D. 1961: Renal arteriography during extracorporeal circulation in dogs with preliminary report upon effects of low molecular weight dextran. *Journal of Thoracic and Cardiovascular Surgery* **41**, 252–60.

Gauss, A., Druck, A., Hemmer, W., Georieff, M. 1994: Abdominal complications following heart surgery. *Anaesthesiol Intensivmed Notfallmed Schmerzther* **29**, 23–9.

German, J.C., Chalmers, G.S., Hirai, J., Mukherjee, N.D., Wakabayashi, A., Connolly, J.E. 1972: Comparison of nonpulsatile and pulsatile extracorporeal circulation on renal tissue perfusion. *Chest* **61**, 65–9.

Gesell, R.A. 1913: On relation of pulse pressure to renal function. *American Journal of Physiology* **32**, 70.

Gibbon, J.H. Jr. 1954: Application of a mechanical heart and lung apparatus to cardiac surgery. *Minnesota Medicine* **37**, 171–85.

Goodyer, A.V.N., Glenn, W.L. 1951: Relation of arterial pulse pressure to renal function. *American Journal of Physiology* **167**, 689–97.

Gourlay, T. 1997: Controlled pulsatile architecture in cardiopulmonary bypass: *in vitro* and clinical studies. PhD thesis, University of Strathclyde.

Gourlay, T., Taylor, K.M. 1994: Pulsatile flow and membrane oxygenators. *Perfusion* **9**, 189–96.

Gourlay, T., Gibbons, M., Taylor, K.M. 1987: Pulsatile flow compatibility of a group of membrane oxygenators. *Perfusion* **2**, 115–26.

Grubhofer, G., Mares, P., Rajek, A., Muller, T., Haisjackl, M., Dworschak, M. *et al.* 2000: Pulsatility does not change cerebral oxygenation during cardiopulmonary bypass. *Acta Anaesthesiological Scandinavica* **44**, 586–91.

Hamel, G. 1889: Dei Bedeutung des pulses fur den blutstrom. *Ztschr Biol NSF*, 474–97.

Hamulu, A., Atay, Y., Yagdi, T., Discigil, B., Bakalim, T., Buket, S. *et al.* 1998: Effects of flow types in cardiopulmonary bypass on gastric intramucosal pH. *Perfusion* **13**, 129–35.

Hata, M., Shiono, M., Orime, Y., Yagi, S., Yamamoto, T., Okumura, H. *et al.* 1999: Clinical use of Jostra Rota Flow centrifugal pump: the first case report in Japan. *Annals of Thoracic and Cardiovascular Surgery* **5**, 230–2.

Hill, J.D., Aguilar, K.J., Baranco, A., de Lanerolle, P., Gerbode, F. 1969: Neuropathological manifestations of cardiac surgery. *Annals of Thoracic Surgery* **7**, 409–19.

Hindman, B.J., Dexter, F., Smith, T., Cutkomp, J. 1995: Pulsatile versus nonpulsatile flow. No difference in cerebral blood flow or metabolism during normothermic cardiopulmonary bypass in rabbits. *Anaesthesiology* **82**, 241–50.

Hooker, D.R. 1910: A study of the isolated kidney: the influence of pulse pressure upon renal function. *American Journal of Physiology* **27**, 24–44.

Hutcheson, I.R., Griffith, T.M. 1991: Release of endothelium-derived relaxing factor is modulated both by frequency and amplitude of pulsatile flow. *American Journal of Physiology* **261**, H257–62.

Inzoli, F., Di Martino, E., Dubini, G., Redaelli, A., Fumero, R. 1996: A new pulsatile blood pump for adult cardiopulmonary bypass: design criteria and preliminary fluid dynamic evaluation. *International Journal of Artificial Organs* **19**, 359–66.

Inzoli, F., Pennati, G., Mastrantonio, F., Fini, M. 1997: Influence of membrane oxygenators on the pulsatile flow in extracorporeal circuits: an experimental analysis. *International Journal of Artificial Organs* **20**, 455–62.

Jacobs, L.A., Klopp, E.H., Seamone, W., Topaz, S.R., Gott, V.L. 1969: Improved organ function during cardiac bypass with a roller pump modified to deliver pulsatile flow. *Journal of Thoracic and Cardiovascular Surgery* **58**, 703–12.

Jansen, N.J., van Oeveren, W., Gu, Y.J., van Vliet, M.H., Eijsman, L., Wildevuur, C.R. 1992: Endotoxin release and tumor necrosis factor formation during cardiopulmonary bypass. *Annals of Thoracic Surgery* **54**, 744–7.

Kaul, T.K., Swaminathan, R., Chatrath, R.R., Watson, D.A. 1990: Vasoactive pressure hormones during and after cardiopulmonary bypass. *International Journal of Artificial Organs* **13**, 293–9.

Kawahara, F., Kadoi, Y., Saito, S., Yoshikawa, D., Goto, F., Fujita, N. 1999: Balloon pump induced pulsatile perfusion during cardiopulmonary bypass does not improve brain oxygenation. *Journal of Thoracic and Cardiovascular Surgery* **118**, 361–6.

Kohlstaedt, L.A., Page, I.H. 1940: The liberation of renin by perfusion of kidneys following reduction of pulse pressure. *Journal of Experimental Medicine* **72**, 201–11.

Komada, T., Maet, H., Imawaki, S., Shiriashi, Y., Tanaka, S. 1992: Hematologic and endocrinologic effects of pulsatile cardiopulmonary bypass using a centrifugal pump. *Nippon Kyobu Geka Zashi* **40**, 901–11.

Kono, M., Orita, H., Shimanuki, T., Fukasawa, M., Inui, K., Wasio, M. 1990: A clinical study of cerebral perfusion during pulsatile and non-pulsatile cardiopulmonary bypass. *Nippon Geka Gakki Zashi* **91**, 1016–22.

Landymore, R.W., Murphy, D.A., Kinley, C.E., Parrott, J.C., Moffitt, E.A., Longley, W.J., Qirbi, A.A. 1979: Does pulsatile flow influence the incidence of postoperative hypertension? *Annals of Thoracic Surgery* **28**, 261–8.

Lau, C.L., Posther, K.E., Stephenson, G.R., Lodge, A., Lawson, J.H., Darling, E.M. *et al.* 1999: Mini-circuit cardiopulmonary bypass with vacuum assisted venous drainage: feasibility of an asanguineous prime in the neonate. *Perfusion* **14**, 389–96.

Levine, F.H., Philbin, D.M., Kono, K., Coggins, C.H., Emerson, C.W., Austin, W.G. *et al.* 1981: Plasma vasopressin levels and urinary sodium excretion during cardiopulmonary bypass with and without pulsatile flow. *Annals of Thoracic Surgery* **32**, 63–7.

Louagie, Y.A., Gonzalez, M., Collard, E., Mayne, A., Gruslin, A., Jamart, J. *et al.* 1992: Does flow character of cardiopulmonary bypass make a difference? *Journal of Thoracic and Cardiovascular Surgery* **104**, 1628–38.

Many, M., Soroff, H.S., Birtwell, W.C., Giron, F., Wise, H., Deterling, R.A. Jr. 1968: The physiologic role of pulsatile and nonpulsatile blood flow. II. Effects on renal function. *Archives of Surgery* **95**, 762–7.

Mathie, R., Desai, J., Taylor, K.M. 1984: Hepatic blood flow and metabolism during pulsatile and non-pulsatile cardiopulmonary bypass. *Life Support Systems* **2**, 303–5.

Matsuda, H., Hirose, H., Nakano, S., Shirakura, R., Ohtani, M., Kaneko, M. *et al.* 1986: Results of open heart surgery in patients with impaired renal function as creatinine clearance below 30 ml/min. The effects of pulsatile perfusion. *Journal of Cardiovascular Surgery* (Torino) **27**, 595–9.

Mavroudis, C. 1978: To pulse or not to pulse. *Annals of Thoracic Surgery* **25**, 259–71.

McLean, J. 1916: The thromboplastic action of cephalin. *American Journal of Physiology* **41**, 250–7.

McMaster, P.D., Parsons, R.J. 1938: The effect of the pulse on the spread of substances through tissues. *Journal of Experimental Medicine* **68**, 377–400.

Minami, K., Korner, M., Vyska, K. 1990: Effects of pulsatile perfusion on plasma catecholamine levels and haemodynamics during and after cardiac operations with cardiopulmonary bypass. *Journal of Thoracic and Cardiovascular Surgery* **99**, 82–91.

Mori, A., Sono, J., Nakashima, M., Minami, K., Okada, Y. 1981: Application of pulsatile cardiopulmonary bypass for profound hypothermia in cardiac surgery. *Jpn Circ J* **45**, 315–22.

Mori, A., Watanabe, K., Onoe, M., Watarida, S., Nakamura, Y., Magara, T. *et al.* 1988: Regional blood flow in the liver, pancreas and kidney during pulsatile and nonpulsatile perfusion under profound hypothermia. *Jpn Circ J* **52**, 219–27.

Mukherjee, N.D., Beran, A.V., Hirai, J. 1973: *In vivo* determination of renal tissue oxygenation during pulsatile and non-pulsatile left heart bypass. *Annals of Thoracic Surgery* **15**, 334–63.

Munster, K., Andersen, U., Mikkelsen, J., Pettersson, G. 1999: Vacuum assisted venous drainage (VAVD). *Perfusion* **14**, 419–23.

Murray, W.R., Mittra, S., Mittra, D., Roberts, L.B., Taylor, K.M. 1982: The amylase creatinine clearance ratio following cardiopulmonary bypass. *Journal of Thoracic and Cardiovascular Surgery* **82**, 248–53.

Mutch, W.A., Lefevre, G.R., Thiessen, D.B., Girling, L.G., Warrian, R.K. 1998: Computer-controlled cardiopulmonary bypass increases jugular venous oxygen saturation during rewarming. *Annals of Thoracic Surgery* **65**, 59–65.

Mutch, W.A., Warrien, R.K., Eschun, G.M., Girling, L.G., Doiron, L., Cheang, M.S. *et al.* 2000: Biologically variable pulsation improves jugular venous oxygen saturation during rewarming. *Annals of Thoracic Surgery* **69**, 491–7.

Nakamura, K., Koga, Y., Sekiya, R., Onizuka, T., Ishii, K., Chiyotanda, S. *et al.* 1989: The effects of pulsatile and non-pulsatile cardiopulmonary bypass on renal bloodflow and function. *Japanese Journal of Surgery* **19**, 334–45.

Nakayama, K., Tamiya, T., Yamamoto, K., Izumi, T., Akimoto, S., Hishizume, S., Limori, T. *et al.* 1963: High amplitude pulsatile pump in extracorporeal circulation with particular reference to hemodynamics. *Surgery* **54**, 798–9.

Ninomiya, J., Shoji, T., Tanaka, I.S., Ikeshita, M., Ochi, M., Yamauchi, S. *et al.* 1994: Clinical evaluation of a new type of centrifugal pump. *Artificial Organs* **18**, 702–5.

Nishida, H., Uesugi, H., Nishinaka, T., Uwabe, K., Aomi, S., Endo, M. *et al.* 1997: Clinical evaluation of pulsatile flow mode of Terumo Capiox centrifugal pump. *Artificial Organs* **21**, 816–21.

Nonoyama, A. 1960: Haemodynamic studies on extracorporeal circulation with pulsatile and non-pulsatile blood flows. *Archives of Japan Chirurgie* **29**, 381–406.

Oelert, H., Eufe, R. 1974: Dog kidney function during total left heart bypass with pulsatile and non-pulsatile flow. *Journal of Cardiovascular Surgery* (Torino) **15**, 674–8.

Ogata, T., Ida, Y., Takeda, J. 1959: Experimental studies on the extracorporeal circulation by use of our pulsatile arterial pump. *Lung* **6**, 381–90.

Ogata, T., Ida, Y., Takeda, J., Saski, H. 1960: A comparative study of the effectiveness of pulsatile and nonpulsatile blood flow in extracorporeal circulation. *Archives of Japan Chirurgie* **29**, 59–65.

Ohri, S.K., Bowles, C.T., Siddiqui, A., Khaghani, A., Keogh, B.E., Wright, G. *et al.* 1994: The effect of cardiopulmonary bypass on gastric and colonic mucosal perfusion, a tonometric assessment. *Perfusion* **9**, 101–8.

Orime, Y., Shiono, M., Hata, H., Yagi, S., Tsukamoto, S., Okumura, H., Nakata, K., Kimura, S., Hata, M., Sezai, A., Sezai, Y. 1999: Cytokine and endothelial damage in pulsatile and nonpulsatile cardiopulmonary bypass. *Artificial Organs* **23**, 508–12.

Pappas, G., Winter, S.D., Kopriva, C.J., Steele, P.P. 1975: Improvement of myocardial and other vital organ functions and metabolism with a simple method of pulsatile flow (IAPB) during clinical cardiopulmonary bypass. *Surgery* 77, 34–44.

Parsons, R.J., McMaster, P.D. 1938: The effect of pulse upon the formtion and flow of lymph. *Journal of Experimental Biology* 68, 353–76.

Philbin, D.M., Levine, F.H., Emerson, C.W., Coggins, C.H., Buckley, M.J., Austen, W.G. 1979: Plasma vasopressin levels and urinary flow during cardiopulmonary bypass in patients with valvular heart disease: effects of pulsatile flow. *Journal of Thoracic and Cardiovascular Surgery* 78, 779–83.

Prior, F.G.R., Moorcroft, V., Gourlay, T., Taylor, K.M. 1995: Further testing of pulse reverse osmosis. A new theory of the maintenance and control of blood pressure. *International Journal of Artificial Organs* 18, 159–70.

Prior, F.G.R., Moorecroft, V., Gourlay, T., Taylor, K.M. 1996: The therapeutic significance of pulse reverse osmosis. *International Journal of Artificial Organs* 19, 487–92.

Reilly, P.M., Bulkey, G.B. 1993: Vasoactive mediators and splanchnic perfusion. *Critical Care Medicine* 21, S55–68.

Riddington, D.W., Venkatesh, B., Boivin, C.M., Elliott, T.S., Marshall, T. et al. 1996: Intestinal permeability, gastric intramucosal pH, and systemic endotoxemia in patients undergoing cardiopulmonary bypass. *JAMA* 275, 1007–12.

Ritter, E.R. 1952: Pressure–flow relations in kidney: alleged effects of pulse pressure. *American Journal of Physiology* 168, 480–9.

Rocke, D.A., Gaffin, S.L., Wells, M.T., Keon, Y., Brock Utine, J.G. 1987: Endotoxaemia associated with cardiopulmonary bypass. *Journal of Thoracic and Cardiovascular Surgery* 93, 832–7.

Rottenberg, D., Sondak, E., Rahat, S., Borman, J.B., Dviri, E., Uretzky, G. 1995: Early experience with a true pulsatile pump for heart surgery. *Perfusion* 10, 171–5.

Runge, T.M., Grover, F.L., Cohen, D.J., Bohls, F.O., Ottmers, S.E. 1989: Preload-responsive, pulsatile flow, externally valved pump: cardiovascular bypass. *Journal of Investigative Surgery* 2, 269–79.

Runge, T.M., Cohen, D.J., Hantler, C.B., Bohls, F.O., Ottmers, S.E., Bricerno, J.C. 1992: Achievement of physiologic pulsatile flow on cardiopulmonary bypass with a 24 French Cannula. *ASAIO Journal* 38, 726–9.

Saggau, W., Baca, I., Ros, E., Storch, H.H., Schmitz, W. 1980: Clinical and experimental studies on pulsatile and continuous flow during extracorporeal circulation. *Herz* 5, 42–50.

Sanderson, J.M., Wright, G., Sims, F.W. 1972: Brain damage in dogs immediately following pulsatile and non-pulsatile blood flows in extracorporeal circulation. *Thorax* 27, 275–86.

Selkurt, E.E. 1951: Effects of pulse pressure and mean arterial pressure modification on renal haemodynamics and electrolyte and water excretion. *Circulation* 4, 541–8.

Shepard, R.B., Kirklin, J.W. 1969: Relation of pulsatile flow to oxygen consumption and other variables during cardiopulmonary bypass. *Journal of Thoracic and Cardiovascular Surgery* 58, 694–702.

Shepard, R.B., Simpson, D.S., Sharp, J.F. 1966: Energy equivalent pressure. *Archives of Surgery* 93, 730–40.

Simpson, J.C. 1981: Cerebral perfusion during cardiac surgery using cardiac bypass. In: Longmore, D., ed. *Towards safer cardiac surgery.* Lancaster: MTP: 287–91.

Starling, E.H. 1896: On adsorbtion of fluids from the connective tissue spaces. *Journal of Physiology* (London) 19, 312–26.

Stinson, E.B., Holloway, E.L., Derby, G.C., Copeland, J.G., Oyer, P.E., Beuhler, D.L. et al. 1977: Control of myocardial performance early after open heart operations by vasodilator treatment. *Journal of Thoracic and Cardiovascular Surgery* 73, 523–30.

Suenaga, E., Naito, K., Cao, Z.L., Suda, H., Ueno, T., Natsuaki, M. et al. 2000: Experimental use of a compact centrifugal pump and membrane oxygenator as a cardiopulmonary support system. *Artificial Organs* 24, 912–15.

Takami, Y., Makinouchi, K., Nakazawa, T., Benkowski, R., Glueck, J., Ohara, Y. et al. 1996: Hemolytic characteristics of a pivot bearing supported Gyro centrifugal pump (C1E3) simulating various clinical applications. *Artificial Organs* 20, 1042–9.

Takeda, J. 1960: Experimental study on peripheral circulation during extracorporeal circulation, with special reference to a comparison of pulsatile flow with non-pulsatile flow. *Archives of Japan Chirurgie* 29, 1407–30.

Tao, W., Zwischenberger, J.B., Nguyen, T.T., Vertrees, R.A., Nutt, L.K., Herndon, D.N. et al. 1995: Gut mucosal ischaemia during normothermic cardiopulmonary bypass results from blood flow redistribution and increased oxygen demand. *Journal of Thoracic and Cardiovascular Surgery* 110, 819–28.

Tayama, E., Nakazawa, T., Takami, Y., Makinouchi, K., Ohtsubo, S., Ohashi, Y. et al. 1997a: The hemolysis test of the Gyro C1E3 pump in pulsatile mode. *Artificial Organs* 21, 675–9.

Tayama, E., Niimi, Y., Takami, Y., Ohashi, Y., Ohtsuka, G., Glueck, J.A. et al. 1997b: Hemolysis test of a centrifugal pump in a pulsatile mode: the effect of pulse rate and RPM variance. *Artificial Organs* 21, 1284–7.

Taylor, K.M. 1980: Effect of pulsatile flow and arterial line filtration on cerebral cellular damage during open heart surgery. Proceedings of Second International Symposium on Psychopathological and Neurological Dysfunction following Open-Heart Surgery.

Taylor, K.M. 1986: Pulsatile perfusion. In: Taylor, K.M., ed. *Cardiopulmonary bypass – principles and management.* London: Chapman & Hall: 85–114.

Taylor, K.M., Bain, W.H., Maxted, K.J., Hutton, M.M., McNab, W.Y., Caves, P.K. 1978: Comparative studies of pulsatile and nonpulsatile flow during cardiopulmonary bypass. I. Pulsatile system employed and its hematologic effects. *Journal of Thoracic and Cardiovascular Surgery* 75, 569–73.

Taylor, K.M., Bain, W.H., Russell, M., Brannan, J.J., Morton, I.J. 1979a: Peripheral vascular resistance and angiotensin II levels during pulsatile and non-pulsatile cardiopulmonary bypass. *Thorax* 34, 594–8.

Taylor, K.M., Wright, G.S., Bain, W.H., Caves, P.K., Beastall, G.H. 1979b: Comparative studies of pulsatile and non-pulsatile flow during cardiopulmonary bypass. III. Anterior pituitary response to thyrotophin-releasing hormone. *Journal of Thoracic and Cardiovascular Surgery* 75, 579–84.

Taylor, K.M., Bain, W.H., Morton, I.J. 1980: The role of angiotensin II in the development of peripheral vasoconstriction during open heart surgery. *American Heart Journal* 100, 935–7.

Taylor, K.M., Bain, W.H., Davidson, K.G., Turner, M.A. 1982: Comparative clinical study of pulsatile and non-pulsatile perfusion in 350 consecutive patients. *Thorax* 37, 324–30.

Townsend, G.E., Wynands, J.E., Whalley, D.G., Wong, P., Bevan, D.R. 1984: Role of renin-angiotensin system in cardiopulmonary bypass hypertension. *Candian Anaesthetists Society Journal* 31, 160–5.

Undar, A., Runge, T.M., Miller, O.L., Felger, M.C., Lansing, R., Korvick, D.L. *et al.* 1996: Design of a physiologic pulsatile flow cardiopulmonary bypass system for neonates and infants. *International Journal of Artificial Organs* **19**, 170–6.

Undar, A., Masai, T., Yang, S.Q., Goddard-Finegold, J., Frazier, O.H., Fraser, C.D. 1999: Effects of perfusion mode on regional and global organ blood flow in a neonatal piglet model. *Annals of Thoracic Surgery* **4**, 1336–42.

Videcoq, M., Desmonts, J.M., Marty, J., Hazebroucq, J., Langlois, J. 1987: Effects of droperidol on peripheral vasculature: use of cardiopulmonary bypass as a study model. *Acta Anaesthesiologica Scandinavica* **31**, 370–4.

Waldenberger, F.R., Vandezande, E., Janssens, P., Morishige, N., Demeyere, R., de Ruyter, E., Wiebalck, A. *et al.* 1997: A new pneumatic pump for extracorporeal circulation: TPP (true pulsatile pump). Experimental and first clinical results. *International Journal of Artificial Organs* **20**, 447–54.

Weinstein, G.S., Zabetakis, P.M., Clavel, A., Franzone, A., Agrawal, M., Gleim, G. *et al.* 1987: The renin–angiotensin system is not responsible for hypertension following coronary artery bypass grafting. *Annals of Thoracic Surgery* **43**, 74–7.

Wesolowski, S.A., Miller, H.H., Halkett, A.E. 1950: Experimental replacement of the heart by a mechanical extracorporeal pump. *Bulletin of the New England Medical Center* **12**, 41–50.

Wilcox, B.R., Coulter, N.A., Peters, R.M., Stacey, R.W. 1967: Power dissipation in the systemic and pulmonary vasculature of dogs. *Surgery* **62**, 25–9.

Williams, G.D., Seifen, A.B., Lawson, N.W., Norton, J.B., Readinger, R.I., Dungan, T.W. *et al.* 1979: Pulsatile perfusion versus conventional high flow non-pulsatile perfusion for rapid core cooling and rewarming of infants for circulatory arrest in cardiac operation. *Journal of Thoracic and Cardiovascular Surgery* **78**, 667–77.

Wright, G. 1989: Factors affecting the pulsatile hydraulic power output of the Stockert roller pump. *Perfusion* **4**, 187–95.

Wright, G. 1997: Mechanical simulation of cardiac function by means of pulsatile blood pumps. *Journal of Cardiothorac Vascular and Anesthesiology* **11**, 299–309.

10

Cardiopulmonary bypass and the brain

G BURKHARD MACKENSEN, HILARY P GROCOTT AND MARK F NEWMAN

KEY POINTS

- In patients undergoing cardiopulmonary bypass for coronary artery bypass surgery the incidence of adverse cerebral outcome is approximately 6 per cent. Type I cerebral injury (focal stroke, stupor or coma) occurs in 3 per cent, and Type II cerebral injury (decline in intellectual function, memory deficit or seizures) in another 3 per cent.
- Cardiopulmonary bypass complicates the normally autoregulated cerebral physiology by introducing factors such as abnormal flow rates and patterns, haemodilution, temperature changes and pH management.
- A major cause of cerebral injury is cerebral emboli, which may be macroemboli (atherosclerotic debris or fat particles) or microemboli (either gaseous or particulate).
- Risk factors associated with adverse cerebral outcomes can be identified and the knowledge used to direct management strategies and clinical decisions.
- The use of neurological monitoring during cardiopulmonary bypass, although promising, has not been widely adopted because of technical difficulties and problems in interpreting its predictive power.
- A large number and variety of agents have been proposed as pharmacological neuroprotection, but clinical investigation of their effectiveness has been difficult, and conclusive evidence of their benefits is still lacking.

INTRODUCTION

The utilization of cardiopulmonary bypass to allow surgery on the heart was first described in the middle part of the last century (Dennis *et al.*, 1951; Gibbon, 1954). Since that time, considerable advancements have been made not only in our understanding of cardiac physiology and surgical technique but also in the technical aspects of cardiopulmonary bypass. This has resulted in an improvement in overall morbidity and mortality as well as overall quality of life after cardiac surgery.

Over the past decade, there has been a change in patient demographics, with a disproportionate increase seen in the number of elderly patients undergoing coronary artery bypass graft surgery (CABG). This reflects both an overall increase in the percentage of the population who are elderly, but also the realization that this patient population may benefit most from cardiac surgery. However, it is this aged patient population that often presents for cardiac surgery with significant comorbidity and organ dysfunction representing significant challenges to peri-operative caregivers. Accordingly, the consequences of cardiopulmonary bypass on neurological and neurocognitive outcomes are significant and remain serious complications of cardiac procedures, particularly in elderly patients (Tuman *et al.*, 1992; Roach *et al.*, 1996; Wolman *et al.*, 1999). These adverse cerebral outcomes after cardiac surgery result in prolonged hospitalization, increased morbidity and mortality as well as increased overall cost (Roach *et al.*, 1996). The incidence of central nervous system (CNS) injury after cardiac surgery varies considerably. The factors associated with this wide variation include how the injury is defined. The incidence of adverse cerebral outcomes after CABG surgery defined as either Type I (focal stroke, stupor or coma) or Type II (decline in intellectual function, memory deficit and seizures) was reported to be 3.1 per cent and 3.0 per cent, respectively (Roach *et al.*, 1996). Wolman *et al.* (1999), in a recent prospective study of patients undergoing intracardiac surgery combined with CABG, reported a 16 per cent incidence of adverse cerebral outcomes with 8.4 per cent Type I outcomes (cerebral death, non-fatal strokes and transient ischaemic attacks (TIA)) and 7.3 per cent Type II outcomes (new intellectual deterioration and seizures). More subtle post-operative cerebral injury, such as neurocognitive dysfunction, has a short-term incidence of approximately 25–80 per cent (Smith *et al.*, 1986; Shaw *et al.*, 1987), a medium-term incidence (6 months) of up to 40 per cent (Borowicz *et al.*, 1996) and a long-term incidence (3–5 years) of 15–42 per cent (Newman *et al.*, 1996a; Newman *et al.*, 2001b).

Known pre-operative risk factors associated with adverse cerebral outcomes in patients undergoing cardiopulmonary bypass surgery, such as cerebrovascular disease, atheromatous disease and other concomitant diseases, have a higher prevalence in the elderly and continue to have a significant impact on long-term outcome and quality of life. Overall, the implications of cardiopulmonary bypass on neurological and neurocognitive outcome and quality of life become even more important if one considers that 800,000 CABG procedures (Roach *et al.*, 1996) as well as more than 200,000 other open-heart procedures (Wolman *et al.*, 1999) are performed annually worldwide. Adverse cerebral outcomes are associated with significantly increased length of hospital and ICU stay, resulting in approximately 6000–10,000 US$ additional in-hospital boarding costs per patient. Roach *et al.* (1996) applied these data to an estimated number of 800,000 annual CABG surgeries worldwide and calculated the additional expense of cerebral injury after cardiopulmonary bypass to be approximately 400 million US$ per year.

This chapter will outline cerebral physiology during cardiopulmonary bypass, define the incidence and implications of central nervous system injury in the context of cardiac surgery and deal with the possible aetiologies of these injuries. Further, it will give an update on current risk stratification and central nervous system monitoring for cardiopulmonary bypass-utilizing procedures. Lastly, this chapter will summarize recent strategies to improve neurological and neurocognitive outcome after cardiac surgery, including a review of important potential approaches to pharmacological neuroprotection.

CEREBRAL PHYSIOLOGY DURING CARDIOPULMONARY BYPASS

It is important to understand the implications of cardiopulmonary bypass on cerebral physiology in order to conceptualize possible aetiologies and mechanisms that would explain cardiopulmonary bypass-related cerebral injury. Under normal conditions, cerebral physiology is principally influenced by cerebral metabolism, as well as the combined interactions of intracerebral cerebral pressure, cerebral perfusion pressure and mean arterial blood pressure on cerebral blood flow. General anaesthesia itself influences several aspects of cerebral physiology, including cerebral metabolic rate of oxygen, cerebral blood flow and electrophysiological function. The unphysiological state of cardiopulmonary bypass, however, further complicates cerebral physiology by introducing important factors, such as cardiopulmonary bypass flow rate, pH management, haematocrit and temperature.

Cerebral blood flow and cerebral metabolism

Generalized cerebral hypoperfusion during cardiopulmonary bypass is theorized to contribute, at least in part, to the adverse neurocognitive outcomes after cardiac surgery. According to several studies investigating the effects of perfusion pressure (principally determined by mean arterial blood pressure) on cerebral blood flow during cardiopulmonary bypass, autoregulation is intact with cerebral blood flow remaining relatively stable within the wide normal range of mean arterial blood pressure (50–100 mmHg) as long as pH and arterial carbon dioxide are kept constant (Rogers *et al.*, 1988; Newman *et al.*, 1996b). This may not be the case, however, for diabetic patients in whom Croughwell *et al.* (1990) showed that cerebral autoregulation is impaired during cardiopulmonary bypass and compensation for an imbalance in adequate oxygen delivery is achieved by increased oxygen extraction. In addition, the autoregulatory curve may be shifted rightward in patients with extensive peripheral vascular disease and a longstanding history of hypertension, thereby making these patients more susceptible to cerebral hypoperfusion during potential hypotensive periods on cardiopulmonary bypass. Because age is a predictor of cognitive function after cardiac surgery, Newman *et al.* (1994) examined if age-related decrements in cognitive function could be associated with impaired cerebral blood flow autoregulation during hypothermic cardiopulmonary bypass. Using the ^{133}Xe clearance method, these authors reported no relationship between the cognitive decline in elderly and age-related changes in autoregulation. In addition, they demonstrated a small but significant effect of mean arterial blood pressure on cerebral blood flow, which they later confirmed to occur at normothermic cardiopulmonary bypass as well (Newman et al., 1994, 1996b). However, because these authors found an association between increased oxygen extraction and some measures of cognitive decline they suggested that an imbalance in cerebral tissue oxygen supply, which is unrelated to age, contributes to acute cognitive decline after cardiac surgery.

According to investigations by Rogers et al. (1988) and Prough et al. (1991), cerebral blood flow during cardiopulmonary bypass declines in a time-dependent fashion despite stable cardiopulmonary bypass flow and tight control of arterial carbon dioxide. However, a more recent study by Croughwell et al. (1998) disputed these results, under similar conditions of mildly hypothermic (35°C) non-pulsatile cardiopulmonary bypass and alpha-stat blood gas management. In their study, cerebral blood flow and cerebral metabolic rate of oxygen were determined in 52 patients undergoing elective CABG surgery, both after initiation of cardiopulmonary bypass and at the end of cardiopulmonary bypass. The experimental results let them conclude that during mildly hypothermic cardiopulmonary bypass, cerebral blood flow does not decrease over time and that the coupling between cerebral blood flow and cerebral metabolic rate of oxygen also remains intact. This is in agreement with experimental data by Hindman et al. (1992) in rabbits and Johnston et al. (1991) in dogs, who demonstrated no time-dependent change of cerebral blood flow after 30, 90 and 150 minutes' hypothermic cardiopulmonary bypass. Theoretically, the discrepancies between the human studies by Rogers et al. (1988) and Prough et al. (1991), on the one side, and Croughwell et al. (1998), on the other, could be because of the fact that the former two groups might have taken their cerebral blood flow measurements before stable cerebral temperatures were reached on cardiopulmonary bypass. Evidence for this theory comes from Grocott et al. (1997), who compared the time course of nasopharyngeal and jugular bulb temperatures during cerebral blood flow in patients undergoing cardiopulmonary bypass procedures. Differences between the two sites were most significant during cooling and rewarming but correlated well during stable cardiopulmonary bypass. During rewarming, jugular bulb temperature exceeded nasopharyngeal temperature by as much as 4°C. The earlier studies may have made their initial measurement at a relatively warmer temperature (and higher cerebral blood flow)

than the later colder temperatures (with lower cerebral blood flow).

Haemodilution

In the early stages of the development of cardiopulmonary bypass, the pump prime was adjusted to provide normal haematocrit levels, thereby avoiding haemodilution. It was only with the introduction of generalized hypothermia that intentional haemodilution during cardiopulmonary bypass became the standard of care. Because hypothermia dramatically increases the viscosity of blood, haemodilution was necessary to improve otherwise compromised microcirculation and thus allow sufficient oxygen transport to the periphery. Shortages and concerns about the safety of the blood supply with the advent of human immunodeficiency virus (HIV) infection and the identification of various hepatitis viruses during the last two decades, resulted in a widely accepted practice of intentional haemodilution (with haematocrit values approaching 18–20 per cent) in order to avoid excessive transfusions. Although this practice has been challenged recently (Fang et al., 1997), the limits of haemodilution during cardiopulmonary bypass in humans are not well defined. Haemodilution itself is known to increase cerebral blood flow compared with baseline non-haemodiluted states. This increase in cerebral blood flow compensates for decreases in arterial oxygen content thereby maintaining sufficient oxygen delivery. If haematocrit drops to critical levels, however, the limits of this compensatory mechanism may be reached and oxygen delivery will be compromised. In a recent dog study, Cook et al. (1998) identified the minimal haematocrit maintaining cerebral oxygen balance over the range of clinically relevant cardiopulmonary bypass temperatures. Although cerebral oxygen demand was maintained at a haematocrit as low as 14 per cent during warm (38°C) cardiopulmonary bypass, physiologically important changes in oxygen supply were noted to occur at a haematocrit of 18 per cent. As expected, cerebral oxygenation was shifted leftward with decreasing cardiopulmonary bypass temperatures in the same model. The authors defined a critical haematocrit of 11 per cent during hypothermic (28°C) cardiopulmonary bypass, but the reduction in critical haematocrit was not proportional to the reduction in cerebral metabolic rate of oxygen. The cerebral response to haemodilution during hypothermic cardiopulmonary bypass was recently investigated in a small number of patients by Sungurtekin et al. (1999). As haemodilution-associated increases in cerebral blood flow compensated for flow reductions observed during hypothermia, these authors did not find any differences in cerebral metabolic rate of oxygen or oxygen delivery when comparing a haemoglobin concentration of 6.2 g/dL with a haemoglobin concentration of 8.5 g/dL. In two recent retrospective reports examining 2862 patients, very low intraoperative haematocrit was not associated with major adverse neurological outcome, such as stroke or increased in-hospital mortality (Hill *et al.*, 2000; van Wermeskerken *et al.*, 2000).

The impact of haemodilution on outcome from cerebral ischaemia has been studied in both human and experimental settings. Results from prospective trials in humans suffering from stroke have been disappointing, and no overall improvement in outcome has been documented (SSSG, 1987; Group TISS, 1988; Group THiSS, 1989). Because of the lack of improvement and potential risk (caused by a reported increase in cerebral oedema) (SSSG, 1988), haemodilution has been abandoned as therapeutic strategy in patients with acute ischaemic stroke (Asplund, 1989). Results from the laboratory have been inconclusive. Cole *et al.* (1994) repeatedly demonstrated improved outcomes and reduced infarct volumes by use of haemodilution with diaspirin cross-linked haemoglobin (DCLHb) in focal cerebral ischaemia models of middle cerebral artery occlusion in rats (Cole *et al.*, 1997). These findings are supported by Belayev *et al.* (1997) in another study of middle cerebral artery occlusion in rats, even when haemodilution was introduced after onset of reperfusion with the use of 20 per cent albumin. Others, such as Reasoner *et al.* (1996) showed that infarct size after middle cerebral artery occlusion in rabbits was increased when critical haemoglobin concentrations at 6 g/dL were reached. Taken together, extrapolation of the findings from the experimental and human stroke literature to the setting of cardiopulmonary bypass is problematic. As long as the impact of severe haemodilution on neurological and neurocognitive outcomes after cardiac surgery using cardiopulmonary bypass has not been investigated in a randomized prospective fashion, there is no conclusive answer to what levels of haemodilution are optimal in order to minimize risk for neurological or neurocognitive decline after cardiopulmonary bypass procedures.

Hyperglycaemia

Cardiopulmonary bypass is known to induce alterations in insulin secretion and resistance, thereby increasing the potential for significant hyperglycaemia (Lanier, 1991). This, compounded by the use of glucose-containing cardioplegia, contributes to the hyperglycaemic response seen with cardiopulmonary bypass. Hyperglycaemia has consistently been shown to worsen neurological outcome after both experimental focal and global cerebral ischaemia (Siesjo, 1988; Warner *et al.*, 1992; Dietrich *et al.*, 1993). This is most likely to be caused by adverse effects of the anaerobic conversion of glucose to lactate,

which ultimately causes intracellular acidosis and impairment of intracellular homeostasis and metabolism (Feerick *et al.*, 1995). In addition, there is a reported increase in the release of excitotoxic amino acids in response to hyperglycaemia and cerebral ischaemia (Siesjo, 1988). Existing data in the human cardiopulmonary bypass literature, however, are less clear. Although Hindman (1995) cautions the use of glucose-containing prime for cardiopulmonary bypass, Metz and Keats (1991) did not find a difference in neurological outcome in patients undergoing cardiopulmonary bypass with a glucose prime (blood glucose during cardiopulmonary bypass of 600–800 mg/dL) versus no glucose prime (blood glucose 200–300 mg/dL). This finding is supported by Nussmeier *et al.* (1999), who recently reported that use of glucose-containing prime was also not a risk factor for cerebral injury or infection in non-diabetic or diabetic patients undergoing CABG procedures. Chaney *et al.* (1999) attempted to maintain normoglycemia during cardiac surgery with the use of an insulin protocol and came to the conclusion that, even with aggressive insulin treatment, hyperglycaemia is resistant, and the strategy may actually predispose to post-operative hypoglycaemia. In the largest retrospective review, outcome data from 2862 CABG patients showed no association between the intraoperative maximum glucose concentration and major adverse neurological outcome or in-hospital mortality (Hill *et al.*, 2000; van Wermeskerken *et al.*, 2000). The appropriate intraoperative glucose management and whether it adversely affects neurological outcome in patients undergoing cardiopulmonary bypass remains uncertain.

Temperature

Manipulation of temperature has been a mainstay of intraoperative management in the setting of cardiac surgery. From the very early days of cardiac surgery, hypothermia during cardiopulmonary bypass has been used as a means to protect the heart, brain and other organs from the adverse sequelae of cardiopulmonary bypass. Although there is a wealth of experimental data supporting the use of hypothermia to protect the brain from injury (Busto *et al.*, 1987; Chen *et al.*, 1991), there is a relative paucity of clinical data supporting its efficacy. Most recently, a controversy has risen with the recent emergence of warm, continuous blood cardioplegia and 'warm cardiopulmonary bypass'. Normothermic cardiopulmonary bypass has been associated with a trend towards a lower incidence of myocardial infarction, a reduced use of intra-aortic balloon pumps and a higher rate of spontaneous defibrillation after cross-clamp removal (Christakis *et al.*, 1992; Kavanagh *et al.*, 1992; Menasche *et al.*, 1992). At the same time, clinical studies have shown varying results of intraoperative temperature management on post-operative stroke and a relative lack of evidence for protection against neurocognitive decline. In a 1995 review of nine trials of warm versus cold cardiopulmonary bypass and antegrade versus retrograde delivery of cardioplegia, the incidence of perioperative stroke and adverse neuropsychological outcomes was independent of temperature (Christakis et al., 1995).

A complicating factor in studying neurological injury during cardiac surgery with respect to temperature has been the definition of hypothermia. The two largest studies have had significantly different results. In a randomized study of 1001 patients by Martin et al. (1994), a hypothermic ($\leqslant 28°C$) group of cardiopulmonary bypass patients was compared with a normothermic ($\geqslant 35°C$) group with respect to the incidence of encephalopathy and stroke. There was a threefold greater incidence of stroke and encephalopathy in the normothermic group. However, in a subset of the same study population, Mora et al. (1996) were unable to show an effect of cardiopulmonary bypass temperature on neurocognitive outcomes. Another large study performed by the Warm Heart Investigators (WHI, 1994) examined the effects of cardiopulmonary bypass temperature management on outcome in 1732 patients. In that study, the incidence of stroke at the time of discharge was not different between the cold (25–30°C) and the warm (33–37°C) group. Consistent with this, another study from that group, by McLean et al. (1996), had similar results. Again, hypothermic bypass was compared with normothermic bypass; however, in the study by McLean et al. (1996), normothermic bypass included patients with temperatures as low as 34–35°C. In fact, these patients were really mildly hypothermic and were compared with the more moderately hypothermic group of 30–32°C; in this particular study there was no difference in either stroke or neurocognitive decline. Although these studies did not look at the same degree of hypothermia versus normothermia, the study by Martin et al. (1994) definitely indicates the risk involved when keeping patients normothermic. The patients in their normothermic group (37°C) were actively warmed, and the blood flow temperature was most certainly greater than 38°C in order to maintain a body temperature of 37°C. This was, in fact, a study of hyperthermia versus hypothermia, thereby highlighting the dangers of hyperthermia. In a prospective randomized trial investigating the effects of normothermic (35.1°C) versus hypothermic (30.4°C) cardiopulmonary bypass on cerebral outcome after CABG surgery at our own institution, we have been unable to detect a difference between the two groups (Grigore et al., 2001).

One of the other issues with regard to temperature and the brain concerns the timing of cerebral insults and the conduct of cardiopulmonary bypass. The times at which the brain is particularly at risk, such as at cannulation and cross-clamp removal, may be occasions when the temperature is not as cool as one would desire. Another issue relates to rewarming. Although, one may very well benefit from hypothermia from a brain prospective, hypothermia necessitates rewarming, during which the brain may be exposed to a number of adverse events. Enomoto et al. (1996) showed an increase in metabolic demand relative to supply in the brain during rapid rewarming that may be caused by a transient abnormality in flow-metabolism coupling. This may increase the risk of cerebral ischaemia, support for which has been shown in a clinical study by Croughwell et al. (1992) where cerebral desaturation was discovered during rewarming from hypothermic cardiopulmonary bypass. The same investigators also showed that patients with the greatest oxygen extraction have the highest incidence of cognitive impairment (Croughwell et al., 1994). According to Haenel et al. (1998), cerebral desaturation observed during rewarming can be avoided by mild hypercapnia, suggesting a better balance between cerebral oxygen supply and demand.

In very recent work from our institution, an association between rate of rewarming and cognitive decline in patients undergoing CABG surgery has been demonstrated (Grigore et al., 2002). Slower rewarming after hypothermia (30–32°C) was associated with less cognitive dysfunction at six weeks after surgery, suggesting that a slower rewarming rate may be an important factor in the prevention of neurocognitive decline after hypothermic cardiopulmonary bypass.

Pulsatile perfusion

Although there are multiple technological differences between various perfusion apparatus, the typical cardiopulmonary bypass apparatus generally incorporates non-pulsatile flow, with either a roller or centrifical pump as a standard mechanism for delivering flow. Although there is no question as to the unphysiological state that non-pulsatile flow creates, there is a relative paucity of data to suggest that pulsatile flow during clinical cardiopulmonary bypass is of benefit to the patient. In the largest double-blind randomized comparison of the effect of pulsatile versus non-pulsatile cardiopulmonary bypass on neurological and neuropsychological outcome ($n = 316$) Murkin et al. (1995) found no significant association between pulsatility in either neuropsychological or neurological outcome. However, because true 'physiological' pulsatility was never accomplished in that study, significant perfusion differences between study groups may have been absent. In a recent study of balloon pump-induced pulsatile perfusion during cardiopulmonary bypass, Kawahara et al. (1999) failed to show any improvements in jugular venous oxygen saturation of regional brain oxygenation. Conflicting results can be obtained from the available experimental data. In a randomized study of pulsatile versus non-pulsatile cardiopulmonary bypass in rabbits, neither cerebral blood flow nor cerebral metabolic rate of oxygen were affected by arterial pulsation (Hindman *et al.*, 1995). Cook *et al.* (1997) also demonstrated that pulsatility has no significant effect on cerebral or renal perfusion over a broad range of cardiopulmonary bypass temperature and flow conditions when investigated in a canine model of cardiopulmonary bypass. However, when introduced after deep hypothermic circulatory arrest in a piglet model, pulsatile perfusion provides superior regional and global cerebral, renal and myocardial blood flow compared with non-pulsatile perfusion (Undar *et al.*, 1999). Interestingly, in a pig model of cardiopulmonary bypass, computer-controlled pulsatile cardiopulmonary bypass was associated with significantly greater jugular venous oxygen saturation during rewarming from hypothermic cardiopulmonary bypass, suggesting that cerebral oxygenation was better preserved with computer-controlled pulsatile cardiopulmonary bypass, which returned biological variability to the flow pattern (Mutch *et al.*, 1998). In summary, in the absence of convincing data in humans proving any beneficial effects on outcome after cardiopulmonary bypass, the need for pulsatile flow during cardiopulmonary bypass does not appear to be warranted. That being said, there is also no evidence suggesting any adverse effects from pulsatility. Therefore, it might be considered if it can be simply performed with no additional costs involved.

pH management

The issue of how to manage the patient's pH during hypothermic cardiopulmonary bypass has been much debated, with opinions on the correct strategy being diametrically opposed (Hindman, 1998). The most common strategy for pH management in adult hypothermic cardiopulmonary bypass is alpha-stat management, in which the pH is uncorrected for temperature. This is opposed to pH-stat management, in which the blood gas is measured at the temperature at which cardiopulmonary bypass is being performed, which amounts to the necessity of adding carbon dioxide to the cardiopulmonary bypass oxygenator fresh gas flow. Under conditions of alpha-stat management cerebral autoregulation is maintained, allowing the coupling of cerebral blood flow to cerebral metabolic rate of oxygen (Taylor, 1998). During pH-stat management with the addition of CO_2, cerebral blood flow is in excess of that needed to maintain metabolism (luxury perfusion) (Schell *et al.*, 1993). Whereas initial studies were unable to show a difference in neurological outcome between the two techniques,

more recent studies have supported an alpha-stat management. Murkin *et al.* (1995), in a double-blind, randomized comparison of alpha-stat and pH-stat management during cardiopulmonary bypass, found that cognitive dysfunction at two months was less prevalent in patients managed with alpha-stat than with pH-stat strategy (27 per cent versus 44 per cent). The reasons for this relative benefit of alpha-stat management may be explained with the luxurious cerebral blood flow that can be seen in pH-stat management, in which the brain may receive more injurious emboli.

The exception to optimal pH management is paediatric cardiac surgery, where patients undergoing profound hypothermic circulatory arrest may benefit from pH-stat management during the cooling phase, in which an increase in cerebral blood flow may allow for more homogeneous cooling of the brain (Kern and Greeley, 1995). Although pH-stat management is commonly used in neonatal cardiac surgery involving deep hypothermic circulatory arrest, this technique potentially has some disadvantages when compared with alpha-stat (Burrows, 1995). Kurth *et al.* (1998), in a piglet model of cardiopulmonary bypass, demonstrated that cortical deoxygenation during hypothermic arrest was slower after pH-stat cardiopulmonary bypass than with alpha-stat management. pH-stat management also increased the pre-DHA cortical oxygen concentration and improved the cortical physiological recovery after deep hypothermic circulatory arrest.

CEREBRAL INJURY AND ITS IMPLICATIONS

Although remarkable advances have been made with respect to myocardial outcomes after CABG and valvular surgery, little progress has been made in protecting the brain during cardiopulmonary bypass. The incidence of stroke and neurocognitive dysfunction after cardiopulmonary bypass even increases as the population ages; the elderly are more susceptible than younger patients to the harmful effects of cardiopulmonary bypass and adverse neurological outcomes are more common. This has been shown by many investigators, including Tuman *et al.* (1992), who demonstrated that the probability of neurological morbidity after CABG surgery increases with patients' age, whereas myocardial protection prevents age-related cardiac morbidity (Fig. 10.1). Further, these authors reported that patients who had a post-operative neurological deficit had a ninefold increase in mortality.

In a landmark study by Roach *et al.* (1996), serious adverse cerebral outcomes, including fatal cerebral injury, non-fatal strokes, new deterioration in intellectual function and new onset of seizures, occurred in 6.1 per cent of 2108 patients and was significantly associated with

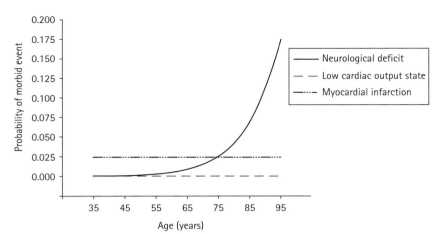

Figure 10.1 *The probability of neurological morbidity after CABG surgery increases with patient age, whereas myocardial protection prevents age-related cardiac morbidity. (Adapted from Tuman, K.J., McCarthy, R.J., Najafi, H., Ivankovich, A.D. 1992: Differential effects of advanced age on neurologic and cardiac risks of coronary artery operations. Cardiovasc Surg **104**, 1510–17 with permission from Mosby Inc.)*

age. These adverse cerebral outcomes were shown to be associated with significantly increased length of hospital and ICU stay resulting in increased medical costs. According to their data, adverse cerebral outcomes were responsible for approximately 6000–10,000 US$ additional in-hospital boarding costs. The present authors applied these data to an estimated 800,000 patients per year who undergo CABG surgery worldwide and estimated the additional expense of cerebral injury to be approximately $400 million per year. Total peri-operative expenses (including complete in-hospital, out-of-hospital and rehabilitation services) were estimated to be as high as $2 to $4 billion annually. In a prospective multicentre study that identified a subgroup of cardiac surgery patients at extraordinary risk of cerebral injury, one out of every six patients (16 per cent) undergoing a combined procedure of CABG surgery and open-heart surgery suffered from serious adverse cerebral outcomes (Wolman *et al.*, 1999). Again, these outcomes commonly result in prolonged in-hospital stays, intensive care and rehabilitation services, all of which increase overall expenses. Given an estimated number of 200,000 patients worldwide undergoing such combined complex procedures annually, the impact of these complications is enormous. Taken together, this information underlines the economical implications of adverse cerebral outcomes with regard to the use of healthcare resources.

Cerebral outcomes after cardiac surgery not only have direct economical implications but also affect the individual quality of life of patients, which indirectly may contribute to overall costs. Although endpoints, such as length of in-hospital stay or time spent in out-of-hospital and rehabilitation services, are frequently determined and reported (Roach *et al.*, 1996; Warner *et al.*, 1997), the assessment of quality of life after cardiac surgery appears to be more complex. In a recent attempt to assess quality of life after cardiac surgery and intensive care therapy, Stoll *et al.* (2000) examined 80 patients. Patients with evidence

of post-traumatic stress disorder showed impaired psychosocial function and life satisfaction compared with those without evidence of post-traumatic stress disorder. As documented by Newman *et al.* (2001a), perception of general health and widely accepted measurements of quality of life are associated with cognitive functioning after cardiac surgery. Further, better cognitive performance at five years after cardiac surgery was associated with a more productive level of working status in that study. Health-related quality of life has also been used as a predictor of mortality after CABG surgery (Rumsfeld *et al.*, 1999).

AETIOLOGY OF CEREBRAL INJURY DURING CARDIOPULMONARY BYPASS

Although the two most common theories regarding the aetiology of central nervous system injuries after cardiac surgery involving cardiopulmonary bypass include the effects of cerebral emboli (both gaseous and particulate) and generalized cerebral hypoperfusion, it is now well accepted that numerous other mechanisms, individually or in combination, may contribute. Besides these two main interrelated aetiological theories other possible factors include systemic inflammation (Butler *et al.*, 1993; Hall *et al.*, 1997, Murkin, 1997), genetic predisposition (APOE) (Newman *et al.*, 1999), cerebral oedema (Harris *et al.*, 1993) and hyperthermia during rewarming or after separation from cardiopulmonary bypass (Cook *et al.*, 1995; Grocott *et al.*, 1997).

Cerebral emboli

Patients undergoing cardiopulmonary bypass can receive considerable numbers of macroemboli (for example, atherosclerotic debris or fat particles) or as many as thousands of microemboli (for example, gaseous bubbles or other

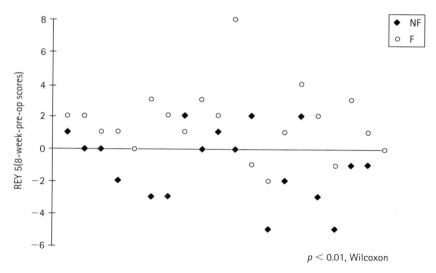

$p < 0.01$, Wilcoxon

Figure 10.2 *Association between the embolic load during cardiopulmonary bypass and neurocognitive outcome represented by the REY auditory verbal learning test in a study evaluating the effects of arterial line filters in patients undergoing cardiopulmonary bypass with bubble oxygenators. The figure shows the verbal memory deficit at eight weeks in the non-filtered (NF) and filtered (F) groups. A negative difference on the vertical axis indicates a deficit in post-operative performance in the test. The filtered bypass group performed significantly better ($p < 0.01$). (Adapted from Pugsley, W., Klinger, L., Paschalis, C. et al. 1990: Microemboli and cerebral impairment during cardiac surgery. Vasc Surg **24**, 34–43 with permission from Westminster Publications.)*

particulate matter) during a typical cardiac procedure (Blauth, 1995; Stump *et al.*, 1996; Barbut *et al.*, 1997a; O'Brien *et al.*, 1997; Grocott *et al.*, 1998). Convincing evidence documenting the embolization of material to the brain during cardiopulmonary bypass procedures includes retinal angiography (Blauth *et al.*, 1986), transcranial Doppler techniques (Padayachee *et al.*, 1987; Grocott *et al.*, 1998; Sylivris *et al.*, 1998) and histological examinations (Moody *et al.*, 1990; Blauth *et al.*, 1992; Moody *et al.*, 1995) as well as magnetic resonance imaging (Toner *et al.*, 1994). The precise composition of these emboli is not clear; however, new developments in transcranial Doppler equipment should ultimately allow the determination of the differential composition of these cerebral emboli *in vivo* (Ries *et al.*, 1998). It is likely that a combination of gaseous emboli and particulate matter is currently being detected by transcranial Doppler equipment. Both particulate and gaseous emboli can cause distal obstruction of end-arterial flow in small cerebral arteries, thereby resulting in ischaemia and neuronal failure. Cerebral arterial gas embolization also leads to migration of gas into very small arteries (with an average diameter of 30–60 μm) and, in addition, causing immediate obstruction and ischaemia; the surface of the gaseous bubble can initiate a foreign-body response and mechanically irritate the vascular endothelium. This can trigger cellular and humoral immune mechanisms, resulting in vasogenic oedema and further impairment of perfusion (Muth and Shank, 2000).

Although a correlation between a given intraoperative cerebral microembolic load and alterations of neurocognitive function has repeatedly been reported (Pugsley

et al., 1994; Clark *et al.*, 1995; Hammon *et al.*, 1977), their clinical relevance has also been questioned by others (Thiel *et al.*, 1997; Jacobs *et al.*, 1998). Pugsley *et al.* (1990) demonstrated a significant association between the embolic load and neurocognitive outcome in a study evaluating the effects of arterial line filters in patients undergoing cardiopulmonary bypass with bubble oxygenators (Fig. 10.2).

Clark *et al.* (1995), using transcranial Doppler techniques during CABG surgery, also showed a positive correlation between the number of intraoperative microemboli and deterioration in cognitive function, detected with a battery of neuropsychologic tests. In a recent study by Hammon *et al.* (1977) of 395 patients undergoing cardiac surgery, neurocognitive decrement was significantly ($p < 0.04$) associated with more than 100 emboli per case. However, Jacobs *et al.* (1998), also in a recent study, found that the number of intraoperative microembolic events during cardiac surgery did not correlate with alterations in neuropsychological function or global cerebral glucose metabolism (CMRGlc) but did correlate with regional changes of global cerebral glucose metabolism. These authors suggested that cognitive changes after cardiac surgery might depend more on the location of emboli-related brain damage than on the absolute number of cerebral emboli alone.

Causes of cerebral macro- and microemboli include patient-related and procedure- or equipment-related sources. Patient-related sources, such as the degree of atheromatous disease of the aorta, intraventricular thrombi or valvular calcification, represent individual risk factors for cerebral embolization and, as a result, post-operative neurological and neurocognitive dysfunction (Blauth *et al.*, 1992; Roach *et al.*, 1996). Procedure-related sources include aortic cannulation and decannulation, initiation of cardiopulmonary bypass (Baker *et al.*, 1995), aortic cross- and side-clamping or clamp removal (Sylvris *et al.*, 1998), ventricular venting and open-chamber surgery Braekken *et al.*, 1997; O'Brien *et al.*, 1997). Another important procedure-related source is the reinfusion of shed blood from cardiotomy suction that has been demonstrated to increase the number of detectable cerebral lipid microemboli sixfold (Fig. 10.3) (Brooker *et al.*, 1998). The duration of cardiopulmonary bypass is also consistently associated with an increase in embolic load (Brown *et al.*, 2000).

Equipment-related factors that have been shown to reduce the intraoperative embolic load include the presence of a 25-μm filter in the aortic inflow line (Padayachee *et al.*, 1988; Pugsley *et al.*, 1994), the use of membrane as opposed to bubble oxygenators (Pearson *et al.*, 1986) and the utilization of 20–40 μm filters in the cardiotomy suction line. Interestingly, the number of gaseous microemboli delivered to the patients may depend on the

cardiopulmonary bypass circuit design and is not necessarily increased by the use of vacuum-assisted venous drainage (Jones *et al.*, 2000). It is important to note, however, that all the equipment-related changes have potentially reduced the general embolic load but clearly cannot eliminate cerebral embolization altogether. This is because a relevant portion of cerebral emboli originates from the ascending aorta where atherosclerotic plaque material is being released secondary to extensive manipulation during aortic cross-clamping, cannulation and decannulation (Moody *et al.*, 1990).

Cerebral hypoperfusion

Cerebral hypoperfusion, be it regional hypoperfusion caused by emboli, or global hypoperfusion caused by the unphysiological effects of cardiopulmonary bypass, or generalized hypotension, has long been thought to be a potential source of post-operative neurological impairment (Gilman, 1965). The majority of discussion surrounding the impact of hypoperfusion relates to the influence of arterial blood pressure. A recent study by Gold *et al.* (1995) supports the concept that a better neurological outcome after cardiopulmonary bypass procedures, at least in patients at high risk, may be related to maintaining higher mean arterial blood pressure. In their study, 248 patients undergoing elective CABG were randomized to either low mean arterial blood pressure (50–70 mmHg) or high mean arterial blood pressure (80–100 mmHg) during cardiopulmonary bypass. Mean arterial blood pressure did not have a significant impact on neurological outcome in patients at low risk for central nervous system injury. However, in patients with high risk for cerebral embolization because of extensive atheromatous disease of the aorta, the higher mean arterial blood pressure resulted in significantly lower risk of poor neurological outcome. Although these results imply that mean arterial blood pressure during cardiopulmonary bypass may have an important effect on collateral perfusion in brain regions that suffer from cardiopulmonary bypass-related emboli, they also support embolization (as opposed to generalized hypoperfusion) as primary source of central nervous system injury after cardiac surgery. In contrast to the findings by Gold *et al.* (1995), van Wermeskerken *et al.* (2000) were unable to demonstrate any advantage of higher mean arterial blood pressure in reducing perioperative stroke, even in high risk patients. In a further study examining the influence of blood pressure during cardiopulmonary bypass, a cardiopulmonary bypass-mean arterial blood pressure of <50 mmHg was similarly not associated with neurocognitive dysfunction (Newman *et al.*, 1995a). The same study, however, found that interactions significantly correlated with neurocognitive decline between a mean arterial blood pressure <50 mmHg during

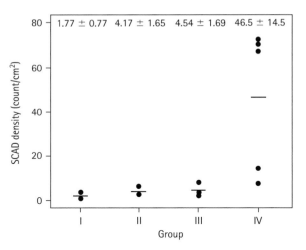

Figure 10.3 *The reinfusion of shed blood from cardiotomy suction increases the number of lipid microemboli significantly. The figure shows the number of small capillary and arterial dilatation (SCAD) counts in an experimental dog study by group: Group I = right-heart cardiopulmonary bypass, Group II = lower extremity cardiopulmonary bypass, Group III = hypothermic cardiopulmonary bypass, and Group IV = hypothermic cardiopulmonary bypass with cardiotomy suction. Dots denote individual dogs, and lines represent the mean for each group. Mean and standard error of the mean for each group are given at the top of the figure. (From Brooker, R.F., Brown, W.R., Moody, D.M. et al. 1998: Cardiotomy suction: a major source of brain lipid emboli during cardiopulmonary bypass.* Annals of Thoracic Surgery **65**, *1651–5, reprinted with permission from The Society of Thoracic Surgeons.)*

cardiopulmonary bypass and age, suggesting that the elderly population might be more susceptible to cerebral hypoperfusion during periods of cardiopulmonary bypass-related hypotension.

Autoregulation of cerebral blood flow remains intact when alpha-stat pH management is used during non-pulsatile cardiopulmonary bypass, even at a mean arterial blood pressure as low as 30 mmHg (Murkin et al., 1987; Taylor, 1998). Murkin et al. (1987) determined the effects of temperature corrected (pH-stat) or non-corrected (alpha-stat) $PaCO_2$ management at 40 mmHg on regulation of cerebral blood flow and flow or metabolism coupling in 38 patients undergoing hypothermic cardiopulmonary bypass. In patients randomized to pH-stat management, cerebral blood flow or cerebral metabolism coupling was not maintained and cerebral blood flow correlated significantly with cerebral perfusion pressure over a wide range (15–95 mmHg). In the alpha-stat group, however, cerebral blood flow regulation was better preserved; that is, cerebral blood flow was independent of pressure changes and dependent upon cerebral oxygen consumption. Interesting evidence regarding the advantage of at least some flow versus no flow during hypothermic cardiac arrest for open-heart surgery can be seen in the paediatric cardiac surgery literature. Newburger et al. (1993) reported from a randomized trial comparing the effects of hypothermic cardiac arrest versus low-flow cardiopulmonary bypass on early postoperative neurological outcomes in young children who underwent arterial switch operations by three months of age. Children assigned to hypothermic cardiac arrest showed a higher incidence of clinical seizures and ictal activity, longer electroencephalographic (EEG) recovery times and greater creatine kinase BB isoenzyme release. At one year of age, the same group of children presented with a higher prevalence of neurological abnormalities, poorer motor function (Bellinger et al., 1995) and expressive language by parental report at 2.5 years of age (Bellinger et al., 1997). In a recent follow-up report on these children, Bellinger et al. (1999) reported that in four-year-old children who underwent arterial switch operations by three months of age, the group that underwent hypothermic cardiac arrest compared with low-flow cardiopulmonary bypass performed significantly worse on assessments of gross motor, fine motor and speech functions.

Inflammation

Cardiopulmonary bypass is known to elicit a widespread systemic inflammation, best described as a 'whole-body' inflammatory reaction (Murkin, 1997). This systemic inflammatory response is initiated and entertained by a number of different processes (Hall et al., 1997), including the contact of blood with the foreign surfaces of the

cardiopulmonary bypass circuit (Kirklin et al., 1983), the development of endotoxaemia because of a reduction in splanchnic blood flow (Kharazmi et al., 1989; Landow and Andersen, 1994) and the development of ischaemia and reperfusion injury. More specifically, this systemic inflammatory response is triggered and propagated by the activation of several cascades within the immune system. Besides activation of various components of the complement cascade (Kirklin et al., 1983), cardiopulmonary bypass has been shown to activate kallikrein-bradykinin, the coagulation, the fibrinolytic and the arachidonic acid cascades. In addition, a variety of pro-inflammatory cytokines, such as tumour necrosis factor-α (TNF-α) (Jansen et al., 1991), interleukin-1 (IL-1), interleukin-6 (IL-6) and interleukin-8 (IL-8) appear to be involved in the cardiopulmonary bypass inflammatory process (Butler et al., 1993; Kawamura et al., 1993). The release of pro-inflammatory cytokines further perpetuates the inflammatory response after cardiopulmonary bypass and results in complex cell-to-cell interactions between activated leukocytes, platelets, and endothelial cells that is mediated by endothelial adhesion molecules (Asimakopoulos and Taylor, 1998). An anti-inflammatory cascade of cytokines is also initiated in response to the pro-inflammatory process (McBride et al., 1995).

Clinically, the whole-body inflammation associated with cardiopulmonary bypass might contribute to the transient cerebral oedema that accompanies cardiac surgery utilizing hypothermic (28°C) and normothermic (37°C) cardiopulmonary bypass (Harris et al., 1993, 1998). However, it is unclear if cerebral oedema after cardiopulmonary bypass contributes to adverse neurological or neurocognitive outcome. In the experimental setting, inflammation is known to contribute to neurological injury or at least to modulate neuronal injury (Garcia et al., 1994; Kogure et al., 1996). As a result of gene expression, cytokines are produced that stimulate the production and expression of adhesion molecules by both endothelial and glial cells. The adhesion molecules stimulate the binding neutrophils to capillary endothelium with subsequent transmigration into the ischaemic tissue. Neutrophils then contribute to damage via their production of free radicals and other cytotoxic substances.

Nandate et al. (1999), using juguloarterial gradients to measure cerebrovascular cytokine production, demonstrated specific and significant IL-8 production in the cerebrovascular bed during cardiopulmonary bypass and suggests that these changes may be suppressed by hypothermia during cardiopulmonary bypass. However, it is uncertain if the IL-8 activation contributes to neurological dysfunction after cardiopulmonary bypass. Hypothermia during cardiopulmonary bypass may significantly attenuate this response. Most difficult to determine is if the inflammatory response seen with cardiopulmonary bypass is merely coincidental (that is, an epiphenomenon) with the cerebral injury or directly contributory to it.

Genetic predisposition

During the last decade, genetic associations have been successfully identified for a number of neurological diseases. In particular, the apolipoprotein 4 (APOE4) gene was found to be associated with sporadic and late-onset Alzheimer's disease (Saunders *et al.*, 1993). This finding started several lines of investigation examining the association of APOE genotype and outcome from acute ischaemic and traumatic central nervous system injury. APOE genotype was subsequently shown to significantly affect outcome and recovery after a number of acute ischaemic insults, including closed head injury (Sorbi *et al.*, 1995; Teasdale *et al.*, 1997), acute stroke (Slooter *et al.*, 1997) and intracerebral haemorrhage (Alberts *et al.*, 1995). These human data find support in large numbers of experimental studies utilizing genetically engineered mice (Sheng *et al.*, 1999). Important, but preliminary information regarding a relationship between the apolipoprotein E genotype and cognitive dysfunction after cardiopulmonary bypass and cardiac surgery came from Tardiff *et al.* (1997). In 65 patients, a significant association between APOE4 and a change in cognitive test score in measures of short-term memory at six weeks post-operatively was detected. These authors suggested that the apolipoprotein E genotype might impact mechanisms of neuronal injury and repair in patients undergoing cardiopulmonary bypass for cardiac surgery. APOE may also affect neurological outcomes by modulating the glial response to inflammatory processes that are associated with ischaemia and reperfusion (Newman *et al.*, 1999). Immunomodulatory properties of APOE have been demonstrated *in vitro* and include the suppression of lymphocyte proliferation and the synthesis of immunoglobulins (Hui *et al.*, 1980; Macy *et al.*, 1983). Indirect mechanisms by which the apolipoprotein genotype may affect neurological outcome after cardiac surgery include the association between APOE and the severity of artherosclerosis that may contribute to the embolic load (Ilveskoski *et al.*, 1999). The association between the APOE4 allele and the percentage of the abdominal and thoracic aorta atherosclerotic involvement has also been confirmed by Hixson (1991) (Fig. 10.4) and Ti *et al.* (2003).

RISK STRATIFICATION

Known pre-operative risk factors associated with adverse cerebral outcomes in patients undergoing cardiopulmonary bypass surgery are similar but not identical for

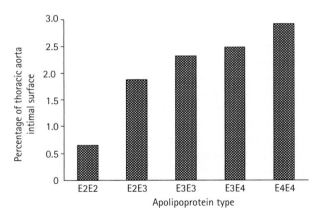

Figure 10.4 *Percentage of the thoracic aorta intimal surface involved with atherosclerotic lesions as a function of APOE genotype for patients in the PDAY study (corrected for age, smoking and serum cholesterol). (Reprinted with permission from Hixson, J.E. 1991: Pathobiological determinants of atherosclerosis in youth research group: apolipoprotein E polymorphisms affect atherosclerosis young males. Arterioscler Throm 11, 1237–44.)*

stroke and other deficits, such as nonfocal encephalopathy or neurocognitive dysfunction. The same is true if adverse cerebral outcomes are separated into Type I (focal stroke, stupor or coma) and Type II (decline in intellectual function, memory deficit and seizures) outcomes (Roach *et al.*, 1996). The concept of risk stratification in patients undergoing cardiac surgery can serve as both an important clinical and scientific tool. First, the identification of relevant risk factors may help to better understand mechanisms of disease. Second, because the incidence of adverse cerebral outcomes is significantly associated with pertinent risk factors, neuroprotective strategies and future pharmacological neuroprotectants, which potentially involve additional cost and their inherent risks, might then only be applied to those patients at risk. Lastly, solid risk stratification can support cardiac surgeons and peri-operative caregivers during difficult clinical decisions.

Risk factors for stroke, stupor or coma (Type I adverse cerebral outcomes)

Identifying risk factors for peri-operative stroke has long been hampered by several important factors, including inadequate sample size, inconsistent variables tested and the lack of a multicentre approach to the problem. This changed when the investigators of the Multicenter Study of Perioperative Ischemia (MCSPI) group presented a new pre-operative stroke risk index based on a prospective, multicentre, observational study that analysed 2207 patients at 24 academic medical centres throughout the

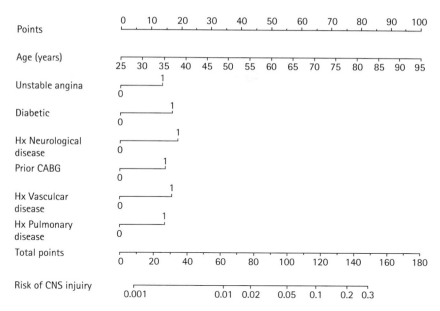

Figure 10.5 *Nomogram for computing risk of central nervous system injury. Neurological risk is determined by assessing points for age and positive history of the predictors listed. The total points for each variable are read from the points line at the top of the nomogram. After computing the total points for an individual patient, the risk of central nervous system injury can be determined by plotting the total points received against the risk score at the bottom of the nomogram. For example, 100 points predict a five percent risk of central nervous system injury. (Reprinted from Newman, M.F., Wolman, R., Kanchuger, M. et al. 1996: Multicenter preoperative stroke risk index for patients undergoing coronary artery bypass graft surgery. Multicenter Study of Perioperative Ischemia (MCSPI) Research Group. Circulation 94, 74–80 (Suppl. 9), with permission from Lippincott, Williams & Wilkins.)*

USA (Newman *et al.*, 1996a). Sixty-eight patients (3.2 per cent) developed major adverse neurological events, defined as cerebrovascular accident, transient ischaemic attack or persistent coma. Figure 10.5 shows that neurological risk is determined by assigning points for patients' age and key predictors, such as unstable angina, diabetes, history of neurologic disease, prior CABG surgery, history of vascular or pulmonary disease. This stroke risk index allows the calculation of individual pre-operative patient's risk for stroke within 95 per cent confidence limits.

Moderate-to-severe atheromatous disease of the ascending aorta, aortic arch and descending aorta presents a known risk factor for stroke cardiac surgical patients and correlates with increasing age. Proximal aortic atherosclerosis, as identified by surgical palpation, was the strongest independent predictor of stroke in the large multicentre study of patients undergoing CABG (Roach *et al.*, 1996). In that study, moderate-to-severe proximal atherosclerosis was associated with a fivefold increase in the incidence of Type I adverse cerebral outcomes compared with patients without significant aortic atherosclerosis. Although intraoperative palpation of the aorta may greatly underestimate the degree of atheromatous disease of the ascending aorta (Ohteki *et al.*, 1990), epi-aortic ultrasonography has been documented to identify significant atheromatous plaques, which may result in a change of the site of aortic cannulation in

patients where surgical palpation does not detect them (Marshall *et al.*, 1989). Transoesophageal echocardiography (TEE) is predominantly being used to grade atheromatous disease of the aorta in cardiac surgical patients. TEE evaluation of the aorta is superior to traditional methods of grading the degree of atheromatous disease in the aortic arch, such as chest X-ray and cardiac catheterization (Marschall *et al.*, 1994). However, interposition of the large airways limits its ability to examine the complete thoracic aorta echocardiographically, whereas parts of the ascending aorta and proximal arch may not be visualized (Konstadt *et al.*, 1994). This is one explanation why epi-aortic ultrasound is superior to TEE in visualizing the entire ascending aorta (Sylivris *et al.*, 1997). Therefore, peri-operative TEE in combination with epi-aortic ultrasound presents a widely used tool to identify patients with higher degrees of aortic atherosclerosis in the operating room (Davila-Roman *et al.*, 1996; Sylivris *et al.*, 1997; Hogue *et al.*, 1999). Hartman *et al.* (1996b), in a prospective study, identified the degree of aortic atheromatous disease as a strong predictor of stroke within one week of CABG surgery and for both stroke and death within six months after CABG surgery (Fig. 10.6). In 189 patients undergoing CABG surgery, the degree of atheromatous disease of the aorta was graded on a scale from I to V by use of TEE and correlated with the incidence of stroke and death. Patients with an

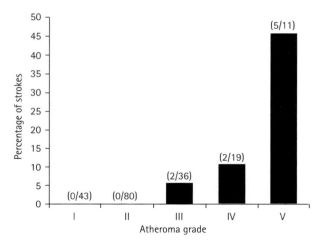

Figure 10.6 *One-week stroke rate as a function of atheroma grade (n = 189). (Reprinted from Hartmann, G.S., Fun-Sun, F.Y., Bruefach, M. et al. 1996: Severity of aortic atheromatous disease diagnosed by transesophageal echocardiography predicts stroke and other outcomes associated with Cardiac artery surgery: a prospective study.* Anesthesia and Analgesia **83**, *701–8, with permission from Lippincott, Williams & Wilkins.)*

atheroma grade V (mobile plaque component) had a stroke rate of 45 per cent.

The severity of aortic atheroma is also associated with significantly prolonged hospitalization after cardiac surgery (Barbut *et al.*, 1997b). Most recently, an association between the atheromatous burden identified by TEE and the cerebral embolic load detected with transcranial Doppler was demonstrated (Mackensen *et al.*, 2003).

A *history of a previous neurological abnormality* (stroke, transient ischaemic attack) has also been identified by several authors as a significant risk factor for Type I outcomes (Tuman *et al.*, 1992; Ricotta *et al.*, 1995; Roach *et al.*, 1996). It has been speculated that a history of neurological disease may result in pathological cerebrovascular conditions, impaired cerebral blood flow during cardiopulmonary bypass, a lack or impairment of autoregulation and inadequate development of collaterals (Roach *et al.*, 1996). Diabetes mellitus has also been shown to expose patients to a greater risk of suffering from Type I adverse cerebral outcomes. Patients with diabetes mellitus suffer from impaired autoregulation during cardiopulmonary bypass (Croughwell *et al.*, 1990) and a generally impaired vascular status that may affect the degree of cerebral vascular atherosclerosis. Further predictors of Type I outcomes in the multicentre study by Roach *et al.* (1996) were the occurrence of unstable angina, the length of cardiopulmonary bypass time, advanced age (≥70 years of age), the surgical technique (left ventricular venting, de-airing techniques, cross-clamp) and the use of an intra-aortic balloon pump.

Risk factors for neurocognitive dysfunction and deterioration in intellectual function, memory deficit or seizures (Type II adverse cerebral outcomes)

The factors thought to contribute to neurocognitive dysfunction include patient age, genetic predisposition, gender, extent of pre-operative cerebrovascular disease, degree of cerebral microembolization, duration of cardiopulmonary bypass, temperature and acid-base management (Arrowsmith *et al.*, 1999). Similar to its predominant role as a peri-operative risk factor for stroke, age is one of the primary risk factors for peri-operative neurocognitive decline (Newman *et al.*, 1994, 1995a). Interestingly, no association between the atheromatous burden of the aorta and encephalopathy or subtle neurocognitive deficits has thus far been demonstrated. Other mechanisms, such as an age-related impairment of cerebral autoregulation or age-related changes in cerebral oxygenation during rewarming after cardiopulmonary bypass, may contribute to an age-dependent cognitive decline. Years of education appears to be another interesting demographic predictor of cognitive decline after cardiac surgery (Newman *et al.*, 1994). Again, as identified in the previously cited study by Roach *et al.* (1996), Type II adverse cerebral outcomes were related to excessive alcohol consumption, postoperative dysrhythmia, a history of CABG surgery and the presence of peripheral vascular disease. Both pulmonary disease and hypertension have been identified as common predictors of Type I and Type II adverse cerebral outcomes.

NEUROPROTECTIVE STRATEGIES

Preventive neuroprotective strategies

As outlined above, risk assessment and stratification of patients undergoing cardiac surgery are essential steps before useful neuroprotective strategies, alteration of surgical management or other interventions can be applied. The flow diagram in Fig. 10.7 shows one reasonable approach to minimizing peri-operative neurologic risk in patients undergoing cardiopulmonary bypass for cardiac surgery. This strategy includes a thorough assessment of the aorta, using TEE as a first, and epi-aortic scan as a second step, followed by a general risk assessment using the stroke risk index as described above (Newman *et al.*, 1996a, 2001a). It seems justified to assume that the patient with a low risk for adverse peri-operative neurologic outcomes by TEE evaluation and history will benefit little neurologically from changes in surgical techniques or cardiopulmonary bypass-related interventions such as temperature management or pressure

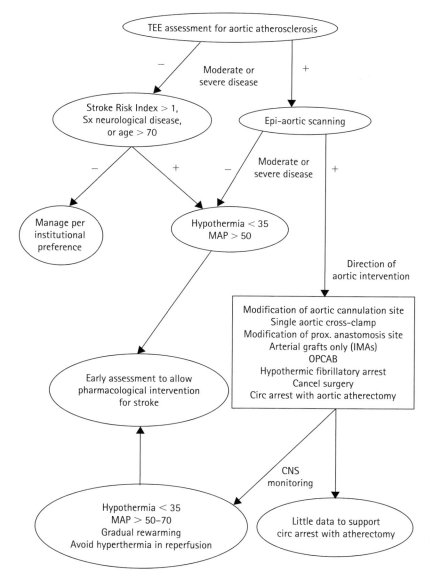

Figure 10.7 *Algorithm for a neurological risk minimization based on assessment of aortic atherosclerosis and pre-operative risk. Recommendations are based on current literature showing temperature and mean aterial pressure effects on neurological outcome in patients at high risk for atherosclerosis. Deep hypothermic circulatory arrest with atherectomy is not recommended in the strategy because of its potential risk and limited data supporting effectiveness. IMA = internal mammary artery; OPCAB = off-pump coronary artery bypass. (Reprinted from Newman, M.F., Stanley, T.O., Grocott, H.P. 2000: Strategies to protect the brain during cardiac surgery. Sem Cardiothor Vasc Anesth 4, 53–64, with permission from W.B. Saunders Company.)*

changes on cardiopulmonary bypass. However, identification of the patient at higher risk for adverse neurological outcomes allows reserving and individually applying cost-intensive strategies for prevention or treatment. Because risk factors for adverse neurological and neurocognitive outcomes possibly overlap but are not identical, the patient at high risk for the development of neurocognitive deficits deserves a different approach that will also be outlined in the following section.

Surgical technique

Atherosclerosis of the proximal aorta has been recognized as one of the major predictors of peri-operative stroke and central nervous system dysfunction after cardiac surgery (Gardner *et al.*, 1985; Hartman *et al.*, 1996a; Roach *et al.*, 1996). Although surgical palpation and even peri-operative

TEE have been shown to underestimate the severity of ascending aortic atheromatous disease, the introduction of epiaortic ultrasound allows a reliable assessment and identification of severe atheromas (Davila-Roman *et al.*, 1996). A major advantage of epi-aortic ultrasound is that it can be performed quickly and non-invasively. Using epi-aortic ultrasound, the incidence of atherosclerosis of the ascending aorta was described to range from 58 per cent to 89 per cent (Marshall *et al.*, 1989; Ohteki *et al.*, 1990). Several investigators have used this information to attempt to reduce central nervous system dysfunction after cardiac surgery by altering either surgical or anesthetic technique. More aggressive changes in surgical technique include the introduction of hypothermic cardiac arrest to allow removal of severe atherosclerotic lesions or to replace the diseased ascending aorta (Wareing *et al.*, 1992, 1993; Kouchoukos *et al.*, 1994). Whereas Wareing *et al.* (1993)

reported a low surgical risk, King et al. (1998), in a more recent study, reported a tenfold increased risk associated with replacement of the ascending aorta for atherosclerotic changes compared with that for aortic aneurysmal disease. The conflicting data, and the lack of a large randomized trial comparing these rather aggressive interventions with a standard approach, point to more conservative alterations of surgical technique. These include changing the site of aortic cannulation, the use of a femoral cannulation or single aortic cross-clamping fibrillatory arrest (King et al., 1998; Newman et al., 2000). Other mechanisms to reduce the manipulation of the diseased aorta include the use of all arterial graphs, such as internal mammary arteries, single aortic cross-clamping or off-pump cardiac surgery, with the use of an aortic side-clamp only (Moshkovitz et al., 1997; Murkin et al., 1999). Avoiding the reinfusion of shed blood from cardiotomy suction that may decrease the number of cerebral lipid microemboli is another surgical contribution to a reduction of the overall embolic load (Brooker et al., 1998). In a recent approach to surgical reduction of particulate embolization, Reichenspurner et al. (2000) describe a new intra-aortic filtration method. In a series of 77 patients undergoing cardiopulmonary bypass, these authors used a novel intra-aortic filter device inserted through a modified aortic cannula immediately before releasing the aortic cross-clamp. Insertion and removal of the filter appeared to be safe, easy and uneventful. Histological analysis of the captured embolic material revealed mostly fibrous atheromatous material and platelet-fibrin. However, it remains to be determined if this new device will affect neurological outcomes after cardiac surgery.

Off-pump CABG surgery, as opposed to conventional CABG procedures using cardiopulmonary bypass, has the potential for lower incidences of neurological and neurocognitive dysfunction (Murkin et al., 1999). One would expect a smaller cerebral embolic load because of the avoidance of aortic cannulation and decannulation, aortic cross clamping and exposure to the pump circuitry. To date, this has only been shown in a small number of patients by Watters et al. (2000), who measured the number of cerebral emboli with transcranial Doppler. However, in a preliminary study, Murkin et al. (1999) showed a significantly lower incidence of cognitive dysfunction in patients undergoing off-pump CABG versus on-pump CABG at five days (66 per cent versus 90 per cent) and three months (5 per cent versus 50 per cent), respectively.

Strategies related to the cardiopulmonary bypass circuit and cardiopulmonary bypass technique

Microembolization during cardiopulmonary bypass has been associated with adverse neurocognitive outcomes (Pugsley et al., 1990; Clark et al., 1995). Preventive measures to reduce the microembolic load during cardiopulmonary bypass that have been shown to be effective include the use of membrane versus bubble oxygenators, the utilization of filters in the aortic inflow line and the use of filters in the cardiotomy suction line of the cardiopulmonary bypass circuits (Pearson et al., 1986; Padayachee et al., 1987; Pugsley et al., 1994). Because an increasing duration of cardiopulmonary bypass is clearly associated with a greater embolic burden (Brown et al., 2000), reserving the use of cardiopulmonary bypass for those parts of cardiac procedures where it is absolutely essential might also contribute to improved outcomes. Another important factor that determines the number of microemboli is the design of the cardiopulmonary bypass circuit, as was shown recently by Jones et al. (2000).

Possible neuroprotective strategies that are related to the physiology of cardiopulmonary bypass, such as temperature management, pH- versus alpha-stat management, perfusion pressure during cardiopulmonary bypass, pulsatile versus non-pulsatile flow and glucose management, have already been discussed in detail earlier in this chapter.

Neurological monitoring

Theoretically, the use of neurologic monitoring in patients at significant risk for adverse cerebral outcomes during cardiac surgery is promising. Significant technical advances led to the development of improved electrophysiological monitoring, the improvement of near-infrared spectroscopy and transcranial Doppler devices. However, because it is difficult to determine the predictive power and value of these neurological monitors in patients undergoing cardiac surgery, their widespread use has not been adopted (Arrowsmith et al., 1999). Although electroencephalography has long been seen as a valuable monitor for intraoperative ischaemia during cardiac surgery, it has not gained wide clinical acceptance. Reasons for this include the electromagnetic environment and electrical noise in the operating room, the requirement for technical support and conflicting results regarding its value in the literature (Bashein et al., 1992; Edmonds et al., 1992).

Transcranial Doppler devices allow the non-invasive measurement of cerebral blood flow velocity and semi-quantitation of embolic events during cardiac surgery. Using transcranial Doppler, the cerebral microembolic load during cardiac surgery has been associated with the degree of neurocognitive dysfunction by several groups (Pugsley et al., 1994; Clark et al., 1995; Hammon et al., 1977). This technique allows comparing different surgical or other interventions to reduce the number of cerebral emboli and, as a result, represents a powerful research tool (Clark et al., 1995; Stump et al., 1996). Further advances in transcranial Doppler equipment should ultimately allow the determination of the composition of cerebral emboli, thereby increasing its utility (Ries *et al.*, 1998). The adequacy of cerebral oxygen cannot be monitored because absolute cerebral blood flow cannot be measured using transcranial Doppler. This, and the fact that transcranial Doppler monitoring is at times technically difficult to perform adequately because of the inability to place the probes securely and to maintain a useful signal, have prevented its widespread use.

Near-infrared spectroscopy has been introduced as another suitable means to monitor the brain at risk for regional ischaemia or critical oxygen desaturation. One limiting factor of this technique is the fact that it can only indicate trends from baseline rather than absolute values. Further, because near-infrared spectroscopy only monitors saturation in small regions, ischaemia in regions other than the one monitored will likely remain undetected. As discussed earlier, cerebral hypoperfusion potentially plays a secondary role after cerebral embolization in the aetiology of neurological and neurocognitive deficits after cardiac surgery with cardiopulmonary bypass. Therefore, a valid monitor of regional or global perfusion could be beneficial in the cardiac surgery setting. Further refinement of this technique and the validation with definite outcomes in larger studies could open the door to its mainstream practice in cardiac surgery because of its ease of use and interpretation (Arrowsmith *et al.*, 1999).

Continuous monitoring of jugular bulb oxygenation presents another more invasive monitor that is being reported during cardiac surgery. Our own data have shown a positive correlation between an increasing arterio-venous oxygen content difference during rewarming and cognitive dysfunction (Croughwell *et al.*, 1994). Although these data were based on intermittent-sampling techniques, obtained during rapid rewarming from hypothermic cardiopulmonary bypass, the continuous monitoring of jugular bulb saturation with fiberoptic devices has been questioned with regard to its accuracy and predictive power (Trubiano *et al.*, 1996). Because of these inherent problems and because of its relatively invasive nature, jugular bulb monitoring has not generally found its way into the mainstream practice of cardiac surgery (Arrowsmith *et al.*, 1999). In summary, further improvements in technical aspects of neurological monitoring devices and additional advances in risk stratification in patients undergoing cardiac surgery should significantly enhance the usefulness of neurological monitoring in the future.

Pharmacological neuroprotection

Experimental animal models of cerebral ischaemic injury have investigated a considerable number of neuroprotective agents. These studies also suggest that many

Table 10.1 *Pharmacological neuroprotectants that have been evaluated in cardiac surgery*

Thiopental
Acadesine
Aprotinin
Nimodipine
GM1-ganglioside
Dextromethorphan
Remacemide
Lidocaine
Beta blockade
Propofol
Etomidate
Pegorgotein
H5G1.1-scFv (Single-chain antibody)
C5 complement inhibitor)

neuroprotectants are only effective if administered either before, during or immediately after the ischaemic insult occurs. In general clinical settings of neurological injury (for example, non-cardiac surgical stroke), patients most often present hours after the ischaemic injury has already occurred. Even the most promising experimental drugs have failed to alter the course of the injury in these patients when given hours after the ischaemic event. In contrast, cardiac surgery represents a unique paradigm in which to both study and ultimately administer neuroprotective agents. The cardiac patient awaiting surgery is an ideal candidate to benefit from prophylactic treatment (Grotta, 1996). Although, to date, there are no FDA-approved pharmacological agents to prevent or treat central nervous system injury during cardiac surgery, a number of agents have been investigated over the past two decades (Table 10.1).

These agents have been targeted both at the presumed aetiologies of cardiopulmonary bypass-associated cerebral injury but more specifically at the ischaemic cascade (Fig. 10.8) (Dirnagl *et al.*, 1999).

The ischaemic cascade

Although the aetiology of cardiac surgery-related cerebral injury is not completely clear, a final common pathway centres on the ischaemic cascade. The ischaemic cascade is a complex network of intracellular pathways during which a number of events then determine if a given neuron follows a pathway towards necrotic or apoptotic cell death or survival (Green and Reed, 1998; Siesjö *et al.*, 1999). Reductions in cerebral blood flow, either globally or regionally, to the point at which the demands of cerebral metabolic rate of oxygen are not met, result in a depletion of cerebral energy stores (ATP and other high-energy phosphates). The resulting membrane ionic pump failure causes a number of detrimental events, including

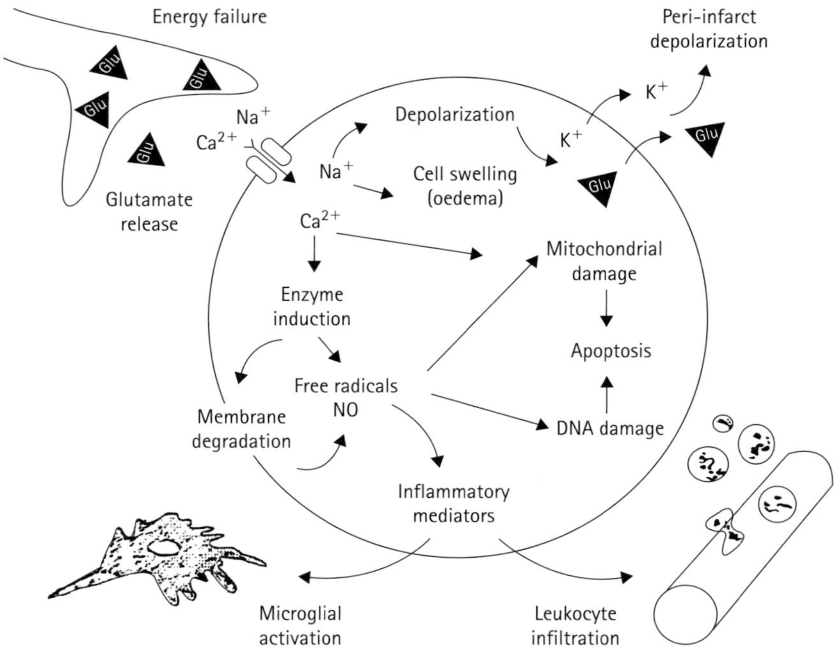

Figure 10.8 *Simplified overview of pathophysiological mechanisms in the focally ischemic brain. Energy failure leads to the depolarization of neurons. Activation of specific glutamate receptors dramatically increases intracellular Ca^{2+}, Na^+ and Cl^- levels, whereas K^+ is released into the extracellular space. Diffusion of glutamate (Glu) and K^+ in the extracellular space can propagate a series of spreading waves of depolarization (peri-infarct depolarizations). Water shifts to the intracellular space via osmotic gradients and cells swell (oedema). The universal intracellular messenger Ca^{2+} overactivates numerous enzyme systems (proteases, lipases, endonucleases, etc.). Free radicals are generated, which damage membranes (lipolysis), mitochondria and DNA, in turn triggering caspase-mediated cell death (apoptosis). Free radicals also induce the formation of inflammatory mediators, which activate microglia and lead to the invasion of blood-borne inflammatory cells. (Reprinted from Dirnagl, U., Iadecola, C., Moskowitz, M. 1999: Pathobiology of ischaemic stroke: an integrated view.* Trends Neurosci **22**, *391–7, with permission from Elsevier Science.)*

the influx of sodium, the opening of voltage-dependent calcium gates, a release of stored intracellular calcium and overall membrane depolarization. The membrane depolarization results in a release of excitatory amino acids (for example, glutamate, aspartate). Activation of specific glutamate receptors results in massive increases of intracellular calcium, sodium and chloride. More specifically, the increase in free cytosolic calcium is caused by an influx of extracellular calcium through plasma membrane channels, and from the release of calcium from intracellular stores such as the endoplasmatic reticulum or mitochondria (Kristian and Siesjö, 1998). At the same time, intracellular potassium is released in the extracellular space, which in combination with the occurrence of extracellular glutamate can initiate spreading waves of peri-infarct depolarizations (Hossman, 1996). The dramatic increase in free cytosolic calcium propagates the cascade further through the activation of a number of calcium-dependent enzymes. The activation of these enzymes, including endonucleases, nitric oxide synthase, various proteases, lipases, protein kinases, and phospholipase activates other intracellular events that ultimately lead to neuronal death. Reactive oxygen species, such as superoxide,

hydroxyl radical and peroxynitrite, are generated, all of which have been shown to contribute to ischaemic brain injury (Fabian *et al.*, 1995; Chan, 1996; Peters *et al.*, 1998). These free radicals further damage membranes, mitochondria and DNA and have been shown to trigger caspase-mediated cell death (apoptosis) (Dirnagl *et al.*, 1999).

To a point, some of these events are potentially reversible, and if reperfusion is established, neuronal recovery may occur. However, with the onset of reperfusion, a number of other destructive pathways can be initiated. The re-establishment of oxygen delivery to areas of previously ischaemic brain provides needed substrate for reactive oxygen species production. In addition, reperfusion may initiate a number of damaging extracellular events, including blood brain barrier breakdown, endothelial swelling and localized thrombosis, which may culminate in microvascular occlusion and further ischaemia. Surviving neurons can also have apoptotic pathways initiated with the transcription and translation of several well-characterized self-destructive proteins. This complexity of events and pathways within the ischaemic cascade is reason for optimism as well as pessimism. The pathways in the ischaemic cascade represent discrete potential targets for neuroprotection. However, the idea that inhibiting any one of these pathways may prevent the destruction of the brain, may be overly optimistic. The redundancy built into the ischaemic cascade insures that the damaged cell is much more than likely to go on to destruction than recovery. That being said, however, the ischaemic cascade remains the foundation for the understanding and development of pharmacological neuroprotective strategies, both in the setting of stroke, as well as cardiac surgery-related cerebral injury.

Thiopental

One of the first agents used as a potential neuroprotective agent for cardiac surgery was the barbiturate, thiopental. In a pioneering study in the early 1980s by Nussmeier *et al.* (1986), thiopental was administered to obtain EEG iso-electricity before cannulation for cardiopulmonary bypass continuing until cardiopulmonary bypass was discontinued. In this landmark study, neurologic complications (post-operative day 10) were significantly reduced in the thiopental group versus control. For a time, this study fundamentally changed the way cardiac anaesthesiology was practised. Although not universally accepted, it became commonplace to use high-dose thiopental for valvular and other open ventricular procedures (considered high risk for neurological injury), based upon the encouraging results of this trial. However, as further investigations into the use of thiopental progressed, it became apparent that this may have been an overly optimistic initial finding. Later studies by Zaidan *et al.* (1991), and further work by Pascoe *et al.* (1996), failed to show a beneficial effect of thiopental on neurological outcome after cardiac surgery. Retrospectively, examining the initial Nussmeier study, the beneficial effects of the thiopental may not have been related to a direct neuroprotective effect but caused by an indirect effect on reducing emboli-containing cerebral blood flow. The well-known cerebral vasoconstricting effects of thiopental (matching cerebral blood flow with a barbiturate-induced reduction in cerebral metabolism) may have resulted in a reduction in embolic load to the brain during cardiopulmonary bypass and, as a result, a beneficial effect on neurological outcome. However, the potential mechanisms for protection from thiopental go beyond a metabolic effect. Barbiturates have also been shown to attenuate the release of excitatory amino acids in response to ischaemia (Zhu *et al.*, 1997), to delay ischaemic depolarization (Verhaegen *et al.*, 1995) and to reduce neurological injury in a model of global ischaemia in gerbils (Amakawa *et al.*, 1996).

Another criticism of all the studies is the fact that the barbiturate was not given at times of highest emboli risk to the brain. The drug is typically given during cardiopulmonary bypass to the point of EEG burst suppression.

This may not be the only time of risk, however. During cannulation, aortic plaques can be liberated and cause stroke. In addition, during both rewarming from cardiopulmonary bypass and decannulation itself, the brain is also at risk. In patients receiving thiopental to the point of burst suppression for neuroprotection, they are rarely electrically silent during these time periods immediately before and just prior to termination of cardiopulmonary bypass. The protective effects of thiopental are not necessarily dependent upon iso-electricity, however. This was demonstrated by Warner *et al.* (1996), in a study of focal ischaemia in the rat.

Acadesine

Further insights into potential neuroprotective agents for cardiac surgery came from investigations by the McSPI group who investigated the adenosine-regulating agent, acadesine (Leung *et al.*, 1994). Acadesine is a purine nucleoside analogue that raises adenosine levels in ischaemic tissues and has primarily been used in clinical trials examining the efficacy of the drug to reduce peri-operative myocardial events in CABG patients. Although these trials, initiated in the early 1990s, focused upon improving myocardial outcome, stroke was examined as a secondary outcome (Mangano, 1995). In a study of 633 patients, post hoc analysis showed a reduction in stroke rate, with nine strokes (4.2 per cent) in the placebo group and two (0.9 per cent) and one (0.5 per cent) strokes in the high- and low-dose acadesine groups, respectively. These results are supported by some data in rodent models of cerebral ischaemia, where adenosine itself also was shown to be protective (Rudolphi *et al.*, 1992; Schubert and Kreutzberg, 1993). However, as the incidence of stroke was not the primary outcome of the study by the McSPI group (that is, the study was not designed a priori to examine neurological outcome), no neuroprotection indication was pursued. There are a number of other adenosine-like agents which, in pre-clinical experimental settings, have provided neuroprotection, and this remains a potentially beneficial class of drugs.

Aprotinin

One of the most intriguing agents which has been receiving attention for quite some time in cardiac surgery is the serine protease inhibitor, aprotinin. This is an old drug, used in the 1950s for the treatment of pancreatitis, which found new uses in the last 20 years, in particular for the prevention of blood loss and transfusion during cardiac surgery. As described earlier, ischaemia invokes an inflammatory reaction that leads to cellular adhesion and activation of neutrophils that invade ischaemic tissue and contribute to cell death via activation of neutrophils.

Indirect evidence suggests that inhibitors of this inflammation may possibly reduce stroke after cardiac surgery. Aprotinin, a non-specific serine protease inhibitor, has shown promise; Aoki *et al.* (1994a) were able to show improvement in cerebral high-energy phosphates following hypothermic circulatory arrest in piglets.

In a large multi-centre trial of aprotinin for primary or 're-do' CABG and valvular surgery, the high-dose (Hammersmith regimen) aprotinin group had a lower stroke rate compared with placebo ($p = 0.032$) (Levy *et al.*, 1995). There has been considerable discussion and investigation as to the potential mechanism for these results. Initial enthusiasm focused upon the non-specific inflammatory effects of this drug on preventing some of the adverse inflammatory sequelae of cerebral ischaemia. However, definitive animal investigations in the setting of cerebral ischaemia failed to show any benefit on either functional or neurohistological outcome after cerebral ischaemia (Grocott *et al.*, 1999). The explanation for these apparently divergent results may be likened to the initial enthusiasm and benefit of thiopental in the preceding decades. That is, the aprotinin may have beneficial effects independent of any direct neuroprotective effect, but through an indirect effect of modulating cerebral emboli. Brooker *et al.* (1998) identified cardiotomy suction as a major source of cerebral emboli during cardiopulmonary bypass. One could extrapolate that if a drug reduces the amount of particulate-containing blood returning from the operative field to the cardiotomy reservoir (by decreasing overall blood loss) then cerebral emboli (and the resulting neurological consequences) might be decreased.

Nimodipine

In the context of the ischaemic cascade, calcium plays a central role in propagating cerebral ischaemic injury. For this reason, as well as a demonstrated beneficial effect of the calcium channel-blocker, nimodipine, in subarachnoid haemorrhage (Barker and Ogilvy, 1996) and experimental cerebral ischaemia (Steen *et al.*, 1983, 1995), a double-blind randomized, single-centre trial to access the effect of nimodipine on neurological, neuro-ophthalmological and neuropsychological outcomes after valvular surgery was initiated (Legault *et al.*, 1996). This study was later suspended by an external review board (after 150 of 400 intended patients) because of a higher number of bleeding complications and deaths in the nimodipine group. Although the reasons for stopping this trial (increased bleeding and death rate in the nimodipine group) presented some controversy and many debates in the literature, there were also no neuropsychological deficit differences between the placebo or nimodipine groups. The true effect of this drug, or similar calcium

channel-blockers, may never truly be known in the setting of cardiac surgery. Bleeding complications have been reported after the use of calcium antagonists in other settings (Pahor *et al.*, 1996; Zuccala *et al.*, 1997; Mykchaskiw *et al.*, 2000).

GM1-ganglioside

Monosialogangliosides are naturally occurring substances in neuronal plasma membranes and have been shown to reduce excitatory amino acid (EAA) toxicity (Skaper *et al.*, 1991). GM1 ganglioside has been employed in a dog hypothermic cardiac arrest model where its administration during cardiopulmonary bypass and hypothermic cardiac arrest led to better neurological recovery and less neuronal injury (Redmond *et al.*, 1993; Baumgartner *et al.*, 1998). Because of its beneficial effects in the setting of spinal cord injury (Geisler *et al.*, 1991), the monosialoganglioside, GM1-ganglioside, was investigated as a potential neuroprotectant during cardiac surgery. In addition to the potential beneficial effects of this type of compound on neuronal membranes, there is also some data to suggest that it has a potential beneficial effect on reducing EAA transmission. In a preliminary (albeit underpowered) cardiac surgery study, there was no beneficial effect demonstrated (Grieco *et al.*, 1996). However, the authors used this pilot trial to describe useful statistical methodology needed to measure differences in neurocognitive outcome, making some of their methodology a template for later trials.

Dextromethorphan

The N-methyl-D-aspartate (NMDA) receptor is known to play a major role in cerebral ischaemic injury. It has also been postulated to play a potential role in cardiopulmonary bypass-associated cerebral injury. Two studies have specifically examined whether antagonism of the NMDA receptor in the setting of cardiac surgery could be protective. The first is remacemide, which will be discussed further in the text. Another agent, dextromethorphan (known for its antitussive activity), has been demonstrated to have some non-specific NMDA antagonism properties. A pilot study examining dextromethorphan in the setting of paediatric cardiac surgery has been performed (Schmitt *et al.*, 1997). This study, involving 12 patients (six in the experimental group), used both EEG and MRI endpoints to determine a difference between treatment groups. Because of the small size of the study, no differences were seen. Overall, however, the drug was well tolerated. To our knowledge, there have been no other studies examining NMDA receptor antagonism in the setting of paediatric cardiac surgery.

Remacemide

Excitotoxicity, modulated by the NMDA receptor, has received much attention in the field of neuroprotection. Although human stroke trials have been limited by distressing side effects, there is a wealth of animal data that suggests that NMDA receptor antagonists are robust neuroprotective agents. EAA pathways in neurological injury have been studied in a piglet model of hypothermic cardiac arrest (Aoki et al., 1994b). Aoki and colleagues were able to show an improvement in cerebral energetics following the administration of dizocilpine (MK-801), an NMDA receptor antagonist. In the same study, these workers showed an adverse response to NBQX (2,3-dihydroxy-6-nitro-7-sulfamoyl-benzo (F) quinoxalione), an AMPA receptor antagonist. Bokesh et al. (2000), testing central nervous system 5161A (cerestat), a novel non-competitive NMDA receptor antagonist, in a neonatal lamb hypothermic cardiac arrest model, were able to show a reduction in c-fos expression, suggesting a potential neuroprotective effect. With this as a background, the anti-epileptic drug, remacemide (remacemide hydrochloride or (±)-2-amino-N-(1-methyl-1,2-diphenyl-ethyl)-acetamide HCl), a non-competitive NMDA antagonist, was assessed for neuroprotection during CABG surgery (Arrowsmith et al., 1998). In this study by Arrowsmith et al. (1998), remacemide was given orally for four days before CABG. A neurocognitive battery was performed one week before and eight weeks after CABG. A deficit was defined as a decrease in one standard deviation (SD) in two or more of the 12 tests within the neurocognitive battery. In addition, patients were evaluated for their learning ability, assessed by subtracting the post-operative neurocognitive score from the pre-operative score (thus formulating a Z score). Although, when one examines the data for the presence or absence of a neurocognitive deficit, there appeared to be no difference ($p = 0.6$), in examining the Z score (a measure of learning ability), there was a beneficial effect in the patients whom received remacemide ($p = 0.028$). This is the first adequately powered study of a neuroprotective agent in the setting of cardiac surgery that has shown a beneficial effect. However, because of the length of time that it took to perform this single-centre trial, initial non-beneficial preliminary results, as well as a prolonged period of data analysis and review for publication, this drug is not currently being developed for this indication.

Lidocaine

Intravenous lidocaine has been recently investigated as a neuroprotectant in cardiac surgery because of its properties as a sodium channel-blocking agent and potential anti-inflammatory effects. In a study of 55 patients undergoing valvular surgery, a lidocaine infusion (in an anti-arrhythmic dose) was begun pre-induction and maintained for 48 hours after surgery (Mitchell et al., 1999). Neurocognitive testing was performed pre-operatively, then 10 days, 10 weeks and six months post-operatively. Compared with placebo, neurocognitive outcome 10 days after surgery was significantly better in the lidocaine group ($p = 0.025$). Although this is a relatively small study, it demonstrates there may be some potential for the use of this drug for neuroprotection in cardiac surgery. Larger more long-term studies of its efficacy are needed before this can be recommended therapy.

Beta–blockade

The use of beta-blockers in patients with cardiac disease is almost a ubiquitous therapy. This therapy, however, has been predominately directed towards the prevention of adverse myocardial events. However, in a recent study of neurological outcomes after cardiac surgery, beta-blockers were demonstrated to be associated with an improvement in neurological outcome (Amory et al., 2002). In this study of over 3000 patients from the Duke Heart Center, the neurological outcomes of stroke, transient ischaemic attack and encephalopathy were studied. Patients receiving beta-blockade therapy had a significantly lower incidence of neurological deficit versus those not receiving beta-blockers. Although, the reasons for this potential benefit are not intuitively obvious, there are several potential reasons why they may be efficacious, including modulating both cerebrovascular tone and cardiopulmonary bypass-related inflammatory events (Savitz et al., 2000).

Propofol

Propofol has similar effects to thiopental on cerebral metabolism and blood flow and has also been shown to have some antioxidant properties as well as some properties of calcium-channel antagonism (Newman et al., 1995b). With supportive data in the setting of experimental cerebral ischaemia, propofol has been evaluated as a neuroprotectant in the cardiac surgery setting. A prospective randomized clinical trial to determine whether propofol-induced EEG burst-suppression would reduce the incidence or severity of cerebral injury during valvular surgery was performed (Roach et al., 1999). In this study, 109 of 215 patients received burst-suppression doses of propofol. There were no differences in two-month neuropsychological outcome between groups. The authors concluded that EEG burst-suppressive doses of propofol, with the resulting cerebral metabolic suppression and reduction of cerebral blood flow, provided no neuroprotection during open ventricular procedures.

Etomidate

Etomidate was one of the first drugs to be studied in the setting of cardiac surgery after the advent of barbiturate cerebral protection (Hempelmann et al., 1982). It was not found to have any significant benefit in that study. This has been confirmed in a recent study examining whether etomidate burst suppression could prevent jugular venous desaturation during rewarming from cardiopulmonary bypass (von Knobelsdorff et al., 1996). This recent study was not able to demonstrate any reduction in desaturation, suggesting that etomidate had no protective properties.

Pegorgotein

The generation of reactive oxygen species is a well-described pathophysiological mechanism of ischaemic reperfusion injury. This, combined with the whole-body inflammatory response associated with cardiopulmonary bypass and its own generation of reactive oxygen species, has opened the field of neuroprotection and cardiac surgery to antioxidant agents. The protective endogenous enzyme, superoxide dismutase, is involved in the catabolism of free radicals. As a result, superoxide dismutase overexpression and mimetics have been used in the setting of experimental ischaemia and reperfusion with promising results (Sheng et al., 2000). Pegorgotein, a covalently linked monomethyoxypolyethyleneglycol to superoxide dismutase, has been shown to be protective against reperfusion-mediated cardiac and neuronal injury in animal studies. A recent study was initiated to examine whether pegorgotein during cardiac surgery would be associated with a reduced number of neurocognitive deficits post-operatively (Butterworth et al., 1999). In this study, 67 patients undergoing primary elective CABG surgery were studied ($n = 22$–23 in each of three groups: placebo; 200 IU/kg pegorgotein; 5000 IU/kg pegorgotein) and no difference in neurocognitive outcome was seen between groups.

Single-chain antibody specific for human complement factor 5

Fitch et al. (1999), in an attempt to prevent the complement activation and tissue injury in patients undergoing cardiopulmonary bypass, examined the effect of a novel single-chain antibody specific for human complement factor 5 (h5G1.1-scFv). Although the drug was found to be safe and well tolerated, it also effectively inhibited the complement activation in patients undergoing cardiopulmonary bypass. Using the sequential mini-mental state examinations (MMSE) the authors demonstrated a reduction in new cognitive deficits at the time of hospital discharge in those patients treated with the highest dose (2 mg/kg). Further studies with this and other anti-inflammatory compounds are warranted to determine the clinical value of this therapeutic strategy.

FUTURE PHARMACOLOGICAL NEUROPROTECTION

There are a number of ongoing investigations of neuroprotection in cardiac surgery, employing both known as well as proprietary agents. Investigations of new pharmacological neuroprotectants face several recurring problems. One of the most obvious has been the size of the trials needed to examine meaningful outcomes. This particular problem is now being addressed in larger multi-centre consortia. Another issue relates to the definition of neurological and neurocognitive outcomes. The determination of the incidence of adverse events is largely dependent upon how one defines that adverse event. Consensus on defining adverse cerebral outcomes is being refined.

One of the biggest problems facing the development of future pharmacological neuroprotectants is the sheer number of potential compounds (several hundreds) in various pre-clinical stages of development. Assuming that a well-designed study to examine neurocognitive outcome needs to enrol a minimum of approximately 400 patients (200 in each group) it becomes apparent that a great deal of resources, both financial and otherwise, are needed to complete these types of studies. If one were to study all the potential compounds, it would take hundreds of millions of dollars and decades to determine which drugs appear to be efficacious. Effective experimental models of cardiopulmonary bypass are needed in order to adequately screen for the drugs most likely to show efficacy in the clinical setting (Grocott et al., 2001; Mackensen et al., 2001).

There are innumerable potential compounds under investigation. Some of the most intriguing potential agents focus upon modulating central nervous system inflammatory events (an obvious target during cardiopulmonary bypass). In addition, advanced generation NMDA receptor antagonists, one of the few classes of drugs with a positive track record in cardiac surgery, are also appearing, and with better side effect profiles. In addition to specific pharmacotherapy, immunological therapy with vaccines aimed at preventing excitotoxicity are now appearing in stroke trials, and could potentially benefit cardiac surgery patients (During et al., 2000). Finally, new targets not previously identified in the ischaemic cascade are also being developed. In particular, anti-apoptotic drugs (aimed at preventing the programmed cell death that occurs after ischaemia) are planned for trial in cardiac surgery. It is only through continued efforts, both experimentally and clinically, that breakthroughs in pharmacological neuro-protection will emerge. However, being realistic, there will be many more failures than successes before the complication of neurological injury is conquered.

REFERENCES

Alberts, M., Graffagnino, C., McClenny, C., DeLong, D., Strittmatter, W., Saunders, A. et al. 1995: ApoE genotype and survival from intracerebral haemorrhage (letter). Lancet 346, 575.

Amakawa, K., Adachi, N., Liu, K., Ikemune, K., Fujitani, T., Arai, T. 1996: Effects of pre- and postischaemic administration of thiopental on transmitter amino acid release and histologic outcome in gerbils. Anesthesiology 85, 1422–30.

Amory, D.W., Grigore, A., Amory, J.K., Gerhardt, M.A., White, W.D., Smith, P.K., et al. 2002: Neuroprotection is associated with beta-adrenergic receptor antagonists during cardiac surgery: evidence from 2,575 patients. Journal of Cardiothoracic and Vascular Anesthesia 16, 270–7.

Aoki, M., Jonas, R.A., Nomura, F., Stromski, M.E., Tsuji, M.K., Hickey, P.R. et al. 1994a: Effects of aprotinin on acute recovery of cerebral metabolism in piglets after hypothermic circulatory arrest. Annals of Thoracic Surgery 58, 146–53.

Aoki, M., Nomura, F., Stromski, M.E., Tsuji, M.K., Fackler, J.C., Hickey, P.R. et al. 1994b: Effects of MK-801 and NBQX on acute recovery of piglet cerebral metabolism after hypothermic circulatory arrest. Journal of Cereberal Blood Flow and Metabolism 14, 156–65.

Arrowsmith, J.E., Harrison, M.J., Newman, S.P., Stygall, J., Timberlake, N., Pugsley, W.B. 1998: Neuroprotection of the brain during cardiopulmonary bypass: a randomized trial of remacemide during coronary artery bypass in 171 patients. Stroke 29, 2357–62.

Arrowsmith, J.E., Grocott, H., Newman, M. 1999: Neurologic risk assessment, monitoring and outcome in cardiac surgery. Journal of Cardiothorac and Vascular Anesthesia 13, 736–43.

Asimakopoulos, G., Taylor, K. 1998: Effects of cardiopulmonary bypass on leucocyte and endothelial adhesion molecules. Annals of Thoracic Surgery 66, 2135–44.

Asplund, K. 1989: Randomized clinical trials of hemodilution in acute ischaemic stroke. Acta Neurol Scand 80, 22–30.

Baker, A.J., Naser, B., Benaroia, M., Mazer, C.D. 1995: Cerebral microemboli during coronary artery bypass using different cardioplegia techniques. Annals of Thoracic Surgery 59, 1187–91.

Barbut, D., Yao, F.S., Lo, Y.W., Silverman, R., Hager, D.N., Trifiletti, R.R. et al. 1997a: Determination of size of aortic emboli and embolic load during coronary artery bypass grafting [see comments]. Annals of Thoracic Surgery 63, 1262–7.

Barbut, D., Lo, Y., Hartman, G., Yao, F., Trifiletti, R., Hager, D. et al. 1997b: Aortic atheroma is related to outcome but not numbers of emboli during coronary bypass. Annals of Thoracic Surgery 64, 454–9.

Barker, F., Ogilvy, C. 1996: Efficacy of prophylactic nimodipine for delayed ischaemic deficit after subarachnoid hemorrhage: a metaanalysis. Journal of Neurosurgery 84, 405–14.

Bashein, G., Nessly, M.L., Bledsoe, S.W., Townes, B.D., Davis, K.B., Coppel, D.B. et al. 1992: Electroencephalography during surgery with cardiopulmonary bypass and hypothermia. Anesthesiology 76, 878–91.

Baumgartner, W.A., Redmond, J.M., Zehr, K.J., Brock, M.V., Tseng, E.E., Blue, M.E. et al. 1998: The role of the monosialoganglioside, GM1 as a neuroprotectant in an experimental model of cardiopulmonary bypass and hypothermic circulatory arrest. Annals of the New York Academy of Science 845, 382–90.

Belayev, L., Busto, R., Zhao, W., Clemens, J.A., Ginsberg, M.D. 1997: Effect of delayed albumin hemodilution on infarction volume and brain oedema after transient middle cerebral artery occlusion in rats. Journal of Neurosurgery 87, 595–601.

Bellinger, D.C., Jonas, R.A., Rappaport, L.A., Wypij, D., Wernovsky, G., Kuban, K.C. et al. 1995: Developmental and neurologic status of children after heart surgery with hypothermic circulatory arrest or low-flow cardiopulmonary bypass. New England Journal of Medicine 332, 549–55.

Bellinger, D.C., Rappaport, L.A., Wypij, D., Wernovsky, G., Newburger, J.W. 1997: Patterns of developmental dysfunction after surgery during infancy to correct transposition of the great arteries. Journal Development Behavioral Pediatrics 18, 75–83.

Bellinger, D.C., Wypij, D., Kuban, K.C., Rappaport, L.A., Hickey, P.R., Wernovsky, G. et al. 1999: Developmental and neurological status of children at 4 years of age after heart surgery with hypothermic circulatory arrest or low-flow cardiopulmonary bypass. Circulation 100, 526–32.

Blauth, J. 1995: Macroemboli and microemboli during cardiopulmonary bypass. Annals of Thoracic Surgery 59, 1300–3.

Blauth, C., Arnold, J., Kohner, E.M., Taylor, K.M. 1986: Retinal microembolism during cardiopulmonary bypass demonstrated by fluorescein angiography. Lancet 2, 837–9.

Blauth, C., Cosgrove, D., Webb, B., Ratliff, N., Boylan, M., Piedmonte, M. et al. 1992: Atheroembolism from the ascending aorta: an emerging problem in cardiac surgery. Journal Thoracic and Cardiovascular Surgery 103, 1104–12.

Bokesh, P.M. Kapural, M., Drummond-Webb, J., Baird, K., Kapural, L., Mee, R.B. et al. 2000: Neuroprotective, anesthetic, and cardiovascular effects of the NMDA antagonist, CNS5161A, in isoflurane-anesthetized lambs. Anesthesiology 93, 202–8.

Borowicz, L., Goldsborough, M., Selenes, O., McKhann, G. 1996: Neuropsychological changes after cardiac surgery: a critical review. Journal of Cardiothorac and Vascular Anesthesia 10, 105–12.

Braekken, S., Russell, D., Brucher, R., Abdelnoor, M., Svennevig, J. 1997: Cerebral microembolic signals during cardiopulmonary bypass surgery: frequency, time of occurence, and association with patient and surgical characteristics. Stroke 28, 1988–92.

Brooker, R.F., Brown, W.R., Moody, D.M., Hammon, J.W. Jr, Reboussin, D.M., Deal, D.D. et al. 1998: Cardiotomy suction: a major source of brain lipid emboli during cardiopulmonary bypass. Annals of Thoracic Surgery 65, 1651–5.

Brown, W.R., Moody, D.M., Challa, V.R., Stump, D.A., Hammon, J.W. 2000: Longer duration of cardiopulmonary bypass is associated with greater numbers of cerebral microemboli. Stroke 31, 707–13.

Burrows, F.A. 1995: Con: pH-stat management of blood gases is preferable to alpha-stat in patients undergoing brain cooling for cardiac surgery [comment]. *Journal of Cardiothoracic and Vascular Anesthesia* **9**, 219–21.

Busto, R., Dietrich, W., Globus, M., Valdés, I., Scheinberg, P., Ginsberg, M. 1987: Small differences in intraischaemic brain temperature critically determine the extent of neuronal injury. *Journal of Cerebreal Blood Flow Metabolism* **7**, 729–38.

Butler, J., Rocker, G., Westaby, S. 1993: Inflammatory response to cardiopulmonary bypass. *Annals of Thoracic Surgery* **55**, 552–9.

Butterworth, J., Legault, C., Stump, D.A., Coker, L., Hammon, J.W. Jr, Troost, B.T. *et al.* 1999: A randomized, blinded trial of the antioxidant pegorgotein: no reduction in neuropsychological deficits, inotropic drug support, or myocardial ischemia after coronary artery bypass surgery. *Journal of Cardiothoracic and Vascular Anesthesia* **13**, 690–4.

Chan, P. 1996: Role of oxidants in ischemic brain damage. *Stroke* **27**, 1124–9.

Chaney, M.A., Nikolov, M.P., Blakeman, B.P., Bakhos, M. 1999: Attempting to maintain normoglycemia during cardiopulmonary bypass with insulin may initiate post-operative hypoglycemia. *Anesthesia and Analgesia* **89**, 1091–5.

Chen, H., Chopp, M., Welch, K. 1991: Effect of mild hyperthermia on the ischaemic infarct volume after middle cerebral artery occlusion in the rat. *Neurology* **41**, 1133–5.

Christakis, G.T., Koch, J.P., Deemar, K.A., Fremes, S.E., Sinclair, L., Chen, E. *et al.* 1992: A randomized study of the systemic effects of warm heart surgery. *Annals of Thoracic Surgery* **54**, 449–57; discussion 457–9.

Christakis, G.T., Abel, J.G., Lichtenstein, S.V. 1995: Neurological outcomes and cardiopulmonary temperature: a clinical review. *Journal of Cardiac Surgery* **10**, 475–80.

Clark, R.E., Brillman, J., Davis, D.A., Lovell, M.R., Price, T.R., Magovern, G.J. 1995: Microemboli during coronary artery bypass grafting. Genesis and effect on outcome [see comments]. *Journal of Thoracic and Cardiovascular Surgery* **109**, 249–57; discussion 257–8.

Cole, D.J., Schell, R.M., Drummond, J.C. 1994: Diaspirin crosslinked hemoglobin (DCLHb): effect of hemodilution during focal cerebral ischemia in rats. *Artif Cells Blood Substit Immobil Biotechnol* **22**, 813–18.

Cole, D.J., Drummond, J.C., Patel, P.M., Reynolds, L.R. 1997: Hypervolemic-hemodilution during cerebral ischemia in rats: effect of diaspirin cross-linked hemoglobin (DCLHb) on neurologic outcome and infarct volume. *Journal of Neurosurgical Anesthesiology* **9**, 44–50.

Cook, D.J., Oliver, W.C. Jr, Orszulak, T.A., Daly, R.C., Bryce, R.D. 1995: Cardiopulmonary bypass temperature, hematocrit, and cerebral oxygen delivery in humans. *Annals of Thoracic Surgery* **60**, 1671–7.

Cook, D.J., Orszulak, T.A., Daly, R.C., Buda, D.A. 1996: Cerebral hyperthermia during cardiopulmonary bypass in adults. *Journal of Thoracic and Cardiovascular Surgery* **111**, 268–9.

Cook, D.J., Orszulak, T.A., Daly, R.C. 1997: The effects of pulsatile cardiopulmonary bypass on cerebral and renal blood flow in dogs. *Journal of Cardiothoracic and Vascular Anesthesia* **11**, 420–7.

Cook, D.J., Orszulak, T.A., Daly, R.C. 1998: Minimum hematocrit at differing cardiopulmonary bypass temperatures in dogs. *Circulation* **98**, 170–4; discussion 175.

Croughwell, N., Lyth, M., Quill, T.J., Newman, M., Greeley, W.J., Smith, L.R. *et al.* 1990: Diabetic patients have abnormal cerebral autoregulation during cardiopulmonary bypass. *Circulation* **82**, 407–12.

Croughwell, N., Frasco, P., Blumenthal, J., Leone, B., White, W., Reves, J. 1992: Warming during cardiopulmonary bypass is associated with jugular bulb desaturation. *Annals of Thoracic Surgery* **58**, 827–32.

Croughwell, N.D., Newman, M.F., Blumenthal, J.A., White, W.D., Lewis, J.B., Frasco, P.E. *et al.* 1994: Jugular bulb saturation and cognitive dysfunction after cardiopulmonary bypass. *Annals of Thoracic Surgery* **58**, 1702–8.

Croughwell, N.D., Reves, J.G., White, W.D., Grocott, H.P., Baldwin, B.I., Clements, F.M. *et al.* 1998: Cardiopulmonary bypass time does not affect cerebral blood flow. *Annals of Thoracic Surgery* **65**, 1226–30.

Davila-Roman, V., Phillips, K., Daily, B., Wareing, T., Murphy, S. 1996: Intraoperative transesophageal echocardiography and epiaortic ultrasound for assessment of atherosclerosis of the thoracic aorta. *J Am Coll Cardiol* **28**, 942–7.

Dennis, C., Spreng, D.J., Nelson, G. 1951: Development of a pump-oxygenator to replace the heart and lungs; an apparatus applicable to human patients and application to one case. *Annals of Thoracic Surgery* **134**, 709–21.

Dietrich, W., Alonso, O., Busto, R. 1993: Moderate hyperglycemia worsens acute blood brain barrier injury after forebrain ischemia in rats. *Stroke* **24**, 111–15.

Dirnagl, U., Iadecola, C., Moskowitz, M. 1999: Pathobiology for ischemic stroke: an integrated view. *TINS* **22**, 391–7.

During, M., Symes, C., Lawlor, P., Lin, J., Dunning, J., Fitzsimons, H. *et al.* 2000: An oral vaccine against NMDR1 with efficacy in experimental stroke and epilepsy. *Science* **287**, 1453–60.

Edmonds, H.L. Jr, Griffiths, L.K., van der Laken, J., Slater, A.D., Shields, C.B. 1992: Quantitative electroencephalographic monitoring during myocardial revascularization predicts post-operative disorientation and improves outcome. *Journal of Thoracic and Cardiovascular Surgery* **103**, 555–63.

Enomoto, S., Hindman, B.J., Dexter, F., Smith, T., Cutkomp, J. 1996: Rapid rewarming causes an increase in the cerebral metabolic rate for oxygen that is temporarily unmatched by cerebral blood flow. A study during cardiopulmonary bypass in rabbits. *Anesthesiology* **84**, 1392–400.

Fabian, R., DeWitt, D., Kent, T. 1995: *In vivo* detection of superoxide anion production by the brain using a cytochrome c electrode. *J Cerebr Blood Metabol* **15**, 242–7.

Fang, W.C., Helm, R.E., Krieger, K.H., Rosengart, T.K., DuBois, W.J., Sason, C. *et al.* 1997: Impact of minimum hematocrit during cardiopulmonary bypass on mortality in patients undergoing coronary artery surgery. *Circulation* **96**, 194–9.

Feerick, A., Johnston, W., Jenkins, L., Lin, C., Mackay, J., Prough, D. 1995: Hyperglycemia during hypothermic canine cardiopulmonary bypass increases cerebral lactate. *Anesthesiology* **82**, 512–20.

Fitch, J.C., Rollins, S., Matis, L., Alford, B., Aranki, S., Collard, C.D. *et al.* 1999: Pharmacology and biological efficacy of a recombinant, humanized, single-chain antibody C5 complement inhibitor in patients undergoing coronary artery bypass graft surgery with cardiopulmonary bypass. *Circulation* **100**, 2499–506.

Garcia, J.H., Liu, K., Yoshida, Y., Lian, J., Chen, S. 1994: Influx of leukocytes and platelets in an evolving brain infarct (Wistar rat). *American Journal of Pathology* **144**, 188–99.

Gardner, T., Horneffer, P., Manolio, T., Pearson, T., Gott, V. 1985: Stroke following coronary artery bypass grafting: a ten year study. *Annals of Thoracic Surgery* **40**, 574–81.

Geisler, F., Dorsey, F., Coleman, W. 1991: Recovery of motor function after spinal-cord injury. A randomized placebo-controlled trial with GM-1 ganglioside. *New England Journal of Medicine* **325**, 1659–60.

Gibbon, J.H.J. 1954: Artificial maintenance of circulation during experimental occlusion of the pulmonary artery. *Archives of Surgery* **34**, 1105–31.

Gilman, S. 1965: Cerebral disorders after open heart operations. *New England Journal of Medicine* **272**, 489–98.

Gold, J., Charlson, M., Williams-Russo, P., Szatrowski, T., Peterson, J., Pirraglia, P. *et al.* 1995: Improvement of outcomes after coronary artery bypass. A randomized trial comparing intraoperative high versus low mean arterial pressure. *Journal of Thoracic and Cardiovascular Surgery* **110**, 1302–14.

Green, D., Reed, J. 1998: Mitochondria and apoptosis. *Science* **281**, 1309–12.

Grieco, G., d'Hollosy, M., Culliford, A.T., Jonas, S. 1996: Evaluating neuroprotective agents for clinical anti-ischaemic benefit using neurological and neuropsychological changes after cardiac surgery under cardiopulmonary bypass. Methodological strategies and results of a double-blind, placebo-controlled trial of GM1 ganglioside. *Stroke* **27**, 858–74.

Grigore, A.M., Mathew, J., Grocott, H.P., Reves, J.G., Blumenthal, J.A., White, W.D. *et al.* Prospective randomized trial of normothermic versus hypothermic cardiopulmonary bypass on cognitive function after coronary artery bypass graft surgery. *Anesthesiology* **95**, 1110–9.

Grigore, A.M., Grocott, H.P., Mathew, J.P., Philips-Bute, B., Stanley, T.O., Landolyo, K.P. *et al.* 2002: The rewarming rate and increased peak temperature after cardiac surgery. *Anesthesia and Analgesia* **94**, 4–10.

Grocott, H.P., Newman, M.F., Croughwell, N.D., White, W.D., Lowry, E., Reves, J.G. 1997: Continuous jugular venous versus nasopharyngeal temperature monitoring during hypothermic cardiopulmonary bypass for cardiac surgery. *Journal of Clinical Anesthesia* **9**, 312–6

Grocott, H., Croughwell, N., Amory, D., White, W., Kirchner, J., Newman, M. 1998: Cerebral emboli and serum S100β during cardiac surgery. *Annals of Thoracic Surgery* **65**, 1645–50.

Grocott, H.P., Mackensen, G.B., Newman, M.F., Warner, D.S. 2001: Neurological injury during cardiopulmonary bypass in the rat. *Perfusion* **16**, 75–81.

Grocott, H.P., Sheng, H., Miura, Y., Sarraf-Yazdi, S., Mackensen, G.B., Pearlstein, R.D. *et al.* 1999: The effects of aprotinin on outcome from cerebral ischemia in the rat. *Anesthesia and Analgesia* **88**, 1–7.

Grotta, J 1996: Rodent models of stroke limitations. What can we learn from recent clinical trials of thrombolysis? *Archives of Neurology* **53**, 1067–69.

Group THiSS 1989: Hypervolemic hemodilution treatment of acute stroke. Results of a randomized multicenter trial using pentastarch. *Stroke* **20**, 1286–7.

Group TISS 1988: Haemodilution in acute stroke: results of the Italian haemodilution trial. Italian Acute Stroke Study Group. *Lancet* **1**, 318–21.

Haenel, F., von Knobelsdorff, G., Werner, C., Schulte am Esch, J. 1998: Hypercapnia prevents jugular bulb desaturation during rewarming from hypothermic cardiopulmonary bypass. *Anesthesiology* **89**, 19–23.

Hall, R., Stafford Smith, M., Rocker, G. 1997: The systemic inflammatory response to cardiopulmonary bypass: pathophysiological, therapeutic, and pharmacological conderations. *Anesthesia and Analgesia* **85**, 766–82.

Hammon, J., Stump, D., Kon, N., Cordell, A., Hudspeth, A., Oaks, T. *et al.* 1977: Risk factors and solutions for the development of neurobehavioral changes after coronary artery bypass grafting. *Annals of Thoracic Surgery* **63**, 1613–18.

Harris, D.N.F., Bailey, S., Smith, P. 1993: Brain swelling in first hour after coronary artery bypass surgery. *Lancet* **342**, 586–7.

Harris, D.N., Oatridge, A., Dob, D., Smith, P.L., Taylor, K.M., Bydder, G.M. 1998: Cerebral swelling after normothermic cardiopulmonary bypass. *Anesthesiology* **88**, 340–5.

Hartman, G., Peterson, J., Konstadt, S., Hahn, R., Szatrowski, T., Charlson, M. *et al.* 1996a: High reproducibility in the interpretation of intraoperative transesophageal echocardiographic evaluation of aortic atheromatous disease. *Anesthesia and Analgesia* **82**, 539–43.

Hartman, G., Yao, F.-S., Bruefach, M., Barbut, D., Peterson, J., Purcell, M. *et al.* 1996b: Severity of aortic atheromatous disease diagnosed by transesophageal echocardiography predicts stroke and other outcomes associated with coronary artery surgery: a prospective study. *Anesthesia and Analgesia* **83**, 701–8.

Hempelmann, G., Dieter, K., Volker, L., Bormann, B. 1982: Cerebral protection in neurosurgery, cardiac surgery, and following cardiac arrest. *Journal of Cerebral Blood Flow and Metabolism* **2**, 66–71.

Hill, S.E., van Wermeskerken, G.K., Lardenoye, J.W., Phillips-Bute, B., Smith, P.K., Reves, J.G. *et al.* 2000: Intraoperative physiologic variables and outcome in cardiac surgery: Part I. In-hospital mortality. *Annals of Thoracic Surgery* **69**, 1070–5; discussion 1075–6.

Hindman, B. 1995: Con: glucose priming solutions should not be used for cardiopulmonary bypass. *Journal of Cardothoracic and Vascular Anesthesia* **9**, 605–7.

Hindman, B.J. 1998: Choice of alpha-stat or pH-stat management and neurologic outcomes after cardiac surgery: it depends. *Anesthesiology* **89**, 5–7.

Hindman, B.J., Dexter, F., Cutkomp, J., Smith, T., Todd, M.M., Tinker, J.H. 1992: Brain blood flow and metabolism do not decrease at stable brain temperature during cardiopulmonary bypass in rabbits. *Anesthesiology* **77**, 342–50.

Hindman, B.J., Dexter, F., Smith, T., Cutkomp, J. 1995: Pulsatile versus nonpulsatile flow. No difference in cerebral blood flow or metabolism during normothermic cardiopulmonary bypass in rabbits. *Anesthesiology* **82**, 241–50.

Hixson, J. 1991: Apolipoprotein E polymorphism affects atherosclerosis in young males. Pathobiological determinants of atherosclerosis in youth (PDAY) research group. *Arteriosclerosis and Thrombosis* **11**, 1237–44.

Hogue, C.W. Jr, Sundt, T.M. 3rd, Goldberg, M., Barner, H., Davila-Roman, V.G. 1999: Neurological complications of cardiac surgery: the need for new paradigms in prevention and treatment. *Semin Thorac Cardiovasc Surg* **11**, 105–15.

Hossman, K.-A. 1996: Periinfarct depolarizations. *Cerebrovascular and Brain Metabolism Reviews* **8**, 195–208.

Hui, D., Harmony, J., Innerarity, T., Mahley, R. 1980: Immunoregulatory plasma lipoproteins. Role of apoprotein E and apoprotein. *Br J Biol Chem* **255**, 1175–81.

Ilveskoski, E., Perola, M., Lehtimaki, T., Laipalla, P., Savolainen, V., Pajarinen, J. *et al.* 1999: Age-dependent association of apolipoprotein E genotype with coronary and aortic atherosclerosis in middle-age men: an autopsy study. *Circulation* **100**, 608–13.

Jacobs, A., Neveling, M., Horst, M., Ghaemi, M., Kessler, J., Eichstaedt, H. *et al.* 1998: Alterations of neuropsychological function and cerebral glucose metabolism after cardiac surgery are not related only to intraoperative microembolic events. *Stroke* **29**, 660–7.

Jansen, N.J., van Oeveren, W., van den Broek, L., Oudemans-van Straaten, H.M., Stoutenbeek, C.P., Joen, M.C. *et al.* 1991: Inhibition by dexamethasone of the reperfusion phenomena in cardiopulmonary bypass. *Journal of Thoracic and Cardiovascular Surgery* **102**, 515–25.

Johnston, W.E., Vinten-Johansen, J., DeWitt, D.S., O'Steen, W.K., Stump, D.A., Prough, D.S. 1991: Cerebral perfusion during canine hypothermic cardiopulmonary bypass: effect of arterial carbon dioxide tension. *Annals of Thoracic Surgery* **52**, 479–89.

Jones, T., Deal, D., Vernon, J., Blackburn, N., Stump, D. 2000: The propagation of entrained air during cardiopulmonary bypass is affected by ciruit design but not by vacuum assisted venous drainage. *Anesthesia and Analgesia* **90**, SCA 39.

Kavanagh, B.P., Mazer, C.D., Panos, A., Lichtenstein, S.V. 1992: Effect of warm heart surgery on peri-operative management of patients undergoing urgent cardiac surgery. *Journal of Cardiothoracic Vascular Anesthesia* **6**, 127–31.

Kawahara, F., Kadoi, Y., Saito, S., Yoshikawa, D., Goto, F., Fujita, N. 1999: Balloon pump-induced pulsatile perfusion during cardiopulmonary bypass does not improve brain oxygenation. *Journal of Thoracic and Cardiovascular Surgery* **118**, 361–6.

Kawamura, T., Wakusawa, R., Okada, K., Inada, S. 1993: Elevation of cytokines during open heart surgery with cardiopulmonary bypass: participation of interleukin-8 and 6 in reperfusion injury. *Canadian Journal of Anesthesia* **40**, 1016–21.

Kern, F.H., Greeley, W.J. 1995: Pro: pH-stat management of blood gases is not preferable to alpha-stat in patients undergoing brain cooling for cardiac surgery. *Journal of Cardiothoracic Vascular Anesthesia* **9**, 215–18.

Kharazmi, A., Andersen, L.W., Baek, L., Valerius, N.H., Laub, M., Rasmussen, J.P. 1989: Endotoxemia and enhanced generation of oxygen radicals by neutrophils from patients undergoing cardiopulmonary bypass. *Journal of Thoracic and Cardiovascular Surgery* **98**, 381–5.

King, R., Kanithanon, R., Shockey, K., Tribble, C.G. 1998: Replacing the atherosclerotic ascending aorta is a high-risk procedure. *Annals of Thoracic Surgery* **66**, 396–401.

Kirklin, J.K., Westaby, S., Blackstone, E.H., Kirklin, J.W., Chenoweth, D.E., Pacifico, A.D. 1983: Complement and the damaging effects of cardiopulmonary bypass. *Journal of Thoracic and Cardiovascular Surgery* **86**, 845–57.

von Knobelsdorff, G., Bischoff, P., Haenel, F., Drogemeier, K., Schulte am Esch, J. 1996: Etomidate induced burst suppression does not attentuate jugular bulb oxygen desaturation during rewarming of cardiopulmonary bypass. *Journal of Neurosurgical Anesthesiology* **8**, 335.

Kogure, K., Yamasaki, Y., Matsuo, Y., Kato, H., Onodera, H. 1996: Inflammation of the brain after ischemia. *Acta Neurochirulgica* **66** (Suppl.), 40–3.

Konstadt, S., Reich, D., Quintana, C., Levy, M. 1994: The ascending aorta: how much does transeophageal echocardiography see? *Anesthesia and Analgesia* **78**, 240–4.

Kouchoukos, N., Wareing, T., Daily, B., Murphy, S. 1994: Management of the severely atherosclerotic aorta during cardiac operations. *Journal of Cardiac Surgery* **9**, 490–4.

Kristian, T., Siesjö, B. 1998: Calcium in ischemic cell death. *Stroke* **29**, 705–18.

Kurth, C.D., O'Rourke, M.M., O'Hara, I.B. 1998: Comparison of pH-stat and alpha-stat cardiopulmonary bypass on cerebral oxygenation and blood flow in relation to hypothermic circulatory arrest in piglets. *Anesthesiology* **89**, 110–18.

Landow, L., Andersen, L. 1994: Splanchnic ischemia and its role in multiple organ failure. *Acta Anaesthesiology Scandinavia* **38**, 626–39.

Lanier, W.L. 1991: Glucose management during cardiopulmonary bypass: cardiovascular and neurologic implications [editorial; comment]. *Anesthesia and Analgesia* **72**, 423–7.

Legault, C., Furberg, C., Wagenknecht, L., Rogers, A., Stump, D., Coker, L. *et al.* 1996: Nimodipine neuroprotection in cardiac valve replacement: report of an early terminated trial. *Stroke* **27**, 593–8.

Leung, J., Stanley III, T., Mathew, J., Curling, P., Barash, P., Salmenpera, M. *et al.* 1994: An initial multicenter, randomized controlled trial on the safety and efficacy of acadesine in patients undergoing coronary artery bypass graft surgery. *Anesthesia and Analgesia* **78**, 420–34.

Levy, J., Pifarre, R., Schaff, H. *et al.* 1995: A multicenter, double-blind, placebo-controlled trial of aprotinin for reducing blood loss and the requirement for donor-blood transfusion inpatients undergoing repeat coronary artery bypass grafting. *Circulation* **92**, 2236–44.

McBride, W.T., Armstrong, M.A., Crockard, A.D., McMurray, T.J., Rea, J.M. 1995: Cytokine balance and immunosuppressive changes at cardiac surgery: contrasting response between patients and isolated cardiopulmonary bypass circuits [see comments]. *British Journal of Anaesthesia* **75**, 724–33.

McLean, R.F., Wong, B.I. 1996: Normothermic versus hypothermic cardiopulmonary bypass: central nervous system outcomes. *Journal of Cardiothoracic and Vascular Anesthesia* **10**, 45–52; quiz 52–3.

Mackensen, G.B., Sato, Y., Nellgard, B., Pineda, J., Newman, M.F., Warner, D.S., Grocott, H.P. 2001: Cardiopulmonary bypass induces neurologic and neurocognitive dysfunction in the rat. *Anesthesiology* **95**, 1485–91.

Mackensen, G.B., Ti, L.K., Philips-Bute, B.G., Mathew, J.P., Newman, M.F., Grocott, H.P. 2003; Cerebral embolization during cardiac surgery: impact of aortic atheroma burden. *British Journal of Anaesthesia* **91**, 656–61.

Macy, M., Okano, Y., Cardin, A. 1983: Suppression of lymphocyte activation by plasma lipoproteins. *Cancer Research* **43**, 2496–502.

Mangano, D. 1995: Effects of acadesine on the incidence of myocardial infarction and adverse cardiac outcomes after coronary artery bypass graft surgery. *Anesthesiology* **83**, 658–73.

Marschall, K., Kanchuger, M., Kessler, K., Grossi, E., Yarmush, L., Roggen, S. 1994: Superiority of transesophageal echocardiography in detecting aortic arch atheromatous disease: identification of patients at increased risk of stroke during cardiac surgery. *J Cardiothorac Vasc Anesth* **8**, 5–13.

Marshall, W., Barzilai, B., Kouchoukos, N., Saffitz, J. 1989: Intraoperative ultrasonic imaging of the ascending aorta. *Annals of Thoracic Surgery* **48**, 339–44.

Martin, T.D., Craver, J.M., Gott, J.P., Weintraub, W.S., Ramsay, J., Mora, C.T. *et al.* 1994: Prospective, randomized trial of retrograde warm blood cardioplegia: myocardial benefit and neurologic threat. *Annals of Thoracic Surgery* **57**, 298–302.

Menasche, P., Peynet, J., Touchot, B., Aziz, M., Haydar, S., Perez, G. *et al.* 1992: Normothermic cardioplegia: is aortic cross-clamping still synonymous with myocardial ischemia? *Annals of Thoracic Surgery* **54**, 472–7; discussion 478.

Metz, S., Keats, A. 1991: Benefits of a glucose-containing priming solution for cardiopulmonary bypass. *Anesthesia and Analgesia* **72**, 428–34.

Mitchell, S., Pellet, O., Gorman, D. 1999: Cerebral protection by lidocaine during cardiac operations. *Annals of Thoracic Surgery* **67**, 1117–24.

Moody, D.M., Bell, M.A., Challa, V.R., Johnston, W.E., Prough, D.S. 1990: Brain microemboli during cardiac surgery or aortography. *Annals of Neurology* **28**, 477–86.

Moody, D.M., Brown, W.R., Challa, V.R., Stump, D.A., Reboussin, D.M., Legault, C. 1995: Brain microemboli associated with cardiopulmonary bypass: a histologic and magnetic resonance imaging study. *Annals of Thoracic Surgery* **59**, 1304–7.

Mora, C.T., Henson, M.B., Weintraub, W.S., Murjin, J.M., Martin, T.D. 1996: The effect of temperature management during cardiopulmonary bypass on neurologic and neuropsychologic outcomes in patients undergoing coronary revascularization. *Journal of Thoracic Cardiovascular Surgery* **112**, 514–22

Moshkovitz, Y., Sternik, L., Paz, Y., Gurevitch, J., Feinberg, M., Smolinsky, A. *et al.* 1997: Primary coronary artery bypass grafting without cardiopulmonary bypass in impaired left ventricular function. *Annals of Thoracic Surgery* **63**, S44–7.

Murkin, J. 1997: Cardiopulmonary bypass and the inflammatory reponse: a role for serine protease inhibitors? *Journal of Cardiothoracic Vascular and Anesthesiology* **11**, 19–23.

Murkin, J.M., Farrar, J.K., Tweed, W.A., McKenzie, F.N., Guiraudon, G. 1987: Cerebral autoregulation and flow/metabolism coupling during cardiopulmonary bypass: the influence of $PaCO_2$. *Anesthesia and Analgesia* **66**, 825–32.

Murkin, J.M., Martzke, J.S., Buchan, A.M., Bentley, C., Wong, C.J. 1995: A randomized study of the influence of perfusion technique and pH management strategy in 316 patients undergoing coronary artery bypass surgery. II. Neurologic and cognitive outcomes. *Journal of Thoracic and Cardiovascular Surgery* **110**, 349–62.

Murkin, J.M., Boyd, W.D., Ganapathy, S., Adams, S.J., Peterson, R.C. 1999: Beating heart surgery: why expect less central nervous system morbidity? *Annals of Thoracic Surgery* **68**, 1498–501.

Mutch, W.A., Lefevre, G.R., Thiessen, D.B., Girling, L.G., Warrian, R.K. 1998: Computer-controlled cardiopulmonary bypass increases jugular venous oxygen saturation during rewarming. *Annals of Thoracic Surgery* **65**, 59–65.

Muth, C., Shank, E. 2000: Primary care: gas embolism. *New England Journal of Medicine* **342**, 476–82.

Mykchaskiw, G., Hoehner, P., Abdel Aziz, A., Heath, B., Eichhorn, J. 2000: Preoperative exposure to calcium channel blockers suggests increased blood product use following cardiac surgery. *Anesthesia and Analgesia* **90**, SCA15.

Nandate, K., Vuylsteke, A., Crosbie, A.E., Messahel, S., Oduro-Dominah, A., Menon, D.K. 1999: Cerebrovascular cytokine responses during coronary artery bypass surgery: specific production of interleukin-8 and its attenuation by hypothermic cardiopulmonary bypass. *Anesthesia and Analgesia* **89**, 823–8.

Newburger, J.W., Jonas, R.A., Wernovsky, G., Wypij, D., Hickey, P.R., Kuban, K.C. *et al.* 1993: A comparison of the perioperative neurologic effects of hypothermic circulatory arrest versus low-flow cardiopulmonary bypass in infant heart surgery. *New England Journal of Medicine* **329**, 1057–64.

Newman, M.F., Croughwell, N.D., Blumenthal, J.A., White, W.D., Lewis, J.B., Smith, L.R. *et al.* 1994: Effect of aging on cerebral autoregulation during cardiopulmonary bypass. Association with post-operative cognitive dysfunction. *Circulation* **90**, 243–9.

Newman, M.F., Kramer, D., Croughwell, N.D., Sanderson, I., Blumenthal, J.A., White, W.D. *et al.* 1995a: Differential age effects of mean arterial pressure and rewarming on cognitive dysfunction after cardiac surgery. *Anesthesia and Analgesia* **81**, 236–42.

Newman, M.F., Murkin, J.M., Roach, G., Croughwell, N.D., White, W.D., Clements, F.M. *et al.* 1995b: Cerebral physiologic effects of burst suppression doses of propofol during nonpulsatile cardiopulmonary bypass. central nervous system Subgroup of McSPI. *Anesthesia and Analgesia* **81**, 452–7.

Newman, M.F., Wolman, R., Kanchuger, M., Marschall, K., Mora-Mangano, C., Roach, G. 1996a: Multicenter preoperative stroke risk index for patients undergoing coronary artery bypass graft surgery. Multicenter Study of Perioperative Ischemia (McSPI) Research Group. *Circulation* **94**, 74–80.

Newman, M.F., Croughwell, N.D., White, W.D., Lowry, E., Baldwin, B.I., Clements, F.M. *et al.* 1996b: Effect of perfusion pressure on cerebral blood flow during normothermic cardiopulmonary bypass. *Circulation* **94**, 353–7.

Newman, M.F., Laskowitz, D.T., Saunders, A.F., Grigore, A.M., Grocott, H.P. 1999: Genetic predictors of perioperative neurologic and neuropsychological injury and recovery. *Sem Cardiothorac Vasc Anesth* **3**, 34–46.

Newman, M.F., Grocott, H.P., Mathew, J.P., White, W.D., Landolfo, K., Reves, J.G. *et al.* 2001a: Report of the substudy assessing the impact of neurocognitive function on quality of life 5 years after cardiac surgery. *Stroke* **32**, 2874–81.

Newman, M., Stanley, T., Grocott, H. 2000: Strategies to protect the brain during cardiac surgery. *Sem Cardiothorac Vasc Anesth* **4**, 53–64.

Newman, M.F., Kirchner, J.L., Philips-Bute, B., Gaver, V., Grocott, H., Jones, R.H. *et al.* 2001b: Longitudinal assessment of neurocognitive function after coronary-artery bypass surgery. *New England Journal of Medicine* **344**, 395–402.

Nussmeier, N.A., Arlund, C., Slogoff, S. 1986: Neuropsychiatric complications after cardiopulmonary bypass: cerebral protection by a barbiturate. *Anesthesiology* **64**, 165–70.

Nussmeier, N., Marino, M., Cooper, J., Green, J., Vaughn, K. 1999: Use of glucose-containing prime is not a risk factor for cerebral injury or infection in nondiabetic or diabetic patients having CABG procedures. *Anesthesiology* **91**, A-122 (abstract).

O'Brien, J., Butterworth, J., Hammon, J., Morris, K., Phipps, J., Stump, D. 1997: Cerebral emboli during cardiac surgery in children. *Anesthesiology* **87**, 1063–9.

Ohteki, H., Itoh, T., Natsuaki, M., Minato, N., Suda, H. 1990: Intraoperative ultrasound imaging of the ascending aorta in ischaemic heart disease. *Annals of Thoracic Surgery* **50**, 539–42.

Padayachee, T., Parson, S., Theobold, R., Linley, J., Gosling, R., Deverall, P. 1987: The detection of microemboli in the middle cerebral artery during cardiopulmonary bypass: a transcranial Doppler ultrasound investigation using membrane and bubble oxygenators. *Annals of Thoracic Surgery* **44**, 298–302.

Padayachee, T., Parsons, S., Theobold, R., Gosling, R., Deverall, P. 1988: The effect of arterial filtration on reduction of gaseous microemobli in the middle cerebral artery during cardiopulmonary bypass. *Annals of Thoracic Surgery* **45**, 647–9.

Pahor, M., Guralnik, J., Furberg, C., Carbonin, P., Havlik, R. 1996: Risk of gastrointestinal haemorrhage with calcium antagonists in hypertensive persons over 67 years old. *Lancet* **347**, 1061–5.

Pascoe, E., Hudson, R., Anderson, B., Kassum, D., Shanks, A., Rosenbloom, M. *et al.* 1996: High-dose thiopentone for open-chamber cardiac surgery: a retrospective review. *Canadian Anaesthetists society journal* **43**, 575–9.

Pearson, D.T., Holden, M.P., Poslad, S.J., Murray, A., Waterhouse, P.S. 1986: A clincial evaluation of the performance characteristics of one membrane and five bubble oxygenators: gas transfer and gaseous microemboli production. *Perfusion* **1**, 15–26.

Peters, O., Back, T., Lindauer, U., Busch, C., Megow, D., Dreier, J. *et al.* 1998: Increased formation of reactive oxygen species after permanent and reversible middle cerebral artery occlusion in the rat. *Journal of Cerebral Blood Flow and Metabolism* **18**, 196–205.

Prough, D., Rogers, A., Stump, D., Roy, R., Cordell, A., Phipps, J. *et al.* 1991: Cerebral blood flow decreases with time whereas cerebral oxygen consumption remains stable during hypothermic cardiopulmonary bypass in humans. *Anesthesia and Analgesia* **72**, 161–8.

Pugsley, W., Klinger, L., Paschalis, C., Aspey, B., Newman, S., Harrison, M. *et al.* 1990: Microemboli and cerebral impairment during cardiac surgery. *Vascular Surgery* **24**, 34–43.

Pugsley, W., Klinger, L., Paschalis, C., Treasure, T., Harrison, M., Newman, S. 1994: The impact of microemboli during cardiopulmonary bypass on neuropsychological functioning. *Stroke* **25**, 1393–9.

Reasoner, D., Ryu, K., Hindman, B., Cutkomp, J., Smith, T. 1996: Marked hemodilution increases neurologic injury after focal cerebral ischemia in rabbits. *Anesthesia and Analgesia* **82**, 61–7.

Redmond, J.M., Gillinov, A.M., Blue, M.E., Zehr, K.J., Troncoso, J.C., Cameron, D.E. *et al.* 1993: The monosialoganglioside, GM1, reduces neurologic injury associated with hypothermic circulatory arrest. *Surgery* **114**, 324–32; discussion 332–3.

Reichenspurner, H., Navia, J., Berry, G., Robbins, R., Barbut, D., Gold, J.P. *et al.* 2000: Particulate emboli capture by an intra-aortic filter device during cardiac surgery. *Journal of Thoracic and Cardiovascular Surgery* **119**, 233–41.

Ricotta, J., Faggioli, G., Castilone, A., Hassett, J. 1995: Risk factors for stroke after cardiac surgery: Buffalo Cardiac-Cerebral Study Group. *Journal of Vascular Surgery* **21**, 359–64.

Ries, F., Tieman, K., Pohl, C., Bauer, C., Mundo, M., Becher, H. 1998: High-resolution emboli detection and differentiation by characteristic postembolic spectral patterns. *Stroke* **29**, 668–72.

Roach, G., Kanchuger, M., Mora Mangano, C., Newman, M. 1996: Adverse cerebral outcomes after coronary bypass surgery. *New England Journal of Medicine* **335**, 1857–63.

Roach, G., Newman, M., Murkin, J., Marztke, J., Ruskin, A., Li, J., Guo, A. *et al.* 1999: Group fTMSoPIMR: ineffectivness of burst suppression therapy in mitigating peri-operative cerebrovascular dysfunction. *Anesthesiology* **90**, 1255–64.

Rogers, A.T., Stump, D.A., Gravlee, G.P., Prough, D.S., Angert, K.C., Wallenhaupt, S.L. *et al.* 1988: Response of cerebral blood flow to phenylephrine infusion during hypothermic cardiopulmonary bypass: influence of $PaCO_2$ management. *Anesthesiology* **69**, 547–51.

Rudolphi, K., Schubert, P., Parkinson, F., Fredholm, B. 1992: Neuroprotective role of adenosine in cerebral ischemia. *TiPS* **13**, 439–45.

Rumsfeld, J.S., MaWhinney, S., McCarthy, M. Jr, Shroyer, A.L., VillaNueva, C.B., O'Brien, M. *et al.* 1999: Health-related quality of life as a predictor of mortality following coronary artery bypass graft surgery. Participants of the Department of Veterans Affairs Cooperative Study Group on Processes, Structures, and Outcomes of Care in Cardiac Surgery. *JAMA* **281**, 1298–303.

Saunders, A.M., Strittmatter, W.J., Schmechel, D., St. George-Hyslop, P.H., Pericak-Vance, M.A., Joo, S.H. *et al* 1993: Association of apolipoprotein E allele ε4 with late-onset familial and sporadic Alzheimer's disease. *Neurology* **43**, 1467–72.

Savitz, S.I., Erhardt, J.A., Anthony, J.V., Gupta, G., Li, X., Barone, F.C. *et al.* 2000: The novel beta-blocker, carvedilol, provides neuroprotection in transient focal stroke. *Journal of Cerebral Blood Flow and Metabolism* **20**, 1197–204.

Scandinavian Stroke Study Group (SSSG) 1987: Multicenter trial of haemodilution in acute ischaemic stroke. I. Results in the total patient population. *Stroke* **18**, 691–9.

Scandinavian Stroke Study Group (SSSG) 1988: Multicenter trial of hemodilution in acute ischaemic stroke. Results of subgroup analyses. *Stroke* **19**, 464–71.

Schell, R.M., Kern, F.H., Greeley, W.J., Schulman, S.R., Frasco, P.E., Croughwell, N.D. 1993: Cerebral blood flow and metabolism during cardiopulmonary bypass. *Anesthesia and Analgesia* **76**, 849–65.

Schubert, P., Kreutzberg, G. 1993: Cerebral protection by adenosine. *Acta Neurochirurgica* **57**, 80–8.

Schmitt, B., Bauersfeld, U., Fanconi, S., Wohlrab, G., Huisman, T.A., Bandtlow, C. *et al.* 1997: The effect of the N-methyl-D-aspartate receptor antagonist dextromethorphan on perioperative brain injury in children undergoing cardiac surgery with cardiopulmonary bypass: results of a pilot study. *Neuropediatrics* **28**, 191–7.

Shaw, P.J., Bates, D., Cartlidge, N.E., French, J.M., Heaviside, D., Julian, D.G. *et al.* 1987: Neurologic and neuropsychological morbidity following major surgery: comparison of coronary artery bypass and peripheral vascular surgery. *Stroke* **18**, 700–7.

Sheng, H., Laskowitz, D.T., Mackensen, G.B., Kudo, M., Pearlstein, R.D., Warner, D.S. 1999: Apolipoprotein E deficiency worsens outcome from global cerebral ischemia in the mouse. *Stroke* **30**, 1118–24.

Sheng, H., Kudo, M., Mackensen, G., Pearlstein, R., Crapo, J., Warner, D. 2000: Mice overexpressing extracellular superoxide dismutase have increased resistance to global cerebral ischemia. *Experimental Neurology* **163**, 392–8.

Siesjo, B. 1988: Acidosis and ischaemic brain damage. *Neurochem Pathol* **9**, 31–87.

Siesjö, B., Hu, B., Kristian, T. 1999: Is the cell death pathway triggered by the mitochondrion or the endoplasmatic reticulum? *Journal of Cerebral Blood Flow and Metabolism* **19**, 19–26.

Skaper, S., Leon, A., Facci, L. 1991: Death of cultured hippocampal pyramidal neurons induced by pathological activation of N-methyl-d-aspartate receptors is reduced by mono-sialogangliosides. *Journal of Pharmacology Experimental Therapeut* **259**, 452–7.

Smith, P., Treasure, T., Newman, S., Joseph, P., Ell, P., Schneidau, A. et al. 1986: Cerebral consequences of cardiopulmonary bypass. *Lancet* **1**, 823–5.

Slooter, A.J., Tang, M.X., van Duijn, C.M., Stern, Y., Ott, A., Bell, K. 1997: Apolipoprotein E ε4 and risk of dementia with stroke, a population based investigation. *JAMA* **227**, 818–21.

Sorbi, S., Nacmias, N., Piacentini, S., Repice, A., Latorraca, S., Forleo, P. et al. 1995: ApoE as a prognostic factor for post-traumatic coma. *Nature Medicine* **1**, 135–7.

Steen, P., Newberg, L., Milde, J., Michenfelder, J. 1983: Nimodipine improves cerebral blood flow and neurologic recovery after complete cerebral ischemia in the dog. *J Cereb Blood Flow Metab* **3**, 38–43.

Steen, P., Gisvold, S., Milde, J., Newberg, L. et al. 1985: Nimodipine improves outcome when given after complete cerebral ischemia in primates. *Anesthesiology* **62**, 406–14.

Stoll, C., Schelling, G., Goetz, A.E., Kilger, E., Bayer, A., Kapfhammer, H.P. et al. 2000: Health-related quality of life and post-traumatic stress disorder in patients after cardiac surgery and intensive care treatment. *Journal of Thoracic and Cardiovascular Surgery* **120**, 505–12.

Stump, D.A., Rogers, A.T., Hammon, J.W., Newman, S.P. 1996: Cerebral emboli and cognitive outcome after cardiac surgery. *Journal of Cardiothoracic Vascular Anesthesiology* **10**, 113–18; quiz 118–19.

Sungurtekin, H., Cook, D.J., Orszulak, T.A., Daly, R.C., Mullany, C.J. 1999: Cerebral response to haemodilution during hypothermic cardiopulmonary bypass in adults. *Anesthesia and Analgesia* **89**, 1078–83.

Sylivris, S., Calafiore, P., Matalanis, G., Rosalion, A., Yuen, H., Buxton, B. et al. 1997: The intraoperative assessment of ascending aortic atheroma: epiaortic imaging is superior to both transesophageal exhocardiography and direct palpation. *Journal of Cardiothoracic Vascular Anesthesiology* **11**, 704–11.

Sylivris, S., Levi, C., Matalanis, G., Rosalion, A., Buxton, B.F., Mitchell, A. et al. 1998: Pattern and significance of cerebral microemboli during coronary artery bypass grafting. *Annals of Thoracic Surgery* **66**, 1674–8.

Tardiff, B.E., Newman, M.F., Saunders, A.M., Strittmatter, W.J., Blumenthal, J.A., White, W.D. et al. 1997: Preliminary report of a genetic basis for cognitive decline after cardiac operations. The Neurologic Outcome Research Group of the Duke Heart Center. *Annals of Thoracic Surgery* **64**, 715–20.

Taylor, K.M. 1998: Brain damage during cardiopulmonary bypass. *Annals of Thoracic Surgery* **65**, S20-6; discussion S27–8.

Teasdale, G., Nicoll, J., Murray, J., Fiddes, M. 1997: Association of apolipoprotein E polymorphism with outcome after head injury. *Lancet* **350**, 1069–71.

Thiel, A., Zimmer, M., Stertmann, W.A., Kaps, M., Hempelmann, G. 1997: Microembolisations during cardiac surgery under extracorporeal circulation. *Anasthesiol Intensivmed Notfallmed Schmerzther* **32**, 715–20.

Ti, L.K., Mackensen, G.B. Grocott, H.P., Laskowitz, D.T., Philips-Bute, B.G., Milano, C.A. et al. 2003: Apolipoprotein E4 increases aortic atheroma burden in cardiac surgical patients. *Journal of Thoracic and Cardiovascular Surgery* **125**, 211–3.

Toner, I., Peden, C.J., Hamid, S.K., Newman, S., Taylor, K.M., Smith, P.L. 1994: Magnetic resonance imaging and neuropsychological changes after coronary artery bypass graft surgery: preliminary findings. *Journal of Neurosurgical Anesthesiology* **6**, 163–9.

Trubiano, P., Heyer, E., Adams, D., McMahon, D., Christiansen, I., Rose, E. et al. 1996: Jugular venous bulb oxyhaemoglobin saturation during cardiac surgery: accuracy and reliability using a continuous monitor. *Anesthesia and Analgesia* **82**, 964–8.

Tuman, K.J., McCarthy, R.J., Najafi, H., Ivankovich, A.D. 1992: Differential effects of advanced age on neurologic and cardiac risks of coronary artery operations. *Journal of Thoracic and Cardiovascular Surgery* **104**, 1510–17.

Undar, A., Masai, T., Yang, S.Q., Goddard-Finegold, J., Frazier, O.H., Fraser, C.D. Jr 1999: Effects of perfusion mode on regional and global organ blood flow in a neonatal piglet model. *Annals of Thoracic Surgery* **68**, 1336–42; discussion 1342–3.

Verhaegen, M., Iaizzo, P., Todd, M. 1995: A comparison of the effects of hypothermia, pentobarbital, and isoflurane on cerebral energy stores at the time of ischemic depolarization. *Anesthesiology* **82**, 1209–15.

Wareing, T.H., Davila-Roman, V.G., Barzilai, B., Murphy, S.F., Kouchoukos, N.T. 1992: Management of the severely atherosclerotic ascending aorta during cardiac operations. A strategy for detection and treatment. *Journal of Thoracic and Cardiovascular Surgery* **103**, 453–62.

Wareing, T., Davila-Roman, V., Daily, B., Murphy, S., Schectman, K., Barzilai, B. et al. 1993: Strategy for the reduction of stroke incidence in cardiac surgical patients. *Annals of Thoracic Surgery* **55**, 1400–8.

Warm Heart Investigators (WHI). 1994: Randomized trial of normothermic versus hypothermic coronary bypass surgery. *Lancet* **343**, 559–63.

Warner, D.S., Gionet, T.X., Todd, M.M., McAllister, A. 1992: Insulin-induced normoglycemia improves ischaemic outcome in hyperglycemic rats. *Stroke* **22**, 1775–81.

Warner, D., Takaoka, S., Wu, B., Ludwig, P., Pearlstein, R., Brinkhous, A. et al. 1996: Electroencephalographic burst suppression is not required to elicit maximal neuroprotection from pentobarbital in a rat model of focal cerebral ischemia. *Anesthesiology* **84**, 475–84.

Warner, C.D., Weintraub, W.S., Craver, J.M., Jones, E.L., Gott, J.P., Guyton, R.A. 1997: Effect of cardiac surgery patient characteristics on patient outcomes from 1981 through 1995. *Circulation* **96**, 1575–9.

Watters, M.P., Cohen, A.M., Monk, C.R., Angelini, G.D., Ryder, I.G. 2000: Reduced cerebral embolic signals in beating heart coronary surgery detected by transcranial Doppler ultrasound. *British Journal of Anaesthesia* **84**, 629–31.

van Wermeskerken, G.K., Lardenoye, J.W., Hill, S.E., Grocott, H.P., Phillips-Bute, B., Smith, P.K. 2000: Intraoperative physiologic variables and outcome in cardiac surgery: Part II. Neurologic outcome. *Annals of Thoracic Surgery* **69**, 1077–83.

Wolman, R.L., Nussmeier, N.A., Aggarwal, A., Kanchuger, M.S., Roach, G.W., Newman, M.F. 1999: Cerebral injury after cardiac surgery: identification of a group at extraordinary risk. *Stroke* **30**, 514–22.

Zaidan, J., Klochany, A., Martin, W., Ziegler, J., Harless, D. *et al.* 1991: Effect of thiopental on neurologic outcome following coronary artery bypass grafting. *Anesthesiology* **74**, 406–11.

Zhu, H.C., Cottrell, J.E., Kass, I.S. 1997: The effect of thiopental and propofol on NMDA- and AMPA-mediated glutamate excitotoxicity. *Anesthesiology* **87**, 944–51.

Zuccala, G., Pahor, M., Landi, F., Gasparini, G., Pagano, F., Carbonin, P. *et al.* 1997: Use of calcium antagonists and need for peri-operative transfusions in older patients with hip fracture. *British Medical Journal* **314**, 643–4.

11

Cardiopulmonary bypass in children with congenital heart disease

CARIN VAN DOORN AND MARTIN ELLIOTT

KEY POINTS

- There are important differences in the use of cardiopulmonary bypass in children with congenital cardiac abnormalities compared with its use in adults with normally connected hearts.
- With a move towards early repair of complex cardiac abnormalities in young children, these differences are related to the effects of cardiopulmonary bypass on immature organ systems, small body size and the need for intracardiac exposure. This requires flexibility in cannulation, and manipulation of temperature and bypass flows to achieve adequate access and a bloodless field.
- Despite extensive research, the complex interactions between cardiac anatomy and physiology, surgical technique, anaesthesia, hypothermia and cardiopulmonary bypass remain poorly understood. Clinically, the use of cardiopulmonary bypass in young children is associated with an exaggerated capillary leak affecting the function of many organ systems.
- More recently, in view of these deleterious effects, there has been a trend towards less haemodilution and, where possible, avoidance of deep hypothermic circulatory arrest. Furthermore,

transcatheter techniques have been developed for repair of selective congenital heart defects without the need for cardiopulmonary bypass.
- Mechanical ventricular assistance in the short and medium term for postcardiotomy myocardial failure, or bridging to recovery or transplantation for cardiomyopathy and myocarditis, may be used in selected cases with a realistic expectation of success.

INTRODUCTION

At present, the most common use of cardiopulmonary bypass is in the treatment of adults with acquired heart disease. The development of this technique, however, was originally driven by the need to perform intracardiac procedures for the correction of congenital heart defects in children. To allow access and visibility within the heart it was necessary to develop blood pumps and techniques for extracorporal oxygenation. After extensive laboratory research, 1953 saw the first successful use of a heart–lung bypass machine in humans by Gibbon (Gibbon, 1954) for the closure of an atrial septal defect (Warden et al., 1954). In 1955, Kirklin and colleagues (Kirklin et al., 1955) reported the first successful clinical series of intracardiac repairs. A further breakthrough came in the 1970s, when

Barrett-Boyes (1973) showed that it was possible to use deep hypothermic total circulatory arrest with cooling and rewarming on bypass to perform complex intracardiac repairs in very small children.

The early applications of cardiopulmonary bypass were associated with high complication rates. Technical developments and improvements in perfusion techniques, with advances in surgical management, have led to a dramatic improvement in survival, particularly for neonates with complex congenital heart disease. Because of these advances, attention is now focusing on post-operative morbidity, much of which is still related to the use of cardiopulmonary bypass. In particular, there is an increasing interest in neurological outcome and its relationship to hypothermia and circulatory arrest.

There are some important differences in the use of cardiopulmonary bypass in children with congenital heart disease compared with its use in adults with structurally normal hearts. These differences are related to the immaturity of organ systems, the small size of the young child, the frequent need for extensive intracardiac access and the presence of abnormal cardiovascular connections. These issues will be discussed in more detail below.

THE EFFECTS OF CARDIOPULMONARY BYPASS ON THE CHILD WITH CONGENITAL HEART DISEASE AND ITS RELATION TO AGE

Repair of a cardiac defect presents multiple sources of stress to the child, including surgical trauma, ischaemia or reperfusion injury, cardiopulmonary bypass, cooling and rewarming, and haemodilution. The differing effects of these various stresses are not known and our current knowledge is limited to the total body inflammatory response that occurs. At the centre of this response is the activation of neutrophils, which is followed by a complex cascade of events that subsequently leads to endothelial damage (Butler et al., 1993). The resulting capillary leak may account for much of the morbidity of cardiopulmonary bypass. This process is exaggerated in neonates and small infants (Finn et al., 1993).

For patients with congenital heart disease the issue is further complicated by the presence of abnormal cardiovascular physiology, usually with cyanosis or heart failure, and the frequent occurrence of abnormalities in other organ systems. In addition, in the young child many organ systems have not yet fully developed at birth and rapid changes in normal physiology occur in the first few weeks of life. Less specialization of organs may mean more resistance to damage and easier repair, but also less sophisticated mechanisms to cope with the effects of cardiopulmonary bypass.

Cardiovascular system

The cardiovascular system and respiratory system are closely integrated and change dramatically at birth with the establishment of a pulmonary circulation and closure of the ductus arteriosus. This raises the oxygen saturation of haemoglobin from approximately 55–60 per cent in foetal blood to 100 per cent post-natally.

The neonatal heart is relatively resistant to ischaemia, but otherwise has very little functional reserve, responding unfavourably to an increase in pre-load and after-load. Post-operative cardiac dysfunction caused by cardiopulmonary bypass is difficult to separate from that due to operative manipulation, but both myocardial oedema and distension of the heart reduce contractility. Cardiac performance may also be affected by congenital heart defects, such as persistent aortopulmonary collaterals, leaking valves and hypoplastic or absent chambers.

Respiratory system

In utero, the lung has no gas exchange and a significant part of lung maturation takes place after the start of respiration with birth. The lung in the foetus and newborn has muscular pulmonary arterioles with increased potential for pulmonary hypertension, but over the first few months of life, the pulmonary vascular resistance drops dramatically. The immature lung is prone to pulmonary oedema, probably related to increased pulmonary capillary permeability and a deficiency of the immature lymphatic system. In premature babies there may also be an alveolar membrane insufficiency caused by lack of surfactant. In neonates and infants, the capillary leak resulting from cardiopulmonary bypass frequently leads to pulmonary oedema, and subsequently to a high ventilation requirement in the early post-operative period.

Because of its close integration with the cardiovascular system, many congenital heart lesions may also involve the lung or may have an important impact on post-natal lung development. This is illustrated by the development of pulmonary vascular hypertension in cardiac defects with pulmonary overflow. In cyanotic conditions there may be persistence of aortopulmonary collateral vessels, which on cardiopulmonary bypass may result in pulmonary shunting with systemic hypotension.

Central nervous system

No new neurons are formed after birth, but the development of the central nervous system continues because of cellular migration, the differentiation of nerve cells and an increase in supporting cells and matrix. The maturation of individual nerve cells remains poorly understood but appears to be a complex process that occurs in close interaction with the supporting tissues. Loss of neurons in the presence of congenital heart disease may be the result of cyanosis or congestive cardiac failure or may be part of a more complex congenital abnormality. The blood brain barrier is poorly developed, making the young brain susceptible to oedema and haemorrhage. The oxygen consumption of the neonatal brain is low and therefore it is more resistant to hypoxic–ischaemic injury than the adult brain.

During normothermic cardiopulmonary bypass, cerebrovascular autoregulation maintains cerebral blood flow at a constant level despite variations in perfusion pressure (Venn, 1989). During moderate hypothermia, cerebrovascular autoregulation is preserved in children, but is lost during deep hypothermia when blood flow becomes dependent on perfusion pressure (Greeley et al., 1989). The vasodilatory effect of increased carbon dioxide levels decreases with lower temperature (Kern et al., 1991). Other factors that may affect the amount and distribution of cerebral blood flow are the rate of cooling and rewarming on cardiopulmonary bypass, acid–base management, air-embolism and hypoperfusion related to aorto-pulmonary collaterals. The predominant substrates for the brain are glucose and oxygen. Research into their metabolism during cardiopulmonary bypass is only just starting and the interpretation of early results is difficult (Bandali et al., 2001).

Neuropsychological injury after cardiopulmonary bypass has been reported as between one per cent and 25 per cent. Damage to the developing brain is difficult to define as some acute neuropsychological changes, such as seizures, may be transient. More subtle changes may only become significant over time and may include learning disabilities, behavioural problems or choreoathetosis. The picture is further clouded by the fact that some congenital heart defects are associated with neuro-developmental disorders or cyanosis.

The brain remains vulnerable in the immediate post-operative period. Mild hypothermia is probably protective after ischaemic injury to the brain, whereas slight hyperthermia can make the damage much worse (Shum-Tim et al., 1998) and care should be taken not to 'overshoot' during rewarming. A low cardiac output state post-operatively may also contribute to further neurological damage.

Other organ systems

The immature renal system in the newborn has a high vascular resistance and low blood flow and glomerulo-filtration rate. Therefore the handling of sodium and regulation of acid–base balance is limited, as is the concentrating and diluting capacity.

Immaturity of the liver may result in coagulopathy. The presence of cyanosis is also associated with a deranged clotting mechanism. It is therefore no surprise that post-operative bleeding is a common problem after cardiopulmonary bypass, in particular in premature infants and newborns and those with cyanotic heart disease. Other factors that contribute to bleeding problems are inadequate haemostasis at the (extensive) suture lines and non-surgical factors, including haemodilution, hypothermia, incomplete reversal of heparin with protamine, platelet dysfunction, activation of the fibrinolytic system and occasionally a consumptive coagulopathy.

Humoral and cellular immune function and inflammatory mediators are present early in life, but the qualitative responses may be subnormal. Prematurity and low birth weight may further compromise the immune function.

PRACTICAL ASPECTS OF CARDIOPULMONARY BYPASS

Despite extensive research, our understanding of cardiopulmonary bypass remains limited and much of the daily routine continues to be based on historical practice. There are wide differences between centres, many of which claim excellent results. General principles on the practical aspects of cardiopulmonary bypass are set out below.

Cardiopulmonary bypass circuit

The purpose of cardiopulmonary bypass is to provide optimal exposure for intracardiac repair while providing adequate perfusion and unobstructed drainage to meet the metabolic needs of the patient. Because the left atrium and pulmonary veins are difficult to access for drainage, the pulmonary circulation is bypassed and extracorporal oxygenation of blood is used. Metabolic need can be reduced by inducing hypothermia and, if deep hypothermic arrest is employed, there is the further advantage that the cannulae can be removed from the operative field, thus improving exposure.

A cardiopulmonary bypass circuit includes arterial and venous cannulae, venous reservoir, oxygenator, heat exchanger and blood pump. In contrast to the use of standard circuits for most adults, cardiopulmonary bypass circuits in children with congenital heart disease have to be individualized to take account of variations in anatomy, surgical repair and size of the patient. The open architecture of the circuit makes it highly adaptable and allows visible monitoring of the various components, but increases blood exposure area and priming volume. The final design may vary considerably between centres.

Cannulation for cardiopulmonary bypass

The ascending aorta is most often cannulated for arterial inflow. For operations in which the right atrium is not entered, or those that are done under deep hypothermic circulatory arrest, venous drainage is via a single cannula in the right atrium. Direct cannulation of the superior and inferior vena cava is performed in most operations that involve access into the right atrium. Flexibility is required, however, to deal with many, sometimes unexpected, anatomical variations. For example, an interrupted aortic arch may require two inflow cannulae, one for the ascending and one for the descending aorta, respectively, to provide total body perfusion. The cannula for lower body perfusion can be placed directly in the descending aorta or in a patent ductus arteriosus, taking care to snare the pulmonary arteries to avoid run off into the pulmonary bed. Alternatively, if the heart is still beating and the duct is open adequate cooling can be achieved with one arterial cannula only. Venous return from a persistent left superior vena cava can be managed with separate cannulation of this vessel or, if it drains to the coronary sinus, with continuous cardiotomy suction via the opened right atrium. In small children, the placement of sufficient cannulae may not be possible and the only option is cooling on cardiopulmonary bypass followed by repair during a period of deep hypothermic circulatory arrest.

During cardiopulmonary bypass in the normally connected circulation there is only a negligible amount of blood returning through the pulmonary circulation. In the presence of congenital heart defects, in particular cyanotic lesions, there may be systemic to pulmonary artery connections that during cardiopulmonary bypass can cause a considerable steal away from the systemic circulation with systemic hypoperfusion and distension of the left side of the heart. Examples include the presence of a patent ductus arteriosus, aorto-pulmonary collaterals or man-made shunts. If possible, these connections should be controlled immediately after initiation of cardiopulmonary bypass and adequate venting of the left heart provided. Hypothermia with reduced flow rate, or ultimately deep hypothermic circulatory arrest, can also be used to manage excessive left heart return.

The size of the cannulae is dictated by the anticipated flow rate, and in small children the correct size is of critical importance. An arterial cannula that is too large may cause left ventricular outflow obstruction; if too small, a high arterial line pressure will be required to achieve adequate flow which will give rise to high shear stress at the cannula tip resulting in increased haemolysis. An adequately sized venous cannula should provide unobstructed drainage by gravity. Vacuum-assisted venous drainage is not widely used in paediatric bypass practice but may allow downsizing of the cannula. Proper positioning and stable fixation of cannulae is extremely important. The choice of cannula design largely depends on individual preference.

Hypothermia and deep hypothermic circulatory arrest

Since oxygen is not stored in the body, the metabolic demand of the cells has to be met continuously. In particular, the brain is very susceptible to hypoxic injury. At normothermia, oxygen delivery depends on flow rate, hematocrit and oxygen saturation of the perfusate. Minimum flow rate under general anaesthesia is age dependent: in neonates 120–200 mL/kg per minute; children up to 10 kg 100–150 mL/kg per minute; older children 80–120 mL/kg per minute and in adults generally up to 2.4 L/min per m^2 (Gaynor et al., 1996). Hypothermia is frequently used to decrease the metabolic rate and allow reduction of pump rate or even circulatory arrest. How much reduction of the metabolism can be achieved without inducing tissue ischaemia is not exactly known, especially because uneven tissue perfusion during cooling, endothelial cell dysfunction and increased blood viscosity may further impair perfusion of the microvasculature. It has been calculated that the critical flow rate at 27°C is 30–35 mL/kg and at 18°C 5–30 mL/kg (Kern et al., 1993). The desired perfusion pressures at these flow rates remain open to debate. In clinical practice, during hypothermia flow rates are often reduced to so-called one-half or one-quarter flow (about 30 mL/kg per minute) to improve visibility in the operative field. The optimal temperature at which deep hypothermic arrest should be carried out is also controversial, but is thought to be somewhere between 14°C and 20°C (Gillinov et al., 1993; Mezrow et al., 1994). Suggested 'safe' ischaemic times are between 11 and 19 minutes at 28°C degrees and between 39 and 65 minutes at 18°C (Greeley et al., 1991). However, even at low temperature, the brain's basal metabolic requirements continue and therefore there is always the risk of neurological injury. Extensive studies have been performed to compare the effects of deep hypothermic circulatory arrest and low flow bypass on neurological function. Although the interpretation of the results is hampered by significant variations in the conductance of cardiopulmonary bypass between centres, the available evidence seems to suggest that circulatory arrest should be avoided where possible.

The rate of core cooling on cardiopulmonary bypass depends on the efficiency of the heat exchanger. To avoid uneven cooling the gradient between water and blood should not exceed more than 10°C. Cooling can further be assisted by surface cooling using a cooling blanket, low theatre room temperature and vasodilators. Full rewarming is important because it significantly reduces the afterload when the patient is weaned off cardiopulmonary bypass, and this is of particular importance for the non-compliant neonatal heart. It also reduces the volume requirement associated with peripheral vasodilatation in the early post-operative period when the patient is otherwise warming up. Peripheral vasodilators and a warming blanket can aid the process, but one should be careful not to 'overshoot' to avoid secondary neurological injury after operative brain ischaemia.

Prime volume and composition

In the young child, the priming volume of the cardiopulmonary bypass circuit is large compared with the circulating body volume, and many children need blood adding to the circuit to avoid extreme haemodilution after initiation of cardiopulmonary bypass. It is only recently that manufacturers started to produce small, low prime circuits to accommodate the shift towards repair at younger age and lower weight.

There is wide variation in prime composition between units. The recipe depends on the following factors (Elliott *et al.*, 1993; Hill *et al.*, 1993):

- desired haematocrit on cardiopulmonary bypass
- perceived requirement for colloid osmotic pressure maintenance during cardiopulmonary bypass
- need for other additives, such as mannitol, sodium bicarbonate, steroids, heparin, and aprotinin
- the temperature at which cardiopulmonary bypass is performed.

The rationale for haemodilution during hypothermic cardiopulmonary bypass is based on the use of hypothermia, which causes a rise in blood viscosity. An added benefit is that the need for blood transfusion is also reduced. Acceptable levels for haemodilution are not specified, but generally a haematocrit between 20 and 30 is used for deep hypothermic arrest. A significant drawback is that haemodilution contributes to the capillary leak associated with cardiopulmonary bypass, but surprisingly little is known about the use of appropriate colloid substitutions to counteract this. Human albumin solution, fresh frozen plasma, and gels and starches are all used. In addition there is a large variation in other additives that may be added to the prime to aid functions such as diuresis, anticoagulation, haemostasis, acid-base balance and control of inflammatory response.

Acid–base balance

At 37°C, intracellular and membrane-based enzyme systems function most efficiently at pH 7.4, and both metabolic and respiratory compensatory mechanisms function to maintain this pH. When hypothermia was first introduced in cardiopulmonary bypass a surprise finding was that cooling moves the blood pH into an alkaline direction. This is related to a shift of the dissociation constant of water so that neutral pH at a body temperature of 20°C is approximately 7.7.

There are currently two schools of thought about how acid-base balance should be managed during hypothermic cardiopulmonary bypass: pH-stat and the more recently developed alpha-stat strategy. Both are based on extrapolating the physiological behaviour of animals that become hypothermic during their normal existence. During hypothermia, hibernating (warm-blooded) animals reduce whole-body oxygen and energy consumption by minimizing flow to non-working areas, such as skeletal muscle, and preserving flow to essential organs, such as the brain. By hypoventilation, they allow a respiratory acidosis to develop, maintaining pH at 7.4 at all temperatures. When the pH-stat strategy is used during cardiopulmonary bypass, carbon dioxide is added during hypothermia. To maintain neutral pH at 17°C this requires a pCO_2 of 4.3 kPa, but if this arterial blood gas sample is analysed at 37°C the pH will be 7.06 and the pCO_2 11.5 kPa, that is, severe respiratory acidosis. In cold-blooded vertebrates body temperature follows ambient temperature. With a decrease in temperature, the ratio (termed alpha) of dissociated to non-dissociated imidazole groups of histidine, an essential component of the protein buffer system, remains constant. This allows an increase in pH parallel to the natural increase in the pH of water. Using the alpha-stat strategy of pH management during cooling, the pCO_2 of arterial blood measured at 37°C is kept constant but the actual CO_2 content falls as a direct function of declining temperature, and pH rises.

There is an ongoing debate about the best pH strategy to protect the brain during hypothermic cardiopulmonary bypass. Advantages of the pH-stat strategy are thought to include improvement of cerebral blood flow, cerebral oxygenation and brain cooling efficiency during cardiopulmonary bypass. This may, however, be at the risk of microembolism and of free radical-mediated damage. Arguments in favour of the alpha-stat strategy are that it preserves cerebral autoregulation and optimizes intracellular enzyme function. The downside may be less metabolic suppression and therefore greater susceptibility to neurological injury. In adults, who stay on full flow with mild to moderate hypothermia, the differences between these strategies may not be that important. The implications, however, may be much greater for neonates undergoing long procedures with low flow or arrest, and possibly periods of reperfusion. Extensive research in this area has been performed, but the interpretation of results is complicated by the multitude of interventions during cardiopulmonary bypass, of which pH management is just one. In addition there are wide variations in pre-morbid neurological conditions and surgical anatomy and no uniform way of measuring neurological injury. Despite a number of excellent studies (Wong *et al.*, 1992; Hiramatsu *et al.*, 1995), the jury is still out.

Ultrafiltration

The use of cardiopulmonary bypass, especially combined with haemodilution and hypothermia, is associated with the development of a capillary leak. This is a particular problem in neonates and can result in severe organ oedema with dysfunction. Ultrafiltration can be used to remove some of the excess body water. During rewarming on cardiopulmonary bypass, blood is shunted from the arterial to the venous side of the circuit through an ultrafilter raising the haematocrit up to 30–35 per cent. An alternate method is modified ultrafiltration (Naik et al., 1991), which is started in the immediate post-bypass period, shunting the blood from the arterial cannula via the filter back to the right atrium, aiming to bring the haematocrit up to 40–45 per cent. Both conventional and MUF have been widely reported and in a recent review of the data there was widespread agreement that the techniques are beneficial in reducing body water, raising haematocrit and colloid osmotic pressure (Elliott, 1999). Ultrafiltration has also been claimed to help reduce the levels of inflammatory mediators induced by cardiopulmonary bypass but these benefits are less clear. Other methods of management of capillary leak in the post-operative period are fluid restriction, diuretics and peritoneal dialysis.

OTHER APPLICATIONS OF MECHANICAL VENTRICULAR SUPPORT

In contrast to the adult population, in whom the development of a permanent total implantable heart is one of the aims, mechanical ventricular assistance in the paediatric population is for short and medium term use only. Indications are post-cardiotomy failure, and bridging to recovery and transplantation for cardiomyopathy. In particular in some children with acute myocarditis, bridge to recovery is a realistic expectation. Furthermore, if this fails it is still possible to accommodate these patients in the transplant programme because, in the paediatric population as opposed to the adult population, there is a relatively good supply of organs, although some children still die before a suitable organ is found (Doyle, 2000).

When considering which device to choose, both the expected length of support and the patient's underlying disease have to be considered. A device used for short-term post-cardiotomy support should be readily available in the operating theatre, its application and management should be easy and its use should do no permanent damage to the heart. If the aim is to bridge to recovery or transplantation, then the time on support may be much longer and degree of physical independence and mobility of the patient becomes important. Complications associated with the use of all the devices include bleeding, infection and neurological complications.

The development of ventricular assist devices for children has been hampered by size limitations. In addition there is a lack of commercial interest because the potential market is small and it is necessary to produce a large range of sizes. The following type of pumps are used in children.

Extracorporal devices: these are essentially centrifugal blood pumps that are normally used in a cardiopulmonary bypass circuit. They can be used either as a left ventricular assist device (LVAD), right ventricular assist device (RVAD) or two pumps in combination for biventricular assist device (BiVAD). The systems are placed at the bedside and are relatively easy to set up and run, but generally require an open chest and are thus for short-term use only. Various different makes of centrifugal pumps are available. Some centres that have experience with extra corporal membrane oxygenation (ECMO) for respiratory failure prefer the use of this technique for cardiac support because it requires only the cannulation of a central artery and vein and sternotomy is not necessary.

In *paracorporeal devices* an external blood pump is placed close to the body and connected to the heart by short cannulae that traverse the skin. Limited mobility is possible as long as the patient remains connected to the power supply. Two devices are available from infant size onwards: the Medos HIA-VAD (Medos Medizintechnik GmbH, Stolberg, Germany) and the Berlin Heart (Mediport Kardiotechnik, Berlin, Germany). For the Thoratec VAD (Thoratec Laboratories, Berkeley, CA, USA) the minimum patient weight is 17 kg. All these devices are driven pneumatically.

Partially implantable devices have a fully implantable pump, but remain dependent for their power supply on a drive line that crosses the skin. The MicroMed/DeBakey (MicroMed Technology Inc., TX, USA) is an electrical axial flow impeller pump for left ventricular assistance from 40 kg onwards. A similar pump, the Jarvik 2000 (Jarvik HEART Inc., NY, USA), has so far been available for adult use only.

CONCLUSIONS

There are important differences in the use of cardiopulmonary bypass in children with congenital cardiac abnormalities compared with its use in adults with normally connected hearts. With a move towards early repair of complex abnormalities in young children, these differences are related to the effects of cardiopulmonary bypass on immature organ systems, small body size and the need for intracardiac exposure. This requires flexibility in cannulation, and manipulation of temperature and bypass flows to achieve adequate access and a bloodless field. Despite extensive research, the consequences of the complex interactions between cardiac anatomy and physiology, surgical technique, anaesthesia, hypothermia and cardiopulmonary bypass remain poorly understood and most of the daily cardiopulmonary bypass routine is based on historical practice. There are widespread differences in management between centres, all claiming excellent results. In general, there is a trend to towards less haemodilution and avoidance of deep hypothermic circulatory arrest. Although cardiopulmonary bypass remains necessary for most repairs of congenital heart disease, we must continue to try to minimize the deleterious effects associated with its use. Furthermore, new transcatheter techniques have been developed that achieve repair of selected congenital cardiac defects without the need for cardiopulmonary bypass.

REFERENCES

Bandali, K.S., Belanger, M.P., Wittnich, C. 2001: Is hyperglycemia seen in children during cardiopulmonary bypass a result of hyperoxia? *Journal of Thoracic and Cardiovascular Surgery* **122**, 753–8.

Barratt-Boyes, B.G. 1973: Complete correction of cardiovascular malformations in the first two years of life using profound hypothermia. In: Barratt-Boyes, B.G., Neutze, J.M., Harris, E.A., eds. *Heart disease in infancy*. Edinburgh, Churchill Livingstone, 1973: 35.

Butler, J., Rocker, G.M., Westaby, S. 1993: Inflammatory response to cardiopulmonary bypass. *Annals of Thoracic Surgery* **55**, 552–9.

Doyle, P. 2000: To pump or not to pump? *Perfusion* **15**, 375–8.

Elliott, M. 1999: Modified ultrafiltration and open heart surgery in children. *Paediatric Anaesthesia* **9**, 1–5.

Elliott, M., Rao, P.V., Hampton, M. 1993: Current paediatric perfusion practice in the United Kingdom. *Perfusion* **8**, 7–25.

Finn, A., Rebuck, N., Strobel, S. *et al.* 1993: Systemic inflammation during paediatric cardiopulmonary bypass: changes in neutrophil adhesive properties. *Perfusion* **8**, 39–48.

Gaynor, J.W. *et al.* 1996: Management of cardiopulmonary bypass in infants and children. In: Baue, Geha, Hammond, Laks, Naunheim, eds. *Glenn's thoracic and cardiovascular surgery* (Sixth edition). New York, NU: Appleton & Lange, Vol. II: 1024.

Gibbon, J.H. Jr. 1954: Application of a mechanical heart and lung apparatus in cardiac surgery. *Minnesota Medicine* **37**, 171–85.

Gillinov, A.M., Redmond, J.M., Zehr, K.J. *et al.* 1993: Superior cerebral protection with profound hypothermia during circulatory arrest. *Annals of Thoracic Surgery* **55**, 1432–9.

Greeley, W.J., Ungerleider, R.M., Smith, L.R., Reves, J.G. 1989: The effects of deep hypothermic cardiopulmonary bypass and total circulatory arrest on cerebral blood flow in infants and children. *Journal of Thoracic and Cardiovascular Surgery* **97**, 737–45.

Greeley, W.J., Kern, F.H., Ungerleider, R.M. *et al.* 1991: The effect of hypothermic cardiopulmonary bypass and total circulatory arrest on cerebral metabolism in neonates, infants, and children. *Journal of Thoracic and Cardiovascular Surgery* **101**, 783–94.

Hill, A.G., Groom, R.C., Akl, B.F., Lefrak, E.A. Karusz, M. 1993: Current paediatric perfusion practice in North America. *Perfusion* **8**, 27–38.

Hiramatsu, T., Miura, T., Forbess, J.M. *et al.* 1995: pH strategies and cerebral energetics before and after circulatory arrest. *Journal of Thoracic and Cardiovascular Surgery* **109**, 948–58.

Kern, F.H., Ungerleider, R.M., Quill, T.J. *et al.* 1991: Cerebral blood flow response to changes in arterial carbon dioxide tension during hypothermic cardiopulmonary bypass in children. *Journal of Thoracic and Cardiovascular Surgery* **101**, 618–22.

Kern, F.H., Ungerleider, R.M., Reves, J.G. *et al.* 1993: Effect of altering pump flow rate on cerebral blood flow and metabolism in infants and children. *Annals of Thoracic Surgery* **56**, 1366–72.

Kirklin, J.W., DuShane, J.W., Patrick, R.T. *et al.* 1955: Intracardiac surgery with the aid of a mechanical pump-oxygenator system (Gibbon type): report of eight cases. *Proceeding of the Staff Meeting of the Mayo Clinic* **30**, 201–206.

Mezrow, C.K., Midulla, P.S., Sadeghi, A.M. *et al.* 1994: Evaluation of cerebral metabolism and quantitative electroencephalography after hypothermic circulatory arrest and low-flow cardiopulmonary bypass at different temperatures. *Journal of Thoracic and Cardiovascular Surgery* **107**, 1006–19.

Naik, S.K., Knight, A., Elliott, M.J. 1991: A successful modification of ultrafiltration for cardiopulmonary bypass in children. *Perfusion* **6**, 41–50.

Shum-Tim, D., Nagashima, M., Shinoka, T., Bucerius, J., Nollert, G., Lidov, H.G. *et al.* 1998: Postischemic hyperthermia exacerbates neurologic injury after deep hypothermic circulatory arrest. *Journal of Thoracic and Cardiovascular Surgery* **116**: 780–92.

Venn, G.E. 1989: Cerebrovascular autoregulation during cardiopulmonary bypass. *Perfusion* **4**, 105–13.

Warden, H.E., Cohen, M., Read, R.C., Lillehei, C.W. 1954: Controlled cross circulation for open intracardiac surgery; physiologic studies and results of creation and closure of ventricular septal defects. *Journal of Thoracic and Cardiovascular Surgery* **28**, 331–41.

Wong, P.C., Barlow, C.F., Hickey, P.R. *et al.* 1992: Factors associated with choreoathetosis after cardiopulmonary bypass in children with congenital heart disease. *Circulation* **86** (5 Suppl), 18–26.

12

Intraoperative myocardial protection

JOHN WC ENTWISTLE III AND ANDREW S WECHSLER

KEY POINTS

- The heart has a constant and high metabolic demand, and a high level of oxygen extraction. Diseased hearts have low energy reserves and are particularly susceptible to further ischaemic injury.
- In order to minimize the injury sustained by the heart, myocardial protection strategies should focus on events occurring before during and after myocardial ischaemia.
- During routine surgery a simple yet effective basic strategy should suffice, but as complexity increases the strategy should be flexible enough to be adapted to provide increased levels of protection.
- Cardioplegia-based techniques remain the basis of myocardial protection, the aims being: rapid induction of diastolic arrest; minimization of energy requirements during ischaemia; prevention of damage caused by absence of blood flow; and prevention of damage caused by reperfusion.
- The list of potential modifications and additives to cardioplegia is extensive, but no 'silver bullet' has yet been identified.
- Experimental studies of myocardial protection are often compromised by the lack of similarity to clinical situations, whilst clinical studies suffer by having necessarily 'soft' endpoints and using surrogate markers of effectiveness.

INTRODUCTION

The goal of any cardiac procedure is to improve or preserve cardiac performance. Paramount to this goal, the cardiac surgeon must avoid unnecessarily imposing further injury upon the heart. This requires a comprehensive myocardial protection policy that encompasses the conduct of the operation before, during and after the period of ischaemia. Failure to protect the heart adequately at any stage may negate the efforts at other times in the procedure and result in myocardial injury and permanent dysfunction. As the patient population has grown progressively older, preoperative myocardial function that once precluded operation is now commonplace and myocardial protective strategies have become increasingly complex. In addition, any cardiac operation may present challenges that require modification of a surgeon's usual protective strategy. Thus, a thorough understanding is required of the available techniques, and the rationale behind them, in order to provide any given individual with the most appropriate myocardial protection for the situation. Although the potential methods for myocardial protection are numerous, only a few strategies are in common use. There are many variations in the details even between similar protocols, but only the most common variables are discussed here.

HISTORY

The earliest cardiac procedures utilized myocardial cooling with concomitant systemic hypothermia to facilitate the conduct of the operation, not necessarily as a form of myocardial protection. In 1955, following the introduction of cardiopulmonary bypass, Melrose began to advocate the use of chemical cardioplegia in order to improve surgical exposure (Melrose *et al.*, 1955). Although infusion of high potassium solutions resulted in myocardial quiescence, this approach was abandoned because the high potassium concentrations produced permanent myocardial injury. The following year, Lillehei proposed the use of retrograde coronary perfusion during aortic valve procedures as a method of intraoperative myocardial protection (Lillehei *et al.*, 1956). Investigations into chemical cardioplegia persisted, predominantly in Europe (Holscher *et al.*, 1961; Bretschneider *et al.*, 1975). Topical myocardial cooling was introduced both by the use of ice cold saline and slush (Hufnagel *et al.*, 1961). Myocardial injury was not specifically associated with poor myocardial protection until Taber *et al.* (1967) and Najafi *et al.* (1969) described myocardial necrosis in post-operative patients who succumbed to low output cardiogenic shock. Subsequently, there were reports of a high rate of peri-operative myocardial infarction in patients undergoing both revascularization (Brewer *et al.*, 1973; Assad-Morell *et al.*, 1975) and open cardiac procedures (Hultgren *et al.*, 1973). Gay and Ebert (1973) reintroduced hyperkalaemic myocardial arrest with lower potassium concentrations than those used by Melrose *et al.* (1955). This led to arrest and myocardial preservation without the untoward effects seen with the higher potassium concentrations. In 1978, Follette and colleagues published their findings, which popularized the use of blood in the cardioplegia (Follette *et al.*, 1978). Over the last two decades, most of the changes in myocardial protection have concentrated on myocardial temperature and the route of cardioplegia administration. In addition, numerous additives to cardioplegia have been proposed and tested to maximize the protective capabilities, with variable results.

PHYSIOLOGY

In order to understand the rationale behind many of the protective techniques available, an understanding of myocardial physiology and energy expenditure is needed. The heart has a high rate of energy expenditure, and thus requires a continuous supply of oxygen during normal conditions. Nutritive blood flow through the coronary arteries is controlled by autoregulation, by which blood flow to the myocardium is varied based on the myocardial energy requirements. It is only functional when the perfusion pressure is within the autoregulatory range. Perfusion of the subendocardium occurs primarily during diastole, when the wall tension of the ventricle is at its least. The perfusion of the myocardium depends on the transmural driving pressure, which is the difference between aortic diastolic pressure and left ventricular end diastolic pressure. Subendocardial perfusion may therefore become insufficient when perfusion pressure decreases or intraventricular pressure increases. The first may occur in the setting of systemic hypotension, or in the presence of significant coronary artery disease that produces pressure drop across a stenotic lesion. Increases in intraventricular pressure may be seen in the hypertrophied ventricle, or when the ventricle acutely distends with blood. The latter may occur in the arrested heart in the presence of aortic insufficiency, when the inflow of blood into the ventricle through the aortic valve has no ready route of egress. Increases in intraventricular pressure can be seen in the fibrillating heart. In addition to the inability of the fibrillating ventricle to empty, the subendocardium is subjected to a relatively sustained state of systole, increasing myocardial wall tension and further decreasing subendocardial perfusion.

The high metabolic demand of the myocardium is demonstrated by the rapid fall in adenosine triphosphate (ATP) content in the presence of ischaemia. The myocardium obtains high-energy phosphates in the form of ATP through aerobic metabolism. In the presence of oxygen, the heart can utilize free fatty acids, glucose, amino acids, pyruvate, acetate and ketone bodies as the source of energy for the formation of ATP. In the presence of oxygen, the heart generates 36 moles of ATP from one mole of glucose. However, under anaerobic conditions, glucose is converted to lactate, and a net of two moles of ATP are generated for every mole of glucose. In addition to this lower level of efficiency, lactate and hydrogen ions accumulate in the tissues, which inhibit glycolysis and many other cellular functions.

The myocardium exhibits a very high, and rather constant, level of oxygen extraction from the blood, and quickly becomes ischaemic when this supply is interrupted. Oxygen consumption is highly dependent upon the contractile state of the heart, heart rate and after-load as well as the temperature of the myocardium. The relationship between myocardial oxygen consumption, temperature and mechanical state is demonstrated in Fig. 12.1. The oxygen consumption in the working ventricle is about 8 mL of O_2 per 100 g of myocardium per minute. This decreases to 5.6 mL of O_2 per 100 g of myocardium in the empty beating heart, and to 1.1 mL of O_2 per 100 g of myocardium per minute in the potassium-arrested heart (Buckberg *et al.*, 1977). Thus, potassium arrest alone is associated with an eightfold decrease in myocardial oxygen consumption. Hypothermia further decreases oxygen utilization by the myocardium in all situations, although the relative contribution of hypothermia is minimized in the setting of hyperkalaemic arrest. In the arrested heart, the relationship between temperature and myocardial oxygen consumption is described by the Q_{10} effect, in which the myocardial oxygen consumption (MVO_2) decreases 50 per cent for each decrease in myocardial temperature of 10°C. Thus, in the

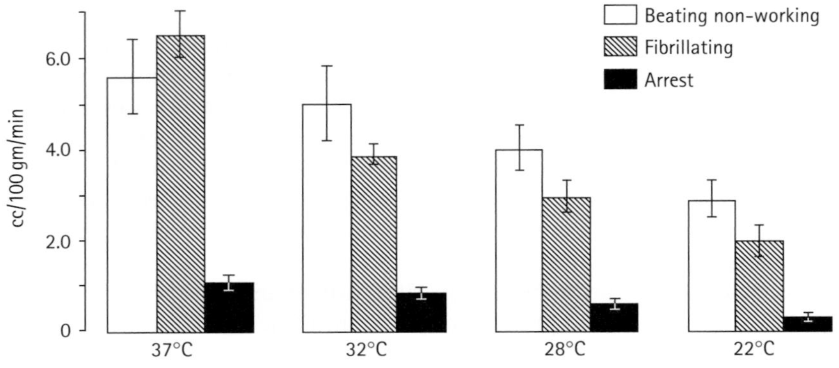

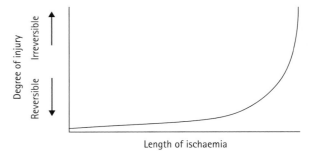

Figure 12.1 *Myocardial oxygen consumption versus cardiac state and temperature. The myocardial oxygen uptake per gram of tissue is displayed relative to the working state of the heart and the temperature of the myocardium. Values are mean ± SEM. (Reprinted from Buckberg et al., 1977, with permission from Elsevier.)*

setting of hyperkalaemic arrest, a decrease in myocardial temperature from 37°C to 22°C results in a further decline in myocardial oxygen consumption from 1.1 mL to 0.3 mL of O_2 per 100 g of myocardium (Buckberg *et al.*, 1977).

ISCHAEMIC INJURY

The mechanisms behind ischaemic myocardial injury are complex. Although damage from the lack of oxygenated blood flow is significant, the injury that occurs as a result of the restoration of blood flow may be equally or more important. The degree of myocardial injury depends upon multiple factors, including the presence of ventricular hypertrophy, pre-ischaemic energy state of the heart, length of the ischaemic interval, level of work imposed upon the ischaemic heart, characteristics of initial reperfusate and the manner in which reperfusion is conducted. In addition, the extent of injury depends on whether the ischaemia is regional or global, the presence of collateral blood flow and numerous other factors. An early manifestation of ischaemic injury is the state of temporary myocardial dysfunction, termed 'stunning'. Myocardial stunning occurs after reperfusion, and is the presence of contractile dysfunction under conditions of normal myocardial oxygen delivery, and in the absence of irreversible structural injury. Stunned myocardium is capable of complete functional recovery if there is no further insult before recovery. In the absence of other confounding factors, the duration of stunning is usually related to the length of the ischaemic interval. Although the recovery of myocardial stunning may occur within hours, severe stunning may persist for a period of days to weeks. As illustrated in Fig. 12.2, the degree of injury varies with the length of the ischaemic interval. In the early period of ischaemia, all of the changes are reversible. However, progression of ischaemic injury results in an irreversible state, accompanied by structural damage and permanent myocardial dysfunction. In general, the transition from reversible to irreversible injury is poorly defined. The histological and biochemical changes in the myocardium

Figure 12.2 *Degree of injury versus length of ischaemia. As the length of the ischaemic interval is increased, the injury becomes progressively irreversible. The transition between reversible and irreversible injury is poorly defined and is influenced by many variables.*

associated with increasing lengths of ischaemia are numerous, and several of the more important changes are listed in Table 12.1. The early events occur within seconds to minutes of the onset of ischaemia, and are completely reversible. Intermediate events occur between minutes and about an hour of ischaemia, and generally occur near the time of transition from reversible to irreversible injury. The late events usually occur after an hour or more of ischaemia, and herald the onset of irreversible changes in the myocardium.

In addition to the length of the ischaemic interval, the degree of myocardial damage is significantly influenced by the conditions upon reperfusion. Potentially salvageable myocardium may be irreversibly injured by inappropriate reperfusion. Similarly, the survival of borderline myocardium may be enhanced through proper reperfusion. Table 12.2 lists some of the variables that may improve myocardial recovery by shifting the injury curve (shown in Fig. 12.2) to the right, or produce additional myocardial necrosis by shifting the curve to the left. Viable myocardium, which would otherwise be labelled as 'stunned', can be converted into infarcted myocardium during reperfusion if the conditions at the end of ischaemia are not optimized. Thus, interventions

Table 12.1 *Important changes in ischaemia*

Early events	Intermediate events	Late events
Anaerobic glycolysis	Increase diastolic $[Ca^{++}]$	Amorphous mitochondrial densities
H^+/lactate accumulation	Release norepinephrine	Break in SR plasmalemma
ATP depletion	Decrease glycogen deposits	Broadening of Z-bands
Contractile arrest	Mild margination of chromatin	

Table 12.2 *Improving myocardial recovery by shifting the injury curve*

Events that shift the curve to the right:
hypothermia
ventricular unloading
pre-ischaemic substrate enhancement
controlled reperfusion
cardioplegia

Events that shift the curve to the left:
pre-ischaemic energy depletion
ventricular fibrillation
ventricular distention
ventricular hypertrophy
uncontrolled reperfusion

taken before, during and after periods of myocardial ischaemia can significantly minimize the injury sustained during an ischaemic interval.

Successful interventions are based upon some of the proposed mechanisms of cellular injury during periods of ischaemia and reperfusion. The timing of reperfusion is also important. As illustrated in Fig. 12.3, early reperfusion can result in complete recovery of contractile function, with no permanent damage. Reperfusion after an intermediate period of ischaemia results in stunning, with diastolic dysfunction generally preceding the onset of systolic dysfunction. Later periods of reperfusion are associated with progressively greater degrees of injury and irreversible damage. Similar to the changes seen with ischaemia, the transition from reversible to irreversible injury is poorly defined, and influenced significantly by the factors listed in Table 12.2.

The mechanisms that lead to myocardial dysfunction after an ischaemic interval are numerous and complex. It is unclear to what extent ischaemia and reperfusion contribute to the process of injury. However, in the setting of cardiac surgery, in which reperfusion is the anticipated consequence of an ischaemic interval, the significance of this distinction is also unclear, and thus all injury sustained during the ischaemia and reperfusion interval can be broadly classified as ischaemic injury. However, it must be kept in mind that there are distinguishing characteristics between ischaemia and reperfusion so the myocardial protective strategy must include properly timed interventions aimed at both sources of injury. Proposed initiating factors behind myocellular ischaemic injury include the depletion of high-energy phosphates, intracellular acidosis, alterations in intracellular calcium homeostasis and direct myocellular injury. Causes of myocellular injury associated with reperfusion include intracellular calcium overload, generation of oxygen-derived free radicals, complement activation, adverse endothelial cell-leukocyte interactions and the development of myocellular oedema. In addition, it is becoming clear that decreased myocardial performance after an episode of ischaemia and reperfusion may represent damage to components of the heart other than the myocytes. This may lead to further myocellular damage or persistent organ dysfunction. Vascular endothelial dysfunction and neutrophil activation occur as a result of ischaemic injury and may be amplified by inflammatory mechanisms induced by cardiopulmonary bypass. These may compound injury already sustained, or can cause myocardial dysfunction through alterations in response to stimuli. Although there are numerous hypotheses concerning ischaemic injury, it is likely that these processes are tightly linked, and that the observed post-ischaemic myocardial dysfunction is related to a combination of these and other processes. Indeed, many of the manipulations designed to decrease ischaemia and reperfusion injury function at several different points on the path to injury. Thus, the application of an intervention to decrease injury must be timed appropriately so that it falls within the therapeutic window for that process.

ATP is the primary high-energy phosphate that fuels contraction and relaxation, and maintains ionic balance. When ATP breaks the actin-myosin cross bridge or fuels an ATP-dependent ionic pump, it is degraded to adenosine diphosphate (ADP). In the presence of oxygen, ATP is reformed with the addition of a phosphate. In the absence of oxygen, anaerobic metabolism cannot replenish these high-energy phosphates rapidly enough, and cellular ATP levels decline. ADP is further degraded to adenosine monophosphate (AMP), which is then broken down to adenosine, inosine, hypoxanthine and then uric acid. These breakdown products are released from the ischaemic cell and washed away during reperfusion, prohibiting the rapid conversion back to ATP (Weisel *et al.*, 1989). Of particular importance is the loss of adenosine, which is actively transported into the interstitial space where degradation to inosine proceeds rapidly. Although such a depletion of high-energy phosphates may contribute

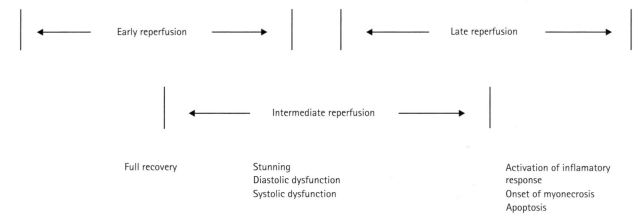

Figure 12.3 *Consequences of reperfusion after varying lengths of ischaemia. Reperfusion is vital to restoring oxygen to the tissues. However, reperfusion may also have detrimental consequences, which increase as the length of ischaemia increases.*

to myocardial dysfunction, evidence demonstrates that stunning may be present with normal levels of high-energy phosphates (Andres *et al.*, 1994).

Oxygen-derived free radicals are highly unstable compounds with an unpaired electron in their outer orbit. They are short-lived, and are formed in abundance upon reperfusion of ischaemic myocardium with oxygenated reperfusate. They cause injury by damaging proteins, nucleic acids, phospholipids and other cellular components. Sources of oxygen free radicals include both enzymatic and non-enzymatic reactions, and involve the generation of the superoxide radical, hydroxyl radical, hypochlorous acid and hydrogen peroxide. Examples of free radical-generating reactions are shown in Table 12.3. Although hydrogen peroxide is not a free radical by itself, it serves as a substrate for the generation of the highly injurious hydroxyl radical for which there are no natural scavengers. In the absence of ischaemia and reperfusion, free radical generation is minimal, and reactive oxygen species are readily eliminated by the actions of endogenous enzymes such as superoxide dismutase, catalase, glutathione and glutathione peroxidase. Some of the elimination pathways of oxygen free radicals are demonstrated in Table 12.4. However, in the setting of reperfusion after ischaemia, the generation of free radicals is dramatically increased because of several factors, and these endogenous systems are quickly overwhelmed. Alterations in enzyme function combine with an increase in free radical precursors to produce the highly reactive oxygen compounds. The Haber–Weiss reaction involves the generation of oxygen free radicals through a reaction catalyzed by iron, which is liberated by red cell hemolysis during cardiopulmonary bypass. Neutrophil activation serves as a potent source of free radicals when oxygen becomes available during reperfusion. To compound the problem, the normal scavengers of oxygen free radicals are depleted during the ischaemic interval, rendering the myocardium more susceptible to injury. Evidence to support the role of oxygen free radical-induced myocardial

Table 12.3 *Examples of free radical-generating reactions*

$2O_2 + NADPH \rightarrow 2O_2^- + NADPH^+$	NADPH oxidase-catalysed formation of superoxide radical
$Fe^{3+} + O_2^- \rightarrow Fe^{2+} + O_2$ $Fe^{2+} + H_2O_2 \rightarrow Fe^{3+} OH + OH^-$ (net) $O_2^- + H_2O_2 \rightarrow O_2 +$ $OH + OH^-$	Haber–Weiss reaction
$H_2O_2 + Cl^- \rightarrow OCl^- + H_2O$	Myeloperoxidase-catalysed formation of hypochlorous acid
$LH + OH \rightarrow L + H_2O$ $L + O_2 \rightarrow LOO$ $LOO + LH \rightarrow LOOH + L$ $L + L \rightarrow L - L$	Initiation and propagation of free radicals

O_2^- = superoxide radical; LH = fatty acid; L = lipid radical; LOO = peroxy radical; OCl^- = hypochlorous acid; LOOH = lipid hydroperoxide.

Table 12.4 *Elimination pathways of oxygen free radicals*

$2O_2^- + 2H^+ \rightarrow H_2O_2 + O_2$	SOD - catalysed dismutation of superoxide radical
$2H_2O_2 \rightarrow O_2 + H_2O$	Catalase - catalysed removal of hydrogen peroxide
$2GSH + LOOH \rightarrow$ $GSSG + LOH + H_2O$	Gluathione peroxidase-catalysed reduction of peroxides

GSH = glutathione; GSSG = oxidized glutathione; LOH = organic alcohol.

damage includes the identification of these species during the early reperfusion period, measurements of the end products of lipid peroxidation, and the ability of exogenously administered free radical scavengers to diminish both the measured free radicals and the resultant myocardial injury. However, not all studies demonstrate such an improvement with free radical scavengers, casting some doubt as to the significance of oxygen species in the origin of myocardial ischaemia and reperfusion injury.

The vascular endothelium is a complex structure that is responsive to, and the producer of, numerous autocoids, cytokines and other small signalling molecules. It is a significant source of adenosine and nitric oxide. Both have potent beneficial effects on coronary perfusion. Adenosine is produced by the endothelium, myocytes and neutrophils. Adenosine has many different actions that are mediated by a family of receptor subtypes. These functions include activation of the ATP-dependent potassium channel (K_{ATP}), inhibition of superoxide generation by neutrophils, and inhibition of neutrophil–endothelial interactions. Nitric oxide (NO) is produced by the vascular endothelium, both constituitively and in response to stimuli such as adenosine, acetylcholine and sheer stress. Both sources of NO release are altered by ischaemia–reperfusion injury (Tsao et al., 1990; Dignan et al., 1992; Nakanishi et al., 1994). This is manifested by an increase in the adherence of neutrophils, and by the impairment of NO-dependent vasodilatation. The vascular endothelium is also responsive to the actions of the vasoconstrictors endothelin and thromboxane. In the presence of endothelial injury, the production of – and responsiveness to – these substances is altered. This results in unregulated levels of myocardial perfusion that may not be adequate to meet the functional myocardial demands. The source of injury to the endothelium is multifold, and includes the same injurious stimuli to the myocytes, such as oxygen free radicals, complement activation and neutrophil migration. In addition, endothelial dysfunction may persist for days to weeks after the initial ischaemic event (Pearson et al., 1995). Endothelial dysfunction also occurs as a consequence of cardiopulmonary bypass itself, without superimposed ischaemia and reperfusion (Feerick et al., 1994).

Neutrophils are intimately involved in the inflammatory response, and they play a large role in the physiological state of the injured myocardium. The injurious effects of neutrophils are mediated through numerous substances and factors, including oxygen-derived free radicals, adhesion molecules and cytokines. Free radical generation is a normal function of the neutrophil in combating infection. However, pathological production of free radicals occurs in response to ischaemia and reperfusion, and these radicals are injurious to the surrounding tissues that have already been exposed to ischaemic injury. A portion of the harmful effects of activated neutrophils requires their adherence to the vascular endothelium. This is mediated by several classes of adhesion molecules, the expression of which is accentuated by the inflammatory state induced by cardiopulmonary bypass and ischaemia–reperfusion injury. The selectins are expressed on the neutrophil surface in response to ischaemia–reperfusion injury (Verrier and Shen, 1993; Kilbridge et al., 1994) and P-selectin results in the initial adherence of the neutrophil to the endothelium. Firm adherence is caused by the interaction of the β_2-integrins (CD11/CD18 complex) on the neutrophil and an activated adhesion molecule (ICAM-1) on the endothelium. Neutrophil accumulation has been demonstrated in myocardium after a period of ischaemia and reperfusion, and may be diminished by neutrophil suppression (Lefer et al., 1993; Nakanishi et al., 1992). This is accompanied by decreased myocardial injury. However, clinical use of neutrophil-depleted blood has not been shown to consistently improve myocardial protection (Browning et al., 1999; Mair et al., 1999).

Calcium homeostasis is intimately linked with proper cellular function. Calcium is present in the cytosol of the resting myocyte at a concentration of approximately 10^{-7} M. Upon cellular depolarization, a limited quantity of calcium enters the cell and triggers the release of calcium stored in the sarcoplasmic reticulum, and the free concentration of calcium is briefly increased to 10^{-5} M. This provides calcium required for myocardial contraction. Myocardial relaxation is associated with rapid uptake of calcium from the cytosol back into the sarcoplasmic reticulum, where it is stored until the next action potential. Despite the cellular dependence upon calcium for normal contraction, calcium is also toxic to the cell when its levels are not tightly controlled. After ischaemia and reperfusion, cytoplasmic calcium levels rapidly increase as calcium is released from the sarcoplasmic reticulum or crosses the plasma membrane through channels such as the sodium–calcium exchanger or the L-type calcium channel. As a result of the ischaemic injury and ATP depletion, the sarcoplasmic reticulum is incapable of maintaining normal cellular calcium levels. The elevation of cytosolic calcium has several harmful effects on the heart, including the activation of enzymes, triggering second messenger cascades and producing alterations in excitation–contraction coupling.

Cellular oedema occurs as a response to ischaemia and reperfusion. The mechanism of its formation is complex, but may depend upon the osmolality of the cardioplegia solution, the use of hypothermia, the accumulation of intracellular sodium ions and the extent of endothelial injury. Oedema is important because it occurs throughout the heart, including myocytes, conduction tissues and vascular endothelium. The impact of cellular oedema is important because it alters the function of these cells. Oedema has been implicated in contractile dysfunction and decreased ventricular compliance. In addition, oedema formation has been linked to the onset of the 'no reflow' phenomenon, in which capillary plugging occurs that inhibits perfusion of the coronary microcirculation when blood flow is restored to the heart.

Numerous mechanisms contribute significantly to myocardial ischaemia and reperfusion injury. The resulting dysfunction reflects alterations in cellular physiology on several different but related fronts. Any myocardial protection strategy must be well organized to address the major proposed sources of myocardial injury. Although some measures, such as the addition of free radical scavengers, combat a defined source of injury, others, such as the use of hypothermia, may offer non-specific protection against a broader range of stimuli. However, not all the proposed mechanisms of myocardial injury are sufficiently significant to justify elaborate measures designed to counteract them. The protective strategy should not be so complex that it interferes unduly with the timely conduct of the operation at hand. During a routine cardiac operation, a surgeon should use a simple, yet complete, basic strategy to provide adequate myocardial protection during the procedure. However, as the complexity of the operation increases, the basic strategy should be sufficiently flexible so that modifications may be made to provide the added level of myocardial protection yet minimize the additional complexity.

CONSEQUENCES OF ISCHAEMIA AND REPERFUSION INJURY

In its mildest form, ischaemia and reperfusion result in mild, temporary myocardial dysfunction known as 'stunning'. Severe injury is associated with irreversible damage and cell necrosis. The physiological manifestations of ischaemia and reperfusion, regardless of the cause, include systolic and diastolic dysfunction, arrhythmias and endothelial dysfunction. Although these forms of dysfunction serve as markers for injury, the clinical significance of these events is suboptimal myocardial performance, and the potential exacerbation of injury already sustained.

Subtle changes in systolic function may be difficult to identify because the measured parameters of left ventricular pressure, ejection fraction, stroke work index and cardiac index are load-sensitive. These measurements, therefore, do not represent the intrinsic function of the heart, but reflect the influence of ventricular load upon myocardial performance. Maximal systolic elastance (E_{max}) is a load-insensitive measurement of systolic function, but requires the creation of pressure–volume loops at different levels of volume loading. This is not generally practical in the clinical setting. Clinically apparent systolic dysfunction can occur after even short periods of ischaemia followed by reperfusion. It is most commonly identified clinically as low cardiac output in the presence of adequate or high filling pressures. In the setting of systolic dysfunction, the myocardium may remain responsive to the addition of exogenous inotropic agents, although this is not universal. The diastolic properties of the ventricular myocardium include the compliance and rate of relaxation of the myocardium. Diastolic function is highly sensitive to ischaemia and reperfusion injury.

Ventricular arrhythmias are usually the manifestation of either ischaemic injury present before the initiation of the operation, injury sustained as a result of poor myocardial protection, or from incomplete revascularization. An example of the first is acute ischaemia necessitating emergent coronary artery bypass grafting (CABG). The frequency of the occurrence of arrhythmias from ischaemic injury follows a bell-shaped curve. Arrhythmias are relatively uncommon after brief ischaemic intervals, increase in frequency as the duration of ischaemia increases and then decrease again with the onset of irreversible injury. Arrhythmias may also be a manifestation of, or exacerbated by, electrolyte abnormalities. The specialized conduction system of the ventricles may be more susceptible to ischaemic injury than are the contractile elements. Arrhythmias may occur after either regional or global injury, and may present as frequent premature ventricular contractions, or life-threatening arrhythmias such as ventricular tachycardia or fibrillation.

Endothelial dysfunction is difficult to assess clinically, but has wide-ranging effects. The damaged endothelium may be the site for complement activation or for neutrophil adherence and transmigration. The endothelium is also a critical component in vascular reactivity. The endothelium is a source of several vasoactive agents, and is responsive to these and substances produced elsewhere. The endothelium regulates the delicate balance between vasorelaxation and vasoconstriction through its production of and response to the relative influences of these vasoactive agents. Active substances include nitric oxide, adenosine, thromboxane and endothelin among others. The myocardial 'no reflow' phenomenon (Kloner et al., 1974) represents areas of myocardium that do not undergo reperfusion at the end of an ischaemic period. The endothelium plays a critical role in the development of areas of no reflow because of the altered function of the damaged endothelium. This is due, at least in part, to altered endothelium-dependent vasorelaxation, capillary plugging from activated neutrophils, increased myocardial diastolic stiffness and capillary compression caused by myocardial oedema.

CRITERIA FOR ASSESSMENT OF MYOCARDIAL PROTECTIVE STRATEGIES

Most methods of myocardial protection undergo rigorous laboratory evaluation before extensive use in human subjects. Initial evaluation is often in the form of studies in the isolated animal heart. Although these data may eventually prove reliable, significant compromises are taken in this situation. The isolated heart is devoid of collateral circulation, which eliminates cardioplegia washout that would otherwise occur. The function of the isolated heart is no longer dependent on neural input, and no longer must respond to alterations in after-load, or variations in systemic catecholamine levels. The isolated heart does not exhibit obstructive coronary artery disease, and thus distribution of experimental cardioplegia may be more uniform than can be expected in the diseased heart. In addition, these initial studies are often performed with crystalloid-based cardioplegia that may have little similarity to the sanguinous cardioplegia used in most clinical settings. Lastly, studies performed with regional ischaemia, as opposed to global ischaemia, may prove highly inaccurate when attempting to project these findings onto a surgical model of global ischaemia. In regional ischaemia, collateral flow may provide some level of oxygenation to the border zone, as well as washout of ischaemic metabolites, both of which are absent during global ischaemia. The choice of endpoints used in the laboratory assessment of myocardial protection requires some degree of compromise. The effectiveness of an intervention in preserving myocardial function must often be based on measurements such as myocardial high-energy phosphate content, contractile force against a given after-load at fixed pre-load or gross estimates on the degree of myocardial infarction. Since these measurements are only approximations of myocardial protection, inaccurate assumptions regarding the effectiveness of a given intervention may result.

Clinical studies of cardioplegia additives may rely on surrogate markers of injury and functional recovery, such as enzyme release, overall myocardial function or patient survival, to gauge the effectiveness of a given agent. Although myocardial function and survival are the most important results, ventricular function is difficult to measure accurately and reliably in the clinical setting. Most patients with good ventricular function will do well with standard protection strategies, and subtle differences will be difficult to detect. However, in patients with poor pre-operative ventricular function, the variability between patients is great enough to make it difficult to achieve statistical significance when studying strategies that offer small degrees of additional protection. In addition, clinically applicable methods of determining myocardial function in the peri-operative setting are often poorly reproducible because of the influence of exogenous catecholamines and other patient-dependent variables upon the results. Subtle variations in myocardial protection strategies between different surgeons may make even single-center studies subject to question since some interventions may not work in the setting of a different overall protection strategy. Thus, it may require numerous patients under the care of a single surgeon to answer accurately some of the questions about myocardial protective techniques, and even then, the applicability of these data to other surgeons, with their own variations in protective strategies, may be in question.

PURPOSE OF CARDIOPLEGIA

Before the invention of an effective method of cardiopulmonary bypass, cardiac procedures were performed upon the beating heart out of necessity. Elaborate techniques were developed to enable surgeons to perform intracardiac procedures, such as suture closure of atrial septal defects, atrial septectomy and valvuloplasty, in the beating heart. However, air embolism was a constant concern whenever the left side of the heart was entered. More complex procedures were made possible through the use of hypothermic circulatory arrest and, later, through cross-perfusion techniques. After the advent of cardiopulmonary bypass, the scope and complexity of cardiac surgical procedures increased, along with the safety of these procedures. The ability to arrest the heart for prolonged periods of time with reliable systemic perfusion required new methods of myocardial protection. Hypothermia alone provided some myocardial protection but was not sufficient for prolonged periods of ischaemia. The advent of cardioplegia provided the route through which the heart could be reliably and rapidly arrested, and the ability to maintain this state with additional doses of cardioplegia.

The goals of myocardial protective strategies are to provide preservation of myocardial function, a bloodless operative field, myocardial quiescence, and to allow for rapid resumption of contractile activity at the conclusion of the procedure. Although numerous strategies have been developed towards this end, there are major differences between them. And, although some components of a given strategy may be broadly applicable and useful when combined with other strategies, others are not readily interchangeable. Indeed, the choice of a warm or tepid temperature for performing an operation dictates the type of cardioplegia and its frequency of administration. Variations in the composition of the cardioplegia may prove disastrous in this setting, despite being advantageous in the setting of a different strategy of myocardial protection. However, all successful myocardial protective strategies recognize the time periods before, during and after the imposed ischaemia in order to lessen the damage to the myocardium.

INTERVENTION BEFORE THE ONSET OF ISCHAEMIA

Myocardial protection begins before the patient arrives in the operating room. Proper planning includes optimization of the patient to best tolerate a cardiac procedure. This may include nutritional intervention, pharmacological manipulation or the placement of an intra-aortic balloon pump to limit ongoing myocardial ischaemia. In addition, the conduct of the operation must be planned around the patient's disease and cardiac status. At times, the best forms of myocardial protection may require the use of beating heart or other non-ischaemic strategies. Alternatively, arrangements may also be required for alterations in the routine protective strategy to take into account unique characteristics of an individual patient, such as ventricular hypertrophy, aortic insufficiency or severe coronary artery disease.

In the elective setting, most hearts have adequate energy stores and are thus able to tolerate a moderate ischaemic interval. However, hearts that are depleted of energy stores have very little reserve, and tolerate ischaemia poorly. Glycogen is an important source of energy for the heart, and a depressed glycogen level is correlated with poor post-operative outcome (Lolley et al., 1985). Glycogen stores may be repleted pre-operatively with the administration of glucose, insulin and potassium (GIK) solution. This has been shown to augment glycogen levels (Lolley et al., 1985; Oldfield et al., 1986) and to improve post-operative myocardial function in both the experimental (McElroy et al., 1989) and clinical (Oldfield et al., 1986) settings. In patients undergoing elective mitral valve replacement, glycogen stores are increased with pre-operative GIK infusion, and these patients experience fewer post-operative complications (Oldfield et al., 1986). However, the mechanism through which GIK infusion works is unclear, and it may represent improved metabolic reserves in the form of glycogen, increased ATP stores from the insulin infusion, or some other mechanism.

Global ischaemia is not always an integral part of cardiac procedures. The recent rebirth of beating heart surgery has been promoted by the growth in technology such as improved myocardial stabilization devices. By improving the exposure and limiting epicardial movement, these devices permit the performance of bypasses previously considered impossible in the beating heart. Intraluminal flow-through devices may be placed through the coronary arteriotomy to permit continuous downstream perfusion during the performance of the anastomosis. With the use of a flow-through device, or the performance of a rapid anastomosis, the period of ischaemia can be limited so that permanent myocardial damage does not ensue. Thus, in such circumstances, the issue of myocardial protection is less critical than in the scenario of prolonged global ischaemia. Another alternative is the performance of cardiac procedures on full cardiopulmonary bypass, but with continuous myocardial perfusion. Procedures using the warm, beating heart with cardiopulmonary support provide continuous myocardial perfusion, yet allow increased manipulation of the heart to access difficult to reach vessels without producing systemic hypotension that might otherwise ensue. With extracorporeal haemodynamic support, the effect of any period of ischaemia is lessened because of the diminished energy consumption achieved with ventricular unloading, since myocardial oxygen consumption decreases to approximately 20 per cent of the energy use at baseline as the work of pumping blood is eliminated. However, ischaemia can occur unwittingly if the heart is distorted to produce kinking of the coronary vessels. In addition, should complications develop and ischaemia ensue, there is little margin of safety since the heart remains warm and unprotected.

Once bypass is initiated, myocardial hypothermia can be used to provide greater safety during intentional or unintentional periods of ischaemia. At low temperatures, ventricular fibrillation often occurs. Hypothermic fibrillatory arrest allows operations to be conducted upon the heart with minimal motion without the interruption of coronary perfusion. Further, since the heart is not beating, the left heart can be entered during the performance of the procedure. As long as the left heart is adequately de-aired at the conclusion of the operation, the risk of systemic air embolism is minimized. However, during the period of fibrillation, subendocardial perfusion pressure is decreased because of high wall tension imposed by the fibrillation, a situation that may be particularly important in the hypertrophied heart (Hottenrott et al., 1973; Sink et al., 1983). Perfusion can be improved by venting the left heart with a sump catheter placed through the right superior pulmonary vein into the left ventricle, and by maintaining higher systemic perfusion pressures. An additional benefit attained through the concomitant use of hypothermia during ventricular fibrillation is the increased protection of the subendocardium from the addition of myocardial cooling. Overall, this technique is not widely used today, although good results have been reported (Akins, 1984; Akins and Carroll, 1987). Intermittent aortic cross-clamping can be used with mild hypothermia and ventricular fibrillation to provide a bloodless field during the performance of the distal anastomoses. In this setting, there has been improved preservation of ventricular diastolic function compared with the use of standard cardioplegic methods (Casthely et al., 1997). The use of ventricular fibrillation in the absence of hypothermia has been attempted in the past, with the use of an alternating current electrical stimulator. One caveat with this approach is the potential for the heart to spontaneously convert to sinus rhythm should the stimulator lose contact with the epicardium. This may be critical during intracardiac procedures where normal electrical activity could lead to the ejection of air into the systemic circulation. More importantly, however, fibrillation with an electrical stimulator at normothermia is very energy-consuming and may result in substantial subendocardial necrosis (Buckberg and Hottenrott, 1975). It is thus not a recommended technique.

An additional source of pre-ischaemic protection can be provided through myocardial pre-conditioning. Classical pre-conditioning refers to the phenomenon through which the myocardium is made able to better tolerate a period of ischaemia shortly after a pre-ischaemic event. It involves the activation of receptors and second messenger systems, as opposed to the 'second window' form of pre-conditioning that occurs much later after a stimulus and involves alterations in gene expression. The initial work on pre-conditioning demonstrated that hearts subjected to a brief period of ischaemia produced smaller areas of infarction when subjected to a subsequent longer period of ischaemia (Murry et al., 1986; Yellon et al., 1992). Pre-conditioning of the myocardium has been induced experimentally through a variety of interventions, and demonstrates that the heart actively participates in protective processes. Classical pre-conditioning has been induced through brief intermittent periods of ischaemia, hyperthermia (Liu et al., 1992) or pre-treatment with a variety of drugs. Bradykinin, nitric oxide, phenylepherine, endotoxin, adenosine (Ely et al., 1985) and potassium channel openers are just a few of the drugs that have been demonstrated to provide a pre-conditioning response. The mechanisms through which these different interventions result in pre-conditioning is unclear, but it is likely to involve activation of second messenger systems and subsequent induction of enzymes that then improve the tolerance of the myocyte to ischaemia and reperfusion. The final common pathway may involve alterations in intracellular calcium concentration. Neither the inhibition mRNA transcription nor protein synthesis blocks the classical pre-conditioning response experimentally, suggesting that the stress response is not required for pre-conditioning (Thornton et al., 1990). The interval between the pre-conditioning stimulus and the final ischaemic event is critical, as there is both a minimum and maximum period of reperfusion, outside of which the protective effect of the pre-conditioning stimulus disappears. In the rat, the minimum period of reperfusion between the pre-conditioning stimulus and ischaemia is between 30 and 60 seconds (Alkhulaifi et al., 1993). The length of the protective effect depends on the species and model, and rarely exceeds two hours. In addition, pre-conditioning is only effective when the length of the subsequent ischaemic interval is limited, as it offers no protection for extensive periods of ischaemia. There is also a threshold to pre-conditioning, beyond which increasing the number of pre-conditioning ischaemic episodes becomes detrimental (Iliodromitis et al., 1997).

Although experimental pre-conditioning has been linked to decreased infarct size in models of regional ischaemia, preservation of high-energy phosphates and improved myocardial function, clinical data regarding pre-conditioning in humans is controversial. In the setting of coronary angioplasty, a period of ischaemia has been associated with less angina, myocardial lactate production and EKG changes if preceded by a brief period of ischaemia followed by five minutes of reperfusion (Deutsch et al., 1990). Similarly, beneficial effects have been demonstrated clinically after a brief period of normothermic ischaemia before a subsequent ischaemic interval, including preservation of ATP levels (Yellon et al., 1993), diminished troponin T release (Jenkins et al., 1997) and diminished ST segment elevations, decreased creatine kinase-MB release and improved myocardial contractility (Lu et al., 1998). However, the benefits of ischaemic pre-conditioning have not been seen universally (Cremer et al., 1997). Differences in the results may reflect the manner in which ischaemic pre-conditioning was induced, since the application of an aortic cross-clamp above a beating heart to induce ischaemia is potentially damaging. Clinically, the benefits of pre-conditioning have been demonstrated most commonly in the setting of unprotected myocardial ischaemia. However, when cardioplegia, hypothermia or other protective methods are employed, pre-conditioning does not usually appear to offer an additional advantage in terms of myocardial preservation (Perrault and Menasche, 1999) despite the positive results seen in the laboratory (Cave and Hearse, 1992). Similarly, pre-conditioning is unlikely to offer any benefit when the injury sustained by the heart is minimal (Faris et al., 1997), a situation analogous to elective coronary surgery. Although the clinical applicability of pre-conditioning remains to be determined for routine cardiac surgery, it will most likely offer benefit in cases where suboptimal myocardial protection is likely. Examples of this include the hypertrophied ventricle, severe coronary artery disease where conventional methods may not provide global protection and off-pump revascularization procedures. Beating heart surgery does not use the most common methods of myocardial protection. Even though the periods of ischaemia are usually brief during the performance of an anastomosis, there is little margin for error. Thus, a pre-conditioning stimulus may offer a small safety net of protection. Although some surgeons routinely use a pre-conditioning period of ischaemia before performing the distal anastomosis, the benefits have yet to be clinically proved.

Lastly, an additional intervention, immediately before the onset of ischaemia, has proved very beneficial. The pre-ischaemic administration of oxygenated warm blood cardioplegia provides oxygen and substrates to the myocardium while the high potassium concentration produces mechanical quiescence. Energy demands of the heart are thus minimized, and the substrates are provided in excess of the metabolic requirements of the heart. In addition, the even distribution of the cardioplegia throughout the myocardium is enhanced since the heart is arrested in diastole. Thus, the cardioplegic solution may serve to direct substrates to the reparative processes that will occur after ischaemia (Rosenkranz et al., 1982, 1983).

INTERVENTION DURING ISCHAEMIA

Most of the efforts directed towards myocardial protection have focused on interventions at the initiation of ischaemia or during ongoing ischaemia. These actions are generally designed to decrease oxygen demand, improve oxygen delivery or ameliorate the harmful effects of ischaemia on substrates, cellular oedema or ionic gradients. There are numerous variations in cardioplegic solutions and techniques. Some of the major variables include the temperature at which the myocardium is maintained, the route of cardioplegia delivery, whether the cardioplegia is crystalloid or blood based and additives to the cardioplegia to produce desired results. If the onset of ischaemia precedes the initiation of protection, much if not all of the benefit of the protective strategy will be lost, as energy demands in the warm active myocardium are very high and the ischaemic myocardium will rapidly develop an energy debt. In the heart with ongoing unprotected ischaemia, the purpose of the myocardial protective strategy must be designed to mitigate the effects of reperfusion since the first dose of cardioplegia will essentially provide a brief period of reperfusion before the onset of surgical ischaemia.

Myocardial temperature

Decreased myocardial temperature reduces oxygen consumption significantly, and the use of hypothermia in myocardial protection is widespread. The protective effects of hypothermia relate to the Q_{10} effect, in which there is a 50 per cent decrease in the myocardial oxygen consumption (MVO_2) for every 10°C decrease in myocardial temperature. Thus, moderate hypothermia, with a decrease in myocardial temperature from 37°C to 25°C, produces a decrease in oxygen consumption in excess of 50 per cent. Further decreases in oxygen consumption are less impressive as the myocardial temperature is decreased below 22°C. Improved protection does occur at lower temperatures, but the relative degree of gain is less as the temperature continues to drop (Rosenfeldt, 1982). Despite the small added gains in myocardial oxygen consumption at lower temperatures, profound myocardial hypothermia to 4°C is relatively safe (Swanson et al., 1980), as evidenced by good myocardial preservation in cardiac transplantation (English et al., 1980). However, myocardial hypothermia has been associated with cellular injury and other detrimental effects. The changes include decreased plasma membrane fluidity and transmembrane transport, increased intracellular oedema and sodium accumulation, altered ionic balance and protein denaturation. The net result may be a delay in recovery of ventricular function (Fremes et al., 1985; Weisel et al., 1989; Yau et al., 1993) despite protection from ischaemic injury.

In addition, oxygen dissociation from haemoglobin is further impaired as myocardial temperature continues to fall. Thus, profound hypothermia is associated with more potential complications without significant added benefit compared with moderate hypothermia. Any potential advantages obtained at these lower temperatures are minimized in the setting of hyperkalaemic myocardial arrest, where the incremental decrease in myocardial oxygen consumption obtained through superimposed hypothermia is less than that seen without arrest.

There are several methods to cool the heart, and the technique of myocardial cooling may influence its effectiveness. Systemic cooling on cardiopulmonary bypass can achieve low myocardial temperatures, although the process is slow because the entire body must also be cooled to the desired myocardial temperature. In addition, the time required to rewarm from profound systemic hypothermia is prolonged for the same reason. When myocardial cooling is used without systemic hypothermia, unintentional myocardial rewarming may occur caused by one of several sources, including direct rewarming from contact along the diaphragmatic and posterior surfaces of the heart, return of systemic blood to the right atrium from the cavae and return of non-coronary collateral perfusion to the right side of the heart. Thus, the advantage of use of systemic hypothermia in conjunction with myocardial cooling is that rewarming of the heart from collateral circulation does not occur to a significant degree. In the absence of profound systemic hypothermia, the frequent administration of cold cardioplegia may be required to avoid regional rewarming and poor protection to those areas.

Topical methods of cooling include the placement of ice, saline slush or a cooling jacket in direct contact with the external surfaces of the heart. The use of ice or slush has several shortcomings. The myocardial temperature may be difficult to control, and areas of the heart may be cooled to temperatures below 0°C (Speicher et al., 1962). This may produce uneven cooling resulting in uneven protection, damage to myocardial tissues that are cooled too deeply, and damage to the phrenic nerve due to prolonged contact with low temperature solutions (Nikas et al., 1998). In addition, the use of ice may cause an increased incidence of post-operative pleural effusions and atelectasis, without an improvement in cardiac enzyme release or inotropic requirements after CABG (Allen et al., 1992). More evenly distributed cooling can be achieved through the continuous application of cold saline irrigation into the pericardium (Lazar and Rivers, 1989) and the use of cold saline has been associated with fewer complications than the use of iced solutions (Allen et al., 1992). External cooling devices have also been developed that allow for continuous cooling with the benefit of decreased bypass time because of the elimination of the need for multidose cardioplegia (Daily et al., 1987). Topical methods of cooling can be used to cool all portions of the heart effectively under optimal conditions. However, the right ventricle is easier to cool through topical means than the left because of the differences in ventricular thickness. This situation may be exaggerated in the presence of left ventricular hypertrophy, and topical cooling is clearly inappropriate as the major method for cooling in this setting. Although external cooling could be used as the sole method of myocardial cooling under normal conditions, it is typically used as an adjunctive measure to other methods of cooling. In combination with mild or moderate systemic hypothermia, topical cooling permits deeper cooling of the myocardium with its attendant benefits, yet minimizes the requirement for deep systemic hypothermia and allows less time for systemic cooling and rewarming.

More commonly, rapid cooling of the heart is attained through the administration of cold cardioplegic solution at a temperature of 4–10°C. Cold cardioplegia may be administered in the antegrade direction through the coronary arteries either by way of the aortic root or through direct ostial cannulation. Alternatively, retrograde administration of hypothermic cardioplegia solution may be used instead of, or in conjunction with, antegrade administration. This is performed through a cannula placed in the coronary sinus. While the use of cardioplegia produces myocardial hypothermia, the myocardial temperature does not necessarily match the temperature of the cardioplegia. In the canine heart, crystalloid cardioplegia delivered at a temperature of 20°C produced a myocardial temperature of 21.5°C. However, when the crystalloid was cooled to 10°C and 4°C, the myocardial temperature declined to only 16.2°C and 15.0°C, respectively (Magovern et al., 1982). In this model, myocardial functional recovery was similar with crystalloid cardioplegia at either 10°C or 4°C and greater compared with cardioplegia at 20°C. When the cooling from the administration of cardioplegia is insufficient, topical cooling may be used as an adjunct to antegrade cardioplegia to increase the rapidity of cooling, or with retrograde cardioplegia to improve cooling of the right ventricle.

Even when the operation is to be conducted under hypothermic conditions, the initial dose of cardioplegia may be either hypothermic or normothermic. When normothermia is used for induction, it must be blood-based cardioplegia, whereas cold cardioplegia may be based on either blood or crystalloid solutions. The advantage of warm induction is that it may lead to greater preservation of myocardial metabolites and thus accelerate functional recovery (Rosenkranz et al., 1982). Part of the rationale for this method is that in the ischaemic heart, the initial administration of cardioplegia may actually represent 'reperfusion' of underperfused tissues, and that they may benefit from the metabolic enhancements made available through warm induction (Rosenkranz et al., 1986). The use of warm cardioplegia produces myocardial arrest,

thus minimizing myocardial oxygen demand. At the same time, oxygen and other metabolic substrates are provided to the myocardium in excess of the demands of the tissue. With warm cardioplegia, the substrates are delivered to the myocardium at a temperature where cellular synthetic processes can occur.

An extension of warm induction has been the use of warm cardioplegia for the duration of the procedure. Clinical studies have demonstrated that continuous warm cardioplegia produces adequate myocardial protection with decreased incidence of peri-operative myocardial infarction (Lichtenstein et al., 1991) and less post-operative low output syndrome (Naylor et al., 1994) or dependence upon intra-aortic balloon pump support (Lichtenstein et al., 1991). When systemic temperatures are allowed to drift downwards during the course of the operation to 33–35°C, and other confounding variables are limited, there also appears to be good neurological protection (Wong et al., 1992; McLean et al., 1994). The use of warm cardioplegia requires the use of blood cardioplegia since oxygen delivery through oxygenated crystalloid cardioplegic methods is insufficient to meet the metabolic needs of the warm myocardium. In addition, since the myocardium is maintained at normothermia, and the metabolic processes of the heart are uninterrupted, the basal energy demands of the heart remain significant. Thus, cardioplegia must be given continuously to avoid the development of anaerobic metabolism and its attendant consequences. Indeed, normothermic cardioplegia provides adequate myocardial protection when delivered at a minimal rate of 80 mL/min with a blood to crystalloid ratio of 4:1 (Yau et al., 1991). A drawback of this technique is that it depends upon good, even distribution of the cardioplegia throughout the myocardium. This is not always possible in the setting of severe coronary vascular disease or ventricular hypertrophy, and the use of warm cardioplegia in this setting may result in unrecognized ischaemic injury.

A recent modification in myocardial temperature has been the use of tepid (29°C) cardioplegia. This was investigated as a manner of providing some degree of myocardial protection obtained through a decrease in temperature, whilst minimizing the deleterious side effects of myocardial hypothermia. Clinical results indicate that cold cardioplegia produces the least anaerobic lactate release and myocardial oxygen consumption, with higher levels of both with tepid cardioplegia, and still higher with warm cardioplegia. In contrast, warm and tepid cardioplegia produce greater left ventricular stroke work index, with immediate return of cardiac function with reperfusion (Hayashida et al., 1994). Thus, tepid cardioplegia results in improved myocardial performance compared with cold cardioplegia while providing improved myocardial protection versus warm cardioplegia. Despite the possible advantages of warm or tepid cardioplegia, myocardial cooling remains superior under some settings. Since warm and tepid cardioplegia are associated with a higher level of myocardial metabolism than cold cardioplegia, they require distribution to all portions of the myocardium to provide adequate protection. This may not be possible in the setting of severe ventricular hypertrophy, severe occlusive coronary artery disease or in the presence of an acute infarction. In the latter, myocardial damage is ongoing at the time of the operation, and acute coronary occlusion lessens the probability of cardioplegic delivery to the ischaemic area. In this setting, continuous retrograde hypothermic cardioplegia results in lower myocardial oxygen consumption in the first hour of reperfusion than either warm or tepid cardioplegia, suggesting that it produces improved ventricular protection (Bufkin et al., 1994). Thus, there are clinical settings where hypothermic delivery is preferred.

Crystalloid and blood cardioplegia

Crystalloid cardioplegia has been studied extensively, and numerous solutions, both commercially available and locally produced, are clinically in use. Blood cardioplegia has gained popularity since the 1980s, and is now the most common type of cardioplegia in use in adult cardiac surgery. One of the major advantages of blood cardioplegia is its simplicity. Blood naturally contains beneficial substances, such as free radical scavengers, buffers, metabolic substrates and haemoglobin for oxygen transport. Despite this, proponents of crystalloid cardioplegia persist, citing the advantages of this method of myocardial protection. Since crystalloid solutions are completely manufactured, all the components of these solutions can be rigorously controlled. In order to achieve the benefits of oxygen delivery to the myocardium at the time of cardioplegia administration, oxygen can be added to crystalloid cardioplegia. Although crystalloid-based solutions do not have the benefit of haemoglobin to augment oxygen-carrying capacity, the amount of oxygen released from haemoglobin at hypothermic temperatures is greatly reduced because of a left shift in the oxygen–haemoglobin dissociation curve. Because of this shift, a significant proportion of the oxygen that is delivered to the tissues is from the oxygen that is dissolved in the plasma and is therefore not bound to haemoglobin. In addition, the metabolic demands of the myocardium are significantly reduced during hypothermia, and the amount of oxygen dissolved in a crystalloid solution and thus available to the myocardium may be sufficient to meet these reduced metabolic needs (Ledingham, 1988). With the use of additives, and under proper clinical conditions, crystalloid cardioplegia can provide very good myocardial protection. However, each additive increases the complexity of the myocardial protective strategy. In most instances,

these additives also serve to make crystalloid cardioplegia more like blood cardioplegia in composition and function, suggesting that it may be simpler to start with a blood-based solution.

In contrast to the tightly controlled composition of crystalloid cardioplegia, blood contains many known and unknown factors that affect its effectiveness as a cardioplegic agent. Many of the components available in blood are the desired substances that are subsequently added to crystalloid cardioplegia, including buffers, metabolic substrates, oxygen free radical scavengers, colloids and oxygen carriers. Thus, it appears that blood is the ideal basis for cardioplegia. Even though blood has many desirable characteristics, it also has some potential shortcomings. The added oxygen-carrying capacity of haemoglobin may not be fully used if very low temperatures are used, because the oxygen available from hypothermic blood is not much greater than that from saline at the same temperature (Digerness et al., 1981). Although it may be clinically insignificant, a major concern about the use of blood cardioplegia relates to the increased viscosity of blood compared with crystalloid solutions. The difference in viscosity is further accentuated in the setting of profound hypothermia. In this setting, the use of blood cardioplegia has been reported to lead to sludging within the coronary microcirculation with occlusion of the capillaries, resulting in unperfused capillary beds and subsequent myocardial ischaemia (Sakai et al.,1988; Gundry et al.,1989). However, clinical use of blood cardioplegia has produced excellent results, negating most of the concerns about sludging in the capillaries. The effect of sanguinous cardioplegia in the setting of critical coronary artery stenosis is controversial. In a canine model of critical coronary stenosis, the use of blood cardioplegia resulted in diminished blood flow to regions supplied by an inflow-restricted coronary vessel. However, flow levels were returned to normal with the use of haemodilution to a hematocrit of 20 vol% (Chitwood et al., 1983). An unfavourable endocardial to epicardial blood flow ratio persisted despite normal regional flow rates, which may have produced unintended endocardial ischaemia. However, in another canine model, blood cardioplegia with a hematocrit of 30 vol% produced higher aortic root pressures during delivery, higher flow distal to a critical stenosis, more rapid myocardial arrest, and more rapid myocardial cooling distal to the stenosis than crystalloid cardioplegia delivered at the same flow rate (Robertson et al., 1983). The improved perfusion of the area of myocardium supplied by the stenotic artery with blood cardioplegia was thought to be caused by diversion of the asanguineous cardioplegia to the regions supplied by normal coronary vessels. To counteract this, crystalloid cardioplegia could be delivered at a similar aortic root pressure to blood cardioplegia, but this could require very large volumes of crystalloid cardioplegia to produce arrest and provide even myocardial protection (Robertson *et al.*, 1983).

Both methods of cardioplegia have strong proponents and opponents, and numerous studies support the safety of either method. Since the 1980s, the use of blood cardioplegia has increased so that it is now the most common type of cardioplegia currently in use. Its popularity rests, in part, with its ease of use and with the beneficial components already present in blood. Despite the widespread use of blood-based cardioplegia, the published data is divided regarding the optimal cardioplegic solution. Blood cardioplegia has been shown to be beneficial compared with crystalloid cardioplegia (Robertson *et al.*, 1983; Vinten-Johansen *et al.*, 1986) in laboratory studies. However, it has also been shown to be of no significant consequence (Rousou *et al.*, 1988) or even detrimental in the setting of profound myocardial hypothermia (Magovern *et al.*, 1982). Clinical studies have similarly shown benefit (Fremes *et al.*, 1984; Iverson *et al.*, 1984; Codd *et al.*, 1985; Christakis *et al.*, 1986a) or no effect (Shapira *et al.*, 1980; Roberts *et al.*, 1982). However, blood cardioplegia has also been shown to have detrimental effects, with decreased right ventricular systolic function after blood cardioplegia (Mullen *et al.*, 1987). Although Roberts and colleagues (Roberts *et al.*, 1982) cited no benefit to blood cardioplegia in the group as a whole, those patients with depressed ejection fraction or longer ischaemic times did show improvement with blood cardioplegia compared with crystalloid cardioplegia. Cited clinical benefits of blood cardioplegia include improved systolic functional recovery, decreased ischaemic injury and decreased myocardial anaerobic metabolism (Fremes *et al.*, 1984). However, long-term follow-up has shown no difference in late post-operative ventricular function (Mullen *et al.*, 1986).

Major difficulties arise when trying to compare blood with crystalloid cardioplegia in either the laboratory or clinical arenas. The composition of blood cardioplegia is complicated by nature because of the numerous constituents present in blood. To make a truly fair comparison, the crystalloid solution should also contain all the components that are already present in blood that have been demonstrated to be important. Thus, in a comparison study, the crystalloid cardioplegia used must represent the optimal formulation available. In addition, the optimal route, rate, frequency, temperature and volume of administration must be used for each type of cardioplegia, and these may be significantly different between the two techniques. For example, while crystalloid cardioplegia given at a temperature of 10°C or 4°C provides superior protection to crystalloid given at 20°C, blood cardioplegia given at 20°C has been shown to be superior to blood cardioplegia given at 4°C (Magovern *et al.*, 1982). Thus, in order to truly compare these two solutions, each under its own presumed optimal conditions, the overall

protection strategies may be sufficiently different to cloud the issue as to whether the benefit of one solution over another is caused by the cardioplegia, or by other differences in the conduct of the operation. There is a strong interrelationship between myocardial temperature, the type of cardioplegia used, and the frequency of cardioplegia administration, as illustrated in Fig. 12.4. At cold temperatures, approaching 4°C, either blood or crystalloid cardioplegia may be used with equivalent results. Similarly, at these colder temperatures, adequate myocardial protection can be achieved in the normal heart with single-dose cardioplegia. However, as the temperature of the myocardium approaches 30°C, the advantages of blood cardioplegia become more apparent. In addition, warmer temperatures require the use of multidose or continuous cardioplegia in order to provide adequate oxygen delivery to the tissues and washout of the metabolites that accumulate during ischaemia.

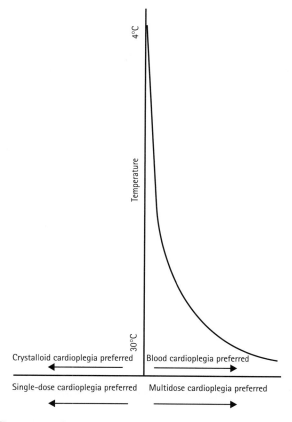

Figure 12.4 *Relationship between myocardial temperature, composition of cardioplegia, and the frequency of administration. As temperatures are increased towards normothermia, crystalloid cardioplegia becomes unacceptable as a protective agent, as oxygen delivery with crystalloid is insufficient to meet the metabolic demands of the warm myocardium. In addition, as the myocardium warms, the frequency of cardioplegia delivery must increase, such that normothermic cardioplegia must be administered continuously.*

Typically, blood cardioplegia is derived by the addition of oxygenated blood from the bypass circuit to a crystalloid base, at a defined ratio (1:1 to 4:1, blood:crystalloid), to produce a final solution with a haematocrit of 16–20 vol%. The ratio of blood to crystalloid is controlled by the ratio of the tubing diameters used for the blood and the crystalloid solution. Both lengths of tubing are run through a single pump head. Since the ratio of the tubing diameters is constant, the ratio of blood to crystalloid is fixed, regardless of the pump rate. The ideal blood:crystalloid ratio is not known, but at normothermia, continuous high-haemoglobin (4:1) cardioplegia produces a significantly lower myocardial oxygen consumption (MVO_2) after cross-clamp release than low-haemoglobin cardioplegia at low flow rates (<80 mL/min). However, this benefit is lost at high flow rates, as either high- or low-haemoglobin cardioplegia produces effective myocardial protection (Yau et al., 1991). With hypothermic arrest, cardioplegia with a haematocrit of either 10 vol% or 20 vol% produces equal metabolic recovery in the canine heart, although the effectiveness of the protection decreases as the temperature of the myocardium increases to 30°C (Rousou et al., 1988). Thus, the ideal blood:crystalloid ratio for a given myocardial protection protocol is likely to depend on the temperature and flow rate of the cardioplegia, as well as other factors.

As blood cardioplegia is used more frequently, many of the myths about it are being dispelled. The safety of increasing ratios of blood to cardioplegia has been documented (Ihnken et al., 1994). A recent addition to the surgeon's armamentarium has been the concept of microplegia, in which the crystalloid component of blood cardioplegia has been virtually eliminated. In this formulation, blood is taken directly from the pump, and minimally modified with the addition of potassium, and sometimes magnesium, to produce a cardioplegic solution (Menasche et al., 1993; Sydzyik et al., 1997). The advantage of minimizing the haemodilution is that the beneficial aspects of blood cardioplegia are preserved, and the resultant cellular oedema is lessened. Clinical results support the efficacy of this strategy of myocardial protection (Menasche et al., 1993).

Route of cardioplegia administration

Cardioplegia may be administered into the coronary circulation in either an antegrade or retrograde fashion. Antegrade administration is most commonly undertaken through the placement of a cardioplegia cannula into the aortic root. Cardioplegia is infused into the root after the cross clamp has been placed on the aorta. The rate of cardioplegia administration is based on the perfusion pressure in the aortic root, and on the stage of the operation. The induction flow rate is based on the body surface area

of the patient, and is often 150 mL/min per m². However, the rate of infusion must be increased to maintain a minimum aortic root pressure, and thus even distribution of the cardioplegia and uniform myocardial protection. The volume of cardioplegia given in the initial dose is approximately 10–15 mL/kg, up to a total dose of 1000 mL. The infusion must be given slowly, over several minutes. Rapid infusion of cardioplegia results in uneven distribution and poor protection (Takahashi et al., 1988, 1989). The antegrade route of cardioplegia delivery given through the aortic root can be inadequate in the presence of critical coronary artery disease or aortic insufficiency. In the former, stenoses in the coronary vessels limit pressure and thus flow through the coronary arteries, and lead to uneven distribution of cardioplegia and thus uneven cooling. In the extreme case of coronary occlusion, areas of underperfused and thus ischaemic myocardium will be poorly protected and subject to greater injury during the period of surgical ischaemia. Topical cooling may serve as a valuable adjunct in this situation. Further, in the case where coronary grafts are to be placed, the underperfused area can be grafted early, and cardioplegia administered through the graft. In the presence of aortic insufficiency, adequate pressure cannot be generated within the aortic root to perfuse the coronary arteries. The problem is compounded by the flow of cardioplegic solution into the left ventricle. As the ventricle distends with solution, the wall tension increases, and this will further diminish the perfusion of the subendocardium. Direct ostial cannulation of the coronary arteries through the open aortic root can be used in this situation to ensure the delivery of cardioplegia and uniform cooling. This technique is somewhat cumbersome in that each ostium must be hand-perfused at the time of initial cooling, and subsequently, in the case of multidose cardioplegia. In addition, direct ostial cannulation can lead to damage of the coronary vessels at the ostia, although this has been diminished through improved cannula designs. Alternative cannula designs permit the ability to secure the cannula tips in the ostia of the coronary arteries for the duration of the ischaemic period to permit either continuous administration of cardioplegia, or multidose administration without the need to reposition the cannulae repeatedly.

The delivery pressure for antegrade cardioplegia is very important. A low aortic root pressure, whether caused by aortic insufficiency or low pump pressure, can produce uneven distribution of the cardioplegia throughout the myocardium (Molina et al., 1989). This is especially important distal to a critical coronary stenosis or in the presence of ventricular hypertrophy. Conversely, high coronary perfusion pressures can also be harmful. While the vascular endothelium is sensitive to elevated perfusion pressures, this is especially critical in the injured heart. High perfusion pressures in the hypoxic neonatal heart (80–100 mmHg) produce significant deterioration in systolic and diastolic function, as well as an increase in myocardial oedema, when compared with the use of perfusion pressures between 30 mmHg and 50 mmHg (Kronon et al., 1998). High perfusion pressure produces similar damage in the ischaemic adult heart (Okamoto et al., 1986), and limitation of the delivery of cardioplegia to pressures of 70 mmHg may result in decreased myocardial injury.

An alternative or supplement to antegrade perfusion is retrograde coronary artery perfusion. This technique was initially proposed by Lillehei in 1956, and has subsequently benefited from advances in cannula design. During retrograde perfusion, cardioplegia is administered into the coronary sinus, and provides flow to the myocardium in a retrograde fashion through the venous system. It permits perfusion of areas of the myocardium inaccessible through the antegrade route because of obstructing coronary artery disease or aortic insufficiency. Retrograde coronary sinus perfusion involves placing a catheter in the coronary sinus through the right atrium. A balloon on the tip is inflated to prevent reflux of the cardioplegia into the right atrium, and the coronary sinus is perfused up to a pressure of 40 mmHg (Menasche and Piwnica, 1987). Complications of this technique include rupture of the coronary sinus from the catheter tip and poor protection of the right ventricle (Partington et al., 1989a, Kaukoranta et al., 1998). The latter is either caused by placing the tip of the catheter beyond the veins draining the right ventricle, or when those veins empty directly into the right atrium. The frequency of this can be decreased by digital pressure or placement of a suture around the coronary sinus as it enters into the right atrium, and using this to snare around the catheter. However, injury to the right coronary artery is a potential complication of this manoeuvre. In the typical elective operation, retrograde perfusion techniques via the coronary sinus have been associated with increased leakage of troponin and creatine phosphokinase MB fraction compared with antegrade perfusion (Kaukoranta et al., 1998), although without apparent clinical consequence. In addition, retrograde cardioplegia may increase the development of myocardial oedema and injury to the microvasculature, even though it may produce improved protection compared with antegrade delivery (Schaper et al., 1985). There is the advantage of convenience in aortic or mitral procedures, where multidose or continuous cardioplegia can be given without significantly interrupting the flow of the procedure. In addition, retrograde techniques may be particularly useful in preserving myocardium in the situation of acute coronary occlusion (Partington et al., 1989b). In this situation, cardioplegia can be delivered distal to an obstructing lesion when collateral flow has not had time to develop. An additional use of retrograde cardioplegia is during all arterial bypass grafting. Antegrade perfusion with cold cardioplegia is not

feasible with the use of in situ arterial grafts (right and left internal mammary arteries, gastro-epiploic artery). When an in situ graft is the last bypass performed in a procedure, additional cardioplegia is not required. However, when multiple in situ grafts are performed, multidose cardioplegia protocols require additional doses between anastomoses. Retrograde cardioplegia is uniquely suited for this situation. However, after each distal anastomosis is completed, the graft must be occluded to prevent the unintentional rewarming in the region supplied by that graft. The use of radial artery grafts allows the use of antegrade cardioplegia, either directly down the graft or through the aortic root after the proximal anastomosis is completed. Additionally, antegrade cardioplegia can be used in the setting of all arterial grafting, even with the use of in situ conduits to perfuse the vascular beds supplied by the native coronary arteries, although the distribution of protection will be limited by the degree of coronary artery disease.

Antegrade and retrograde techniques can be used independently or together, depending on the needs of the patient and the preference of the surgeon. Often, when the retrograde route is to be used as the primary method of cardioplegia delivery, the myocardium is arrested with an initial dose of cardioplegia given through the antegrade route. This is followed by subsequent doses given in a retrograde fashion while the root of the aorta is vented either actively or passively. The combined use of both techniques provides the benefits of both approaches and maximizes even cardioplegia distribution (Partington et al., 1989b). When the initial dose of cardioplegia is administered through the antegrade route and subsequent dosing is via the retrograde route with additional antegrade cardioplegia given down each completed bypass graft, there is improved lactate washout and ventricular function after reperfusion (Rao et al., 1998). This demonstrates that different regions of myocardium are perfused with the two techniques. However, in clinical practice, the potential benefits of the combined routes administration of cardioplegia may not be readily appreciable in patients undergoing first-time elective CABG (Cernaianu et al., 1996). As opposed to only providing the initial dose of cardioplegia through the antegrade route, both routes may be used throughout the course of the procedure. When both antegrade and retrograde routes of cardioplegia are used together, they can be administered in an alternating or simultaneous manner. In the first, retrograde cardioplegia is interrupted periodically after the completion of each anastomosis for the administration of cardioplegia down each graft and through the aortic root. In contrast, simultaneous administration of antegrade and retrograde cardioplegia uses continuous retrograde cardioplegia, with a brief dose of antegrade cardioplegia down each completed graft (Ihnken et al., 1994). Besides minimizing maldistribution with the combined delivery of cardioplegia, simultaneous administration decreases the time spent delivering cardioplegia compared with sequential administration. Because of the presence of veno-venous collaterals that drain much of the coronary sinus infusion, venous hypertension does not occur when retrograde and antegrade cardioplegia are administered simultaneously. The clinical outcomes are similar between the alternate and simultaneous methods, but the simultaneous method offers the advantage of simplicity (Shirai et al., 1996). In this situation, the aortic root does not need to be de-aired between doses of cardioplegia, and it minimizes the number of times that the cardioplegia must be turned off and on.

Cardioplegia administration can either be continuous or intermittent. Typically, intermittent administration is performed because it allows optimal visualization during the course of the procedure. In addition, in the hypothermic setting, the metabolic demands of the myocardium are greatly reduced, and the intermittent administration of oxygenated cardioplegia can provide the vast majority of the substrates required during the subsequent ischaemic interval. When intermittent dosing is used, each dose of cardioplegia is essentially a brief period of reperfusion. Since high initial reperfusion pressures promote reperfusion injury, each dose should be administered at a low pressure to minimize this source of injury. Continuous administration offers uninterrupted oxygen delivery and metabolite washout. This may be the most important when hypothermia is avoided or minimized, and myocardial metabolic demands remain significant. However, visualization is hindered in some procedures, such as bypass or valve replacement. An additional disadvantage of continuous cardioplegia may be cardioplegic overdose. In continuous administration, large doses of cardioplegia are used. In crystalloid-based solutions, or blood containing solutions that are diluted with crystalloid, this can result in significant haemodilution with its attendant consequences. Further, when continuous administration is used to facilitate warm myocardial preservation, myocardial electromechanical activity will resume if potassium concentrations are decreased. In order to prevent this, potassium concentrations in the cardioplegia are maintained at supranormal levels, resulting in a larger potassium load to the patient. In the setting of continuous cardioplegia, positioning of the heart may affect the distribution of the cardioplegia, and parts of the heart may be unwittingly left unprotected despite continuous delivery. Regardless of these concerns, studies have shown that continuous retrograde cardioplegia may better preserve myocardial pH, and thus may lead to better protection (Bomfim et al., 1981; Khuri et al., 1988). In contrast to the hypothermic heart, the warm heart continues to use substrate at a rapid rate, and may benefit from continuous administration of cardioplegia. Continuous or near-continuous techniques are particularly considered when warmer cardioplegic temperatures are employed.

Frequency of cardioplegia administration

Cardioplegia can be administered either as a single dose, multiple doses or continuously, as the clinical situation and myocardial protection strategy dictate. As a general rule, the frequency of administration varies directly with the temperature of the myocardium. The relationship between myocardial temperature, the composition of the cardioplegia and the frequency of cardioplegia administration is illustrated in Fig. 12.4, as previously discussed.

With the use of myocardial cooling, the metabolic demands of the heart are markedly diminished and the frequency of cardioplegic administration can be decreased. Although an operation may be conducted after the administration of a single dose of cardioplegia, there are several benefits to multidose regimens. In the setting of coronary artery disease, the induction dose of cardioplegia may not be well distributed throughout the myocardium. Additional cardioplegia, given down each completed graft, serves to better protect these areas of the heart. During an ischaemic interval, the myocardium is depleted of its high-energy phosphates, anaerobic metabolism occurs and cellular acidosis ensues. Repeated doses of cardioplegia provide oxygen to the tissues and wash out the harmful metabolites and lactate. With the use of cold blood cardioplegia, ATP levels are replenished with each successive infusion of cardioplegia and remain stable after reperfusion, whereas they steadily decline during ischaemia and remain depressed during reperfusion with the use of crystalloid cardioplegia (Catinella et al., 1984). The advantages of multidose cardioplegia seen in the adult heart do not hold true in the immature myocardium, where multidose cardioplegia may be detrimental during hypothermia (Murashita and Hearse, 1991).

When warm or tepid cardioplegia is used, the metabolic demands of the heart remain high, and any period of ischaemia is accompanied by rapid utilization of metabolic reserves. If the ischaemic interval is lengthened, there is the subsequent onset of acidosis and myocellular injury. Thus, the administration of cardioplegia should be frequent at a minimum, or preferably continuous. During CABG, the only feasible route for continuous cardioplegia is retrograde. However, during the construction of the distal anastomosis, visualization is often impaired because of the flow of cardioplegia through the arteriotomy, necessitating interruption of the cardioplegia until the anastomosis is completed. Thus, even in the setting of 'continuous' retrograde cardioplegia, there is no cardioplegia delivered for approximately 20–30 per cent of the ischaemic time (Hayashida et al., 1994).

Additives to cardioplegia

All regimens of cardioplegia involve the use of additives as a means of achieving myocardial arrest and protection from ischaemic injury. The choice of additives depends on many factors, including the base of the cardioplegia solution (crystalloid versus blood), the length of the operation, the temperature at which the operation will occur and patient factors, among others. Interestingly, most of the additives available for clinical use are present in some form in blood. These include buffers, free radical scavengers, metabolic substrates, osmotic agents and oxygen-carrying molecules. Thus, the use of additives with crystalloid-based cardioplegia serves to produce a substance that closely resembles blood in many different respects, suggesting that blood-based cardioplegia may require only minimal manipulation to produce the optimal cardioplegic solution.

The list of potential additives to any cardioplegic solution is extensive. Even the basic electrolyte composition of the cardioplegia is a subject of investigation and debate. To date, no 'silver bullet' has been identified that offers perfect myocardial protection in any situation, and no strategy is optimized for all possible situations. Thus, a myocardial protection strategy must balance the complexity, cost, reproducibility and degree of benefit that each alteration in the cardioplegia produces. Most healthy hearts will tolerate a reasonable period of ischaemia and reperfusion under any modern strategy of myocardial protection. The difficulty comes when determining the best strategy for the borderline ventricle. In this situation, one must remember that the goal is to perform an operation to improve or preserve myocardial function, and that the delivery of cardioplegia is just a means to that end. Thus, a sufficiently complex system of cardioplegic administration may produce more harm than benefit by adding to the overall time of ischaemia without producing much improvement in myocardial preservation.

Electrolyte composition of cardioplegia

The primary purposes of cardioplegia include the ability to produce rapid myocardial arrest, to maintain electro-mechanical asystole, to prevent myocardial oedema and to provide a mechanism for the effective manipulation of myocardial temperature. The electrolyte composition of the cardioplegia plays an important role in the first three of these goals. Cardioplegia can broadly be categorized as either 'intracellular' or 'extracellular' based on the overall electrolyte composition. Intracellular solutions are crystalloid-based by definition, and consist of low sodium, low calcium and high potassium concentrations. The main mechanism of action is that by mimicking the intracellular environment, little energy is expended to maintain ionic homeostasis across the extracellular membrane. A benefit of the low sodium concentration is that it leaves an osmotic gap that can be filled with other protective agents without creating a hyperosmolar solution. A well-known example of an intracellular solution is Bretschneider's solution. Cardiac arrest is induced by eliminating the high $[Na]_o/[Na]_i$ ratio, and thereby eliminating phase zero of the action potential (that attributed to rapid sodium influx). With the widespread popularity of blood cardioplegia in adult cardiac surgery, the use of intracellular solutions has become much less frequent, and is becoming of historical interest only, except in the field of cardiac transplantation where most centres use an intracellular solution for donor organ preservation.

In contrast to the intracellular solutions, extracellular cardioplegia contains an electrolyte composition similar to serum. This solution is then modified with the addition of potassium in order to produce myocardial quiescence. Additional agents are then added to the extracellular solution as required to offer additional protective benefits.

Potassium was originally introduced as a cardioplegic agent because of its ability to rapidly induce electro-mechanical quiescence. However, the high potassium concentration in the initial studies also induced myocellular injury, and was thus abandoned. It was reintroduced when it was discovered that arrest could be initiated with much lower potassium concentrations and that myocardial recovery was possible. Potassium induces electro-mechanical quiescence through depolarization of the cellular membrane. With initial depolarization, voltage-gated sodium channels open to allow for the influx of sodium across the cellular membrane. This leads to further depolarization and phase zero of the action potential. Shortly after these channels open, they close through a time-dependent mechanism, and cannot open again until the membrane has repolarized. Thus the cell is unexcitable, in a state of diastolic arrest. Despite mechanical inactivity of the heart, electrical activity can continue for a short period of time. Although this does not result in contraction, it does serve to deplete energy stores as ATP-dependent pumps attempt to counteract the flux of ions across the cellular membrane. Thus, the administration of cardioplegia must continue until there is electrical silence. The concentration of potassium required to produce arrest is related to the temperature of the myocardium, so that less potassium is needed during hypothermia. In general, potassium concentrations of 8–30 mM are usually sufficient to induce electro-mechanical arrest. In the presence of hypothermia, myocardial inactivity can be preserved even if the potassium concentration in subsequent doses of cardioplegia is reduced to a much lower level. This strategy decreases the total amount of potassium given to the patient. Indeed, under the micoplegia protocol, the potassium concentration in the cardioplegia can be decreased after induction to a point low enough to just maintain arrest. Other mechanisms of producing myocardial arrest have included the use of hypocalcemia, or the addition of magnesium or local anesthetics. However, because of its simplicity and effectiveness, hyperkalaemia has remained the most common method of inducing asystole.

Calcium is an extremely important cation in relation to both myocardial function and protection. It plays a critical role in the plateau phase of the action potential, and it is important in excitation–contraction coupling, among other functions. Its intracellular levels are regulated through several pumps and channels. The sodium–calcium exchange pump is particularly important in that small changes in calcium concentration may have important implications on sodium transport, and thus on intracellular ionic concentrations and the development of oedema. The optimal calcium concentration in a cardioplegic solution varies significantly with the type of cardioplegia used. Because of the broad range of effects that calcium has on cellular function, both significant hypocalcaemia and hypercalcaemia are harmful to the myocardium. Cardioplegia solutions without calcium will produce myocardial arrest caused by the lack of calcium influx across the plasma membrane. However, absent (Jynge et al., 1977) or very low calcium levels are detrimental, as they predispose the heart to damage through the 'calcium paradox'. In this situation, extracellular hypocalcaemia leads to the depletion of calcium from the myocyte. Upon reperfusion, there is an influx of calcium back into the myocyte, and subsequent contracture and cellular damage. In clinical practice, it is difficult to lower calcium concentrations sufficiently to produce a 'calcium paradox'. One method of combating high calcium levels associated with ischaemia and reperfusion is through the use of calcium channel blockers. The addition of verapamil or nifedipine to crystalloid cardioplegia results in improved functional recovery. However, verapamil is associated with a hypocontractile state in the early reperfusion period (Yamamoto et al., 1985). Clinically, the use of diltiazem in crystalloid cardioplegia preserves high-energy phosphates and improves myocardial metabolism, but it is a powerful negative inotropic agent and produces prolonged periods of electromechanical arrest after reperfusion (Christakis et al., 1986b). This may be important during the use of the radial artery as a conduit, as diltiazem is often used intraoperatively and post-operatively in an attempt to reduce conduit spasm.

Magnesium is a divalent ion that interacts with many of the enzymes and channels that normally use and transport calcium. The presence of magnesium within a cardioplegic solution greatly influences the activity of calcium within the myocyte. Magnesium provides improved myocardial recovery after hyperkalaemic arrest (Hearse et al., 1978; Reynolds et al., 1989). The benefits of magnesium in cardioplegia depend on the concentration of calcium within the cardioplegia, and magnesium seems to offer no benefit with the use of calcium-free cardioplegia. The percentage of recovery in aortic flow after cardioplegic arrest depends on the relative concentrations of magnesium and calcium within a cardioplegic solution (Takemoto et al., 1992). The addition of magnesium to cardioplegia appears to protect the heart from the potentially deleterious presence of calcium within the cardioplegia. When blood cardioplegia is used, the addition of magnesium prevents the production of lactate during ischaemia, and prevents the fall in ATP and amino acid levels that otherwise occurs during reperfusion (Caputo et al., 1998a). Thus, the use of magnesium in blood cardioplegia may eliminate the need to control calcium levels within the blood cardioplegia.

Buffer

Cellular function and enzymatic processes occur with maximum efficiency within a narrow pH range. In the heart, deviation away from this leads to poor energy utilization, and decreased responsiveness to inotropic stimulation. Under normal situations, the pH of the cell is tightly controlled by both intracellular and extracellular processes. However, during ischaemia, the products of metabolism, including the hydrogen ion, accumulate rapidly. As the pH falls, cellular function deteriorates and contractile dysfunction ensues. To combat this, cardioplegia must contain buffers to minimize the accumulation of hydrogen ions and the fall in pH. Blood-based cardioplegia contains natural buffering systems, such as the histidine and imidazole groups of proteins. Optimal buffers must be capable of buffering large amounts of hydrogen ion. In addition, the optimal buffer should have a pKa within the vicinity of 7.4. Buffers that are particularly favourable include THAM, Tris and histidine.

The method in which the pH is monitored is also important during hypothermia. Since pH measurements are temperature dependent, the manner in which the pH is interpreted can have a significant impact on the management of acid–base balance. During hypothermia, the pH of blood normally rises, and may achieve values of 7.8–7.9 at very low temperatures. Utilizing the α-stat protocol, the pH of the blood sample is corrected to 37°C, to provide a pH value that is independent of patient temperature. In contrast, under the pH-stat protocol, the pH value is measured at the temperature of the patient, and is corrected to 7.4 through the addition of CO_2 into the perfusion circuit. In this situation, the pH that the hypothermic patient experiences represents a relative acidosis and may impair myocardial performance. Indeed, the addition of CO_2 to return the pH to 7.4 is associated with poor ventricular function when compared with allowing the pH to rise appropriately (Becker *et al.*, 1981). The end result under the pH-stat strategy is impaired ventricular function and recovery when compared with management under the α-stat protocol. However, a significant advantage to pH-stat management may be improved cerebral protection. The addition of CO_2 leads to a reflexive increase in cerebral blood flow, and thus improved oxygen delivery. This results in improved cerebral metabolism and protection (Kirshbom *et al.*, 1996).

Osmolality

Oedema is detrimental to myocardial function. One method to limit the formation of oedema is through the regulation of the osmolality of the cardioplegia solutions. The osmolality of most solutions currently used places them in the range from mild hypotonicity to mild hypertonicity, although blood cardioplegia with several additives may be significantly hypertonic. The osmolality of the solution is affected by its ionic concentration, as well as by the addition of osmotically active agents. Popular additives to cardioplegia to alter the osmolality include mannitol, glucose and albumen. The addition of mannitol to cardioplegia to produce a hyperosmolar solution results in less myocellular oedema after cardioplegic arrest (Folgia *et al.*, 1979) and produces enhanced contractility of the left ventricle (Goto *et al.*, 1991). The osmotic agents normally present in blood minimize the need to adjust osmolality when using blood cardioplegia at a high blood to crystalloid ratio.

Glutamate–aspartate

After a period of ischaemia, the heart is depleted of its high-energy phosphates and many substrates involved in the reformation of ATP. The amino acids glutamate and aspartate are intermediates in the Kreb's cycle, and theoretically can be used to restore high-energy phosphate levels in the myocardium after a period of ischaemia. In an isolated working rat heart model, the addition of glutamic acid to the cardioplegic solution produces better preservation of tissue ATP and aspartate levels than unmodified cardioplegia (Pisarenko *et al.*, 1983), demonstrating the beneficial effect of substrate enhancement. In a similar study, the addition of glutamate alone does not result in improved functional recovery, but the addition of aspartate, either alone or with glutamate, produces significant improvements in post-ischaemic recovery of myocardial function, under both normothermic and hypothermic conditions (Pisarenko *et al.*, 1995). In hearts subjected to warm global ischaemia before a period of protected ischaemia, the addition of glutamate alone (Rosenkranz *et al.*, 1984), or with aspartate (Rosenkranz *et al.*, 1986), to blood cardioplegia produces improved oxygen uptake

and functional recovery. However, substrate enhancement does not appear to always improve myocardial preservation. In the setting of normal myocardium undergoing a period of ischaemia and reperfusion under hypothermic arrest, the addition of glutamate does not improve the degree of functional recovery (Robertson *et al.*, 1984). Thus, in damaged myocardium, which is energy-depleted before the onset of surgical ischaemia, and may be less capable of tolerating the ischaemic stress, the use of substrate enhancement may be beneficial. This may also extend to the myocardial damage associated with the onset of brain death in organ donors. Aspartate and glutamate, added to the induction cardioplegia used before organ harvesting, produces preservation of creatine kinase and glutamate levels, and a reduction in myocardial lactate content (Tixier *et al.*, 1991).

INTERVENTION DURING REPERFUSION

The period of reperfusion is as critical to the myocardium as is the ischaemic interval. Although ischaemia is clearly injurious, data support the concept that damage can be compounded during the reperfusion period. Upon reperfusion, critically injured myocytes undergo rapid development of cellular oedema, mitochondrial oedema, disruption of the tissue lattice and development of contraction bands. Cells that undergo this constellation of changes demonstrate irreversible myocardial injury and cell death. In the absence of reperfusion, the same cells would slowly undergo changes consistent with cellular necrosis. While the end result in both cases is myocellular death, the process of reperfusion clearly alters the manner in which the cellular death occurs. The point at which myocytes become irreversibly injured is indistinct, and no test can accurately determine when a myocyte has suffered irreversible injury. However, it is very apparent that poorly controlled reperfusion can produce lethal injury in potentially salvageable myocytes, and that these cells then undergo the rapid changes characteristic of irreversible myocardial injury. In addition, interventions during this period can significantly lessen this damage and improve myocardial performance. An important caveat of this is that each time that cardioplegia is given in a multidose protocol, the heart is essentially undergoing a brief period of reperfusion. Therefore, the criteria for successful reperfusion at the end of the case must also be adhered to throughout the operation. Similarly, additives to the cardioplegia solution to prevent reperfusion injury may provide additional benefit if included earlier. The corollary is that with frequent reperfusion, the ischaemic injury is minimized.

The pressure at which a reperfusate is delivered is an important variable that the surgeon has the ability to regulate closely, and which appears to play a role in the development of the no-reflow phenomenon. During the ischaemic interval, the endothelium is damaged and its vasoregulatory capacities are markedly diminished. This injury can be worsened by high reperfusion pressures (Okamoto et al., 1986; Sawatari et al., 1991) but may not occur if the initial reperfusion pressures are limited (Vinten-Johansen et al., 1992; Sato et al., 1997). Controlled reperfusion of infarcting tissue decreases myocardial oedema, limits infarct size and preserves inotropic–responsive systolic function compared with uncontrolled reperfusion (Okamoto et al., 1986). In order to limit the myocardial damage associated with reperfusion, the initial perfusion pressure should be limited to approximately 30 mmHg for the first one to two minutes of reperfusion. Subsequently, the perfusion pressure can be increased gradually, but the pressures should still be tightly controlled, with a mean pressure of approximately 70 mmHg or less. Myocardial blood flow at these pressures should be adequate because of the myocardial hyperaemic response. These perfusion pressures should remain in this range for at least the first 30 minutes of reperfusion.

At the conclusion of an ischaemic period, the heart is energy-depleted and in a vulnerable state. If the metabolic demands upon the heart are too great during this period, the rate of recovery is diminished and irreversible injury may ensue. Therefore, the initial period of reperfusion should be designed to provide maximal energy delivery yet allow continued myocardial relaxation. Controlled reperfusion with the heart in a non-working state will lessen the oxygen requirements of the ischaemic muscle and improve functional recovery (Allen et al., 1986b). Several techniques may provide this. If the heart is kept cold initially, potassium can be removed from the reperfusion solution and mechanical quiescence will remain. This will allow for the washout of metabolic byproducts, and provide oxygen and substrates for the myocardium at a time when metabolic demands are at a minimum. As the heart is allowed to rewarm, electro-mechanical activity will slowly resume in a controlled fashion. Alternatively, terminal warm hyperkalaemic blood cardioplegia ('hot shot') may be given at the onset of reperfusion as a method of preventing metabolic derangement at the time of reperfusion. This method preserves intracellular ATP and amino acid levels when compared with the use of cold hyperkalaemic blood cardioplegia (Caputo et al., 1998b). In the clinical setting, terminal warm blood cardioplegia produces preservation of glycogen and ATP concentrations, and improved metabolic recovery (Teoh et al., 1986).

The post-ischaemic heart is particularly vulnerable to injurious stimuli, and the contractile state of the heart during the early period of reperfusion is critical. Ventricular fibrillation leads to rapid depletion of energy stores and impaired subendocardial blood flow. It should therefore be treated aggressively with cardioversion to minimize substrate utilization and allow maximal subendocardial blood flow. The ventricle can be further protected by allowing the heart to remain empty during the early stages of reperfusion. Since the empty beating heart consumes less energy than the heart performing mechanical work, the heart can use this period for substrate repletion. In addition, it prevents the occurrence of ventricular distention that may otherwise result if the ventricle cannot function immediately.

An important adjunct to all of the protective manoeuvres undertaken for myocardial preservation is the de-airing process. Although air emboli have significant systemic consequences, they also lead to abnormalities in myocardial perfusion. Coronary air emboli may come from a variety of sources, and are particularly common when performing CABG. The right coronary artery is vulnerable to emboli because of its anterior position in the aortic root. In addition, bypass grafts often have proximal anastomoses on the anterior surface of the aorta. Although venting the aorta will remove most of the air from the aortic root, it is difficult to remove all the air. Air may also be introduced into the coronary circulation at the time of performing the distal bypass, when initially flushing the vein graft with cardioplegia, or it may be entrained into the coronary arteries from active suction on the aortic root. All of these sources must be minimized to avoid this source of injury.

Oxygen-derived free radicals are highly reactive oxygen species that contribute to the myocardial damage associated with ischaemia and reperfusion. The intrinsic free radical scavengers block many of the injurious effects of the free radicals that are formed under normal conditions; they may be rapidly overwhelmed during times of myocardial stress. The primary time of oxygen-derived free radical-induced damage is at the time of reperfusion. At this time, production of the free radicals is at a maximum, and the endogenous defense mechanisms are significantly weakened. Thus, interventions aimed at the prevention of free radical-induced injury must be targeted towards the time of reperfusion. However, it can be argued that earlier intervention may also be beneficial for two independent reasons. First, each period of cardioplegia administration during the course of an operation is essentially a brief period of reperfusion, and can be associated with the production of free radicals. Second, early administration may permit the scavenger to be at the site of free radical production before reperfusion, and thus before the burst of free radical production. Since free radicals are short-lived, there are many different species that are injurious and damage occurs in close proximity to the place in which the radicals are generated, any intervention against oxygen-derived free radicals must be targeted against species formed early in the chain reaction, must include scavengers of several different free radicals and must be available at the site of generation. The latter may require that the agent against the free radical be intracellular if this is where they are formed. This limits the applicability of enzymes, such as exogenous superoxide dismutase, which do not readily cross the cell membrane.

Clinical studies involving the use of free radical scavengers have produced mixed results, in part because of the large numbers of variables involved. One major factor in the effectiveness of free radical scavengers is the base composition of the cardioplegic solution. Crystalloid solutions have no inherent anti-free radical activity, whereas blood-based cardioplegia contains scavengers in the plasma (urate, plasma proteins, ascorbate, vitamin E) and in the red blood cells (catalase, superoxide dismutase, glutathione). In a canine model, diminished myocardial recovery occurred when scavengers were omitted from oxygenated crystalloid cardioplegia, or when the inherent scavengers in blood were blocked (Julia *et al.*, 1991). However, blood appears to offer sufficient free radical-scavenging activity to minimize the amount of free radical-induced damage at the time of reperfusion. Therefore, it may be more difficult to demonstrate an advantage of exogenous free radical scavengers in the setting of blood cardioplegia, and their routine use in blood cardioplegia is controversial at best.

Hypercalcaemia is detrimental to the heart during the reperfusion period, and methods to decrease this may diminish the harmful effects of reperfusion. In an experimental model of regional ischaemia, the use of hypocalaemic (150 μmol/L) substrate-enhanced blood cardioplegia with diltiazem (300 μg/kg) produces improved functional and histological recovery when compared with reperfusion with normocalcaemic blood cardioplegia (Allen *et al.*, 1986a).

FUTURE DIRECTIONS

There are many new strategies in myocardial protection on the horizon that have undergone the initial phases of laboratory investigation, but have not yet begun or completed the initial stages of human investigation. Discussion of these will focus on what is known about them, and will project their usefulness in the future.

Although potassium provides rapid myocardial arrest in diastole, it is a depolarizing agent. It produces a membrane potential that is less negative than the normal resting potential. Arrest ensues because the voltage-dependent sodium channels cannot reactivate and action potentials cannot propagate. An alternative is the initiation of hyperpolarized myocardial arrest with a class of drug termed 'potassium channel openers'. These agents include aprikalim and pinacidil, and they open the ATP-sensitive potassium channels (K_{ATP}). The presumed mechanism of action for these agents is through hyperpolarization of the cell membrane. In this state, the action potential cannot propagate. At a more negative resting membrane potential, the other ionic channels that normally open during depolarization remain closed, and the ionic imbalances that occur with depolarized arrest do not occur. This results in less energy expenditure to restore ionic balance, and less cellular oedema at the conclusion of the ischaemic period. However, these agents may be pro-arrhythmic. In addition, they are not readily washed out like potassium, and this results in less control over the restoration of regular myocardial contractile function at the conclusion of the procedure.

Current methods of myocardial protection are dependent upon the intrinsic state of the myocardium for proper function. Manipulation of the characteristics of the myocardium and endothelium may provide a mechanism by which the heart may be made more resistant to ischaemia and reperfusion injury. Although the techniques of gene therapy are still in their infancy, genetic alteration of the heart has been demonstrated under experimental conditions. Using the ability to focally modulate the genetic make-up of some or all of the cells within the heart, surgeons may one day be able to improve myocardial protection. Potential mechanisms for this include limiting the endothelial–neutrophil interaction, manipulation of endogenous free radical scavenger levels and modulation of the number of adrenergic receptors, to name a few. Such changes could limit the degree to which the inflammatory process is activated, provide additional protection from the harmful effects of reperfusion or alter the responsiveness of the myocardium to inotropic stimulation. However, the usefulness of gene therapy is limited by the ability to target and efficiently transfect the cells of interest, the availability of specific gene sequences of interest and the ability to control the expression of the inserted gene. Thus, while gene therapy is an attractive and evolving technology, too many unresolved questions remain before it is clinically applicable towards improving myocardial protection. However, the tools of gene therapy may prove extremely useful in the experimental validation of other novel approaches to myocardial protection.

The ability to capture the endogenous elements involved in myocardial protection is much more likely to result in a clinically applicable method to enhance myocardial protection. Although ischaemic pre-conditioning has shown potential in producing these results, the data are somewhat conflicting and the ability to induce ischaemic pre-conditioning somewhat cumbersome. Chemical pre-conditioning represents an alternative method for inducing these same protective mechanisms, without the requirement of subjecting the heart to a potentially injurious ischaemic insult.

REFERENCES

Akins, C.W. 1984: Noncardioplegic myocardial preservation for coronary revascularization. *Journal of Thoracic and Cardiovascular Surgery* **88**, 174–81.

Akins, C.W., Carroll, D.L. 1987: Event-free survival following nonemergency myocardial revascularization during hypothermic fibrillatory arrest. *Annals of Thoracic Surgery* **43**, 628–33.

Alkhulaifi, A.M., Pugsley, W.B., Yellon, D.M. 1993: The influence of the time period between preconditioning ischaemia and prolonged ischaemia on myocardial protection. *Cardioscience* **4**, 163–9.

Allen, B.S., Okamoto, F., Buckberg, G.D. *et al.* 1986a: Reperfusate composition: benefits of marked hypocalcemia and diltiazem on regional recovery. *Journal of Thoracic and Cardiovascular Surgery* **92**, 564–72.

Allen, B.S., Okamoto, F., Buckberg, G.D. *et al.* 1986b: Effects of 'duration' of reperfusate administration versus reperfusate 'dose' on regional functional, biochemical, and histochemical recovery. *Journal of Thoracic and Cardiovascular Surgery* **92**, 594–604.

Allen, B.S., Buckberg, G.D., Rosenkranz, E.R. *et al.* 1992: Topical cardiac hypothermia in patients with coronary disease. An unnecessary adjunct to cardioplegic protection and cause of pulmonary morbidity. *Journal of Thoracic and Cardiovascular Surgery* **104**, 626–31.

Andres, J., Flameng, W., van Belle, H. 1994: Energetic state of the postischaemic myocardium and its relation to contractile failure. *Journal of Physiology and Pharmacology* **45**, 91–103.

Assad-Morell, J.L., Wallace, R.B., Elveback, L.R. *et al.* 1975: Serum enzyme data in diagnosis of myocardial infarction during or early after aorta-coronary saphenous vein bypass graft operations. *Journal of Thoracic and Cardiovascular Surgery* **69**, 851–7.

Becker, H., Vinten-Johansen, J., Buckberg, G.D. *et al.* 1981: Myocardial damage caused by keeping pH 7.40 during systemic deep hypothermia. *Journal of Thoracic and Cardiovascular Surgery* **82**, 810–21.

Bomfim, V., Kaijser, L., Bendz, R. *et al.* 1981: Myocardial protection during aortic valve replacement. Cardiac metabolism and enzyme release following continuous blood cardioplegia. *Scandinavian Journal of Cardiothoracic Surgery* **15**, 141–7.

Bretschneider, J., Hubner, G., Knoll, D. *et al.* 1975: Myocardial resistance and tolerance to ischemia: physiological and biochemical basis. *Journal of Cardiovascular Surgery* **16**, 241–60.

Brewer, D.L., Bilbro, R.H., Bartel, A.G. 1973: Myocardial infarction as a complication of coronary bypass surgery. *Circulation* **47**, 58–64.

Browning, P.G., Pullan, M., Jackson, M., Rashid, A. 1999: Leucocyte-depleted cardioplegia does not reduce reperfusion injury in hypothermic coronary artery bypass surgery. *Perfusion* **14**, 371–7.

Buckberg, G.D., Hottenrott, C.E. 1975: Ventricular fibrillation. Its effect on myocardial flow, distribution, and performance. *Annals of Thoracic Surgery* **20**, 76–85.

Buckberg, G.D., Brazier, J.R., Nelson, R.L. *et al.* 1977: Studies of the effects of hypothermia on regional myocardial blood flow and metabolism during cardiopulmonary bypass. I. The adequately perfused beating, fibrillating, and arrested heart. *Journal of Thoracic and Cardiovascular Surgery* **73**, 87–94.

Bufkin, B.L., Mellitt, R.J., Gott, J.P. *et al.* 1994: Aerobic blood cardioplegia for revascularization of acute infarct: effects of delivery temperature. *Annals of Thoracic Surgery* **58**, 953–60.

Caputo, M., Bryan, A.J., Calafiore, A.M. *et al.* 1998a: Intermittent antegrade hyperkalemic warm blood cardioplegia supplemented with magnesium prevents myocardial substrate derangement in patients undergoing coronary artery bypass surgery. *European Journal of Cardiothoracic Surgery* **14**, 596–601.

Caputo, M., Dihmis, W.C., Bryan, A.J. *et al.* 1998b: Warm blood hyperkalemic reperfusion ('hot shot') prevents myocardial substrate derangement in patients undergoing coronary artery bypass surgery. *European Journal of Cardiothoracic Surgery* **13**, 559–64.

Casthely, P.A., Shah, C., Mekhjian, H. *et al.* 1997: Left ventricular diastolic function after coronary artery bypass grafting: a correlative study with three different myocardial protection techniques. *Journal of Thoracic and Cardiovascular Surgery* **114**, 254–60.

Catinella, F.P., Cunningham, J.N., Spencer, F.C. 1984: Myocardial protection during prolonged aortic cross-clamping. *Journal of Thoracic and Cardiovascular Surgery* **88**, 411–23.

Cave, A.C., Hearse, D.J. 1992: Ischaemic preconditioning and contractile function: studies with normothermic and hypothermic global ischaemia. *Journal of Molecular and Cellular Cardiology* **24**, 1113–23.

Cernaianu, A.C., Flum, D.R., Maurer, M. *et al.* 1996: Comparison of antegrade with antegrade/retrograde cold blood cardioplegia for myocardial revascularization. *Texas Heart Institute Journal* **23**, 9–14.

Chitwood, W.R., Hill, R.C., Kleinman, L.H., Wechsler, A.S. 1983: Transmural myocardial flow distribution during hypothermia: effects of coronary inflow restriction. *Journal of Thoracic and Cardiovascular Surgery* **86**, 61–9.

Christakis, G.T., Fremes, S.E., Weisel, R.D. *et al.* 1986a: Reducing the risk of urgent revascularization for unstable angina: a randomized clinical trial. *Journal of Vascular Surgery* **3**, 764–72.

Christakis, G.T., Fremes, S.E., Weisel, R.D. *et al.* 1986b: Diltiazem cardioplegia. A balance of risk and benefit. *Journal of Thoracic and Cardiovascular Surgery* **91**, 647–61.

Codd, J.E., Barner, H.B., Pennington, D.G. *et al.* 1985: Intraoperative myocardial protection: a comparison of blood and asanguinous cardioplegia. *Annals of Thoracic Surgery* **39**, 125–31.

Cremer, J., Steinhoff, G., Karck, M. *et al.* 1997: Ischemic preconditioning prior to myocardial protection with cold blood cardioplegia in coronary surgery. *European Journal of Cardiothoracic Surgery* **12**, 753–8.

Daily, P.O., Pfeffer, T.A., Wisniewski, J.B. *et al.* 1987: Clinical comparisons of methods of cardiac cooling. *Journal of Thoracic and Cardiovascular Surgery* **93**, 324–36.

Deutsch, E., Berger, M., Kussmaul, W.G. *et al.* 1990: Adaptation to ischemia during PTCA: clinical, hemodynamic, and metabolic features. *Circulation* **82**, 2044–51.

Digerness, S.B., Vanini, V., Wideman, F.E. 1981: *In vitro* comparison of oxygen availability from asanguinous and sanguinous cardioplegic media. *Circulation* **64** (Suppl. II), II-80–II-83.

Dignan, R.J., Dyke, C.M., Abd-Elfattah, A.S. *et al.* 1992: Coronary artery endothelial cell and smooth muscle dysfunction after global myocardial ischemia. *Annals of Thoracic Surgery* **5**, 311–17.

English, T., Cooper, D.K.C., Medd, R., Wheeldon, D. 1980: Orthotopic heart transplantation after 16 hours of ischaemia. *British Heart Journal* **43**, 721–2.

Ely, S.W., Mentzer, R.M. Jr., Lasley, R.D. *et al.* 1985: Functional and metabolic evidence of enhanced myocardial tolerance to ischemia and reperfusion with adenosine. *Journal of Thoracic and Cardiovascular Surgery* **90**, 549–56.

Faris, B., Peynet, J., Wassef, M. *et al.* 1997: Failure of preconditioning to improve postcardioplegia stunning of minimally infarcted hearts. *Annals of Thoracic Surgery* **64**, 1735–41.

Feerick, A.E., Johnston, W.E., Steinsland, O. *et al.* 1994: Cardiopulmonary bypass impairs vascular endothelial relaxation: effects of gaseous microemboli in dogs. *American Journal of Physiology* **267**, H1174–H1182.

Folgia, R.P., Steed, D.L., Follette, D.M. *et al.* 1979: Iatrogenic myocardial edema with potassium cardioplegia. *Journal of Thoracic and Cardiovascular Surgery* **78**, 217–22.

Follette, D.M., Mulder, D.G., Maloney, J.V., Buckberg, G.D. 1978: Advantages of blood cardioplegia over continuous coronary perfusion or intermittent ischemia. Experimental and clinical study. *Journal of Thoracic and Cardiovascular Surgery* **76**, 604–19.

Fremes, S.E., Christakis, G.T., Weisel, R.D. *et al.* 1984: A clinical trial of blood and crystalloid cardioplegia. *Journal of Thoracic and Cardiovascular Surgery* **88**, 726–41.

Fremes, S.E., Weisel, R.D., Christakis, G.T. *et al.* 1985: Myocardial metabolism and ventricular function following cold potassium cardioplegia. *Journal of Thoracic and Cardiovascular Surgery* **89**, 531–46.

Gay, W.A., Ebert, P.A. 1973: Functional, metabolic, and morphologic effects of potassium-induced cardioplegia. *Surgery* **74**, 284–90.

Goto, R., Tearle, H., Steward, D.J., Ashmore, P.G. 1991: Myocardial oedema and ventricular function after cardioplegia with added mannitol. *Canadian Journal of Anaethesia* **38**, 7–14.

Gundry, S.R., Sequeira, A., Coughlin, T.R., McLaughlin, J.S. 1989: Post-operative conduction disturbances: a comparison of blood and crystalloid cardioplegia. *Annals of Thoracic Surgery* **47**, 384–90.

Hayashida, N., Ikonomidis, J.S., Weisel, R.D. *et al.* 1994: The optimal cardioplegic temperature. *Annals of Thoracic Surgery* **58**, 961–71.

Hearse, D.J., Stewart, D.A., Braimbridge, M.V. 1978: Myocardial protection during ischemic cardiac arrest. The importance of magnesium in cardioplegic infusates. *Journal of Thoracic and Cardiovascular Surgery* **75**, 877–85.

Holscher, B., Just, O.H., Merker, H.J. 1961: Studies by electron microscope on various forms of induced cardiac arrest in dog and rabbit. *Surgery* **49**, 492–9.

Hottenrott, C.E., Towers, B., Kurkji, H.J. *et al.* 1973: The hazard of ventricular fibrillation in hypertrophied ventricles during cardiopulmonary bypass. *Journal of Thoracic and Cardiovascular Surgery* **66**, 742–53.

Hufnagel, C.A., Conrad, P.W., Schanno, J., Pifarre, R. 1961: Profound cardiac hypothermia. *Annals of Surgery* **153**, 790–6.

Hultgren, H.N., Miyagawa, M., Buch, W., Angell, W.W. 1973: Ischemic myocardial injury during cardiopulmonary bypass surgery. *American Heart Journal* **85**, 167–76.

Iliodromitis, E.K., Kremastinos, D.T., Katritsis, D.G., Papadopoulos, C.C., Hearse, D.J. 1997: Multiple cycles of preconditioning cause loss of protection in open-chest rabbits. *Journal of Molecular and Cellular Cardiology* **29**, 915–20.

Ihnken, K., Morita, K., Buckberg, G.D. 1994: New approaches to blood cardioplegic delivery to reduce hemodilution and cardioplegic overdose. *Journal of Cardiac Surgery* **9**, 26–36.

Iverson, L.I.G., Young, J.N., Ennix, C.L. Jr. *et al.* 1984: Myocardial protection: a comparison of cold blood and cold crystalloid cardioplegia. *Journal of Thoracic and Cardiovascular Surgery* **87**, 509–16.

Jenkins, D.P., Pugsley, W.B., Alkulaifi, A.M. *et al.* 1997: Ischemic preconditioning reduces troponin T release in patients undergoing coronary artery bypass surgery. *Heart* **77**, 314–18.

Julia, P.L., Buckberg, G.D., Acar, C. *et al.* 1991: Studies of controlled reperfusion after ischemia. XXI. Reperfusate composition: superiority of blood cardioplegia over crystalloid cardioplegia in limiting reperfusion damage – importance of endogenous oxygen free radical scavengers in red blood cells. *Journal of Thoracic and Cardiovascular Surgery* **101**, 303–13.

Jynge, P., Hearse, D.J., Braimbridge, M.V. 1977: Myocardial protection during ischemic cardiac arrest. A possible hazard with calcium-free cardioplegic infusates. *Journal of Thoracic and Cardiovascular Surgery* **73**, 848–55.

Kaukoranta, P.K., Lepojarvi, M.V., Kiviluoma, K.T. *et al.* 1998: Myocardial protection during antegrade versus retrograde cardioplegia. *Annals of Thoracic Surgery* **66**, 755–61.

Khuri, S.F., Warner, K.G., Josa, M. *et al.* 1988: The superiority of continuous cold blood cardioplegia in the metabolic protection of the hypertrophied human heart. *Journal of Thoracic and Cardiovascular Surgery* **95**, 442–54.

Kilbridge, P.M., Mayer, J.E. Jr., Newburger, J.W. *et al.* 1994: Induction of intracellular adhesion molecule-1 and E-selectin mRNA in heart and skeletal muscle of pediatric patients undergoing cardiopulmonary bypass. *Journal of Thoracic and Cardiovascular Surgery* **107**, 1183–92.

Kirshbom, P.M., Skaryak, L.R., DiBernardo, L.R. *et al.* 1996: pH-stat cooling improves cerebral metabolic recovery after circulatory arrest in a piglet model of aortopulmonary collaterals. *Journal of Thoracic and Cardiovascular Surgery* **111**, 147–55.

Kloner, R.A., Ganote, C.E., Jennings, R.B. 1974: The 'no-reflow' phenomenon after temporary coronary occlusion in the dog. *Journal of Clinical Investigation* **54**, 1496–508.

Kronon, M., Bolling, K.S., Allen, B.S. *et al.* 1998: The importance of cardioplegic infusion pressure in neonatal myocardial protection. *Annals of Thoracic Surgery* **66**, 1358–64.

Lazar, H.L., Rivers, S. 1989: Importance of topical hypothermia during hetergeneous distribution of cardioplegic solution. *Journal of Thoracic and Cardiovascular Surgery* **98**, 251–7.

Ledingham, S.J.M. 1988: Intraoperative protection of the paediatric myocardium. *Current Opinion in Cardiology* **3**, 741–7.

Lefer, D.J., Nakanishi, K., Johnston, W.E., Vinten-Johansen, J. 1993: Antineutrophil and myocardial protecting actions of a novel nitric oxide donor after acute myocardial ischemia and reperfusion of dogs. *Circulation* **88**, 2337–50.

Lillehei, C.W., DeWall, R.A., Gott, V.L., Varco, R.L. 1956: The direct vision correction of calcific aortic stenosis by means of a pump oxygenator and retrograde coronary sinus perfusion. *Diseases of the Chest* **30**, 123–7.

Lichtenstein, S.V., Ashe, K.A., El Dalati, H. *et al.* 1991: Warm heart surgery. *Journal of Thoracic and Cardiovascular Surgery* **101**, 269–74.

Liu, X., Engelman, R.M., Moraru, I.I. *et al.* 1992: Heat shock. A new approach for myocardial preservation in cardiac surgery. *Circulation* **86** (Suppl. II), II-358–II-363.

Lolley, D.M., Myers, W.O., Ray, J.F. *et al.* 1985: Clinical experience with preoperative myocardial nutrition management. *Journal of Cardiovascular Surgery* **26**, 236–43.

Lu, E.X., Chen, S.X., Hu, T.H. *et al.* 1998: Preconditioning enhances myocardial protection in patients undergoing open heart surgery. *Thoracic and Cardiovascular Surgery* **46**, 28–32.

McElroy, D.D., Walker, W.E., Taegtmeyer, H. 1989: Glycogen loading improves left ventricular function of the rabbit heart after hypothermic ischemic arrest. *Journal of Applied Cardiology* **4**, 455–65.

McLean, R.F., Wong, B.I., Naylor, C.D. *et al.* 1994: Cardiopulmonary bypass, temperature, and central nervous system dysfunction. *Circulation* 90 (Suppl. II), II-250–II-255.

Magovern, G.J. Jr., Flaherty, J.T., Gott, V.L. *et al.* 1982: Failure of blood cardioplegia to protect myocardium at lower temperatures. *Circulation* 66 (Suppl. I), I-60–I-67.

Mair, P., Hoermann, C., Mair, J. *et al.* 1999: Effects of a leucocyte depleting arterial filter on perioperative proteolytic enzyme and oxygen free radical release in patients undergoing aortocoronary bypass surgery. *Acta Anaesthesiologica Scandinavica* **43**, 452–7.

Melrose, D.G., Dreyer, B., Bentall, H.H., Baker, J.B.E. 1955: Elective cardiac arrest. Preliminary communication. *Lancet* **2**, 21–2.

Menasche, P., Piwnica, A. 1987: Retrograde cardioplegia through the coronary sinus. *Annals of Thoracic Surgery* **44**, 214–16.

Menasche, P., Fleury, J.P., Veyssie, L. *et al.* 1993: Limitation of vasodilation associated with warm heart operation by a 'mini-cardioplegia' delivery technique. *Annals of Thoracic Surgery* **56**, 1148–53.

Molina, J.E., Galliani, C.A., Einzig, S. *et al.* 1989: Physical and mechanical effects of cardioplegic injection on flow distribution and myocardial damage in hearts with normal coronary arteries. *Journal of Thoracic and Cardiovascular Surgery* **97**, 870–7.

Mullen, J.C., Christakis, G.T., Weisel, R.D. *et al.* 1986: Late post-operative ventricular function after blood and crystalloid cardioplegia. *Circulation* **74** (Suppl. III), III-89–III-98.

Mullen, J.C., Fremes, S.E., Weisel, R.D. *et al.* 1987: Right ventricular function: a comparison between blood and crystalloid cardioplegia. *Annals of Thoracic Surgery* **43**, 17–24.

Murashita, T., Hearse, D.J. 1991: Temperature-response studies of the detrimental effects of multidose versus single-dose cardioplegic solution in the rabbit heart. *Journal of Thoracic and Cardiovascular Surgery* **102**, 673–83.

Murry, C.E., Jennings, R.B., Reimer, K.A. 1986: Preconditioning with ischemia: a delay of lethal cell injury in ischemic myocardium. *Circulation* **74**, 1124–36.

Najafi, H., Henson, D., Dye, W.S. *et al.* 1969: Left ventricular hemorrhagic necrosis. *Annals of Thoracic Surgery* **7**, 550–61.

Nakanishi, K., Vinten-Johansen, J., Lefer, D.J. *et al.* 1992: Intracoronary L-arginine during reperfusion improves endothelial function and reduces infarct size. *American Journal of Physiology* **263**, H1650–H1658.

Nakanishi, K., Zhao, Z.-Q., Vinten-Johansen, J. *et al.* 1994: Coronary artery endothelial dysfunction after ischemia, blood cardioplegia, and reperfusion. *Annals of Thoracic Surgery* **58**, 191–9.

Naylor, C.D., Lichtenstein, S.V., Fremes, S.E., Warm Heart Investigators. 1994: Randomised trial of normothermic versus hypothermic coronary bypass surgery. *Lancet* **343**, 559–63.

Nikas, D.J., Ramadan, F.M., Elefteriades, J.A. 1998: Topical hypothermia: ineffective and deleterious as adjunct to cardioplegia for myocardial protection. *Annals of Thoracic Surgery* **65**, 28–31.

Okamoto, F., Allen, B.S., Buckberg, G.D. *et al.* 1986: Studies of controlled reperfusion after ischaemia. XIV. Reperfusion conditions: importance of ensuring gentle versus sudden reperfusion during relief of coronary occlusion. *Journal of Thoracic and Cardiovascular Surgery* **92**, 613–20.

Oldfield, G.S., Commerford, P.J., Opie, L.H. 1986: Effects of pre-operative glucose–insulin–potassium on myocardial glycogen levels and on complications of mitral valve replacement. *Journal of Thoracic and Cardiovascular Surgery* **91**, 874–8.

Partington, M.T., Acar, C., Buckberg, G.D. *et al.* 1989a: Studies of retrograde cardioplegia. I. Capillary blood flow distribution to myocardium supplied by open and occluded arteries. *Journal of Thoracic and Cardiovascular Surgery* **97**, 605–12.

Partington, M.T., Acar, C., Buckberg, G.D., Julia, P.L. 1989b: Studies of retrograde cardioplegia. II. Advantages of antegrade/ retrograde cardioplegia to optimize distribution in jeopardized myocardium. *Journal of Thoracic and Cardiovascular Surgery* **97**, 613–22.

Pearson, P.J., Schaff, H.V., Vanhoutte, P.M. 1995: Long-term impairment of endothelium-dependent relaxation to aggregating platelets after reperfusion injury in canine coronary arteries. *Circulation* **81**, 1921–7.

Perrault, L.P., Menasche, P. 1999: Preconditioning: can nature's shield be raised against surgical ischemic–reperfusion injury? *Annals of Thoracic Surgery* **68**, 1988–94.

Pisarenko, O.I., Solomatina, E.S., Studneva, I.M. *et al.* 1983: Protective effect of glutamic acid on cardiac function and metabolism during cardioplegia and reperfusion. *Basic Research in Cardiology* **78**, 534–43.

Pisarenko, O.I., Rosenfeldt, F.L., Langley, L. *et al.* 1995: Differing protection with aspartate and glutamate cardioplegia in the isolated rat heart. *Annals of Thoracic Surgery* **59**, 1541–8.

Rao, V., Cohen, G., Weisel, R.D. *et al.* 1998: Optimal flow rates for integrated cardioplegia. *Journal of Thoracic and Cardiovascular Surgery* **115**, 226–35.

Reynolds, T.R., Geffin, G.A., Titus, J.S. *et al.* 1989: Myocardial preservation related to magnesium content of hyperkalemic cardioplegic solutions at 8 degrees C. *Annals of Thoracic Surgery* **47**, 907–13.

Roberts, A.J., Moran, J.M., Sanders, J.H. *et al.* 1982: Clinical evaluation of the relative effectiveness of multidose crystalloid cardioplegia and cold blood potassium cardioplegia in coronary artery bypass graft surgery: a nonrandomized matched-pair analysis. *Annals of Thoracic Surgery* **33**, 421–33.

Robertson, J.M., Buckberg, G.D., Vinten-Johansen, J., Leaf, J.D. 1983: Comparison of distribution beyond coronary stenoses of blood and asanguineous cardioplegic solutions. *Journal of Thoracic and Cardiovascular Surgery* **86**, 80–6.

Robertson, J.M., Vinten-Johansen, J., Buckberg, G.D. *et al.* 1984: Safety of prolonged aortic clamping with blood cardioplegia. I. Glutamate enrichment in normal hearts. *Journal of Thoracic and Cardiovascular Surgery* **88**, 395–401.

Rosenfeldt, F.L. 1982: The relationship between myocardial temperature and recovery after experimental cardioplegic arrest. *Journal of Thoracic and Cardiovascular Surgery* **84**, 656–66.

Rosenkranz, E.R., Vinten-Johansen, J., Buckberg, G.D. *et al.* 1982: Benefits of normothermic induction of blood cardioplegia in energy-depleted hearts with maintenance of arrest by multidose cold blood cardioplegic infusions. *Journal of Thoracic and Cardiovascular Surgery* **84**, 667–77.

Rosenkranz, E.R., Buckberg, G.D., Laks, H., Mulder, D.G. 1983: Warm induction of cardioplegia with glutamate-enriched blood in coronary patients with cardiogenic shock who are dependent on inotropic drugs and intraaortic balloon support. *Journal of Thoracic and Cardiovascular Surgery* **86**, 507–18.

Rosenkranz, E.R., Okamoto, F., Buckberg, G.D. *et al.* 1984: Safety of prolonged aortic clamping with blood cardioplegia. II. Glutamate enrichment in energy-depleted hearts. *Journal of Thoracic and Cardiovascular Surgery* **88**, 402–10.

Rosenkranz, E.R., Okamoto, F., Buckberg, G.D. *et al.* 1986: Safety of prolonged aortic clamping with blood cardioplegia. III. Aspartate enrichment of glutamate–blood cardioplegia in energy-depleted hearts after ischemic and reperfusion injury. *Journal of Thoracic and Cardiovascular Surgery* **91**, 428–35.

Rousou, J.A., Engelman, R.M., Breyer, R.H. *et al.* 1988: The effect of temperature and hematocrit level of oxygenated cardioplegic solutions on myocardial preservation. *Journal of Thoracic and Cardiovascular Surgery* **95**, 625–30.

Sakai, A., Miya, J., Sohara, Y. *et al.* 1988: Role of red blood cells in the coronary microcirculation during cold blood cardioplegia. *Cardiovascular Research* **22**, 62–6.

Sato, H., Jordan, J.E., Zhao, Z.-Q. *et al.* 1997: Gradual reperfusion reduces infarct size and endothelial injury but augments neutrophil accumulation. *Annals of Thoracic Surgery* **64**, 1099–107.

Sawatari, K., Kadoba, K., Bergner, K.A. *et al.* 1991: Influence of the initial reperfusion pressure after hypothermic cardioplegic ischemia on endothelial modulation of coronary tone in neonatal lambs. Impaired coronary vasodilator response to acetylcholine. *Journal of Thoracic and Cardiovascular Surgery* **101**, 777–82.

Schaper, J., Walter, P., Scheld, H., Hehrlein, F. 1985: The effects of retrograde perfusion of cardioplegic solution in cardiac operations. *Journal of Thoracic and Cardiovascular Surgery* **90**, 882–7.

Shapira, N., Kirsh, M., Jochim, K., Behrendt, D.M. 1980: Comparison of the effect of blood cardioplegia to crystalloid cardioplegia on myocardial contractility in man. *Journal of Thoracic and Cardiovascular Surgery* **80**, 647–53.

Shirai, T., Rao, V., Weisel, R.D. *et al.* 1996: Antegrade and retrograde cardioplegia: alternate or simultaneous? *Journal of Thoracic and Cardiovascular Surgery* **112**, 787–96.

Sink, J.D., Hill, R.C., Attarian, D.E., Wechsler, A.S. 1983: Myocardial blood flow and oxygen consumption in the empty-beating, fibrillating, and potassium-arrested hypertrophied canine heart. *Annals of Thoracic Surgery* **35**, 372–9.

Speicher, C.E., Ferrigan, L., Wolfson, S.K. *et al.* 1962: Cold injury of the myocardium and pericardium in cardiac hypothermia. *Surgery, Gynecology and Obstetrics* **114**, 659–65.

Swanson, D.K., Dufek, J.H., Kahn, D.R. 1980: Improved myocardial preservation at 4°C. *Annals of Thoracic Surgery* **30**, 518–26.

Sydzyik, R.T., Stammers, A.H., Zavadil, D.P. *et al*, 1997: Evaluation of a new generation cardioplegia administration system. *Journal of Extra Corporeal Technology* **29**, 145–53.

Taber, R.F., Morales, A.R., Fine, G. 1967: Myocardial necrosis and the postoperative low-cardiac-output syndrome. *Annals of Thoracic Surgery* **4**, 12–27.

Takahashi, A., Chambers, D.J., Braimbridge, M.V., Hearse, D.J. 1988: Optimal myocardial protection during crystalloid cardioplegia. Interrelationship between volume and duration of infusion. *Journal of Thoracic and Cardiovascular Surgery* **96**, 730–40.

Takahashi, A., Chambers, D.J., Braimbridge, M.V., Hearse, D.J. 1989: Cardioplegia: relation of myocardial protection to infusion volume and duration. *European Journal of Cardiothoracic Surgery* **3**, 130–3.

Takemoto, N., Kuroda, H., Mori, T. 1992: The reciprocal protective effects of magnesium and calcium in hyperkalemic cardioplegic solutions on ischemic myocardium. *Basic Research in Cardiology* **87**, 559–69.

Teoh, K.H., Christakis, G.T., Weisel, R.D. *et al.* 1986: Accelerated myocardial metabolic recovery with terminal warm cardioplegia. *Journal of Thoracic and Cardiovascular Surgery* **91**, 888–95.

Thornton, J., Striplin, S., Liu, G.S. *et al.* 1990: Inhibition of protein synthesis does not block myocardial protection afforded by preconditioning. *American Journal of Physiology* **259**, H1822–H1825.

Tixier, D., Matheis, G., Buckberg, G.D., Young, H.H. 1991: Donor hearts with impaired hemodynamics. Benefit of warm substrate-enriched blood cardioplegic solution for induction of cardioplegia during cardiac harvesting. *Journal of Thoracic and Cardiovascular Surgery* **192**, 207–13.

Tsao, P.S., Aoki, N., Lefer, D.J. *et al.* 1990: Time course of endothelial dysfunction and myocardial injury during myocardial ischemia and reperfusion in the cat. *Circulation* **82**, 1402–12.

Verrier, E.D., Shen, I. 1993: Potential role of neutrophil anti-adhesion therapy in myocardial stunning, myocardial infarction, and organ dysfunction after cardiopulmonary bypass. *Journal of Cardiac Surgery* **8**, 309–12.

Vinten-Johansen, J., Edgerton, T.A., Breyer, R.H. *et al.* 1986: Surgical revascularization of acute (1 hour) coronary occlusion: blood versus crystalloid cardioplegia. *Annals of Thoracic Surgery* **42**, 247–54.

Vinten-Johansen, J., Lefer, D.J., Nakanishi, K. *et al.* 1992: Controlled coronary hydrodynamics at the time of reperfusion reduces postischaemic injury. *Coronary Artery Disease* **3**, 1081–93.

Weisel, R.D., Mickle, D.A.G., Finkle, C.D. *et al.* 1989: Delayed myocardial metabolic recovery after blood cardioplegia. *Annals of Thoracic Surgery* **48**, 503–7.

Wong, B.I., McLean, R.F., Naylor, C.D. *et al.* 1992: Central-nervous-system dysfunction after warm or hypothermic cardiopulmonary bypass. *Lancet* **339**, 1383–4.

Yamamoto, F., Manning, A.S., Crome, R. *et al.* 1985: Calcium antagonists and myocardial protection: a comparative study of the functional, metabolic and electrical consequences of verapamil and nifedipine as additives to the St. Thomas' cardioplegic solution. *Thoracic and Cardiovascular Surgery* **33**, 354–9.

Yau, T.M., Weisel, R.D., Mickle, D.A.G. *et al.* 1991: Optimal delivery of blood cardioplegia. *Circulation* **84** (Suppl. III), III-380–III-388.

Yau, T.M., Ikonomidis, J.S., Weisel, R.D. *et al.* 1993: Ventricular function after normothermic versus hypothermic cardioplegia. *Journal of Thoracic and Cardiovascular Surgery* **105**, 833–43.

Yellon, D.M., Alkhulaifi, A.M., Browne, E.E., Pugsley, W.B. 1992: Ischemic preconditioning limits infarct size in the rat heart. *Cardiovascular Research* **26**, 983–7.

Yellon, D.M., Alkhulaifi, A.M., Pugsley, W.B. 1993: Preconditioning the human myocardium. *Lancet* **342**, 276–7.

13

Blood conservation

MIKE CROSS

KEY POINTS

- The use of blood for cardiac surgery varies widely between centres.
- Strict criteria for blood transfusion are poorly defined.
- Blood conservation requires a multidisciplinary approach.
- Blood conservation requires a multifaceted approach.
- A blood transfusion protocol should be used in all cardiac surgical centres.

INTRODUCTION

Blood conservation should be routine practice in any centre undertaking cardiac surgery because of the well-documented risks and costs of transfusion. The incidence of transfusion varies between centres, and it has been proposed that one reason for this is a lack of teaching and education in blood conservation (Goodnough et al., 1991). The aim of this chapter is to address this problem.

Techniques used to conserve blood can broadly be divided into those that can be used pre-operatively, those that are used in the operating room and those that are used post-operatively. Although there will inevitably be some overlap in this classification it is a useful framework with which to start.

Before discussing the current techniques available to conserve blood and blood products it is important to consider the indications for a blood transfusion as well as the risks involved in transfusing blood or blood products.

INDICATIONS FOR, RISKS OF AND ALTERNATIVES TO BLOOD AND BLOOD PRODUCT TRANSFUSION

Indications for red cell transfusion

By the end of the 1920s the complexities of blood typing and anticoagulation were largely understood and by the time of World War II blood transfusion was considered an essential part of casualty resuscitation. Clinical experience at this time gave rise to the general rule that a haemoglobin concentration of 10 g/dL or a haematocrit of 30 per cent was acceptable (Dacie and Homer, 1946). These numbers were confirmed as being 'optimal' in the late 1960s when it was shown that any decrease in oxygen-carrying capacity caused by a fall in the haematocrit was compensated for by an increase in viscosity-related flow as long as the haematocrit did not fall below 30 per cent (Crowell and Smith, 1967). The relative oxygen

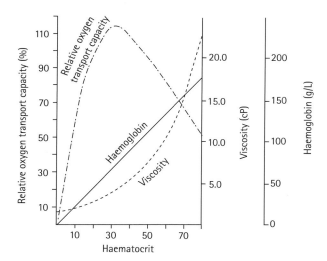

Figure 13.1 *Influence of packed cell volume and therefore viscosity on the relative oxygen transport capacity of blood. The relative oxygen transport capacity is maximal at approximately 30 per cent. (Reproduced with permission from Wood, J.H., Kee, D.B. 1995: Hemorheology of the cerebral circulation in stroke.* Stroke **16**, 765–72.)

transport capacity was shown, therefore, to be maximal at a haematocrit of 30 per cent (Fig. 13.1).

The concept of the 'optimal haematocrit' was used and not questioned until 1983, when an epidemiological link demonstrated between AIDS and transfused blood. This caused an abrupt change in transfusion practice and very rapidly the concept of the 'lowest acceptable haematocrit' was developed.

More recently, financial constraints as well as problems of availability have reinforced the concept of the lowest acceptable haematocrit. The availability of blood and blood products in the UK is being affected by the emergence of variant Creutzfeld–Jacob disease (vCJD). Fears that vCJD may be transmitted by blood transfusion, as recently demonstrated with bovine spongiform encephalopathy (BSE) in sheep (Houston *et al.*, 2000), mean that the donor population may be restricted to those who have not received a blood transfusion when BSE was prevalent (1980–1996). This change would mean that 10 per cent of the donor population would be removed and, at present levels of use, blood demand would outstrip supply. Development of a blood test of donors for the prion would reduce the donor population to a much greater extent and the introduction of such a test is likely within the next two years. Blood conservation on grounds of availability is becoming imperative.

Patients presenting for cardiac surgery will have different requirements for transfusion depending upon whether they are compromised by disease before cardiopulmonary bypass, whether they are hypothermic during cardiopulmonary bypass or whether they have had their myocardial disease corrected by surgery.

INDICATIONS FOR TRANSFUSION IN THE PATIENT COMPROMISED BY MYOCARDIAL DISEASE BEFORE CARDIOPULMONARY BYPASS

Different organs in the body vary in their ability to maintain adequate oxygen consumption as the haematocrit falls. The heart is the organ with the highest oxygen extraction ratio (55 per cent) during resting conditions, and there is little ability to increase this further as the haematocrit falls. Oxygen consumption in the heart is maintained as the haematocrit falls by an increase in blood flow. The increased flow occurs by a combination of increased cardiac output (mainly increased stroke volume), decreased viscosity and vasodilation. Vessels that are stenosed by atherosclerosis are already maximally vasodilated and for this reason tolerance of a low haematocrit is much reduced in this population. Animal work in this area suggests that a haematocrit of 20–24 per cent is tolerated before biochemical or contractile evidence of dysfunction occurs, although significant intersubject variability occurs even in the animal population (Spahn *et al.*, 1993). Translating these findings into clinical guidance is difficult because most animal models are of single-vessel disease with little development of collateral circulation. Studies of acute normovolaemic haemodilution in patients presenting for coronary artery surgery suggest that a haemoglobin concentration of 9.9 g/dL is safe in this population (Spahn *et al.*, 1996), although many clinicians will allow the haematocrit to fall below this in the lower risk patient if there is no evidence of clinical instability. It seems that a haematocrit of 25–28 per cent is adequate in the patient with cardiovascular disease when anaesthetized before revascularization. Fortunately, such a low haematocrit is not very common and pharmacological treatment with iron or erythropoietin is often possible prior to surgery.

INDICATIONS FOR TRANSFUSION DURING CARDIOPULMONARY BYPASS

Hard evidence for a transfusion threshold during cardiopulmonary bypass is nearly as poor as it is in the preoperative period, but there is no doubt that transfusion is not indicated until the haematocrit has fallen significantly below acceptable pre-cardiopulmonary bypass levels.

A lower haematocrit can be tolerated for a number of reasons: 'cardiac output' can be controlled during cardiopulmonary bypass; hypothermia during cardiopulmonary bypass decreases the body's oxygen requirements by approximately seven per cent per degree Celsius; general anaesthesia will decrease the metabolic rate and any fall in temperature increases the amount of dissolved oxygen that can be carried in the blood. The advantages of hypothermia, however, are offset by the fact that hypothermia increases blood viscosity. This can lead to microvascular sludging and end organ damage. The question therefore is: At what haematocrit is the advantage of haemodilution with respect to viscosity outweighed by the disadvantages with respect to oxygen delivery? What is the minimum safe haematocrit during cardiopulmonary bypass?

Anecdotal evidence has consistently pointed to a haematocrit of 15–18 per cent being well tolerated during cardiopulmonary bypass using moderate hypothermia. Indeed, it has been shown in a randomized study of 300 patients that a transfusion trigger of 15 per cent rather than 21 per cent might be beneficial with respect to morbidity and mortality (Jones *et al.*, 1991). Although such a low haematocrit may be acceptable, certain caveats need to be applied when allowing the haematocrit to fall to these very low levels during cardiopulmonary bypass. In a study of more than 2500 patients Fang and colleagues (Fang *et al.*, 1997) showed that in the absence of significant risk factors it was not until the haematocrit had been allowed to fall to 14 per cent that there was an increase in mortality. However, the threshold for transfusion should be raised to 18 per cent in the presence of a number of risk factors, such as unstable angina, congestive heart failure, renal failure, peripheral vascular disease or advanced age, if increased mortality is to be avoided. Although diabetes was not found to be a risk factor in the latter study, most people would include it as a risk factor of increased morbidity. These levels should all be revised upwards if normothermia is used during cardiopulmonary bypass. Although most clinicians will allow the haematocrit to fall below 20 per cent during cardiopulmonary bypass, recent evidence has suggested that this may not be beneficial. A large study using a database of cardiac surgery performed in New England has suggested that the mortality after cardiac surgery may double if the minimum haematocrit during cardiopulmonary bypass is allowed to fall below 19 per cent compared with a haematocrit of 24 per cent (Defoe *et al.*, 2001). Whether this is a real effect or whether the low haematocrit during cardiopulmonary bypass is a surrogate marker for the need for a post-operative transfusion, with its associated problems, is a question that has not yet been resolved.

INDICATIONS FOR TRANSFUSION AFTER CARDIOPULMONARY BYPASS

Although many patients will complete their cardiac operation with a haematocrit higher than most accepted transfusion thresholds it is during the post-operative period when most blood is transfused. Continued bleeding after surgery means that decisions need to be made on a daily basis about the need for red cell, platelet, fresh frozen plasma and cryoprecipitate transfusion. It is during this period that it is most important to have a clear understanding about the concept of a lowest acceptable haematocrit.

Much of the evidence that underlies the decision to transfuse patients in the post-operative period is anecdotal in nature. Different groups have shown 'successful outcomes' or 'good clinical results' with a transfusion trigger haematocrit of 22–24 per cent. In a small study (Johnson *et al.*, 1992) comparing a restrictive transfusion policy, where transfusion occurred only if the haematocrit was less than 25 per cent, with a liberal transfusion policy, where the aim was to maintain a haematocrit of 32 per cent, there was no significant difference between the groups in the recovery of the patients. Many people have suggested that patients have 'less energy' post-operatively when a restrictive transfusion policy is used, but this study included an exercise test on the fifth post-operative day.

More recently, two significant studies have emerged suggesting that a liberal transfusion policy may in fact be detrimental (Spiess *et al.*, 1998; Hebert *et al.*, 1999). Spiess *et al.* (1998) showed that the haematocrit upon admission to the intensive care unit is an independent predictor of the likelihood of having a peri-operative myocardial infarction. These workers compared patients who had a haematocrit of less than 24 per cent on admission to the intensive care unit with those who had a haematocrit of greater than 34 per cent. The infarction rate was 3.6 per cent in the first group and 8.3 per cent in the second. Even more marked was the finding that the mortality in patients who had surgery for unstable angina was 3.7 per cent in the first group and 10.4 per cent in the second. The results were somewhere between these figures in the group who had an admission haematocrit of 24–34 per cent. It is unclear from the work of Spiess *et al.* (1998) whether it was the higher haematocrit *per se* or the blood transfusion that probably accompanied the high haematocrit that gave rise to the findings. Hebert *et al.* (1999) showed that a restrictive strategy of red cell transfusion in critically ill patients was at least as effective as, and perhaps superior to, a liberal strategy with the possible exception of those with clinically significant cardiac disease or those with advanced age. This was a large, randomized, controlled trial and it has reopened the debate about blood transfusion in the intensive care unit.

If the haematocrit value alone is not able to determine accurately the need for a transfusion are there any other easily measured but more physiological markers of the need for transfusion?

The oxygen extraction ratio and the mixed venous saturation (SvO_2) are both indices of oxygen utilization that can easily be measured on the intensive care unit. It has been proposed that transfusion triggers might be determined by these values. An oxygen extraction ratio of less than 30 per cent despite a haematocrit of 15 per cent has been shown to be safe with regard to haemodynamic and biochemical markers of myocardial ischaemia (Mathru et al., 1992). SvO_2 is known to be a sensitive indicator of overall oxygen consumption and transfusion algorithms have been written that have included SvO_2 data, but there is no hard evidence that this additional information can in any way alter outcome (Goodnough et al., 1995).

Risks of allogeneic blood transfusion

The epidemiological evidence that blood transfusion may increase mortality and morbidity is only just starting to emerge (Spiess et al., 1998; Hebert et al., 1999; Engoren et al., 2002). Engoren et al. (2002) demonstrated a 70 per cent increase in five-year mortality, which after correction for co-morbidities and other factors is attributable to blood transfusion. The risks of viral infection from blood are now well recognized and are becoming more remote. The advent of nucleic acid amplification technology (NAT), which identifies the nucleic acids of viruses, will soon reduce the risk of infection with hepatitis C or HIV. The risk may fall to one in 1,000,000 as the donor window, which is the time between infection and development of a marker of infection, falls from approximately 50 days to one day. Although hepatitis C is well recognized, 'new' viruses are being described and the significance of these is not yet known. Transfusion transmissible virus (TTV) was first described in 2000 and is now known to be present in 50 per cent of the population in the USA (Handa et al., 2000). The significance of this finding is, as yet, unknown. Of much greater concern is bacterial infection acquired from blood, or more commonly platelets, because there is no accepted test to identify blood products that have bacterial contamination. The estimated risk of bacterial contamination of platelets is one in 12,000 (Dodd, 1994). This is increased sevenfold if pooled platelets from multiple donors are used. The estimated mortality from platelet-related sepsis is 26 per cent (Goldman and Blajchman, 1991), which makes this the most common cause of transfusion-related death. The risks of fresh frozen plasma-related infections are decreasing with the introduction of new techniques. Solvent detergent treatment of fresh frozen plasma will destroy the lipid envelopes of viruses such as HIV or hepatitis C. Donor retesting after the period of the donor window, before issue of the fresh frozen plasma, is also reducing the risk of infection.

Transfusion-mediated immunomodulation can be demonstrated in all patients receiving a blood transfusion, and a recent meta-analysis suggested that the rate of post-operative infection and cancer recurrence increases with exposure to allogeneic blood (Vamvakas, 1996). The risks are probably related to exposure to leucocytes and this can be reduced by leucoreduction of transfused blood. Leucoreduction of blood and blood products has become universal in Europe. Leucoreduction of blood and blood products was made mandatory in the UK during the late 1990s because of the theoretical risk that BSE may be transmitted by blood and that leucoreduction may decrease this possibility. The process has not yet become routine practice in the USA, mainly because of the cost implications (Table 13.1).

Risks of autologous blood transfusion

Prima facie, there are no infective or immunological risks associated with an autologous transfusion, although the risk of bacterial contamination at the time of collection still exists. The most common reason for a blood transfusion reaction, however, is clerical error when the wrong unit of blood is given to a patient. This risk is identical whether an autologous or an allogeneic blood transfusion is given. Errors are less likely when an autologous unit collected by acute normovolaemic haemodilution is reinfused than when it is collected by pre-operative autologous donation because of the short time period between donation and reinfusion.

Indications for transfusion of platelets, fresh frozen plasma and cryoprecipitate

After cardiac surgery there is almost always some degree of coagulopathy if cardiopulmonary bypass has been used. The fact that the incidence of blood product transfusion varies between institutions (Goodnough et al., 1991) suggests that transfusion of blood products to control bleeding that may accompany this coagulopathy is not optimal in all centres. Whereas it is possible to use a single number (the haematocrit) to decide whether a red cell transfusion is required, it is much more difficult to find a good indicator that a transfusion of platelets or fresh frozen plasma is required. A combination of rate of bleeding and the INR, APTT and platelet count is often used. Rates in excess of 300 mL during the first postoperative hour, or 150 mL for each of the first two hours, is a commonly used protocol. Units that have developed protocols for transfusion of blood products vary in the tests that they use to help them make a decision to transfuse. Although all units will have the ability to determine the INR, the APTT and the platelet count after surgery, not all units will have thromboelastography. Recently, it has been shown that blood product transfusion can be reduced by inclusion of thromboelastography data in a transfusion protocol (Shore-Lesserson et al., 1999). What is clear beyond doubt is that any transfusion protocol is better than no protocol. All units should have a protocol in place.

Table 13.1 *Risks of blood transfusion; the advent of nucleic acid amplification techniques will probably reduce the risk of infection from hepatitis C and HIV even further*

Risk factor	Estimated frequency		No. of deaths per million units
	Per actual unit	Per 10^6 units	
Infection			
Viral			
Hepatitis A	1/1,000,000	1	0
Hepatitis B	1/30,000 to 1/250,000	7–32	0–0.14
Hepatitis C	1/30,000 to 1/150,000	4–36	0.5–17
HIV	1/200,000 to 1/2,000,000	0.5–4	0
HTLV types I and II	1/250,000 to 1/2,000,000	0.5–4	0
Parvovirus B19	1/10,000	100	0
Bacterial contamination:			
Red cells	1/500,000	2	0.1–0.25
Platelets	1/12,000	83	21
Acute haemolytic reactions	1/250,000 to 1/1,000,000	1–4	0.67
Delayed haemolytic reactions	1/1000	1000	0.4
Transfusion-related acute lung injury	1/5000	200	0.2
Transfusion immunomodulation (e.g. infection or tumour recurrence)	Unknown	Unknown	Unknown

Adapted with permission from Goodnough, L.T. *et al.* 1999: Transfusion article, Medical progress article. *New England Journal of Medicine* **340**, 438–47.

It is unclear what volume of blood products should be given once the decision to give that blood product has been made. Each unit of platelets contains approximately 5.5×10^{10} platelets and a therapeutic dose is generally considered to be 2.75×10^{11}, which means that most units empirically transfuse four or six units of platelets once the decision to transfuse has been made. Some units will use a dosing regimen of one unit per 10 kg of body-weight. Six units of platelets will contain approximately the same concentration of coagulation factors as one unit of fresh frozen plasma and for this reason if blood products are to be given in sequence depending upon results some would argue that platelets should be given first. The transfusion of fresh frozen plasma is another situation where the optimal volume to transfuse is not well defined. A volume of 10 mL/kg or four units is generally adequate to correct clotting factor deficiencies (BCSH, 1992), but many patients who are bleeding with a prolonged INR will respond to much smaller volumes. Two units of fresh frozen plasma is often the empiric dose once the decision to transfuse has been taken. Cryoprecipitate is usually reserved for patients who continue to bleed despite therapy with platelets and fresh frozen plasma. The evidence that cryoprecipitate is useful in this situation is poor unless the fibrinogen concentration is less than 80 mg/dL (BCSH, 1992).

Alternatives to allogeneic blood transfusion

It is now more than 50 years since the hypothesis that a haemoglobin solution can act as an oxygen carrier was tested (Amberson *et al.*, 1949). The advantages of a red cell substitute are not only that the risks of infection or immunomodulation are removed but also the need for cross-matching is eliminated. A long shelf-life is also a desirable attribute. Work within this field has followed two distinct paths. Haemoglobin preparations and per-fluorocarbon emulsions are the most likely pharmacological approaches to intravascular gas transport. Despite the passage of time, neither approach has led to routine clinical use of these agents but it appears likely that this will change during the next 10 years.

Guidelines for red cell transfusion

In summary, the lowest acceptable haematocrit in any individual patient depends upon a number of factors and there is no generally valid transfusion threshold. Table 13.2 gives a broad indication of the lowest acceptable haematocrit below which there is evidence of increased biochemical or clinical morbidity. A patient suffering from one or more of the conditions listed in the right-hand column will require transfusion at a higher haematocrit than the same patient who does not, particularly in the presence of clinical signs or symptoms.

Protocol for blood and blood product transfusion

Although it would be impossible to describe a generally accepted protocol for transfusion, there is universal

Table 13.2 *Guidelines for a lowest acceptable haematocrit during the peri-operative period*

Time period	Lowest acceptable haematocrit	Reasons for increasing the lowest acceptable haematocrit
Pre-operative or pre-cardiopulmonary bypass	28%	Ongoing ischaemia Haemodynamic instability Small body size

Cardiopulmonary bypass	15%
	18% in the presence of risk factors
		Risk factor to raise haematocrit to 18%:
		    unstable angina
		    congestive heart failure
		    peripheral vascular disease
		    renal failure
		    advanced age

Post-cardiopulmonary bypass or post-operative	24%	Incomplete revascularization Low cardiac output Respiratory failure Myocardial ischaemia Cerebral ischaemia

agreement that a protocol that is acceptable to all the clinicians involved is better than no protocol at all, and development of a transfusion protocol should be central to all units' efforts to conserve blood.

PRE-OPERATIVE BLOOD CONSERVATION TECHNIQUES

Maximum surgical blood order schedule

The maximum surgical blood order schedule is a table of elective surgical procedures that lists the number of units of blood routinely cross-matched for them pre-operatively. The maximum surgical blood order schedule is hospital-specific, occasionally surgeon-specific and should be published after discussion between surgeons, anaesthetists and blood bank personnel. The schedule is based on a retrospective analysis of actual blood usage associated with an individual surgical procedure and aims to correlate as closely as possible the amount of blood cross-matched (C) with the amount of blood transfused (T). Because it is rare for large amounts of blood to be required within a very short period of time, a C:T ratio of 2:1 is generally considered acceptable for cardiac surgery, providing that the laboratory can provide additional blood in a reasonable time period (30–45 minutes). Use of the maximum surgical blood order schedule within a hospital permits efficient use of blood stocks and reduces wastage caused by date expiry. Some hospitals have now replaced individual cross-matching with computerized cross-matching when patients are electronically cross-matched with all group-identical units in the blood fridge for the operating rooms or the intensive care unit. This system will allow even less wastage and significantly fewer emergency additional cross-match requests (Chan *et al.*, 1996).

Pre-operative autologous donation

Pre-operative autologous donation is a technique of blood conservation in which patients who are scheduled for surgery in the near future donate their own blood on a number of occasions, depending upon the number of units required. The blood is screened and stored and is then available for reinfusion during the peri-operative period. Although it is generally accepted to be a safe and effective blood conservation measure provided that the technique is applied in a logical way (Owings *et al.*, 1989), the risks associated with autologous donation exceed those of the healthy volunteer donor population (Popovsky *et al.*, 1995). Central to the principle of pre-operative autologous donation is the fact that red cell regeneration in patients receiving oral iron supplementation takes approximately two weeks per unit of blood removed. If any shorter time period is allowed to elapse between donations or between donation and surgery, the effectiveness of pre-operative autologous donation is reduced. In fact, the patient will instead have undergone a form of normovolaemic haemodilution, a technique which is often performed safely, more effectively and with less expense at the time of surgery.

PATIENT SELECTION

Not all patients presenting for cardiac surgery will be suitable for pre-operative autologous donation. Any patient who cannot wait two weeks for surgery is, by definition not suitable for pre-operative autologous donation because of the lack of time for red cell regeneration.

Patients may be unsuitable for pre-operative autologous donation for a number of medical reasons. Those patients with unstable or crescendo angina, symptomatic left main stem disease or congestive heart failure will not be suitable for pre-operative autologous donation because they may be unable to tolerate the reduction in oxygen carrying capacity and/or the hypovolaemia that may be involved in this procedure. Aortic stenosis has been suggested as a contraindication, but it has been shown that pre-operative autologous donation can be safely performed in this group of patients (Dzik *et al.*, 1992). Active endocarditis should be considered a contraindication because the storage period will allow time for bacterial replication in a contaminated unit. Haemoglobinopathies, such as sickle cell trait, are contraindications. Pre-operative anaemia is a contraindication to pre-operative autologous donation. A haematocrit of less than 34 per cent or a low red cell mass should lead to an investigation of the anaemia rather than inclusion in a pre-operative autologous donation programme.

Old age is not considered a contraindication to pre-operative autologous donation because the incidence of adverse reactions to donation is similar to the younger population (Garry *et al.*, 1991).

OPTIMAL DURATION AND DONATION INTERVAL OF PRE–OPERATIVE AUTOLOGOUS DONATION

Pre-operative autologous donation should commence at a time before surgery so that the selected number of units of blood can be collected with full red cell regeneration prior to surgery. If less than two weeks elapses between donations before surgery, the haematocrit at the time of surgery will be lower than it would have been without pre-operative autologous donation. The chance of an autologous transfusion with all its attendant risks will then be increased. The time period between the first donation and surgery is limited by the maximum storage time for blood. In general this is 42 days. The maximum number of units of blood, therefore, that can be removed with full red cell regeneration is three, assuming that surgery is scheduled exactly 42 days after the first donation. Are there any ways to reduce the time period for red cell regeneration? Oral iron supplementation should always be given from the time of commencing pre-operative autologous donation, with vitamin C to increase gastrointestinal absorption of iron. Any variability in times for red cell regeneration appears to depend on the iron stores of the patient when pre-operative autologous donation commences. Parenteral iron has been proposed as a method of increasing the speed of red cell regeneration. Although this may increase the speed of regeneration the incidence of anaphylaxis is too high for it to be a technique that is used regularly.

Erythropoeitin therapy in combination with pre-operative autologous donation has been shown to be an effective method of reducing the time for red cell regeneration. A dose of 600 U/kg on days 14 and 7 pre-operatively allows two units of blood to be removed during this period while still having the haematocrit return to baseline at the time of surgery (Watanabe *et al.*, 1991). The safety of this treatment is well established, but the main objection to its much wider use is the cost involved. The recommended price in the UK in 2003 for the treatment regimen used by Watanabe *et al.* (1991) is £700 per patient.

OPTIMAL NUMBER OF UNITS OF BLOOD COLLECTED

If too many units of blood are collected from a patient, the additional blood in excess of that required will be wasted and the cost-effectiveness of the technique will be diminished. In order to collect the appropriate number of units it is important to know the average transfusion risk for that patient. The calculation should include not only the type of operation to be undertaken but also factors such as the weight, haematocrit and drug history of the patient (for example, history of aspirin therapy).

COST–EFFECTIVENESS OF PRE–OPERATIVE AUTOLOGOUS DONATION

Even the remotest risk of death during pre-operative autologous donation will negate its potential benefits. It has been estimated that pre-operative autologous donation of two units of blood before cardiac surgery had an estimated cost of $500,000 per quality-adjusted life-year (QALY) compared with many surgical interventions that have a cost of less than $50,000 per QALY (Birkmeyer *et al.*, 1994). The decreasing incidence of viral infection from allogeneic blood transfusion will increase the cost per QALY still further, although the evidence that allogeneic blood transfusion is associated with an increased risk of post-operative infection or cancer recurrence may offset this.

TRANSFUSION THRESHOLD FOR PRE–OPERATIVE AUTOLOGOUS DONATION BLOOD

The risks of transfusion of autologous blood and blood products are significantly less than those associated with allogeneic transfusion. For this reason there is a tendency to change the threshold for reinfusion of pre-operative autologous donation blood. However, there are risks associated with any transfusion. The risks are mainly caused by clerical error resulting in the transfusion of the incorrect unit. Other risks, such as bacterial contamination of the unit, air embolus or volume overload, must also be considered. The threshold for transfusion should be based on clinical need rather than influenced by the increased safety of pre-operative autologous donation blood.

Erythropoietin

Erythropoietin is an endogenous glycoprotein hormone that is the main stimulus for red blood cell production. It is produced by the kidney in response to tissue hypoxia, which may be caused by decreased oxygen carrying capacity (anaemia), decreased oxygen tension (hypoxia) or increased oxygen affinity of the blood (alkalosis or low red cell 2,3 DPG levels). Recombinant erythropoietin is produced by a tumour cell line after transfection with the erythropoietin gene. It is virtually identical to endogenous erythropoietin.

Erythropoietin administered before cardiac surgery has been shown to be an effective adjunct to blood conservation (Laupacis and Fergusson, 1998). It may be used to reduce the time for red cell regeneration and therefore to improve the effectiveness of pre-operative autologous donation, to correct pre-operative anaemia or to cause acute pre-operative marrow stimulation so that the patient presents for surgery with a relatively high haematocrit. Subcutaneous injection is the preferred route of administration because it leads to more prolonged raised erythropoietin levels. A similar effect can therefore be obtained with a lower, less costly dose.

Concerns that acute pre-operative marrow stimulation may increase thrombotic complications were raised when it was shown that a higher death rate occurred in patients receiving erythropoietin compared with control subjects (D'Ambra et al., 1997). This increased rate failed to reach statistical significance but it emphasizes the need for further research before erythropoietin is introduced into general clinical practice, which may occur when the patent expires.

BLOOD CONSERVATION TECHNIQUES IN THE OPERATING ROOM

Acute normovolaemic haemodilution

Acute normovolaemic haemodilution is a technique that has been used by many clinicians to help reduce the need for allogeneic blood transfusion. It involves the removal of blood from a patient during the early stages of an operation (before any significant blood loss) with simultaneous replacement with a non-blood fluid to maintain normovolaemia. The blood is stored in a preservative, such as CPDA-1. Blood that is lost during the operation therefore contains less red cells than it would have done without acute normovolaemic haemodilution. The autologous blood, which contains a full complement of clotting factors and effective platelets, can be reinfused when the operation is complete or sooner if clinically indicated. In cardiac surgery, blood is removed during the pre-bypass period and generally reinfused at the end of the operation.

EFFICACY OF ACUTE NORMOVOLAEMIC HAEMODILUTION

Blood transfusion requirements during cardiac surgery have changed greatly over the last 20 years with the introduction of pharmacological agents to reduce blood loss, the development of modern cardiopulmonary bypass circuits and the movement towards lower transfusion thresholds. This has meant that many of the older studies assessing the effectiveness of acute normovolaemic haemodilution are no longer valid. It is unlikely that new studies will appear from the USA because in many states physicians are obliged to offer some form of autologous blood provision and research has therefore centred on a comparison of pre-operative autologous donation with acute normovolaemic haemodilution. Modern, prospective, randomized, controlled studies of the use of acute normovolaemic haemodilution in cardiac surgery that are not open to criticism, are almost non-existent (Gillon et al., 1999). Mathematical modelling of acute normovolaemic haemodilution performed in the non-cardiac setting has suggested that the procedure is unlikely to be effective unless the surgical blood loss is substantial (more than 3000 mL) and the transfusion threshold is approximately 25 per cent (Goodnough et al., 1997). Until appropriate studies are completed, advocates of acute normovolaemic haemodilution must rely upon older and less robust data to support their practice. If acute normovolaemic haemodilution is to be undertaken it is important that the practicalities and risks of 'optimal' acute normovolaemic haemodilution are understood.

PATIENT SELECTION

Patients who are deemed unsuitable for pre-operative autologous donation for medical reasons will in general be unsuitable for acute normovolaemic haemodilution. The time for red cell regeneration is not an issue for acute normovolaemic haemodilution and therefore patients who might have been excluded from pre-operative autologous donation purely on grounds of time will be suitable for acute normovolaemic haemodilution.

TIMING OF ACUTE NORMOVOLAEMIC HAEMODILUTION

Patients presenting for cardiac surgery will always require central venous cannulation. The side arm of a pulmonary artery catheter introducer is a suitable route for removal of blood. Even with a pulmonary artery catheter in situ a 8.5F introducer is generally large enough to allow drainage by gravity to occur at a reasonable rate of 10–15 minutes per unit, with the aim of completion before heparinization.

Concerns that heparin may impair platelet function in the collected blood (John *et al.*, 1993) mean that most clinicians now aim to complete acute normovolaemic haemodilution before this point.

STORAGE OF BLOOD

Guidelines have recently been produced covering many of the concerns about collection, labelling, storage and reinfusion or disposal of autologous blood (Napier, 1997). Blood is collected into a standard collection bag identical to those used by the Blood Transfusion Service. Ideally, a rocker scale should be used so that the correct volume of blood can be added to each bag to maintain the correct anticoagulant ratio and so that complete mixing occurs. The collection line is knotted twice before removal of the integral needle and the bag is labelled so that it can be checked before reinfusion. Storage of acute normovolaemic haemodilution blood should be in the operating room so that the risk of a clerical error leading to an incorrect reinfusion is kept to a minimum. Storage of platelets at room temperature is optimal for preservation of function and the short time period that the blood is stored for means that the risk of bacterial contamination or replication is minimal.

OPTIMAL ACUTE NORMOVOLAEMIC HAEMODILUTION

If acute normovolaemic haemodilution is to be effective it is important that an optimal volume of blood is removed. If 50 mL of blood is removed from a 70 kg patient presenting for cardiac surgery it is unlikely that any benefit of acute normovolaemic haemodilution, in terms of haematocrit level at discharge or allogeneic blood transfusion, will be demonstrated. The maximum volume of blood that can safely be removed should always be removed if the technique is to be an effective one. When discussing the transfusion threshold before or during cardiopulmonary bypass it was suggested that a haematocrit of 25–28 per cent before cardiopulmonary bypass or 15–18 per cent during cardiopulmonary bypass is generally considered safe. Using these figures and by estimating the blood volume of the patient and knowing the priming volume of the cardiopulmonary bypass circuit, it is possible to calculate the volume of blood that can be withdrawn without exceeding either of the transfusion thresholds. In practice, this calculation is complicated by the fact that only whole units of blood should be removed so that the blood:anticoagulant ratio is maintained in the blood that is removed.

In Figure 13.2 the first equation is used to calculate the haematocrit immediately before cardiopulmonary bypass that will give rise to a haematocrit of 18 per cent during cardiopulmonary bypass. If, using the first equation, the calculated haematocrit immediately before cardiopulmonary bypass that will give rise to a haematocrit

$$(1)\ HCT_{pre\text{-}CPB} = \frac{HCT_{during\ CPB} \times (EBV + CPB\ priming\ vol.)}{EBV}$$

$$(2)\ ANH\ blood\ volume = \frac{EBV \times (HCT_{initial} - HCT_{pre\text{-}CPB})}{HCT_{initial}}$$

Figure 13.2 *Formulae used to calculate the volume of blood removed by ANH, which will give rise to a haematocrit of 15–18 per cent during cardiopulmonary bybass. $HCT_{pre\text{-}CPB}$ = the haematocrit before CPB that, when an allowance is made for the CPB priming volume and the estimated blood volume, will give rise to a given HCT during CPB. It is usually limited by clinical circumstances to 25–28%; $HCT_{during\ CPB}$ = either the target HCT to be achieved on CPB (15–18%) or the HCT that will be achieved during CPB when the HCT before CPB is not allowed to fall below 25–28%; EBV is the estimated blood volume of the patient, calculated from the patient's weight, height and sex; CPB priming vol. = the priming volume of the CPB circuit after removal of any pre-bypass filter that is being used. It will vary between institutions and will vary between patients if retrograde autologous priming of the CPB circuit is used; ANH blood vol. = the volume of blood that may be removed by acute normovolaemic haemodilution that will either give rise to a target HCT before CPB (25–28%) or that will give rise to a target HCT during CPB (15–18%); $HCT_{initial}$ = the first HCT that is measured in the operating room after induction of anaesthesia and the fluid administration that usually accompanies induction of anaesthesia.*

of 18 per cent during cardiopulmonary bypass is more than 25–28 per cent then the calculated value should be used in the second equation when calculating the volume of blood to be removed. If the figure calculated is less than 25–28 per cent then we must accept that the minimum acceptable haematocrit before cardiopulmonary bypass is 25–28 per cent and this number must be used in the second equation to calculate the acute normovolaemic haemodilution blood volume to be removed rather than the lower haematocrit calculated.

To understand the practicalities of these calculations two worked examples are given.

Example 1
Assume initial haematocrit = 40 per cent, EBV = 5000 mL, cardiopulmonary bypass circuit priming volume = 1500 mL. The estimated haematocrit$_{pre\text{-}CPB}$ that will give rise to a haematocrit$_{during\ CPB}$ of 18 per cent is:

$$haematocrit_{pre\text{-}CPB} = \frac{18 \times (5000 + 1500)}{5000}$$

$$= 23.4\ per\ cent.$$

Clearly, this is an unacceptable haematocrit in the pre-cardiopulmonary bypass period and therefore a figure of 25–28 per cent must be used in the second calculation.

Assuming that a haematocrit of 27 per cent is considered acceptable:

$$\left.\begin{array}{l}\text{Acute normovolaemic}\\\text{haemodilution}\\\text{blood volume}\end{array}\right\} = \frac{5000 \times (40 - 27)}{40}$$

$$= 1625\,\text{mL}.$$

By rearranging the first equation this will give rise to an estimated haematocrit$_{\text{during CPB}}$ of 20.7 per cent.

Example 2

Assume initial haematocrit = 34 per cent, EBV = 3800 mL, cardiopulmonary bypass circuit priming volume = 2300 mL. The estimated haematocrit$_{\text{pre-CPB}}$ that will give rise to a haematocrit$_{\text{during CPB}}$ of 18 per cent is:

$$\text{haematocrit}_{\text{pre-CPB}} = \frac{18 \times (3800 + 2300)}{3800}$$

$$= 28.9\,\text{per cent}.$$

This figure is safe before cardiopulmonary bypass and therefore can be used in the second calculation:

$$\left.\begin{array}{l}\text{Acute normovolaemic}\\\text{haemodilution}\\\text{blood volume}\end{array}\right\} = \frac{3800 \times (34 - 28.9)}{34}$$

$$= 570\,\text{mL}.$$

REINFUSION OF ACUTE NORMOVOLAEMIC HAEMODILUTION BLOOD

Reinfusion of acute normovolaemic haemodilution blood should take place during cardiopulmonary bypass if the haematocrit falls to an unacceptably low level (below 15–18 per cent). This should only occur after blood that may have been collected by cell salvage is returned to the cardiopulmonary bypass circuit and all blood available by cardiotomy suction from the mediastinum and pleural spaces is also returned. The bag of acute normovolaemic haemodilution blood that has been collected last with the lowest concentration of platelets and clotting factors should be used first.

After cardiopulmonary bypass blood should not be reinfused until administration of protamine is complete unless a low haematocrit at this time makes it obligatory. Again, when blood is returned it should be given in the reverse order to that in which it was collected. It will reduce the chance of a clerical error if all the acute normovolaemic haemodilution blood is reinfused before the end of surgery, or at least connected to the patient by this time.

Intraoperative platelet–rich plasmapheresis

Platelet-rich plasmapheresis is a technique that has been used in the pre-cardiopulmonary bypass period to reduce the need for allogeneic blood transfusion. The aim of the procedure is to minimize the post-cardiopulmonary bypass bleeding by providing the patient with autologous functional platelets and coagulation factors that have not been exposed to the cardiopulmonary bypass circuit. The technique involves removal of blood from the patient via a large-bore central line and mixing it with an anticoagulant, such as ACDA-1. The blood then passes into a centrifuge where it is spun to separate the red cells from the plasma and the platelets. The red cells are returned to the patient and the platelet rich plasma is stored ready for reinfusion after cardiopulmonary bypass. The technique is not one of preserving red cells but one of reducing the coagulopathy that often follows cardiopulmonary bypass. If the tendency to bleed is reduced so the likelihood of an allogeneic transfusion is reduced.

EFFICACY OF PLATELET–RICH PLASMAPHERESIS

The success of platelet-rich plasmapheresis in limiting exposure to allogeneic blood transfusion has been mixed. Early studies published in the late 1980s (Giordano et al., 1988) suggested that allogeneic blood transfusion could be reduced by 50 per cent using this technique. This landmark study has been open to much criticism because of a number of factors. Historically, control subjects were used; the control group received a mean platelet transfusion of six units and the mean post-operative chest tube drainage approached 1500 mL in both groups. Clearly, these last two factors mean that the findings are of questionable relevance today. Following this, a prospective, randomized study of 100 patients using standardized transfusion criteria was performed, which showed a 60 per cent reduction in transfusion requirements (Jones et al., 1990). This reduction occurred without any significant difference in post-operative blood loss. More recent studies have, in general, failed to show any significant blood-sparing effect (Ereth et al., 1993), although these studies have also been open to criticism with the median platelet yield obtained by platelet-rich plasmapheresis being that which many people would consider inadequate. Apart from the issues of transfusion protocols, platelet yield and blinding of studies there may be other reasons that platelet-rich plasmapheresis is not effective. The storage of platelets in CPDA-1 may damage the platelet membrane (Wallace et al., 1976) and the plateletpheresis process itself may activate platelets, making them less effective when reinfused (Ford et al., 1999). In 1998, a meta-analysis of the effect of platelet-rich plasmapheresis upon transfusion requirements was published which suggested that platelet-rich plasmapheresis could reduce the proportion of patients receiving an allogeneic blood transfusion (Rubens et al., 1998). However, the poor methodological quality of most of the trials and the marked heterogeneity of the results make it very difficult to determine the true efficacy of platelet-rich plasmapheresis. The use of platelet-rich plasmapheresis will preclude the use of optimal acute normovolaemic haemodilution, a technique with a larger body of supportive evidence, and for this reason its use should be limited to large, well-controlled, prospective clinical trials.

PRACTICALITIES OF PLATELET–RICH PLASMAPHERESIS

Platelet-rich plasmapheresis requires a dedicated large (8-Fr) internal jugular catheter. After induction of anaesthesia, blood is removed from this catheter using a roller pump. Blood is immediately mixed with an anticoagulant in a fixed ratio and then passes into a centrifuge chamber, which will hold approximately 250 mL. The blood is then spun at 3500 rpm to separate the red cells from the plasma and the platelets. When the centrifuge is full of red cells and they are starting to spill into the collection bag containing the platelet-rich plasmapheresis product the centrifuge automatically stops and the red cells are returned to the patient. The platelet-rich plasmapheresis product should have a haematocrit of approximately five per cent because the largest most active platelets are contained in the layer, which is very close to the red cell layer in the centrifuge. Depending upon the haematocrit of the patient the process will remove aliquots of approximately 400 mL before the centrifuge chamber fills with 250 mL of red cells. The process is repeated until an adequate number of platelets have been collected (3×10^{11} is generally considered adequate, which depending upon the platelet count of the patient usually equates to a platelet-rich plasmapheresis product volume of 1000–1500 mL). The process, which often takes an hour to complete, should be finished before heparinization of the patient and for this reason if it is to be performed effectively may actually prolong the operation. The removal of blood must be matched by an infusion of colloid or crystalloid to maintain normovolaemia. The infusion rate must be varied depending upon whether the platelet-rich plasmapheresis process is removing or reinfusing blood. The complex nature of the technique means that a dedicated technician always performs it. Close co-ordination between anaesthetist and technician is essential if the technique is to be performed safely. The platelet-rich plasmapheresis product should be stored at room temperature in the operating room and reinfused at the end of the operation after reversal of heparin.

Intraoperative cell salvage

Intraoperative cell salvage has been widely used during cardiac surgery for the last 20 years. The process involves collection of blood from the surgical field with immediate mixing with heparin so that coagulation does not occur. The heparinized blood then passes through a 25 µm filter into a collection reservoir. From there, when

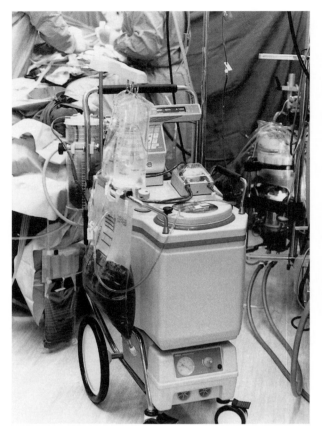

Figure 13.3 *Intraoperative cell salvage is widely used during cardiac surgery. The cost of cell salvage per case is approximately the same as a single unit of homologous blood.*

an adequate volume has been collected, the blood passes into a centrifugal bowl where the red cells are separated by differential centrifugation and then washed in normal saline solution. The waste from this bowl, which contains plasma, platelets, free haemoglobin, heparin and debris from the operating field, passes into a waste collection bag after which the remaining red cells suspended in a normal saline solution with a haematocrit of approximately 55 per cent are pumped into a reinfusion bag (Fig. 13.3; Fig. 13.4).

Cell salvage can also be used to concentrate the residual blood left in the cardiopulmonary bypass machine. However, not only is the heparin removed by the washing process, but so are all the clotting factors and platelets that would be returned to the patient if reinfusion of unaltered blood is used. The red cells that are reinfused have a survival which is equal to that of the patient's own or homologous blood, the morphology is unchanged, the levels of 2,3 DPG are higher than homologous blood and the osmotic fragility is unchanged. All evidence suggests that the washed product from a cell salvage system is equal or superior to homologous blood. The ability of intraoperative cell salvage to reduce the need for homologous

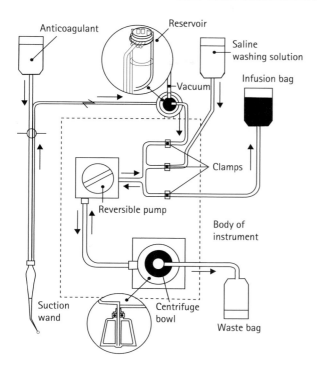

Figure 13.4 *The design of a cell salvage device. The instrument includes a dual-lumen suction wand, a reservoir for the aspirated blood, infusion bags for the washed blood and the waste, as well serial tubing clamps controlled by a microprocessor. Adapted from Williamson and Taswell (1991).*

blood transfusion after cardiac surgery is well-documented (Hall *et al.*, 1990). The cost-effectiveness of cell salvage has changed dramatically over the last 12 months as the cost of blood in the UK has risen sharply with the introduction of leucodepletion. The cost of cell salvage per case is now little more than the cost of a single unit of concentrated red cells. Using this fact alone, intraoperative cell salvage should be used for all cases where the median blood loss intraoperatively and blood use post-operatively is in excess of one unit. This will vary from centre to centre and therefore local cost benefit analyses should be made before universal introduction for low risk cases.

Ultrafiltration

Ultrafiltration during cardiopulmonary bypass has now become common practice for reversing pulmonary and tissue oedema in patients presenting with overloaded circulatory volume (Magilligan, 1985) and it is an effective method of haemoconcentrating patients during or after cardiopulmonary bypass (Boldt *et al.*, 1989). Ultrafiltration is a convective process. The driving force for ultrafiltration is the hydrostatic pressure differential occurring across a membrane. The membrane of the ultrafiltration device contains pores that are irregular in shape and size varying between 10 and 35 angstroms.

Removal of the solutes is determined by the pore size of the membrane with all molecules smaller than the smallest pore in the membrane being of equal concentration on both sides of the membrane. Pharmacological agents with low molecular weights, such as heparin or aprotinin, will also pass through the ultrafilter and, with respect to the former, activated clotting times should be monitored more frequently when used during cardiopulmonary bypass. The filter can easily be introduced into the circuit during cardiopulmonary bypass when it is required. The main advantage of ultrafiltration over cell salvage as a means of haemoconcentrating residual blood from the cardiopulmonary bypass machine is that there is little or no loss of platelets or clotting factors using this technique (Boldt *et al.*, 1989).

Cardiopulmonary bypass circuit design and oxygenator type

The cardiopulmonary bypass is circuit the major contributor to haemodilution during cardiac surgery. Manufacturers of membrane oxygenators and blood cardioplegia devices have addressed this issue and developed components with lower priming volumes. Careful consideration to the design of the cardiopulmonary bypass circuit and position of its individual components can also help to minimize haemodilution.

TUBING

The adult bypass circuit generally comprises 3/8-inch arterial and 1/2-inch venous polyvinyl chloride tubing. This combination, using gravity drainage, can cope with blood flow rates of up to 6 L/min. However, to minimize haemodilution in the smaller patient, requiring blood flow rates of less than 4.5 L/min, the venous line can be reduced to 3/8-inch tubing. The priming volume of tubing in relation to the diameter is shown in Table 13.3.

From Table 13.3 it can be seen that reducing the length of 1/2-inch venous tubing by 50 cm will reduce the priming volume by nearly 60 mL/m, or changing from 1/2-inch to 3/8-inch tubing in the case of the smaller patient will reduce the priming volume by

Table 13.3 *Volume of fluid in tubing*

Tubing size (ID) inch	Tubing size (ID) mm	Volume (mL/m)
3/16	4.5	15
1/4	6.0	30
3/8	9.0	65
1/2	12	115
3/4	18	255

ID = internal diameter.

Table 13.4 *Membrane oxygenators; the priming volume of hollow fibre oxygenators varies between 220 and 290 mL*

Manufacturer	Oxygenator name	Surface area (m²)	Priming volume (mL)
Cobe	CML Duo*	2.6	460
Cobe	Optima	1.7	260
Medtronic	Affinity	2.5	270
Medtronic	Maxima Forte	2.4	295
Terumo	Capiox Sx 18	1.8	270
Minntech	Biocor 200	1.9	255
Jostra	Quadrox	1.8	250
Bard	Quantum	1.9	274
Sorin	Monolyth	2.2	290
Dideco	D903 Avant	1.7	250
Gish	Vision	2.5	280
Baxter	Univox	1.8	220

*Flat plate membrane oxygenator.

50 mL/m. The complications of varying the components of the cardiopulmonary bypass circuit with the weight of the patient may not be worth the risk that is inherent in not using a standard circuit.

OXYGENATOR

There are three types of oxygenator available for use within the bypass circuit: the bubble oxygenator; the flat sheet membrane oxygenator; and the hollow fibre membrane oxygenator. Membrane oxygenators are used more generally than bubble oxygenators. Studies have shown the membrane oxygenator to be superior with respect to blood compatibility (Nilsson *et al.*, 1990), blood gas control and lower levels of gaseous microemboli generation (Pearson, 1988). In recent years, oxygenator manufacturers have moved away from the flat plate membrane oxygenator towards the hollow fibre membrane oxygenators offering lower membrane surface area, a reduced priming volume with no detriment to haemocompatibility or gas transfer. A flat plate membrane oxygenator that attempts to overcome the problem of high priming volume is the Cobe Duo (Cobe Laboratories, Denver, USA). This oxygenator has two equally divided membrane compartments. For larger patients both compartments are used; however, in the smaller patient only one compartment is used, reducing the priming volume by 50 per cent.

Priming volumes of current membrane oxygenators are shown in Table 13.4. A substantial reduction in priming volume can be achieved by changing from the flat plate technology to that of the hollow fibre; however, the reduction in priming volume is minimal between oxygenators of similar design.

BLOOD CARDIOPLEGIA DEVICES

The majority of modern single pass blood cardioplegia devices that are produced contribute little to patients'

haemodilution with priming volumes, excluding the tubing, ranging from 35 mL to 55 mL. The use of blood cardioplegia rather than crystalloid cardioplegia will help to minimize haemodilution during cardiopulmonary bypass because there is significantly less clear fluid added to the circuit.

PUMP CONSOLE

Having chosen a low prime hollow fibre oxygenator, its position on the pump console should allow for good visualization of the blood reservoir level while being close to the arterial pump head to minimize tubing lengths. By positioning the oxygenator at the rear of the pump console between the arterial pump head and the operating table tubing lengths can be kept to a minimum.

A 1/2-inch venous line, 1.6 m in length can be used routinely for all adult cases. This only requires an additional 80 mL more priming volume than the 3/8-tubing, whilst ensuring that drainage will not be restricted because of the diameter of the tubing. Decreased venous return caused by excessive negative pressure while using a 1/2-inch venous line, as reported in the literature (DeBois and Krieger, 1998), can be avoided by partial occlusion of the venous line with a clamp.

The priming volume for the entire circuit incorporating an Avant D905 oxygenator (Sorin Biomedica, Mirandola, Italy), arterial line filter (Pall Biomedical, Portsmouth, UK) and blood cardioplegia device (Sorin Biomedica, Mirandola, Italy) is 1600 mL. Attempts to further significantly reduce the degree of haemodilution of the patient are achieved by retrograde autologous priming at the onset of cardiopulmonary bypass, reducing the overall priming volume to between 600 mL and 700 mL.

Heparin–bonded circuits

One technique that has been developed to try and reduce the inflammatory response to cardiopulmonary bypass is to coat all the plastic surfaces of the cardiopulmonary bypass machine with heparin. This may be done either through a covalent or an ionic linkage. There is evidence that this modification of the cardiopulmonary bypass circuit leads to a reduction in complement (Velthius *et al.*, 1996) and leucocyte activation (Borowiec *et al.*, 1992) as well as a reduction in thrombin production (Muehrcke *et al.*, 1996). It has been postulated that this may reduce the coagulopathy that accompanies cardiopulmonary bypass and therefore decrease post-operative bleeding. Clinical studies that have tried to answer this question can be divided into two groups: those that have used a reduced dose of heparin when using heparin-bonded circuits (typically an ACT of 200–300s during cardiopulmonary bypass) and those that have used normal ACTs (typically 480s during cardiopulmonary bypass). By the use of a reduced dose of heparin, studies have shown a reduction in bleeding and transfusion (Aldea *et al.*, 1996); however, case reports of intracardiac clot formation using a reduced heparin dose (Muehrcke *et al.*, 1995), evidence of increased thrombin production using a reduced heparin dose (Gorman *et al.*, 1996) and the lack of any studies that have been sufficiently powered to detect neurological sequelae suggest that the combination of heparin-bonded circuits and reduced heparin dose may not be as safe as was originally postulated. The use of heparin-bonded circuits and full dose heparin appears to reduce the inflammatory response to cardiopulmonary bypass, leading to reduced post-operative complications and reduced hospital stay (Ovrum *et al.*, 1996), but this combination does not appear to reduce bleeding or blood transfusion. The role of heparin-bonded circuits as part of a blood conservation protocol is still controversial and it may be that in combination with a reduction in systemic anticoagulation they eventually find a place in the management of cardiopulmonary bypass in patients at high risk of significant bleeding (Woolf and Mythen, 1998).

Retrograde autologous priming of the cardiopulmonary bypass circuit

Retrograde autologous priming or prime displacement of the cardiopulmonary bypass circuit is a technique employed to reduce the priming volume of the circuit. The reduced haemodilution that therefore occurs at the onset of cardiopulmonary bypass allows a higher haematocrit to be maintained throughout cardiopulmonary bypass. As discussed earlier, it could be that a higher haematocrit during cardiopulmonary bypass may be beneficial (Defoe *et al.*, 2001). After cardiopulmonary bypass, the higher haematocrit means that the patient is less likely to reach a transfusion threshold and therefore receive a blood transfusion. Although a method of autologously priming the cardiopulmonary bypass circuit was first described in 1960 (Panico and Neptune, 1960), the technique did not prove popular until much later when, in the1990s, numerous authors published modifications of the technique of priming the cardiopulmonary bypass circuit (Cromar and Wolk, 1998). Reductions in homologous blood usage as a result of this modification have recently been demonstrated (Balachandran *et al.*, 2002).

The technique of retrograde autologous priming in adult cardiac surgery can differ between cardiac centres, as pump configurations and cardiopulmonary bypass circuit designs are not standardized. However, whatever method is used the primary aim is to displace the clear fluid prime with autologous blood and reduce haemodilution at the onset of cardiopulmonary bypass.

The following technique may be undertaken using the circuit shown in Figure 13.5. The D905 Avant oxygenator (Sorin Biomedica, Mirandola, Italy), with integral isolated cardiotomy reservoir, allows any blood lost during cannulation to be collected before retrograde autologous priming, kept separate from the clear fluid in the venous reservoir, and then returned to the patient's circulation once full cardiopulmonary bypass has been established. Before aortic cannulation the recirculation line is clamped and clamps are applied at positions A, B and C. After aortic cannulation, the clamp at position A is removed and the aortic pressure is confirmed. Once aortic and right atrial cannulation has been achieved, 50–100 μg phenylephrine may be administered to maintain the patient's systolic blood pressure greater than 100 mmHg during the retrograde autologous priming process. The clamp is slowly removed from position C, allowing the blood to flow retrograde from the patient's aorta, displacing approximately 100 mL of prime into the prime bag. Once the arterial blood has reached the clamp at position B, an arterial line clamp is reapplied at position A and then the clamp is removed from position B. At the commencement of cardiopulmonary bypass, the variable occlusion clamp on the venous line is slowly released, allowing blood to drain from the patient and simultaneously the arterial pump is slowly rotated at a sufficient flow (600–800 mL/min) to maintain a constant level in the venous reservoir. Once the venous blood has displaced the clear fluid priming solution in the reservoir, oxygenator and arterial line filter and has reached the recirculation line, the arterial line clamp is removed from position A and reapplied at position C. The venous clamp is then fully opened and the pump flow increased to establish full cardiopulmonary bypass. In the event of the patient's mean arterial blood pressure falling below 50 mmHg the procedure is stopped and full cardiopulmonary bypass initiated. Although this technique works well with a roller pump, great care must be taken if using a centrifugal pump that the venous reservoir level does not fall excessively. When using a centrifugal pump an alternative technique may be used, where there is greater prime displacement via the aortic cannula (Rosengart *et al.*, 1998).

After termination of cardiopulmonary bypass and removal of cannulae the prime solution is returned to the circuit, displacing the patient's blood, which is then collected for reinfusion by the anaesthetist. Alternatively, cell salvage may be used to concentrate the blood remaining in the cardiopulmonary bypass circuit at the end of cardiopulmonary bypass.

Prime displacement using this technique is achieved in less than two minutes, reducing the priming volume from 1600 mL to approximately 600 mL. Table 13.5 shows how retrograde autologous priming will reduce haemodilution during cardiopulmonary bypass. The smaller, anaemic patient with a pre-cardiopulmonary bypass haematocrit of 30 per cent using a normal prime would have an on-cardiopulmonary bypass haematocrit of 20 per cent; however, by using the retrograde autologous priming technique the haematocrit would be 25 per cent. With a larger patient or with a higher haematocrit before cardiopulmonary bypass the technique should be

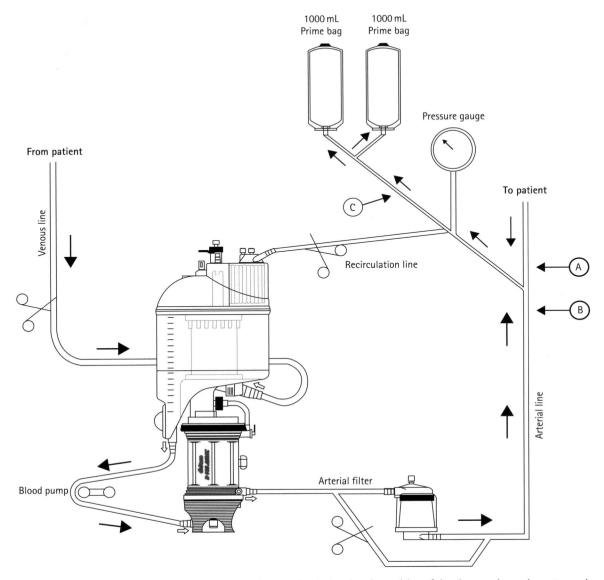

Figure 13.5 *Schematic drawing of the cardiopulmonary bypass circuit showing the position of the clamps when using retrograde autologous priming of the circuit. (See text for detail.)*

Table 13.5 *The effect of retrograde autologous priming of the cardiopulmonary bypass circuit on the on-cardiopulmonary bypass haematocrit*

Pre-cardiopulmonary bypass haematocrit	On-cardiopulmonary bypass haematocrit prime 1600 mL (patient's weight, kg)					On-cardiopulmonary bypass haematocrit prime 600 mL (patient's weight, kg)				
	50	60	70	80	90	50	60	70	80	90
40	27	28	30	31	31	34	35	35	36	36
35	23	25	26	27	27	30	30	31	31	32
30	20	21	22	23	24	25	26	27	27	27

*A haematocrit in excess of 28 per cent may be undesirable when using hypothermia and the technique should be combined with ANH to overcome this problem.
Calculations based on blood volume 65 mL/kg.

combined with acute normovolaemic haemodilution to prevent a high haematocrit during cardiopulmonary bypass. It is not known whether the problem of a relatively high haematocrit during hypothermic cardiopulmonary bypass with the high viscosity that may occur in this situation is clinically significant.

MONITORING OF COAGULATION AND ANTICOAGULATION FOR CARDIAC SURGERY

Monitoring of coagulation in the peri-operative period is an integral part of cardiac surgery. Pre-operative abnormalities of coagulation are outside the scope of this chapter and will not be discussed further. The gold standard of care, with regard to coagulation, for many years has been the measurement of the platelet count, the prothrombin time or INR, the APTT and the activated clotting time (ACT). Treatment both during and after surgery has been based on these results. Newer tests, including functional assays of heparin concentration and thromboelastography are emerging, which are proving to be valuable if used as part of a treatment algorithm.

Platelet count, APTT and INR

Thrombocytopaenia exists, by definition, if the platelet count falls to less than 150,000/mL. In practice there is no evidence of any increased bleeding during or after cardiac surgery at levels much lower than this providing that the platelet function is normal. A platelet count of less than 100,000/mL is considered to be a cut-off point below which platelets should be administered if there is clinically significant bleeding and there is no information about platelet function. The APTT and the INR are both measures of protein cascade function, and it has never been intended that they should be used to determine the likelihood of coagulopathic bleeding after surgery. Algorithms that use these three tests have been shown to reduce blood product use after cardiac surgery (Despotis et al., 1994). The likelihood, however, is that any algorithm for blood transfusion is better than no algorithm and it is unlikely that this is an optimal protocol to follow now that whole blood tests of clot viscoelasticity, such as thromboelastography, are available.

Activated clotting time and heparin concentration measurement

Anticoagulation is essential if cardiac surgery is to be undertaken using cardiopulmonary bypass. Unfractionated heparin is used to anticoagulate the patient. Empirical heparin therapy may result in excessive or inadequate anticoagulation, and monitoring of its effect is necessary to ensure that anticoagulation is adequate during cardiopulmonary bypass and that reversal is complete afterwards. The ACT is a functional assay that demonstrates the individual response to anticoagulation. The ACT was introduced into general cardiac practice in 1975 when Bull and colleagues (Bull et al., 1975) showed that there was a linear relationship between the heparin dose and the ACT and that the slope of the relationship varied between patients. These workers also showed that at an ACT of 300s there was no clot formation in the residual blood after discontinuation of cardiopulmonary bypass. The value of 480s, which is often quoted as being adequate, was based on this finding with an additional safety margin. The automated ACT is generally performed using one of two devices. The Hemochron ACT device (International Technidyne) requires 2 mL of whole blood to be placed in a pre-warmed glass tube containing a magnet and celite (diatomaceous earth) or kaolin (aluminium silicate) as a contact activator. The tube is placed into a rotating well within a heated block (Fig. 13.6).

The magnet remains in the lower part of the tube until the formed clot lifts the magnet from the lower part of the tube. This displacement activates a switch and stops the timer.

The Hemotec device (Medtronic/Hemotec Inc.) uses 0.4 mL of whole blood added to a pre-warmed cartridge containing kaolin. Mixing occurs by means of a plunger. As clotting occurs descent of the plunger is impeded and this is detected by an optical sensor, which stops the timer (Fig. 13.7).

Use of the ACT (with an adequate ACT for cardiopulmonary bypass defined as 480s) is now almost universal. Many investigators have tried to improve upon this technique with the aim of better control of anticoagulation during cardiopulmonary bypass and more accurate reversal of heparin after cardiopulmonary bypass, so that bleeding and the use of blood or blood products is reduced. Given the variability of the ACT, its imprecision and its response to factors unrelated to heparin dose, heparin concentration monitoring has been suggested as an alternative. Quantitative assays of heparin concentration using chromogenic substrates for factor Xa are complicated and impractical for use in the operating room. A functional assay using protamine titration is more commonly used. The principle involved is that a clot will form earliest in the presence of an optimal neutralizing ratio of protamine. Excess protamine or heparin will prolong clot formation. Assuming that the optimal neutralizing ratio is 10 µg protamine to one unit of heparin, the heparin concentration can be calculated. Used alone and without any reference to an associated ACT, it has been shown that the use of heparin concentration to monitor anticoagulation during cardiopulmonary bypass may actually lead to an increased blood loss after surgery (Gravlee et al., 1990). This technique has, therefore, been abandoned. When a combination of ACT monitoring and heparin

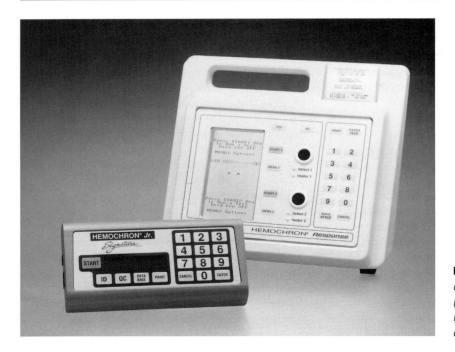

Figure 13.6 *The Haemochron Response and the Haemochron J ACT device (International Technidyne Corporation L) used for monitoring anticoagulation during cardiac surgery.*

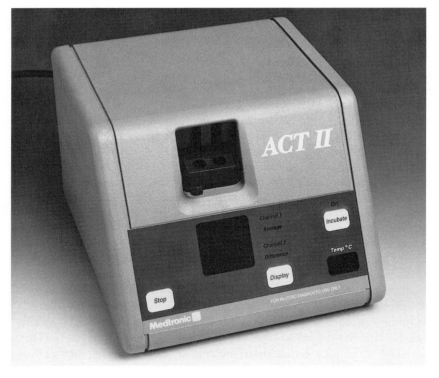

Figure 13.7 *The Hemotec ACT II device (Medtronic/Hemotec Inc.) used for monitoring anticoagulation during surgery.*

concentration monitoring is used the improved control of anticoagulation during cardiopulmonary bypass and reversal of heparin leads to reductions in blood loss and blood product use during the post-operative period.

The *Hepcon* (Medtronic/Hemotec Inc.) is an automated device that measures the ACT with incremental doses of heparin, allowing a heparin dose–response curve to be constructed (Fig. 13.8). This enables an individual dose of heparin to be given, which will produce an

adequate ACT (for example, 480 s) before cardiopulmonary bypass. The heparin concentration that results from this dose of heparin can then be calculated using a protamine titration assay. During cardiopulmonary bypass it is important that the ACT is maintained at or above the target value and that the heparin concentration is maintained at approximately the previously calculated value. If either level falls then additional heparin should be administered. At the end of cardiopulmonary

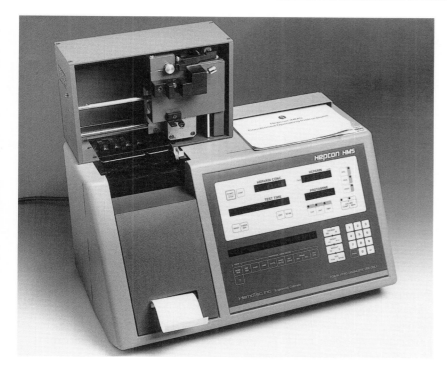

Figure 13.8 *The* Hepcon *heparin management system (Medtronic/ Hemotec Inc.) measures the ACT with incremental doses of heparin, allowing a dose–response curve to be constructed. A specific dose of heparin can therefore be given before cardiopulmonary bypass. It will also permit accurate dosing with protamine after cardiopulmonary bypass.*

bypass the protamine titration assay can be used to calculate the appropriate dose of protamine. Using this system a number of authors have demonstrated that, despite higher doses of heparin and lower doses of protamine, significant savings can be made with respect to blood loss and blood product administration during the post-operative period (Despotis and Joist, 1999). Although 480 s is generally accepted as an adequate ACT, in most patients this must be modified in the presence of aprotinin. Aprotinin is known to artifactually prolong the celite ACT (Wang *et al.*, 1992) so that a very low heparin level may accompany an ACT of 480 s. This problem can be overcome either by using an ACT of 750 s as the cut-off for further heparin administration or by using a kaolin activated ACT. Kaolin absorbs nearly all the aprotinin as soon as it is mixed in the tube and therefore the result will be unaffected by the presence of aprotinin.

Thromboelastography

The thromboelastogram is a test of whole blood clot formation and strength. Although first introduced into the laboratory more than 50 years ago, it is only recently that thromboelastography has been introduced into clinical practice. The system uses a small disposable plastic cup, which is placed in a heated block. A small disposable plastic pin is lowered into the cup but it does not touch the sides or bottom (Fig. 13.9).

The pin is maintained in a stable position by an electromagnetic field. The cup moves through an arc of 4.5° once every second, pauses for one second and then moves

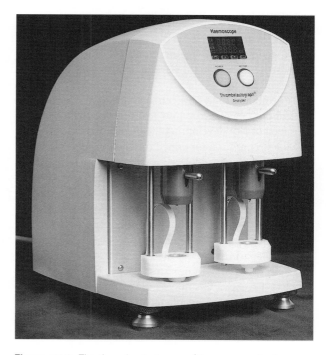

Figure 13.9 *The thromboelastogram (Haemoscope Inc.) can provide data about four aspects of coagulation: how fast a clot starts to form, the speed of clot development; clot strength; and whether a clot breaks down abnormally rapidly.*

back through the same arc in the opposite direction. When blood is added to the cup (0.36 mL) no deflection of the pin occurs when the cup moves through the arc until the blood starts to clot. When the blood does start to clot, the rotational motion of the cup is transferred to the

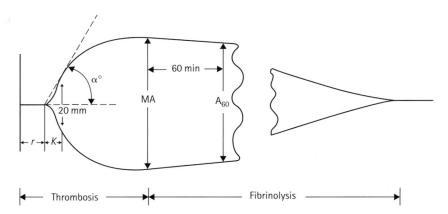

Figure 13.10 *Quantification of thromboelastograph variables. Analysis of the thromboelastograph tracing.* r = *reaction time (time from sample placement in the cuvettte until the thromboelastograph tracing amplitude reaches 2 mm; normal range = 6–8 min). In the absence of evidence of residual heparin a prolonged r time in the presence of excessive bleeding is often treated with fresh frozen plasma.* K = *clot formation time (time from r time until the amplitude of the tracing reaches 20 mm; normal range = 3–6 min). Alpha angle* $\alpha°$ = *angle formed by the slope of the thromboelastograph tracing from the r time to the K time. It represents the speed at which the clot forms; normal range = 50–60°. Maximum amplitude = greatest amplitude on the thromboelastograph tracing. It represents the strength of the fibrin clot; normal range = 50–60 mm. The maximum amplitude is decreased by quantitative or qualitative abnormalities of platelets. A decreased maximum amplitude in the presence of excessive bleeding is often treated with platelets.* A_{60} = *thromboelastograph amplitude 60 minutes after maximum amplitude. It represents clot lysis; normal range = maximum amplitude − 5 mm. Adapted from Ford et al. (1999).*

pin and the force exerted is displayed as a computer trace showing clot strength against time. The thromboelastography trace has standard parameters (Fig. 13.10), which can be measured.

Thromboelastography can answer four major questions about coagulation: how fast the clot starts to form; the speed of clot development; clot strength; and whether the clot strength is maintained or whether it breaks down abnormally rapidly (clot lysis). If all four aspects of the thromboelastogram are normal there will be no coagulopathy and any post-operative bleeding will be surgical bleeding. Which particular part of the thromboelastography trace is deranged can be used to help guide transfusion therapy. In general a prolonged *r* time that is not caused by residual heparin is best treated with fresh frozen plasma and a decreased maximum amplitude is best treated with platelets. Excessive fibrinolysis may sometimes be treated with aprotinin. It is possible to detect residual heparin by the addition of heparinase to the cup. By performing two tests in parallel, one with and one without heparinase, it is possible to determine whether a prolonged *r* time is caused by residual heparin. A number of studies have shown that thromboelastography is the best predictor of abnormal post-operative bleeding (Spiess *et al.*, 1987), and it has also been shown that inclusion of thromboelastogram parameters in a transfusion algorithm can reduce transfusions in complex cardiac surgery (Shore-Lesserson, 1999). Thromboelastography can also be used to determine whether desmopressin will be an effective drug to reduce bleeding after cardiopulmonary bypass for it appears that

it is only effective in patients who have a reduced maximum amplitude (Mongan and Hosking, 1992).

The practicalities of thromboelastography are not straightforward. The equipment requires training to use, and extreme attention to detail is needed when using the equipment. Critical quality control must be performed on a regular basis if meaningful results are to be obtained. Providing that these criteria can be met thromboelastography is proving in many respects to be a useful adjunct to blood conservation.

PHARMACOLOGICAL APPROACHES TO BLOOD CONSERVATION

There are three main areas where pharmacological therapy may be of relevance with respect to blood conservation. Pre-operatively, the withdrawal of anticoagulants, such as aspirin or warfarin, at an appropriate interval before surgery must be addressed. Peri-operatively, the choice of heparin type or dose may be important, and the use of antifibrinolytic agents or other drugs may be beneficial with regard to blood conservation.

Withdrawal of anticoagulants before surgery

Anticoagulation of one form or another is almost universal in patients presenting for heart surgery, and a considered withdrawal of therapy is often appropriate. A risk analysis is important in all patients before stopping drugs before surgery, but the benefits of decreased bleeding and the reduced exposure to allogeneic blood in the peri-operative period often outweigh the disadvantages of short-term cessation of anticoagulation.

ASPIRIN

Aspirin therapy is used in many patients presenting for coronary artery bypass grafting (CABG) because it has been shown to reduce the incidence of myocardial infarction (Flapan, 1994). The disadvantage of continuing aspirin therapy until the day of operation is that there is an increased risk of blood loss and blood transfusion (Puga, 1990). This risk, however, must be weighed against the improved graft patency rate that occurs in patients who continue aspirin throughout the peri-operative period (Goldman *et al.*, 1988). For this reason few people will delay an operation because a patient is still taking aspirin but, if time allows, aspirin is generally stopped one week pre-operatively to allow the effects of aspirin on platelet function to disappear.

TICLOPIDINE, CLOPIDOGREL

Ticlopidine, clopidogrel and other platelet receptor antagonists, often used when coronary artery stents are placed, will also increase the risk of bleeding and should be stopped pre-operatively if possible.

WARFARIN

Warfarin is now considered first-line treatment for patients with atrial fibrillation and for this reason many patients presenting for cardiac surgery will be taking the drug. It should be stopped several days before surgery so that the INR can fall to 2.0 prior to surgery.

LOW MOLECULAR WEIGHT HEPARIN

Low molecular weight heparin is used as a treatment for unstable angina and therefore many patients presenting for urgent CABG will be taking the drug. The drug is incompletely inactivated by protamine and for this reason there may be increased bleeding after surgery. There is, however, no good evidence to support this in clinical practice.

HEPARIN TYPE AND DOSE

Unfractionated heparin consists of a mixture of polyanionic polysaccharides with a molecular weight ranging from 2000 to 30,000 daltons. It is obtained commercially from either bovine lung or porcine intestine. There is significant variation in composition and activity. Bovine heparin is more highly sulphated and therefore requires more protamine for neutralization. It has less variability with regard to concentration than porcine heparin, its half-life is slightly shorter and it may cause more thrombocytopenia. The bioassay to determine the potency of heparin ensures that bovine heparin contains at least 140 U/mg, whereas porcine contains at least 120 U/mg. Because heparin is marketed in 1000 or 5000 U/mL concentrations, the potency of each lot may vary considerably. Porcine heparin is more commonly used and a dose of heparin is chosen to raise the ACT above 480 s before cardiopulmonary bypass. The dose generally required is 300–400 U/kg. Further dosing is either by ACT monitoring or by heparin concentration monitoring. A heparin concentration during cardiopulmonary bypass of 3 U/mL is considered adequate.

PROTAMINE

Calculation of the appropriate dose of protamine at the end of cardiopulmonary bypass is difficult and many formulae exist. The use of empirical doses that depend upon the initial or total dose of heparin are simple and common, but usually result in an excessive dose of protamine. The use of a heparin dose–response curve drawn before cardiopulmonary bypass allows a more accurate dose of protamine to be given. This process can be automated and it has been shown that by use of this system protamine dose can be reduced by 40 per cent. The effectiveness of this technique translates into significant reductions in blood loss and blood transfusion (Jobes *et al.*, 1995). It is not clear, however, if it is the precision of anticoagulation or heparin reversal that is important in this process of blood conservation.

Haemostatic drugs

A number of haemostatic drugs have been used during cardiac surgery to try and reduce bleeding and blood transfusion after cardiac surgery. These include: the antifibrinolytic amino acids, tranexamic acid and aminocaproic acid; the polypeptide, aprotinin; and the arginine vasopressin analogue, desmopressin.

TRANEXAMIC ACID AND AMINOCAPROIC ACID

These amino acids are both lysine analogues. They both work by competing to bind to plasminogen and prevent its conversion to plasmin, thereby suppressing fibrinolysis. They are given intravenously. The dosing regimens used vary widely but the following have been suggested: for tranexamic acid, 10 mg/kg as a bolus at the beginning of the operation followed by 1 mg/kg per hour (Horrow *et al.*, 1995). For aminocaproic acid, 15 mg/kg at the beginning of the operation followed by 15 mg/kg per hour (Vander Salm *et al.*, 1996). Most studies have shown that with these drugs it is possible to reduce chest drain loss after cardiac surgery by 30–40 per cent. It has been much more difficult to show that the incidence of blood transfusion can be reduced. A meta-analysis of prophylactic drug treatment in the prevention of post-operative bleeding (Fremes et al., 1994) failed to show any benefit with regard to exposure to post-operative transfusion, although the volume of transfusion and the mean chest drain loss were both significantly reduced. Studies that have been large enough to include safety data have not been conducted and, for this reason, answers to the questions that have been asked about the safety of aprotinin are not available for tranexamic acid or aminocaproic acid. It has been suggested that the use of tranexamic acid or aminocaproic acid should be reserved for the low-risk cases that comprise the majority of the workload, so that the aprotinin, which is much more expensive, can be used in the high-risk cases (Hardy and Belisle, 1994).

APROTININ

Aprotinin is a basic polypeptide with a molecular weight of 6500 daltons, which is isolated from bovine lung. It is a broad-spectrum serine protease inhibitor that will inhibit proteases such as trypsin, plasmin, kallikrein, elastase and thrombin. Besides the protease activity of aprotinin, evidence is starting to emerge to suggest that it may have direct platelet-protective properties (Shore-Lesserson, 1999). It is this broad spectrum of activity that distinguishes it from the lysine analogues.

The efficacy of aprotinin in patients having operations that use cardiopulmonary bypass is now well established. Not only is the chest drain loss reduced by 50 per cent but the exposure to homologous blood transfusion, as well as the volume of blood transfused, is significantly reduced. The superiority of aprotinin over the lysine analogues is established without doubt for complex or 're-do' surgery, but a number of studies have failed to show any extra benefit in primary coronary artery surgery. The cost-effectiveness also becomes an issue in this group of patients. Because of the cost implications, various dosing regimens have been developed. Early studies used what is now accepted as high dose or 'Hammersmith dose' (the hospital in London where it was first introduced). This consists of 2,000,000 KIU before cardiopulmonary bypass, 2,000,000 KIU added to the pump prime and 500,000 KIU/h as an infusion after the initial loading dose (Royston et al., 1987). Low-dose or half-dose regimens have been developed, which use exactly half the Hammersmith dose and, lastly, pump prime regimens have been developed which involve adding 2,000,000 KIU to the pump prime without any loading dose or infusion. Numerous studies have been performed comparing these dosing regimens, but only one study has compared all three dosing regimens with a placebo (Levy et al.,

1995). This study was performed in patients undergoing repeat coronary artery surgery and showed that both the high- and low-dose regimens were equally effective and significantly better than the pump prime dose, which again was more effective than placebo. The transfusion rates were 54 per cent, 46 per cent, 72 per cent and 75 per cent, respectively, with mean transfusion volumes of 1.6 units, 1.6 units, 2.5 units and 3.4 units, respectively. No similar study has been performed for primary cardiac surgery, and studies comparing lysine analogues with aprotinin have often been open to criticism. The meta-analysis of prophylactic drug treatment (Fremes et al., 1994) concluded that aprotinin (mainly using the high-dose regimen) was as effective as tranexamic acid or aminocaproic acid (in a population consisting of a mixture of primary and repeat coronary artery surgery, valve surgery or CABG and valve surgery) at reducing chest drain loss and mean transfusion volume. Aprotinin did, however, appear to be superior when it came to reducing exposure to blood. When cost is added to the equation it would seem sensible to use a lysine analogue for primary surgery and to use the low-dose aprotinin regimen for repeat or complex surgery. It is important, however, to consider the safety profile of aprotinin when deciding whether it should be used routinely. The safety of aprotinin has been studied extensively. The decreased level of fibrinolysis that is associated with aprotinin has raised concerns that it may be a pro-thrombotic agent and influence the incidence of myocardial infarction, graft patency, stroke or renal dysfunction.

Reports of an increased incidence of myocardial infarction associated with aprotinin use appeared in 1992 (Cosgrove et al., 1992). The heparin control in this study suggested that some of the patients were inadequately anticoagulated using celite ACTs of 480 s before further heparin administration. Three large studies have failed to show an increased incidence of myocardial infarction with aprotinin (Levy et al., 1995; Alderman et al., 1998; Lemmer et al., 1996), and it is now generally accepted that aprotinin is safe in this respect. The issue of graft occlusion is more complicated. Although early studies suggested that aprotinin did not influence the incidence of graft occlusion (Bidstrup et al., 1993; Lemmer et al., 1994), the IMAGE trial (Alderman et al., 1998) showed a trend towards increased graft occlusion after the data was adjusted for risk factors associated with vein graft occlusion. The results were possibly skewed by large intercentre differences and after two centres were removed from the analysis there was no evidence of increased graft occlusion. It may be reasonable to conclude that aprotinin is safe except for the population at risk of vein graft occlusion, namely female sex, lack of prior aspirin therapy and poor quality or small distal vessels.

Concerns about the increased risk of stroke that may accompany the use of aprotinin have not been borne out by a large multicentre trial (Levy *et al.*, 1995). In fact, this study showed a reduced incidence of stroke with aprotinin, a finding that has been supported by pooled data from the Bayer database.

There is no evidence that aprotinin affects the incidence of renal failure in patients undergoing coronary artery surgery. Evidence that aprotinin may influence the incidence of renal failure in patients undergoing aortic surgery requiring cardiopulmonary bypass and circulatory arrest comes from a study using retrospective control subjects with different heparin management in each group (Sundt *et al.*, 1993).

DESMOPRESSIN

Desmopressin is a synthetic analogue of vasopressin that is devoid of significant antidiuretic or vasopressor effects. It has been shown to be effective at reducing blood loss in some studies, but this is not always the case, and a meta-analysis failed to confirm its efficacy (Fremes *et al.*, 1994). Although it is known that desmopressin will increase levels of factor VIII and von Willebrand factor after cardiopulmonary bypass, it is uncertain if this is its mechanism of action. It may have other direct platelet-preserving effects. Desmopressin will consistently decrease post-operative bleeding if there is platelet impairment as demonstrated by the thromboelastography (Mongan and Hosking, 1992). An algorithm for its use, which includes measurement of the maximum amplitude by thromboelastography and exclusion of hypofibrinogenaemia and thrombocytopenia, will probably prove to be the most appropriate way of using the drug.

RECOMBINANT FACTOR VIIA

Recombinant factor VIIa is approved for treatment of haemorrhage in haemophiliacs who develop inhibitors to factor VIII or IX. It has been used to control bleeding after cardiac surgery, when its mechanism of action appears to be for the rVIIa to bind to tissue factor exposed at sites of vessel injury. The TF-fVIIa complex initiates the coagulation cascade on activated platelet surfaces. A number of case reports have appeared in the literature (Al Douri *et al.*, 2000) but at the moment no randomized studies have been conducted.

SURGICAL TECHNIQUES AS AN ADJUNCT TO BLOOD CONSERVATION

All efforts to conserve blood will be to no avail if there is anything except a meticulous surgical technique throughout the operation. Many texts have been published on this subject, and effective surgical haemostasis must be the mainstay of blood conservation. This can hardly be stressed strongly enough.

Post-operative techniques in blood conservation

Blood conservation in the intensive care unit centres on reducing the amount of bleeding from the patient, or reinfusing into the patient blood that is lost from the chest drains.

HYPOTHERMIA

Normal coagulation requires both adequate number and adequate function of platelets. Although the platelet count can fall quite markedly before there is an influence on the blood loss after cardiac surgery, this is not the case with platelet function. Platelet function is nearly always deranged after cardiac surgery and this will be made worse in the presence of hypothermia (Khuri *et al.*, 1992). Detection of the influence of hypothermia on platelet function is particularly difficult in the peri-operative period because the thromboelastography, which is the best bedside monitor of platelet function, operates at 37°C and therefore fails to detect the influence of temperature. Clotting factor levels are not significantly affected by moderate hypothermia and because the simple tests of coagulation are all performed at 37°C the PT, APTT and the thrombin time will often be reported as normal when there is indeed a coagulopathy in the hypothermic patient. Clotting tests, performed on normal human plasma at temperatures of less than 35°C, show a significant slowing of clotting factor function (Reed *et al.*, 1990). Convective warming is an effective means of warming patients and this should be used in all cases. The development of pre-packed sterile convective warming blankets means that this technique can now be used in the operating room as soon as the leg wound has been closed to prevent the fall in temperature that nearly always occurs in the post-cardiopulmonary bypass period.

REINFUSION OF SHED MEDIASTINAL BLOOD

The collection of shed mediastinal blood is usually performed using a collection chamber designed for the purpose, often the cardiotomy reservoir from the cardiopulmonary bypass circuit. Blood is allowed to drain into this from the chest drains, and from there it is either continuously reinfused using a pump or it is intermittently emptied into a collection bag and then reinfused into the patient. The use of a continuous system means that precautions must be taken to avoid an air embolus, whereas the intermittent system is more labour intensive for the intensive care unit nursing staff. A maximum volume for reinfusion of 500–750 mL or time for reinfusion of 6 hours is usually stipulated when using the technique.

The efficacy of reinfusion of shed mediastinal blood has been debated since it was first demonstrated that a 50 per cent reduction in homologous blood use after cardiac surgery was possible using the technique (Schaff et al., 1978). Although a number of studies have been published to support this finding, there is an equal body of evidence that has failed to demonstrate a significant reduction in homologous red cell transfusion (Body et al., 1999). A recent meta-analysis of 12 studies of reinfusion of shed mediastinal blood suggested that, at best, the technique was only marginally effective (Huet et al., 1999). Given the divided opinion about the efficacy of reinfusion of shed mediastinal blood, it is important to consider the safety of the technique as well as any developments that may improve its efficacy.

Although the main aim of reinfusion of shed mediastinal blood is to reduce exposure to homologous blood and blood products, it may do this with a risk of increased post-operative bleeding and abnormalities of coagulation (De Haan et al., 1993). Shed mediastinal blood is a thrombocytopenic, defibrinogenated product with a haematocrit of approximately 20 per cent. The haematocrit may vary, depending on the rate of bleeding. Red cell haemolysis is common and plasma-free haemoglobin levels as high as 4 g/L may be found. Although this is high, the total exposure to plasma-free haemoglobin is not enough to cause renal failure. Tissue plasminogen activator and fibrin degradation products are both elevated in shed mediastinal blood and, although raised levels may be found systemically after reinfusion of shed mediastinal blood, this is unlikely to be a reflection of a systemic response. Some studies have demonstrated bacterial contamination of shed mediastinal blood, although this has not been associated with evidence of sepsis.

Most studies of reinfusion of shed mediastinal blood have been with an unwashed product. The reason for this is that it is fast, easy to use, inexpensive and the volume of shed mediastinal blood obtained may be insufficient to fill a bowl for washing and centrifugation. Washing shed mediastinal blood will remove the tissue plasminogen activator and fibrin degradation products, but in light of the fact that nearly all studies have failed to demonstrate increased bleeding without washing, few centres support this approach.

PATIENT POSITIONING AND VENTILATION

Sensible positioning of the patient in the intensive care unit can in theory reduce venous bleeding. As soon as haemodynamic stability has been confirmed elevating the head of the bed by 10° will help to reduce venous pressure.

Most patients are ventilated for several hours after cardiac surgery, usually with a small amount of positive end expiratory pressure (PEEP). Increasing the level of PEEP to 7.5 or 10 cmH$_2$O, if haemodynamic stability allows, will help to tamponade venous bleeding and may be considered in the presence of excessive bleeding.

BLOOD SAMPLING WASTE VOLUME

Regular blood sampling for blood gas, electrolyte and coagulation analysis, as well as full blood and platelet counts, occurs during the post-operative period. Two aspects of this process can be altered in an attempt to reduce blood loss at this time. Appropriate positioning of a three-way tap close to the arterial cannula can reduce the volume of blood wasted when blood is sampled from an arterial line. The size of tube that is used for transport of blood to the laboratory can be reduced. Paediatric tubes are readily available and are usually used for blood sampling from children. There is rarely any good reason not to use the same tubes for adults, using the philosophy that every bit counts.

CONCLUSION

Blood conservation should begin as soon as a patient is referred for cardiac surgery and it will always be a multidisciplinary task. Haematologists, the Blood Transfusion Service, anaesthetists, surgeons, perfusionists and intensive care unit staff all have a role to play and until the use of homologous blood is replaced by artificial oxygen carriers this co-ordinated effort must continue.

ACKNOWLEDGEMENT

The author would like to thank Steven Hansbro, Department of Clinical Perfusion, The Yorkshire Heart Centre, Leeds, UK for his assistance in preparation of the manuscript.

REFERENCES

Al Douri, M., Shafi, T., Al Khudairi, D. et al. 2000: Effect of the administration of recombinant activated factor VII (fFVIIa; NovoSeven) in the management of severe uncontrolled bleeding in patients undergoing heart valve replacement surgery. Blood, Coagulation and Fibrinolysis 11 (Suppl. 1), S121–7.

Aldea, G.S., Doursounian, M., O'Gara, P. et al. 1996: Heparin-bonded circuits with a reduced anticoagulation protocol in primary CABG: a prospective, randomized study. Annals of Thoracic Surgery 62, 41–7.

Alderman, E.L., Levy, J.H., Rich, J.B. et al. 1998: Analyses of coronary graft patency after aprotinin use: results from the International Multicenter Aprotinin Graft patency Experience (IMAGE) trial. Journal of Thoracic and Cardiovascular Surgery 116, 716–30.

Amberson, W.R., Jennings, J.J., Rhode, C.M. 1949: Clinical experience with hemoglobin–saline solutions. Journal of Applied Physiology 1, 469–89.

Balachandran, S., Cross, M.H., Karthikeyan, S. et al. 2002: Retrograde autologous priming of the cardiopulmonary bypass circuit reduces blood transfusion after coronary artery surgery. *Annals of Thoracic Surgery* **73**, 1912–18.

Bidstrup, B.P., Underwood, S.R., Sapsford, R.N. *et al.* 1993: Effects of aprotinin (Trasylol) on aorta-coronary bypass graft patency. *Journal of Thoracic and Cardiovascular Surgery* **105**, 147–53.

Birkmeyer, J.D., AuBuchon, J.P., Littenberg, B. *et al.* 1994: Cost-effectiveness of pre-operative autologous donation in coronary artery bypass grafting. *Annals of Thoracic Surgery* **57**, 161–9.

Body, S.C., Birminham, J., Parks, R. *et al.* 1999: Safety and efficacy of shed mediastinal blood transfusion after cardiac surgery: a multicenter observational study. *Journal of Thoracic and Cardiovascular Anesthesia* **13**, 410–16.

Boldt, J., Kling, D., von Bormann, B. *et al.* 1989: Blood conservation in cardiac operations. Cell separation versus hemofiltration. *Journal of Thoracic and Cardiovascular Surgery* **97**, 832–40.

Borowiec, J., Thelin, S., Bagge, L. *et al.* 1992: Heparin-coated circuits reduce activation of granulocytes during cardiopulmonary bypass. A clinical study. *Journal of Thoracic and Cardiovascular Surgery* **104**, 642–7.

British Committee for Standards in Haematology 1992: Guidelines for the use of fresh frozen plasma. *Transfusion Medicine* **2**, 57–63.

Bull, B.S., Korpman, R.A., Huse, W.M. *et al.* 1975: Heparin therapy during extracorporeal circulation. *Journal of Thoracic and Cardiovascular Surgery* **69**, 674–84.

Chan, A.H.C., Chan, J.C.M., Wong, L.Y.F., Cheng, G. 1996: From maximum blood order schedule to unlimited computer crossmatching: evolution of blood transfusion for surgical patients at a tertiary hospital in Hong Kong. *Transfusion Medicine* **6**, 121–4.

Cosgrove, D., Heric, B., Lytle, B.W. *et al.* 1992: Aprotinin therapy for reoperative myocardial revascularization: a placebo controlled study. *Annals of Thoracic Surgery* **54**, 1031–6.

Cromer, M.J., Wolk, D.R. 1998: A minimal priming technique that allows for a higher circulating haemoglobin on cardiopulmonary bypass. *Perfusion* **13**, 311–13.

Crowell, J.W., Smith, E.E. 1967: Determinant of the optimal hematocrit. *Journal of Applied Physiology* **22**, 501–4.

Dacie, J.V., Homer, G.F. 1946: Blood-loss in battle casualties. Use of transfusion fluids. *Lancet* **1**, 371–7.

D'Ambra, M.N., Gray, R.J., Hillman, R. *et al.* 1997: Effect of recombinant erythropoietin on transfusion risk in coronary artery bypass patients. *Annals of Thoracic Surgery* **64**, 1686–93.

DeBois, W., Krieger, K.H. 1998: The influence of oxygenator type and priming volume on blood requirements. In: Krieger, K.H., Isom, O.W., eds. *Blood conservation in cardiac surgery*. New York, NY: Springer Verlag; 327–71.

Defoe, G.R., Ross, C.S., Olmstead, E.M. *et al.* 2001: Lowest hematocrit on bypass and adverse outcomes associated with coronary artery bypass grafting. Northern New England cardiovascular study group. *Annals of Thoracic Surgery* **71**, 769–76.

De Haan, J., Schonberger, J., Haan, J. *et al.* 1993: Tissue-type plasminogen activators and fibrin monomers synergistically cause platelet dysfunction during retransfusion of shed blood after cardiopulmonary bypass. *Journal of Thoracic and Cardiovascular Surgery* **106**, 1017–23.

Despotis, G.J., Joist, J.H. 1999: Anticoagulation and anticoagulation reversal with cardiac surgery involving cardiopulmonary bypass; an update. *Journal of Cardiothoracic Vascular Anesthesia* **13** (Suppl. 1), 18–29.

Despotis, G.J., Santoro, S.A., Spitznagel, E. *et al.* 1994: Prospective evaluation and clinical utility of on-site monitoring of patients undergoing cardiac operation. *Journal of Thoracic and Cardiovascular Surgery* **107**, 271–9.

Dodd, R.Y. 1994: Adverse consequences of blood transfusion: quantitative risk estimates. In: Nance, S.T., ed. *Blood supply: risks, perceptions and prospects for the future*. Besthesda, MD: American Association of Blood Banks: 1–24.

Dzik, W.H., Fleischer, A.G., Ciavarella, D. *et al.* 1992: Safety and efficacy of autologous blood donation before elective valve operation. *Annals of Thoracic Surgery* **54**, 1177–81.

Engoren, M.C., Habib, R.H., Zacharias, A. *et al.* 2002: Effect of blood transfusion on long term survival after cardiac operation. *Annals of Thoracic Surgery* **74**, 1180–6.

Ereth, M.H., Oliver, W.C. Jr, Beynen, F.M.K. *et al.* 1993: Autologous platelet-rich plasma does not reduce transfusion of homologous blood products in patients undergoing repeat valvular surgery. *Anesthesiology* **79**, 540–7.

Fang, W.C., Helm, R.E., Krieger, K.H. *et al.* 1997: Impact of minimum hematocrit during cardiopulmonary bypass on mortality in patients undergoing coronary artery surgery. *Circulation* **96** (Suppl. II), II-194–II-199.

Flapan, A.D. 1994: Management of patients after their first myocardial infarction. *British Medical Journal* **309**, 1129–34.

Ford, S.M.S, Unsworth-White, M.J., Aziz, T. *et al.* 1999: Haemostatic function of pheresed platelets during cardiac surgery. *British Journal of Anaesthesia* **82** (Suppl. 2), A.64.

Fremes, S.E., Wong, W.I., Lee, E. *et al.* 1994: Metaanalysis of prophylactic drug treatment in the prevention of postoperative bleeding. *Annals of Thoracic Surgery* **58**, 1580–8.

Garry, P.J., Vanderjagt, D.J., Wayne, S.J. *et al.* 1991: A prospective study of blood donations in healthy elderly persons. *Transfusion* **31**, 686–92.

Gillon, J., Desmond, M., Thomas, M.J.G. 1999: Acute normovolaemic haemodilution. *Transfus Med* **9**, 259–64.

Giordano, G.F., Rivers, S.L., Chung, G.K.T. *et al.* 1988: Autologous platelet-rich plasma in cardiac surgery: effect on intraoperative and postoperative transfusion requirements. *Annals of Thoracic Surgery* **46**, 416–19.

Goldman, M., Blajchman, M.A. 1991: Blood product-associated bacterial sepsis. *Transfusion Medicine Reviews* **5**, 73–83.

Goldman, S., Copeland, J., Moritz, T. *et al.* 1988: Improvement in early saphenous vein graft patency after coronary artery bypass surgery with antiplatelet therapy: results of a Veterans Administration Cooperative Study. *Circulation* **77**, 1324–32.

Goodnough, L.T., Johnston, M.F.M., Toy, P.T.C.Y. 1991: The variability in transfusion practice in coronary artery bypass surgery. *Journal of the American Medical Association* **265**, 86–90.

Goodnough, L.T., Despotis, G.J., Hogue, C.W., Ferguson, T.B. 1995: On the need for improved transfusion indicators in cardiac surgery. *Annals of Thoracic Surgery* **60**, 473–80.

Goodnough, L.T., Monk, T.G., Brecher, M.E. 1997: Acute normovolemic hemodilution in surgery. *Hematology* **2**, 413–20.

Gorman, R.C., Ziats, N., Rao, A.K. *et al.* 1996: Surface-bound heparin fails to reduce thrombin formation during clinical cardiopulmonary bypass. *Journal of Thoracic and Cardiovascular Surgery* **111**, 1–11.

Gravlee, G.P., Haddon, W.S., Rothberger, H.K. *et al.* 1990: Heparin dosing and monitoring for cardiopulmonary bypass. A comparison of techniques with measurement of subclinical plasma coagulation. *Journal of Thoracic and Cardiovascular Surgery* **99**, 518–27.

Hall, R.I., Schweiger, I.M., Finlayson, D.C. 1990: The benefit of the Haemonetics cell saver apparatus during cardiac surgery. *Canadian Anaesthetists Society Journal* **37**, 618–23.

Handa, A., Dickstein, B., Young, N.S. et al. 2000: Prevalence of the newly described circovirus, TTV in United States blood donors. *Transfusion* **40**, 245–51.

Hardy, J., Belisle, S. 1994: Natural and synthetic antifibrinolytics in adult cardiac surgery: efficacy, effectiveness and efficiency. *Canadian Anaesthetists Society Journal* **41**, 1104–12.

Hebert, P.C., Wells, G., Blajchman, M.A. et al. 1999: A multicenter, randomized, controlled clinical trial of transfusion requirements in critical care. *New England Journal of Medicine* **340**, 409–17.

Horrow, J.C., Van Riper, D.F., Strong, M.D. et al. 1995: The dose response relationship of tranexamic acid. *Anesthesiology* **82**, 383–92.

Houston, F., Foster, J.D., Chong, A. et al. 2000: Transmission of BSE by blood transfusion in sheep. *Lancet* **356**, 999–1000.

Huet, C., Salmi, R., Fergusson, D. et al. 1999: A meta-analysis of the effectiveness of cell salvage to minimize perioperative allogeneic blood transfusion in cardiac and orthopedic surgery. *Anesthesia and Analgesia* **89**, 861–9.

Jobes, D.R., Aitken, G.L., Shaffer, G.W. 1995: Increased accuracy and precision of heparin and protamine dosing reduces blood loss and transfusion in patients undergoing primary cardiac operations. *Journal of Thoracic and Cardiovascular Surgery* **110**, 36–45.

John, L.C.H., Rees, G.M., Kovacs, I.B. 1993: Inhibition of platelet function by heparin. An etiologic factor in post bypass hemorrhage. *Journal of Thoracic and Cardiovascular Surgery* **105**, 816–22.

Johnson, R.G., Thurer, R.L., Kruskall, M.S. et al. 1992: Comparison of two transfusion strategies after elective operations for myocardial revascularization. *Journal of Thoracic and Cardiovascular Surgery* **104**, 307–14.

Jones, J.W., McCoy, T.A., Rawitscher, R.E., Lindsley, D.A. 1990: Effects of intra-operative plasmapheresis on blood loss in cardiac surgery. *Annals of Thoracic Surgery* **49**, 585–90.

Jones, J.W., Rawitscher, R.E., McLean, T.R. et al. 1991: Benefit from combining blood conservation measures in cardiac surgery. *Annals of Thoracic Surgery* **51**, 541–6.

Khuri, S.F., Wolfe, J.A., Josa, M. et al. 1992: Hematologic changes during and after cardiopulmonary bypass and their relationship to the bleeding time and nonsurgical blood loss. *Journal of Thoracic and Cardiovascular Surgery* **104**, 108–16.

Laupacis, A., Fergusson, D. 1998: Erythropoietin to minimize perioperative blood transfusion: a systematic review of randomized trials. *Transfusion Medicine* **8**, 309–17.

Lemmer, J.H., Stanford, W., Bonney, S.L. et al. 1994: Aprotinin for coronary bypass surgery: efficacy, safety and influence on early saphenous vein graft patency. *Journal of Thoracic and Cardiovascular Surgery* **107**, 543–53.

Lemmer, J.H. Jr, Dilling, E.W., Morton, J.R. et al. 1996: Aprotinin for primary coronary artery bypass grafting: a multi-center trial of three dose regimens. *Annals of Thoracic Surgery* **62**, 1659–68.

Levy, J.H., Pifarre, R., Schaff, H. et al. 1995: A multicenter, placebo-controlled, double-blind trial of aprotinin for reducing blood loss and requirement for donor-blood transfusion in patients undergoing repeat coronary artery bypass grafting. *Circulation* **92**, 2236–44.

Magilligan, D.J. 1985: Indications for ultrafiltration in the cardiac surgical patient. *Journal of Thoracic and Cardiovascular Surgery* **89**, 183–9.

Mathru, M., Kleinman, B., Blakeman, B. et al. 1992: Myocardial metabolism and adaptation during extreme hemodilution in humans after coronary revascularization. *Critical Care Medicine* **20**, 1420–5.

Mongan, P.D., Hosking, M.P. 1992: The role of desmopressin acetate in patients undergoing coronary artery bypass surgery. A controlled clinical trial with thromboelastographic risk stratification. *Anesthesiology* **77**, 38–46.

Muehrcke, D.D., McCarthy, P.M., Stewart, R.W. et al. 1995: Complications of extracorporeal life support systems using heparin-bound surfaces. The risk of intracardiac clot formation. *Journal of Thoracic and Cardiovascular Surgery* **110**, 843–51.

Muehrcke, D.D., McCarthy, P.M., Kottke-Marchant, K.K. et al. 1996: Biocompatibility of heparin-coated extracorporeal bypass circuits: a randomized, masked, clinical trial. *Journal of Thoracic and Cardiovascular Surgery* **112**, 472–83.

Napier, J.A. 1997: Red cell replacement in surgery. *Transfusion Medicine* **7**, 265–8.

Nilsson, L., Bagge, L., Nystrom, S.O. 1990: Blood cell trauma and postoperative bleeding: comparison of bubble and membrane oxygenators and observations on coronary suction. *Scandinavian Journal of Thoracic and Cardiovascular Surgery* **24**, 65–9.

Ovrum, E., Am, H.E., Tangen, G., Ringdal, M.A. 1996: Heparinized cardiopulmonary bypass and full heparin dose marginally improve clinical performance. *Annals of Thoracic Surgery* **62**, 1128–33.

Owings, D.V., Kruskall, M.S., Thurer, R.L., Donovan, L.M. 1989: Autologous blood donation prior to elective cardiac surgery. Safety and effect on subsequent blood use. *Journal of the American Medical Association* **262**, 1963–8.

Panico, F.G., Neptune, W.B. 1960: A mechanism to eliminate the donor blood prime from the pump oxygenator. *Surgical Forum* **10**, 605–9.

Pearson, D.T. 1988: Blood gas control during cardiopulmonary bypass. *Perfusion* **3**, 113–33.

Popovsky, M.A., Whitaker, B., Arnold, N.L. 1995: Severe outcomes of allogeneic and autologous blood donations: frequency and characterization. *Transfusion* **35**, 734–7.

Puga, F.J. 1990: Risk of preoperative aspirin in patients undergoing coronary artery bypass surgery. *J Am Coll Cardiol* **15**, 21–2.

Reed, R.L., Johnston, T.D., Hudson, J.D. et al. 1990: Hypothermia and blood coagulation: dissociation between enzyme activity and clotting factor levels. *Circulatory Shock* **32**, 141–52.

Rosengart, T.K., DeBois, W., O'Hara, M. et al. 1998: Retrograde autologous priming for cardiopulmonary bypass: a safe and effective means of decreasing haemodilution and transfusion requirements. *Journal of Thoracic and Cardiovascular Surgery* **115**, 426–39.

Royston, D., Taylor, K.M., Bidstrup, B.P. et al. 1987: Effect of aprotinin on need for blood transfusion after repeat open-heart surgery. *Lancet* **2**, 1289–91.

Rubens, F.D., Fergusson, D., Wells, P.S. et al. 1998: Platelet-rich plasmapheresis in cardiac surgery: a meta-analysis of the effect on transfusion requirements. *Journal of Thoracic and Cardiovascular Surgery* **116**, 641–7.

Schaff, H.V., Hauer, J.M., Gardner, T.J. *et al.* 1978: Autotransfusion of shed mediastinal blood after cardiac surgery: a prospective study. *Journal of Thoracic and Cardiovascular Surgery* **75**, 632–41.

Shore-Lesserson, L. 1999: Aprotinin has direct platelet protective properties: fact or fiction? *Journal of Cardiothoracic and Vascular Anesthesia* **13**, 379–81.

Shore-Lesserson, L., Manspeizer, H.E., DePerio, M. *et al.* 1999: Thromboelastography-guided transfusion algorithm reduces transfusions in complex cardiac surgery. *Anesthesia and Analgesia* **88**, 312–19.

Spahn, D.R., Smith, L.R., Veronee, C.D. *et al.* 1993: Acute isovolemic hemodilution and blood transfusion. Effects on regional function and metabolism in myocardium with compromised coronary blood flow. *Journal of Thoracic and Cardiovascular Surgery* **105**, 694–704.

Spahn, D.R., Schmid, E.R., Seifert, B., Pasch, T. 1996: Hemodilution tolerance in patients with coronary artery disease who are receiving chronic β-adrenergic blocker therapy. *Anesthesia and Analgesia* **82**, 687–94.

Spiess, B.D., Tuman, K.J., McCarthy, R.J. *et al.* 1987: Thromboelastography as an indicator of post-cardiopulmonary bypass coagulopathies. *Journal of Clinical Monitoring* **3**, 25–30.

Spiess, B.D., Ley, C., Body, S.C. *et al.* 1998: Hematocrit value on intensive care unit entry influences the frequency of Q-wave myocardial infarction after coronary artery bypass grafting. *Journal of Thoracic and Cardiovascular Surgery* **116**, 460–7.

Sundt, T.M., Kouchoukos, N.T., Saffitz, J.E. *et al.* 1993: Renal dysfunction and intravascular coagulation with aprotinin and circulatory arrest. *Annals of Thoracic Surgery* **55**, 1418–24.

Vamvakas, E.C. 1996: Transfusion-associated cancer recurrence and postoperative infection: meta-analysis of randomized, controlled trials. *Transfusion* **36**, 175–86.

Vander Salm, T.J., Kaur, S., Lancey, R.A. *et al.* 1996: Reduction of bleeding after heart operations through the prophylactic use of epsilon-aminocaproic acid. *Journal of Thoracic and Cardiovascular Surgery* **112**, 1098–107.

Velthius, H., Jansen, P.G.M., Hack, C.E. *et al.* 1996: Specific complement inhibition with heparin-coated extracorporeal circuits. *Annals of Thoracic Surgery* **61**, 1153–7.

Wallace, H.W., Brooks, H., Stein, T.P., Zimmerman, N.J. 1976: The contribution of anticoagulants to platelet dysfunction with extracorporeal circulation. *Journal of Thoracic and Cardiovascular Surgery* **32**, 735–41.

Wang, J.S., Lin, C.Y., Hung, W.T. *et al.* 1992: *In vitro* effects of aprotinin on activated clotting time measured with different activators. *Journal of Thoracic and Cardiovascular Surgery* **104**, 1135–40.

Watanabe, Y., Katsuo, F., Konoshi, T. *et al.* 1991: Autologous blood transfusion with recombinant human erythropoietin in heart operations. *Annals of Thoracic Surgery* **51**, 767–72.

Williamson, K.R., Taswell, H.F. 1991: Intraoperative blood salvage: a review. *Transfusion* **31**, 662–75.

Woolf, R.L., Mythen, M.G. 1998: Con: Heparin-bonded cardiopulmonary bypass circuits do not represent a desirable and cost-effective advance in cardiopulmonary bypass technology. *Journal of Thoracic Cardiovascular Anesthesia* **12**, 710–12.

14

Mechanical circulatory support

STEPHEN WESTABY AND SATOSHI SAITO

KEY POINTS

- The aim of mechanical circulatory support is to support the circulation and reduce the work of the ischaemic or damaged heart while recovery of cardiac metabolism and function occurs.
- The intra-aortic balloon pump is the most commonly used form of support and, properly used, has a high degree of success and an acceptable level of device-related complications.
- Extracorporeal devices used for short-term support in acute situations have approximately 30 per cent survival rates, but a high incidence of haemorrhagic complications.
- Implantable devices for longer term use have high incidences of infective and other complications, as well as difficulties with power delivery and portability.
- Second-generation implantable devices have shown promise in overcoming some of the problems of earlier models.
- The development of a satisfactory total artificial heart remains a major challenge.

HISTORICAL BACKGROUND

Mechanical systems to support the circulation evolved soon after the first use of cardiopulmonary bypass by Gibbon in 1953. At that time, myocardial protection was poor and many patients required one or two hours of coronary reperfusion before they could be successfully separated from the extracorporeal circuit. Patients with persisting myocardial dysfunction always died and surgeons were convinced that a more prolonged and less damaging form of cardiac support was required.

In 1965, Spencer described four patients with post-cardiotomy heart failure, who were supported for prolonged periods with femoro-femoral cardiopulmonary bypass (Spencer *et al.*, 1965). One patient survived and was discharged from the hospital. Hall and colleagues (Hall *et al.*, 1964) developed an intrathoracic left ventricular bypass pump, implanted into the left hemithorax, to connect the left atrium and descending thoracic aorta. The device consisted of an inner blood chamber surrounded by a reinforced silicone rubber air tube into which pulses of compressed air were supplied to expel blood from the lumen. Ball valves at the inlet and outlet provided unidirectional flow and the pump was triggered by the R-wave of the electrocardiogram. The system was used in 1963 and established the basic principles of mechanical circulatory support. Unfortunately, the patient died from cerebral injury sustained before the device was employed. DeBakey (1971) was the first to achieve survival using a left ventricular bypass pump in 1966 (Fig. 14.1). The pump was placed extracorporeally to connect the left atrium and axilliary artery and was removed without opening the chest. In this case, the female patient was supported for 10 days with flows up to 1200 mL/min. She survived and left hospital despite severe post-cardiotomy heart failure after double valve replacement.

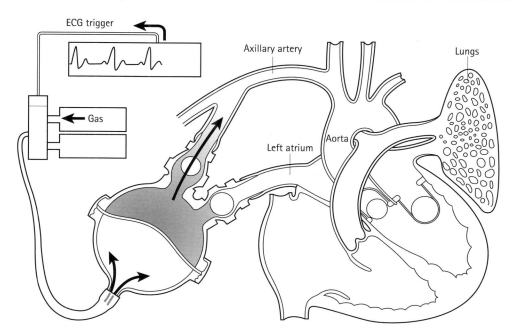

Figure 14.1 *Diagram of DeBakey's first successful left ventricular assist device in patients after double valve replacement.*

The intra-aortic balloon pump was developed in the late 1960s and emerged to be the most frequently used form of cardiac assistance. Moulopoulos *et al.* (1962) reported the use of a latex balloon placed in the descending thoracic aorta in 1962. This was inflated during diastole and deflated during systole. With further development, Kantrowitz and colleagues successfully applied the intra-aortic balloon pump for post-myocardial infarction cardiogenic shock (Westaby, 1997). In 1973, Buckley and colleagues (Buckley *et al.*, 1973) reported the use of the intra-aortic balloon pump to support patients who could not be weaned from cardiopulmonary bypass.

The National Heart, Lung, and Blood Institute (NHLBI) became actively involved in mechanical circulatory support research after the formation of the Artificial Heart Programme in 1964. In 1970, the Artificial Heart Programme became the Medical Devices Applications Branch of the NHLBI, with long-term objectives to:

- produce emergency cardiac assist systems that could treat acute circulatory insufficiency
- provide temporary cardiac assist systems that could support the circulation for days to months until the patient's clinical condition was stabilized
- provide permanent heart assist systems on a lifetime basis
- develop implantable artificial hearts that could completely replace irreparably damaged natural hearts.

This strategy was stimulated by the left ventricular assist device conference of 1972, which emphasized the development of long-term systems. In 1977, two requests

for proposals were issued by John Watson, the newly appointed Director of the Devices and Technology Branch of the NHLBI, one for the development of left heart assist blood pumps and the other for production of electrical energy converters to power and control left ventricular assist device systems. These initiatives were followed in 1988 by another for the development of an implantable integrated electrically powered left heart assist system designed to provide circulatory support for more than two years. These proposals laid the foundation upon which the entire field of mechanical circulatory support evolved. In particular, they gave rise to the ABIOMED and Thoratec extracorporeal bi-ventricular support systems and the implantable Novacor and HeartMate left ventricular assist devices, which have been the mainstay of circulatory support strategies until the introduction of axial flow impeller pumps in the late 1990s.

As blood pumps evolved from short-term external devices to fully implantable systems, the applications of circulatory support also changed. Early success with post-cardiotomy recovery led to their employment in the management of acute cardiac failure through myocarditis or myocardial infarction. The feasibility of long-term support, with the introduction of cyclosporin and immunosuppression, led to the widespread adoption of mechanical support as a bridge to transplantation. The progressive decrease in donor organ availability eventually led to trials of permanent mechanical circulatory support versus continued medical therapy (Rose *et al.*, 2001). Recognition of improving left ventricular function during unloading introduced the possibility of a mechanical bridge to myocardial recovery (Westaby *et al.*, 2000).

A wide variety of temporary and long-term mechanical support devices is now available in affluent healthcare systems. These allow salvage of an ever increasing proportion of heart failure patients by left ventricular assist device or bi-ventricular assist device support with or without cardiac transplantation.

DEVICES USED FOR SHORT-TERM CIRCULATORY SUPPORT

The intra-aortic balloon pump

The intra-aortic balloon pump has advantages over other assist devices in terms of ease of insertion and removal, but it cannot substantially increase systemic blood flow. The balloon is positioned in the descending thoracic aorta with its tip just distal to the left subclavian artery. It is programmed to inflate during diastole and to deflate just before left ventricular ejection (Fig. 14.2). By deflating in the aorta immediately before left ventricular ejection, the intra-aortic balloon pump functions to reduce after-load, thereby decreasing left ventricular work and myocardial oxygen consumption. Balloon inflation increases diastolic pressure and augments perfusion of the coronary arteries (Fig. 14.3). By using transoesophageal echocardiography, peak diastolic coronary flow velocity increases by a mean of 117 per cent, with an increase in mean flow velocity integral of 87 per cent. Moreover, blood flow velocities of 1.5 times to twice baseline have been measured in the stenosed left anterior descending coronary arteries of patients supported by intra-aortic balloon pumps. Factors that determine the effectiveness of intra-aortic balloon pump support include balloon volume, location in the aorta, rate of inflation and deflation, and synchrony relative to the events during the cardiac cycle. The optimal inflation or deflation timing has been shown to be with inflation slightly preceding the diacrotic notch and deflation bordering on isovolumetric systole. Modern intra-aortic balloon pump controllers are designed to optimize timing during sinus rhythm and in the presence of cardiac arrhythmias. The intra-aortic balloon pump also has the capacity to improve right heart function through ventricular interdependence mechanisms and augmentation of right coronary blood flow. Although the intra-aortic balloon pump provides a small increase in antegrade carotid flow during diastole, there is no net improvement in cerebral blood flow caused by flow reversal in early systole. This probably occurs through balloon deflation before ejection of blood into the aorta.

INDICATIONS FOR INTRA-AORTIC BALLOON PUMP USE

Five to 10 per cent of patients hospitalized with acute myocardial infarction will develop cardiogenic shock. For

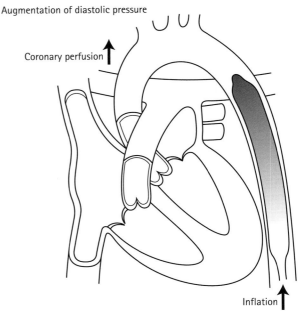

Augmentation of diastolic pressure

Coronary perfusion

Inflation

(a) Diastole: Inflation

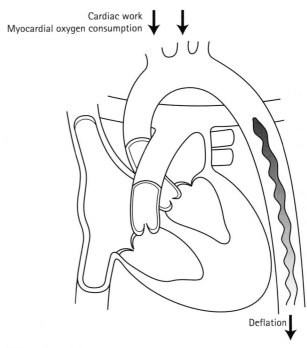

Decreased after-load

Cardiac work
Myocardial oxygen consumption

Deflation

(b) Systole: Deflation

Figure 14.2 *Principles of aortic balloon pump support: (a) during diastole; (b) during systole.*

these patients, the intra-aortic balloon pump is used to decrease myocardial oxygen consumption (by reducing after-load) as well as increasing blood flow during diastole. The same principles apply to patients with unstable angina

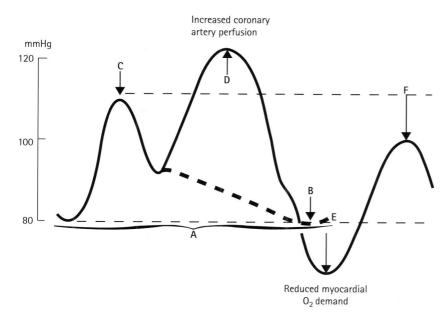

Figure 14.3 *Influence of the intra-aortic balloon pump on arterial trace. A = one complete cardiac cycle; B = unassisted aortic end diastolic pressure; C = unassisted systolic pressure; D = diastolic augmentation; E = reduced aortic end diastolic pressure; F = reduced systolic pressure.*

and myocardial ischaemia refractory to medical therapy, in which case the intra-aortic balloon pump is inserted by the cardiologist during cardiac catheterization. Between 10 and 15 per cent of patients undergoing cardiac surgery receive an intra-aortic balloon pump either pre-operatively, to reduce risk, or post-operatively, to support the patient after weaning difficulties.

Pre-operative intra-aortic balloon pump placement allows stabilization of patients with acute coronary syndromes before revascularization. In one series of coronary bypass patients with ejection faction <25 per cent, 30-day mortality with pre-operative intra-aortic balloon pump placement was 2.7 per cent compared with 11.9 per cent for unsupported patients (Dietl *et al.*, 1996).

Baldwin and colleagues (Baldwin *et al.*, 1993) developed a model for predicting post-cardiotomy intra-aortic balloon pump survival for patients who required assistance during weaning from cardiopulmonary bypass. The overall mortality was 48 per cent. If present before or within 10 minutes of the first attempt at weaning from cardiopulmonary bypass, the following variables were predictors of mortality:

- complete heart block and the need for pacing
- advanced age
- elevated pre-operative blood urea nitrogen
- female gender.

Christenson *et al.* (1995) reported 48 per cent mortality for intra-aortic balloon pump patients with post-cardiotomy heart failure. They identified pre-operative myocardial ischaemia and combined cardiac surgical procedures as risk factors for mortality. In a large series of intra-aortic balloon pump patients from the Massachusetts General Hospital, multivariate predictors of death in medical and surgical patients included intra-aortic balloon pump insertion in the operating room or intensive care unit, transthoracic insertion, advanced age, procedures other than coronary artery bypass grafting (CABG) or percutaneous transluminal coronary angioplasty and insertion for cardiogenic shock (Torchiana *et al.*, 1997). In this series, predictors of death were great age, mitral valve replacement, prolonged cardiopulmonary bypass, urgent or emergency operation, pre-operative renal dysfunction, complex ventricular dysrhythmias, right ventricular failure and emergency resumption of cardiopulmonary bypass.

TECHNICAL ASPECTS OF BALLOON PUMP USE

Percutaneous, and subsequently sheathless, intra-aortic balloon pump insertion were important developments that allowed for extended indications for use by both surgeons and by cardiologists. On occasion, however, when atherosclerotic disease or extreme tortuosity of the aorto-iliac system does not allow passage from the femoral vessels, it is necessary to place the balloon directly into the ascending aorta. This requires balloon insertion and removal through an open chest, although on occasion a prosthetic graft can be sewn to the aorta to convey the balloon catheter through the right second intercostal space.

When the intra-aortic balloon pump is used pre-operatively, intravenous heparin is mandatory. In patients who have intra-aortic balloon pumps placed for heart failure, anti-coagulation with warfarin is also used. Patients who leave the operating room with an intra-aortic balloon pump after cardiopulmonary bypass are not maintained on intravenous heparin but may be given intravenous low molecular weight dextran at a rate of 20 mL/h. This is initiated after chest tube drainage rates have decreased to acceptable levels. In a small set of patients who require an intra-aortic balloon pump for four or five days, low molecular weight dextran is changed to subcutaneous low molecular weight heparin or intravenous heparin to maintain the APPT at twice normal.

There are three sources for a balloon pump synchronization signal, namely: R-wave sensing from the electrocardiogram; arterial pulse detection from the arterial trace and R-wave sensing of implanted atrial or ventricular pacing wires. The detection of the R-wave initiates intra-aortic balloon pump deflation so that the balloon will be fully deflated during ventricular systole. Before removing the balloon catheter, it is necessary to determine that the patient can maintain haemodynamic stability by carefully weaning the support. Commonly, the intra-aortic balloon pump is switched from a 1:1 augmentation frequency to 1:2 then 1:4 and, lastly, to 1:8, whilst reviewing the patient's haemodynamic status. Reduction in the augmentation volume may also be used as a means of weaning support. The duration of time spent on these settings should be minimized, as there is an increased risk of thrombosis on the balloon surface with lower inflation rates. Once haemodynamic stability is established, the intra-aortic balloon pump should be placed back in the 1:2 mode to lower the likelihood of thrombosis until it can be removed. Heparin should be discontinued before intra-aortic balloon pump removal in order to normalize the APTT. In general, coagulation should be normal before intra-aortic balloon pump removal, with a platelet count $>100,000$ per mm^3 and prothrombin time of less than 15 s.

COMPLICATIONS OF INTRA-AORTIC BALLOON PUMP USE

Vascular complications are the most frequent cause of morbidity for percutaneous intra-aortic balloon pumps, with rates between nine per cent and 36 per cent (Busch *et al.*, 1997). Femoral cannulation may be complicated by peripheral ischaemia caused by mechanical occlusion, thrombosis or embolism. It is therefore important to enter the common femoral and not the superficial femoral artery in order to minimize complications. Factors predisposing to lower extremity ischaemia include female gender, diabetes mellitus and pre-existing peripheral vascular disease. Injury to the aorta may include intramural haematoma, dissection, arterial perforation and arterial thrombus and embolism. Patients at greatest risk of ischaemic complications are those with a history of peripheral vascular disease, cardiogenic shock as the indication for intra-aortic balloon pump use and a history of smoking (Vilacosta *et al.*, 1995). Intra-aortic balloon pump use is also a risk factor for mesenteric ischaemia after cardiac surgery, and acute pancreatitis may occur possibly as a result of athero-emboli in the coeliac axis. Neurological complications are much less frequent than

vascular complications, but paraplegia has occurred secondary to aortic dissection or adventitial haematoma producing spinal cord infarction. Stroke has occurred after balloon rupture and cerebral helium embolization. Hyperbaric oxygen therapy can minimize the severity of the neurological deficit. Balloon rupture has been reported in 0.5–6 per cent of patients (Vilacosta *et al.*, 1995). Rupture may result in balloon entrapment because blood leaks into the system and forms clots, which block full deflation and extraction.

The intra-aortic balloon pump may be the only mechanical support device available in non-transplant cardiac centres. This is largely because blood pumps have been used predominantly for bridge to cardiac transplantation. It is likely that the intra-aortic balloon pump will continue its important role because of its ease of insertion and capacity to unload the left ventricle and improve coronary blood flow. Nevertheless, there is increasing justification to provide all cardiac centres with more advanced systems to support the circulation on a temporary basis.

Extracorporeal centrifugal blood pumps

Centrifugal pumps impart momentum to fluid by means of fast-moving blades, impellers or concentric cones (Fig. 14.4). Fluid enters the pump axially from an inlet pipe or tubing and is caught up between veins or stages and whirled outwards. Rotation of the impeller causes the

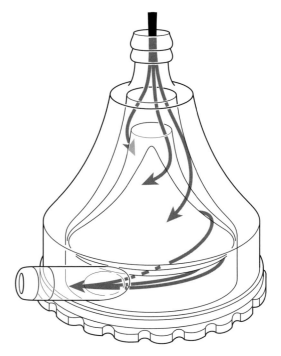

Figure 14.4 *Centrifugal blood pump.*

velocity of blood to change while it moves towards the periphery of the pump. As blood exits through the outlet port, pressure is increased. Centrifugal pumps can provide high flow rates with low pressure rises, but are particularly sensitive to after-load. Centrifugal pumps have been used for extracorporeal membrane oxygenization in left heart bypass during surgery on the thoracic aorta, post-cardiotomy or myocarditis left ventricular failure, bridge to transplantation, right heart assist after cardiac transplantation and as a bridge to more sophisticated pulsatile assist devices (Pagani *et al.*, 2001). In extracorporeal membrane oxygenization, centrifugal pumps are less destructive to blood cellular elements than are roller pumps. For any clinical application that would require longer than four hours of mechanical assist a centrifugal pump is preferable to a roller pump (Hoerr *et al.*, 1987).

The major indication for centrifugal mechanical assistance is failure to wean from cardiopulmonary bypass secondary to left, right or bi-ventricular failure. After the unsuccessful attempt at weaning, the heart is allowed to rest on cardiopulmonary bypass while it is determined whether the surgical repair can be improved. Low-dose inotropic agents are then initiated and, if repeat separation from cardiopulmonary bypass is unsuccessful, intra-aortic balloon pump support is instituted. If subsequent weaning efforts with high-dose multiple intropes prove unsuccessful, and death is imminent, the centrifugal blood pump is applied for salvage. Usual haemodynamic criteria include a cardiac index $<1.8\,L/m^2$, a blood pressure $<90\,mmHg$, atrial pressures $>20\,mmHg$, systemic vascular resistance $>2100\,dynes/s$ per cm^{-5} and low urine output.

Three centrifugal pumps commonly in use are the Medtronic Biomedicus, the Sarns3M and the St Jude models. A number of different sites are available for both left and right heart cannulation. For left-heart support, blood is extracted from the left atrium (superior pulmonary vein, left atrial appendage or dome of the left atrium) or left ventricular apex. The pump returns blood to the ascending aorta, arch, subclavian or femoral arteries. For right-heart bypass, blood is removed from the right atrial appendage or free wall (with ventricular cannulation through the tricuspid valve) and returned to the pulmonary artery. The preferred right atrial site is the junction of the inferior vena cava and right atrium, orientating the tip of the 36F cannula superiorly. This allows the cannula direct exit from the mediastinum inferiorly through the abdominal wall without kinking.

Post-operative bleeding is common with centrifugal blood pumps, the most common source being the cannulation sites. Concentric purse string sutures are employed at all cannulation sites with the innermost tied to prevent bleeding and the outermost left to be secured at the time of cannula removal. It is important to avoid movement at the cannulation sites post-operatively. Exiting directly through the intercostal spaces should be avoided if possible because chest wall movement during ventilation and the use of a sternal retractor can cause disruption of the cannulation site. The aortic cannula is generally brought through the median sternotomy incision superior to the sternum. The right and left atrial cannulas exit inferiorly to the right costal margin and the pulmonary artery cannula exits inferior to the left costal margin. It is usually easier to pass the cannulae through the abdominal wall before inserting them into the left and right atria and pulmonary artery. A plastic T-connector with Luer lock is used to join the cardiac cannulae and the bypass tubing. This facilitates priming and air removal when elective or urgent device exchange is necessary.

Incorporation of a haemofiltration system in the centrifugal tubing circuit is an expedient technique for removal of excess intravascular volume. The ultrafiltration rate is controlled by passing the effluent through an infusion pump that controls the egress and avoids large intravascular volume shifts. Left-heart bypass is always started slowly initially, and right ventricular function is assessed. Increased delivery of blood to the right heart may precipitate right ventricular dilatation and failure. The centrifugal pump speed is set at the lowest rpm that will accomplish the flow prescribed (3–6 L/min). Central venous pressure is maintained in the physiological range by addition of fluids or blood.

Flow at any given centrifugal pump speed is pre-load and after-load (blood pressure) dependent. In the absence of adequate pre-load, the atrium will collapse around the inlet cannula causing cessation of pump flow. The atrium then fills but, with inadequate volume, the process repeats itself rapidly and must be managed by decreasing the rpm or administering fluid to the patient. A sudden fall in flow may suggest an abrupt increase in after-load, for instance if the patient wakes up, or a kinked outflow tube. After-load reduction or correction of the technical problem restores pump flow. In the event of right-sided bypass with pulmonary hypertension, nitric oxide is used to reduce pulmonary vascular resistance.

For post-cardiotomy centrifugal support, coagulopathy is invariable and bleeding common. The preferred anticoagulation strategy is to completely reverse heparin with protamine in the operating room then begin a heparin infusion post-operatively when the PTT drops below 60 s. This rarely occurs during the first 24 hours. The PTT is then maintained in the range between 40 and 60 s. Although it is preferable to close the sternum, this must be left open in many cases to avoid cardiac compression and tamponade. If sternal closure is impractical, skin closure is preferred either by direct apposition or with a transparent silicone sheet sutured to the edges and covered with an adhesive drape to produce an airtight seal. In the event of late tamponade, mediastinal exploration is performed in the intensive care unit, thereby avoiding a return trip to the operating room. Renal failure and pulmonary oedema are common in this setting and are managed with the haemofilter.

Because of durability problems, centrifugal pumps are designed to be used for no more than five days, though we have successfully exceeded this limit. The system must be supervised by trained personnel and the pump components should be replaced every 48–96 hours. In addition, the externalized cannulae pose a risk of infection. Despite the use of heparin-bonded circuits and connectors, the pump's electromagnetic elements are potential sites for thrombus and fibrin formation. To minimize embolic risk and troublesome bleeding through heparinization, the goal is to remove the device as soon as haemodynamic competence and stability return. This rarely takes less than 24 hours.

Weaning from centrifugal mechanical assistance is straightforward. As left ventricular function recovers, pulse pressure will be observed during full flow and amplified as pump speed is decreased. Thermodilution cardiac output measurements allow right ventricular output to be measured. By subtracting pump flow, the portion of cardiac output contributed by the recovering left ventricle is determined. When a right ventricular index of 2.0–2.2 L/m^2 is obtained with minimal inotropic support and the pump at low flow, on and off trials are performed and repeated every eight hours until recovery is confirmed. Timing of weaning from bi-ventricular support is more difficult and requires echocardiographic assessment of ventricular function. Pulmonary arterial mixed venous saturation less than 50 per cent reflects inadequate tissue perfusion. If perfusion is adequate, both devices are temporarily decreased to the lowest rpm that will prevent flow reversal after which on and off trials are observed. In practice, there is a finite window of opportunity for device removal between myocardial recovery and device-related complications. In general, around 50 per cent of patients recover sufficient myocardial function to be weaned, of whom half will survive to leave hospital.

THE ABIOMED BVS 5000

This was the first cardiac assist device approved by the Food and Drug Administration in 1992 for support of post-cardiotomy patients. After the intra-aortic balloon pump, it is the second most popular system and has been used in more than 4000 patients (Samuel *et al.*, 2001). The BVS 5000 (Fig. 14.5) is an external pulsatile assist device that is capable of providing short-term left, right or bi-ventricular support. Although designed for a maximum use of two weeks, it has been successfully employed in transplant candidates for much longer periods. The system components include trans-thoracic cannulae, disposable external pumps and a microprocessor-controlled pneumatic drive console. Each pump has an upper chamber (atrium) that collects blood by means of gravity and a lower chamber (ventricle) that propels blood out of the pump. Two tri-leaflet valves, one located between the two

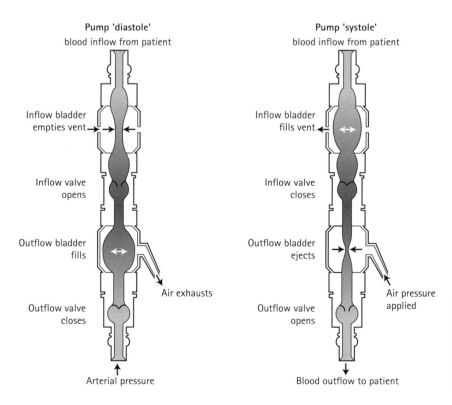

Figure 14.5 *Schematic of the ABIOMED BVS 5000 blood pump, showing the pump in systole (right) and diastole (left). The ventricular (outflow) bladder collapses during pump systole and fills during pump diastole.*

chambers and the other located in the outflow portion of the lower chamber, produce one-way flow. Blood drains from the collecting chamber into the blood pump by gravity. This passive filling avoids native atrial collapse, inflow cannula suction of air and haemolysis. Each chamber contains a smooth-surfaced 100 mL polyurethane bladder. Compressed air enters the blood pump's ventricular chamber during pump systole, causing bladder collapse and thus returning the blood to the patient. During diastole, air is vented through the console to the atmosphere allowing ventricular bladder filling. A single system supports one side of the heart. The collecting bladders operate in a 'fill to empty' mode. Adequate intravascular volume is mandatory for optimal device flow. Inadequate filling occurs if the external blood pump position is too high, whereas prolonged filling may occur if the blood pump position is too low or if the patient is volume-overloaded. Filling of the collecting chamber can be inspected visually at the bedside and the pump height adjusted as required. Typical height is approximately 25 cm below the patient's atria. In some bi-ventricular assist cases, it is necessary to adjust right and left pump heights independently. It is important to balance the flows to prevent excessive right-sided flow and pulmonary overload.

Depending on the type of support required, the inflow cannulae are placed in the right and/or left atrium. The outflow cannulae are anastomosed to the pulmonary artery or the aorta via an Angioflex-coated Dacron graft. The cannulae exit from the patient sub-costally and are covered with Dacron velour at the exit sites. The sub-costal positioning of the cannulae permits sternal closure, which is not always possible with other devices. The Dacron velour interface between the cannulae and skin promotes the growth of fibrotic tissue, reducing infection and increasing the stability and security of the junction. Power is supplied by the pneumatic drive console, which is connected to the lower chamber by means of a drive-line. The console automatically maintains the stroke volume at 82 mL and monitors passive filling, thereby adjusting the pump rate as needed to provide flows of up to 4 L/min. Pumping is not synchronized with the patient's own heart. The automated control system of the BVS 5000, with on and off operation, automatically adjusts for changes in the patient's pre-load and after-load, and requires minimal operator intervention. This simplicity renders the device easier for nurses to manage than an intra-aortic balloon pump and, unlike other external devices, it requires no added personnel for management. The two-valve design mimics a natural heart and fully decompresses the ventricle while providing pulsatile flow at physiological levels to the major organs. During support the pump allows withdrawal of inotropes to reduce myocardial oxygen demand. The mechanism is after-load sensitive so that the outflow graft must not be kinked or impaired.

Implantation is usually performed with the patient on cardiopulmonary bypass. The outflow cannulae are anastomosed first to the main pulmonary artery and infero-lateral aspect of the aorta. Once the outflow cannulae are inserted, the inflow cannulae are placed in the mid-right atrial wall and either the left atrium or left ventricular apex. The choice depends on ease of insertion and the presence of a mitral prosthesis. Left ventricular cannulation is used if the left atrium is not accessible because of small size or scarring from previous operations. If there is a mechanical mitral prosthesis, left ventricular cannulation is preferred to maintain flow across the prosthesis and reduce the risk of thromboembolism.

Once the patient is weaned from cardiopulmonary bypass and BVS 5000 support has been initiated, the heparin is completely reversed in order to achieve a normal activated clotting time. All cannulation sites are inspected for bleeding and then the chest closed if possible to maintain body temperature and prevent infection. The patient can then be extubated during mechanical support. The device can be used for all forms of recoverable heart failure, including acute myocardial infarction, myocarditis, chest trauma and right ventricular support with an implantable left ventricular assist device. If recovery does not occur, the BVS 5000 can be used as a bridge to an implantable left ventricular assist device for long-term support or transplantation. After recovery of the coagulation system, the pump requires full anticoagulation, as thrombi may form in the sinuses of the valves if the patient is sub-optimally anticoagulated.

From ABIOMEDs' Worldwide Registry, 63 per cent of users have been post-cardiotomy patients with an average age of 56 years and a mean duration of five days' support (Jett, 1996). Fifteen per cent of patients had dilated cardiomyopathy, seven per cent acute myocardial infarction, nine per cent failed transplantation, two per cent myocarditis and four per cent other indications. Fifty-two per cent of patients had bi-ventricular assist, 34 per cent left ventricular assist and 14 per cent isolated right ventricular assist. Although most dilated cardiomyopathy patients had bi-ventricular assist, myocarditis patients survived on left ventricular assist alone. Post-cardiotomy support resulted in 30 per cent survival, whereas the acute myocardial infarction hospital discharge rate is 33 per cent. When the device was inserted within three hours of the decision to implant, survival was 60 per cent, versus 20 per cent when insertion was delayed. Success with left ventricular assist alone was better with earlier implantation. The longest duration of support has been 90 days.

THE AB 180 CIRCULATORY SUPPORT SYSTEM

The AB 180 is an implantable centrifugal blood pump originally designed to provide temporary ventricular assist (up to 14 days) for patients who fail to wean from

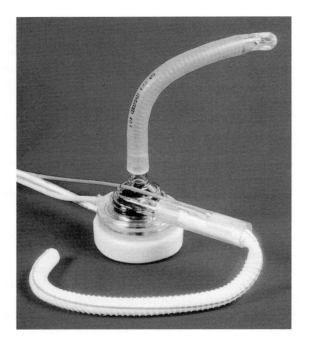

Figure 14.6 *AB 180 centrifugal blood pump.*

cardiopulmonary bypass (Fig. 14.6) (Magovern *et al.*, 2001). The inflow cannula is inserted into the left atrium and conveys blood to a polysulfone upper housing of 5 mL functional volume. An expanded PTFE vascular graft is attached to the outflow port of the upper housing. A polysulfone six-bladed 25 mm diameter impeller rotates within the upper housing at speeds of 2500–4500 rpm. The pump has two features not previously used in an implantable circulatory assist device. The first is an infusion system that pumps sterile water at 10 mL/h into the base of the lower housing to provide a fluid dynamic bearing to all rotating surfaces. Heparin (60–90 IU/mL) is used as a regional anticoagulant that does not raise the patient's PTT above normal limits. The second feature is a balloon-occluding mechanism that operates in the event of unexpected pump stoppage. This prevents backflow from the aorta to the left atrium, which would result in rapid left ventricular distension.

The controller is a microprocessor-based device that contains an isolation transformer, a battery to provide power during transportation of the patient, a constant low flow infusion pump, an air pump for the balloon occluder, an audio alarm and associated circuit boards. The only knob is for speed control. Blood flow is calculated from a graph that plots blood flow as a function of pump speed and the mean arterial pressure minus the left atrial pressure. A variety of alarms are included to safeguard the patient. In the event of post-cardiotomy failure to wean from cardiopulmonary bypass, the AB 180 is placed within the right pleural cavity with the inflow cannula within the left atrium and the outflow graft anastomosed to the

ascending aorta. The pump driveline is brought percutaneously under the right sub-costal margin or from the lower end of the sternotomy wound since re-sternotomy is required to remove the pump. Blood flow is non-pulsatile until myocardial recovery provides ejection through the left ventricular outflow tract.

After initial success with a small number of post-cardiotomy and myocarditis patients, the AB 180 has been modified for percutaneous use in the catheter laboratory. Access to the left atrium is obtained via Seldinger technique and puncture of the interatrial septum. A thin-walled inflow cannula is then inserted through the septum and pump flow is returned to the femoral artery. With continued ventilation of the lungs, this system provides temporary circulatory support for cardiogenic shock of varying aetiology (Westaby *et al.*, 1998).

DEVICES USED TO BRIDGE TO CARDIAC TRANSPLANTATION OR RECOVERY

For patients with chronic heart failure, several devices are available for extended bridge to transplantation. These include the Thoratec extracorporeal system, the Novacor left ventricular assist device and the Thermocardiosystem HeartMate implantable blood pumps. In some cases, the quality of life provided by these systems is similar to that of heart transplant recipients.

Thoratec ventricular assist device

Introduced clinically in 1982, the Thoratec ventricular assist device (Thoratec Corporation, Berkeley, CA, USA) is an external pulsatile pneumatic system that offers left, right or bi-ventricular support (Fig. 14.7) (Farrar 2000). The pump's polycarbonate housing contains a flexible, seamless, segmented polyurethane sac. Bjork–Shiley concave–convex tilting-disc valves in the inlet and outlet cannulae assure one-way flow. For left ventricular support, the inflow cannula is placed in the left atrium or left ventricular apex, and the outflow cannula is inserted into the ascending aorta via a Dacron graft. For right ventricular support, the inflow and outflow cannulae are placed in the right atrium and pulmonary artery, respectively. After exiting from the skin sub-costally, the cannulae enter the blood pump, which rests against the abdomen. The external console provides alternating positive and negative pressure to the pump via a pneumatic driveline. To maintain physiological blood flow, the volume (or fill to empty) mode of operation allows the pump to change speed as needed.

The operator can choose from three pumping modes:

- *fixed-rate mode* depends upon a pre-set pattern independent of the patient's natural heart rate

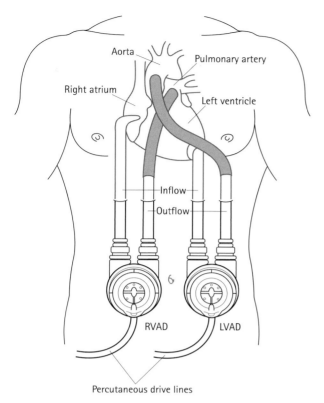

Figure 14.7 *Thoratec para-corporeal bi-ventricular system.*

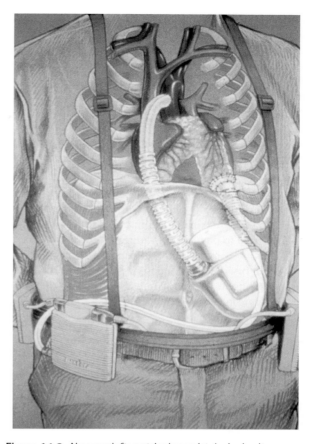

Figure 14.8 *Novacor left ventricular assist device in situ.*

- *synchronous mode* is attuned to the patient's ECG, so that flow ejection is triggered by the R-wave
- *asynchronous fill-to-empty mode* provides continuous maximal flow as regulated by the pump's filling rate.

For patients who need bi-ventricular support, excessive pulmonary congestion is prevented by adjusting right-sided flow so that it is somewhat less than left-sided flow.

Because of the long established safety record and versatility of Thoratec, the system is used widely for supporting critically ill patients, as a bridge to either transplantation or cardiac recovery. Drawbacks include limited patient mobility and the need for external cannulae. To prevent thrombus formation within the pump sac, patients must undergo continuous anticoagulation. Although the device can be used for adult patients with a wide range of body habitus (body surface area 0.73–2.5 m^2), it is too large for paediatric support.

In a large multicentre study, 74 per cent of left ventricular assist device patients and 58 per cent of bi-ventricular assist device patients survived to transplantation, with a hospital discharge rate of 89 per cent and 81 per cent, respectively (Frazier *et al.*, 1992). The most common complications were bleeding (42 per cent), renal failure (35 per cent), infection (36 per cent), hepatic failure (24 per cent), haemolysis (19 per cent), respiratory failure (17 per cent), multiorgan failure (16 per cent) and neurological events

(22 per cent). It may not be possible, pre-operatively, to predict which patients will need bi-ventricular support. Those with clinically severe right heart failure, elevated pulmonary vascular resistance and intractable ventricular dysrrhythmias are most likely to require a right ventricular assist device when systemic venous return increases during left ventricular assist device support.

Two other extracorporeal pneumatic displacement blood pumps have been developed in Europe and provide small size suitable for the paediatric population. The Berlin Heart and Medos systems employ similar cannulation strategies and have been used for prolonged (weeks or months) bridge to transplantation or recovery.

NOVACOR LEFT VENTRICULAR ASSIST DEVICE

The Novacor left ventricular assist device (Baxter Healthcare Corporation, Novacor Division, Oakland, CA, USA) is an implantable pusher plate blood pump that provides pulsatile left ventricular support (Fig. 14.8) (Portner *et al.*, 2001). The fibreglass-reinforced housing contains a seamless polyurethane pump sac and dual pusher plates. An external electric console, with the aid of an electromagnetic energy converter, powers the device. Compression by the pusher plates ejects blood from the pump sac.

Pump systole yields a stroke volume of 70 mL and a maximal output of 10 L/min. Both the inflow and outflow cannulae contain a bioprosthetic valve that maintains unidirectional flow. The inflow cannula is inserted into the left ventricular apex, and the outflow graft anastomosed to the ascending aorta. The pump and external console are connected by a percutaneous driveline that exits from the patient's right flank. The driveline transmits the electrical power cable and an air vent power to the pump but also permits venting. Transducers within the pump transmit signals to the console, thereby regulating blood flow. Three pumping modes are available:

- *synchronized mode*, which depends upon the patient's ECG signal, maximizes cardiac unloading and allows the pump to be filled with minimal effort
- *fill-to-empty mode*, which maximizes the pump's output by adjusting the pumping rate automatically in response to the filling rate
- *fixed-rate mode*, which depends upon a constant pre-set pumping rate.

Implantation of the Novacor left ventricular assist device is by median sternotomy and an extended midline abdominal incision. Positioned within the abdominal wall anterior to the posterior rectus sheath, the pump rests between the left iliac crest and the costal margin. During placement of the inflow and outflow cannulae, cardiopulmonary bypass is required.

HeartMate left ventricular assist device

The HeartMate left ventricular assist device (Thermocardiosystems Inc., Woburn, MA, USA) is available in an implantable pneumatic and a vented electric version (Frazier *et al.*, 2001a). The two versions have identical blood pumps, which differ mainly with respect to pump actuation. The pumping mechanism consists of a flexible polyurethane diaphragm within a titanium alloy outer housing (Fig. 14.9). The Dacron inflow and outflow conduits each contain a 25 mm porcine xenograft valve. To promote the formation of a pseudo-neointimal layer, all of the blood-contacting surfaces (except the valves) are textured. The titanium surfaces contain sintered titanium microspheres, and the diaphragm contains fibrils extruded from a polyurethane base. Each pump has a maximum

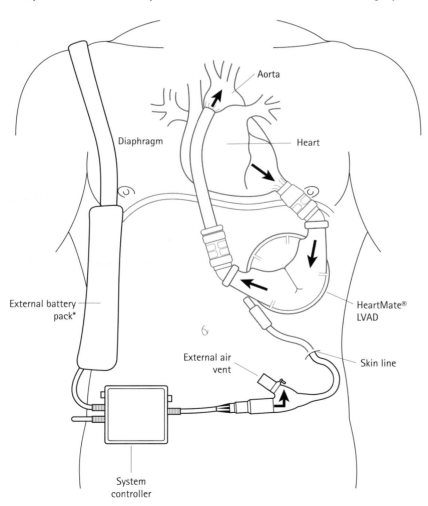

Figure 14.9 *The Thermocardiosystems externally vented pusher plate left ventricular assist device. *Left-side battery omitted for clarity.*

effective stroke volume of 8 mL. Implantation necessitates an extended median sternotomy incorporating a midline abdominal incision. In October 1994, the US government approved the implantable pneumatic left ventricular assist device for bridge to transplantation. Clinical trials of the vented electric left ventricular assist device are continuing.

IMPLANTED PNEUMATIC LEFT VENTRICULAR ASSIST DEVICE

The pneumatic blood pump weighs 570 g and produces flows of up to 12 L/min. It is regulated by a microprocessor-based drive console linked to the pump by a 18 mm Dacron-covered driveline, which exits above the patient's left iliac crest. In response to pneumatic pulses, the diaphragm moves upwards and ejects from the blood sac. The stroke volume depends upon the position of the diagphragm, which is continuously monitored by a sensor in the pump housing. The implanted pneumatic left ventricular assist device offers three modes of operation:

- *fixed-rate mode* (generally used when the patient is at rest), pumping relies on a pre-selected rate
- *automatic mode*, which depends upon the pump's filling status, flow is continually maximized to achieve an average stroke volume of 75 mL
- *external synchronous mode*, pumping is co-ordinated with the patient's ECG signals.

The 33 kg drive console is light enough to be pulled on a cart. Alternatively, internal batteries can permit 40 minutes of tether-free ambulation. Recently, an 8.5 kg portable driver became available for clinical use. Because it can be worn on a shoulder strap or pulled on wheels, this driver greatly enhances patients' quality of life. With battery power, unlimited mobility is possible for up to eight hours at a time. Patients can live at home and lead a fairly normal life while awaiting transplantation.

VENTED ELECTRIC LEFT VENTRICULAR ASSIST DEVICE

The major advantages of the vented electric left ventricular assist device are its portability and ease of use. Because the system requires only a small controller and a pair of batteries, it offers almost unlimited freedom. After discharge from hospital, patients use the portable driver (when maximal mobility is desired) or a battery charger and 60 m power cable (when restricted mobility is acceptable). The patient and family members can easily operate and maintain the device. The fixed-rate or automatic pumping modes are selected with a toggle switch. Other operating parameters can be changed with the aid of a personal computer or a display-monitoring unit. If an abnormal operating condition arises, the patient is alerted by visual and audible alarms.

These first-generation left ventricular assist devices, originating in the 1970s, have been very effective in the bridge to transplant setting. In the absence of a donor organ some Novacor patients have survived for four years. This success has set the procedure for the use of mechanical assistance as an alternative to cardiac transplantation in selected patients.

Complications in first-generation implantable left ventricular assist devices

The pusher plate left ventricular assist devices are large, space-occupying foreign bodies with direct connection to the skin via their drive line. Infection is common, particularly in patients who leave hospital, and has serious implications for their permanent use. Reported infection rates range from 20 per cent to 75 per cent, although not all the infections described are device-related (McCarthy et al., 1996). Staphylococcal organisms are responsible for the majority of percutaneous driveline infections (Argenziano et al., 1997). Infection generally leads to re-hospitalization, septic embolism and re-operations, including revision of the percutaneous driveline or removal or exchange of the infected device. These morbidities have a significant negative effect on quality of life and lead to increased cost of left ventricular assist device treatment. Long-term antibiotic treatment and acquired immunosuppression have led to a surprising incidence of fungal infections. Candida infections within the device are commonly complicated by conduit occlusion, endocarditis and stroke (Goldstein et al., 1995). Candida colonization is a late event, after left ventricular assist device implantation, that is seldom experienced after implantation of other devices, such as mechanical prosthetic valves, implantable defibrillators or pacemakers. The Columbia University group studied the prevalence of disseminated candida infection in NYHA Class IV patients who received either the Thermocardiosystem HeartMate left ventricular assist device or medical management (Frazier et al., 1995). Disseminated candida infection developed in 28 per cent of left ventricular assist device recipients by three months after implantation, and in 44 per cent by nine months, compared with only three per cent in control studies. This appeared to be caused by progressive development of defects in T-cell immunity, since left ventricular assist device recipients demonstrated more than 70 per cent lower T-cell proliferative responses after activation of the T-cell receptor complex as compared with control subjects (Ankersmith et al., 1999). T-cells from left ventricular assist device recipients had higher levels of spontaneous apoptosis than control subjects, revealing a progressive defect in cellular immunity and increased risk for opportunistic infection. This worrying iatrogenic cause of activation-induced

T-cell death has similar features to the human immuno-deficiency virus type I (HIV-I).

The major consequences of consumptive coagulopathy in the pusher plate left ventricular assist devices are bleeding, thromboembolism and coagulation factor deficiencies, particularly of platelets and the soluble coagulation proteins. A weak overall thrombotic stimulus, through continuous fibrinolysis, permits long-term support without warfarin. If anticoagulants can be avoided, late bleeding complications disappear. When warfarin is required, bleeding can be expected to occur at approximately the same incidence as for a mechanical prosthetic valve. The incidence of thromboembolism and stroke varies markedly between current blood pumps. The Heart-Mate left ventricular assist device appears to produce the weakest overall thrombotic stimulus with a 2–4 per cent incidence of clinical thromboembolism without anti-coagulation (Slater et al., 1996). The Novacor left ventricular assist device has a higher incidence, and generally requires long-term anticoagulation first with heparin then with both warfarin and platelet inhibitors (Schmid et al., 1998a). In patients taking warfarin, Pennington and colleagues (Pennington et al., 1994) observed thrombus formation in 28 per cent and a stroke rate of 20 per cent. Others have documented up to 47 per cent incidence of cerebral embolization in anticoagulated patients on the Novacor left ventricular assist device. However, when platelet inhibitors are added to the anticoagulation protocol, the incidence of stroke decreases to one per cent without increasing bleeding. Pennington et al. (1994) found a thrombosis rate of 15 per cent and a stroke rate of three per cent in 106 anticoagulated patients on the Thoratec system. These rates are for clinically detected thromboembolism to the brain even though the brain receives only 14 per cent of the cardiac output. In fact, autopsies reveal a much higher incidence of systemic emboli.

Pusher plate left ventricular assist devices also generate asymptomatic microemboli. The origin of these particles is not precisely defined, but they are probably aggregates of platelets, white cells and fibrin produced by contact with non-endothelialized surfaces. By use of an ultrasound probe placed over the middle cerebral artery and random 30-minute monitoring sessions (350 in all) in eight patients over a total of 990 days of Novacor left ventricular assist device support, Schmid et al. (1998b) observed 231 suspected microemboli. The rate of embolization did not decrease with time, and events were recorded in two-thirds of the monitoring sessions. Using similar technology, Moazami observed 19 incidences of embolization during 35 monitoring sessions (54 per cent) in 14 patients with the HeartMate left ventricular assist device (Moazami et al., 1997). The majority of events were concentrated in three patients, one of whom died of a stroke; nine patients (64 per cent) had none. These substantial rates of micro- and macroembolism are related to the extent of blood foreign surface interaction, with major sources of thromboembolism being long inflow cannulae and degeneration of prosthetic heart valves. New blood pumps designed with very small blood foreign surface interaction, no inflow cannula or prosthetic valves already seem to have eliminated this complication.

Numerous other complications can occur with the pusher plate left ventricular assist devices. Porcine xenografts fail rapidly when subject to the substantial pressure differentials within the mechanical environment. Constant movement of these large devices within the abdominal pocket can lead to graft erosion and profound haemorrhage. Mechanical failure has occurred in a small proportion of patients predominantly with the Thermo-cardiosystem left ventricular assist device. Device noise and its effect on the patient and their relatives cannot be ignored.

Second–generation left ventricular assist devices

The design characteristics thought necessary to permit widespread application of a new cardiac assist device are regarded as follows:

- small size and weight, which allows the pump to be implanted within the thoracic cavity in patients of all sizes
- small biocompatible blood contact surface area to decrease activation of the contact system of plasma
- simple, silent blood propulsion system with few movable parts, capable of providing the whole left-sided output (but should be able to be turned down safely to work synergistically with the native left ventricle)
- reliable control and power delivery system mechanism that is easily portable and manageable by patients and their relatives, and with a high probability of freedom from infection.

For many years, powerful miniaturized continuous flow pumps have been available for fluids, such as oil and water, but it was thought that rapid acceleration of blood through a narrow channel would result in haemolysis or thrombosis. The axial flow impeller pumps that have been developed over the last 10 years attempt to address the physiological and biocompatibility requirements of a second-generation left ventricular assist device.

THE JARVIK 2000 HEART

The Texas Heart Institute (USA) and the Oxford Heart Centre (UK) are collaborating to evaluate the Jarvik 2000 Heart (Jarvik Heart Inc., NY) (Frazier et al., 2001b). This compact device is inserted through an apical cuff into the body of the left ventricle. An impervious Dacron graft conveys blood to the descending thoracic aorta. The adult model measures 2.5 cm in diameter and is 5.5 cm in length. The weight is 85 g and the displacement volume 25 mL. The size approximates to that of the inflow cannula of the Thermocardiosystem left ventricular assist device. A smaller paediatric model under development measures 1.4 cm in diameter and is 5 cm in length. One-fifth of the size of the larger model, it weighs only 18 g with a displacement volume of 5 mL. The electromagnetic pump consists of a rotor with impeller blades encased in a titanium shell supported at each end by blood immersed ceramic bearings <1 mm in diameter. The rotor is the sole moving part and all blood contact surfaces are titanium. Coils embedded in the titanium shell generate a magnetic field that powers the impeller across the gap through which the blood flows. Power is delivered from external batteries by a fine percutaneous wire and is regulated by a pulse width or modulated, brushless, DC motor controller that determines pump speed. *In vitro* studies show the adult device to provide up to 10 L/min blood flow at 12,000 rpm. At normal operating speeds of 9000–12,000 rpm, flow rates of between 4 L/min and 6 L/min are obtained at a mean aortic pressure of 80 mmHg and a power requirement of 7–10 watts. The device is silent to the unassisted ear, but can be heard through a stethoscope.

The external batteries and controller are carried on a belt and are of similar size and weight to a portable telephone. The Houston group is pursuing a totally implantable system that uses transcutaneous energy delivery (Westaby *et al.*, 1997; Frazier *et al.*, 2001b). For bridge to transplantation, power is supplied by a simple velour-covered cable, which exits the abdominal wall. In an innovative approach to power delivery for permanent implants, the Oxford Group bring the internal electric wires through the left pleural cavity to the apex of the chest and then subcutaneously across the neck to the skull. Here, a rigidly fixed percutaneous titanium pedestal transmits the fine electric wires through the skin of the scalp (Jarvik *et al.*, 1998). The impetus for this approach is recognition of the reduced risk of infection in long-standing cochlear implant technology, because of a combination of immobility and highly vascular scalp skin.

Both laboratory and clinical experience suggest that the intraventricular position of the Jarvik 2000 Heart has distinct advantages. The device is virtually completely surrounded by the left ventricular cavity, so there is no external pocket with the potential for haematoma formation and infection. Only the left pleural cavity is entered, and the vascular graft delivers blood to the descending aorta. This leaves the anterior mediastinum untouched pending transplantation. Because there is no inflow cannula, the device itself remains well aligned within the ventricle even when the heart is decompressed and changes position. Other devices with an inflow cannula, a tethered

apex and an external pocket have suffered malalignment and severe haemolysis when the shape and position of the ventricle changes.

Retrograde flow to the upper body ending in the coronary arteries is less likely to produce the 'blind pocket' syndrome in the aortic root than when an ascending aortic graft directs blood flow towards the head. A continuously closed aortic valve has the propensity for fusion of the cusps and thrombus formation in the aortic sinuses. For this reason, the speed of the Jarvik impeller is regulated to allow antegrade ejection through the aortic valve as well as offloading through the pump.

Clinical experience began with bridge to transplant patients in Houston (USA), and permanent implants for non-transplant eligible patients in Oxford (UK). To date there have been 37 implants with survival to two years in the first permanent implant patient with dilated cardiomyopathy (Westaby *et al.*, 2000, 2002).

During weaning from cardiopulmonary bypass, inhaled nitric oxide is used to reduce the pulmonary vascular resistance, and milrinone or dobutamine infusion as an inotrope for the right ventricle. Transoesophageal echocardiography is used to assess left ventricular offloading and right ventricular function. After-load is carefully regulated to promote systemic blood flow. The patient soon learns to regulate pump speed according to physiological requirements and to change the batteries. With the pump switched off for five minutes, aortic regurgitation retrogradely through the vascular graft is about 10 per cent of total cardiac output and is usually well tolerated.

Continued medical management is important. Both beta-blockade and ACE inhibitors are used to reduce after-load. Warfarin is given to maintain the INR between 2.5 and 3.5. Hospital discharge is usually possible between three and four weeks post-operatively. All cardiomyopathy patients have improvement in native heart function, and left ventricular contraction transmits pulse to the systemic circulation (Jarvik *et al.*, 1998). The internal components of the system are said to be imperceptible to patients.

Of the 37 patients implanted, 13 (35 per cent) have been successfully transplanted after a mean support time of 274 days and among these patients there has been no infection, thromboembolism or device failure. Fourteen patients (39 per cent) died during support, 12 from multi-organ failure and two from adult respiratory syndrome. These were not device-related events. Two patients died from stroke, and two from myocardial infarction and must be considered device-related deaths.

THE MicroMed DeBakey LEFT VENTRICULAR ASSIST DEVICE

This axial flow pump was developed jointly by the National Aeronautic and Space Administration (NASA) and Baylor College of Medicine after a NASA engineer underwent cardiac transplantation at Baylor College (Noon *et al.*, 2001). The device is a miniaturized electromagnetically actuated titanium axial flow pump, which propels blood from the left ventricle into the ascending aorta. A titanium inflow cannula connects the pump to the apex of the left ventricle and an impervious vascular graft connects the outflow conduit to the ascending aorta. The pump itself is small (30 × 76 mm; 93 g) and may provide flow in excess of 10 L/min. It consists of a flow straightener, inducer or impeller, and diffuser, which are fully enclosed in a titanium flow tube and are driven by a brushless direct current motor stator that is contained in the stator housing. The impeller is the only moving part of the pump. It spins at 7500–12,500 rpm, powered by an extracorporeal controller that is connected with the pump via a percutaneous cable. Two external 12-watt DC batteries provide six to eight hours of operation. A transit time flow meter placed around the outflow conduit provides a continuous readout of pump flow. The measured pump flow is displayed either on the external left ventricular assist device controller or on the clinical data acquisition system, with pump speed, power consumption and current signals from the pump.

The method of implantation is usually via a median sternotomy using normothermic cardiopulmonary bypass via femoral arterial and venous cannulation. The left hemidiaphragm is detached in its anterior portion to provide a pre-peritoneal pocket for the pump. With the heart beating, the sewing ring is attached to the left ventricular apex with interrupted sutures. A coring tool is then used to excise the segment of myocardium within the sewing ring and then the inflow cannula is inserted into the left ventricle, taking care to achieve an optimal position free of any trabecular obstructions. The inflow cannula should point straight to the aortic valve to provide an unimpeded blood inflow during ventricular contraction. The Dacron graft is connected to the ascending aorta and the device de-aired before switching on. The patient is then weaned from cardiopulmonary bypass and the left ventricular assist device pump speed increased. Inhaled nitric oxide is used to reduce pulmonary vascular resistance, although effective left ventricular offloading causes the pulmonary arterial pressure to fall. The aortic valve usually remains closed. Inotropic support may be required for the right ventricle. Heparin is given six to eight hours after the end of the operation when surgical bleeding is under control (15,000 U/day). Oral warfarin therapy is used to achieve an INR of 3.0–3.5. This is usually supplemented with aspirin 100 mg/day.

The DeBakey left ventricular assist device has been used in Europe and the USA for bridge to transplantation with mixed results. The outcome for the first 47 implants was presented by Turina, at the European Society of Cardiothoracic Surgery in September 2000 (Wieselthaler *et al.*, 2001). At that time, 44 pumps had been used in Europe and three at Baylor College. Hospital mortality exceeded 30 per cent. The average assist period was 63 (±2) days. The pump speed was usually set at 9000–10,500 rpm and kept constant. The average pump flow in an awake supine patient was 4.8 (±0.88) L/min. Indices of haemolysis in the Zurich patients showed average plasma-free haemoglobin of 13 mg/dL and an LDH of 1776 U/L. Severe haemolysis in some patients was probably related to an adverse position and partial obstruction of the inflow cannula within the left ventricle.

With fully ambulatory patients, stress exercise has been performed and demonstrates that the pump can practically double the flow rate without adjustment of pump speed. This occurs through increased ventricular filling. Indices of heart failure including renal hepatic and neurological function normalized rapidly in survivors with normal pump function. A positive nitrogen balance was achieved after four to six weeks.

To date about 150 Micromed pumps have been implanted and the device has recently been modified to include heparin coating.

HeartMate II Left Ventricular Assist System

This device originated in 1991 with a research partnership between the Nimbus Company and the University of Pittsburgh. The HeartMate II left ventricular assist device is an axial flow pump with a percutaneous power lead, external power source and system driver (Fig. 14.10) (Griffiths *et al.*, 2001). It is designed for long-term use rather than bridge to transplantation.

The small, 124 mL left ventricular assist device is cradled between the inlet and outlet elbow connectors, and lies parallel to the diaphragm. It may be placed within the muscles of abdominal wall or pre-peritoneally. This reduces the amount of dissection required to create the nesting pocket. The pump has only one moving part, a rotor that spins on inlet and outlet ball-and-cup bearings. The motor is contained in the pump housing and creates a magnetic field that spins the rotor and imports torque to the internal cylindrical magnet. Blood flows from the inlet cannula into a 12 mm titanium blood path, past three neutral airfoil-shaped guided vanes.

The inlet and outlet cannulae are made of woven Dacron and require pre-clotting. The inlet cannula is very flexible, just before its union screwing to the titanium 90° elbow joining the pump. The flexible portion was added to reduce the risk of malalignment of the long intraventricular rigid portion, which had caused septal erosions. The outflow graft is made entirely of woven Dacron and is sheathed by a polypropylene 'bend relief'. The end of the outflow graft is sutured to the side of the ascending aorta and screw-connected to the pump by a rigid elbow.

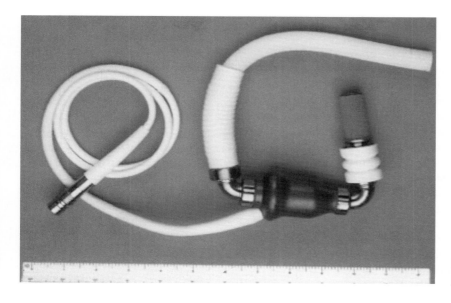

Figure 14.10 *HeartMate II axial flow pump with inlet and outlet conduits.*

The HeartMate II motor is commutated using electro-magnetic field sensing, which maintains pump speed independent of rotor torque. This results in a linear current–pump flow relationship between pump speed and motor current that has been used to formulate an algorithm for prediction of flow. The HeartMate II has a two-speed control mode. The manual speed control can be accessed only by a technical operator and is for use intraoperatively and peri-operatively. Pump rates of 8000–9000 rpm, with pressure differentials of 80–100 mmHg and flows of 3–4 L/min have been most effective. For auto mode a unique control algorithm is drawn from the HQI interrelationship. The rotational speed of the pump is managed to maintain a prescribed pulsatility during the cardiac cycle. This sensorless auto speed con-trol is perhaps the most distinguishing feature of the HeartMate II.

The system was tested in more than 40 calves since 1997 (Thomas *et al.*, 1997). In 2001/2002 human implants were carried out in Israel, Germany and the UK, but have been suspended.

TOTALLY ARTIFICIAL HEART

The concept of total heart replacement with a mechanical device has been around since the late 1960s. The Jarvik 7 (later Cardiowest) total artificial heart was successfully used for bridge to transplantation in about 350 patients between 1980 and 2000.

ABIOCOR IMPLANTABLE REPLACEMENT HEART

The AbioCor implantable replacement heart has been developed by ABIOMED and the University of Louisville (Dowling *et al.*, 2001). The AbioCor implantable replacement heart is an electrohydraulically actuated device capable of providing a cardiac output in excess of 9 L/min. The thoracic unit consists of an energy converter and two blood pumps that approximate the shape and volume of the natural heart. This is implanted in the pericardium vacated by the excised natural heart. All blood-contacting surfaces, including the two blood pumps (stroke volume of 60 mL) and the four tri-leaflet valves (24 mm internal diameter) are fabricated from polyurethane.

The blood pumping membranes are driven hydraul-ically by a high efficiency miniature centrifugal pump driven by a brushless direct current motor. This centrifu-gal pump operates unidirectionally, whereas hydraulic flow reversal is achieved through two valves that alternate the direction of hydraulic fluid flow between the left and right pumping chambers. There is a one-to-one corres-pondence between blood and hydraulic fluid displace-ment. An atrial flow balancing chamber attached to the left inflow conduit is located between the left inflow port and left inflow valve and is used to control the left–right blood flow balance. The pump motor impellers and the valves are essentially the only moving parts of the energy converter. The thoracic unit is connected to an internal controller, battery and secondary transcutaneous energy transfer coil. External components of the AbioCor implantable replace-ment heart consist of the primary transcutaneous energy transfer coil, batteries and portable electronics.

Animal experience with the AbioCor at the University of Louisville began in 1998 (Dowling *et al.*, 2001). Nineteen animals underwent implantation of the device for a pro-posed 30-days' duration. There were six deaths, none related to device malfunction. All animals demonstrated satisfactory haemodynamics, with normal pressure in the aorta, pulmonary artery, left atrium and right atrium. There was no significant haemolysis and all animals had normal end organ function.

Initial clinical experience with the AbioCor implantable replacement heart was presented at the 2002 American Association for Thoracic Surgery meeting by Robert D. Dowling (Dowling *et al.*, 2002). Six male adult patients with severe, irreversible bi-ventricular failure (more than 80 per cent predicted mortality), who were not candidates for transplantation, met the study criteria and had cardiac replacement of the AbioCor implantable replacement heart. At operation the internal transcutaneous energy transfer coil, battery and controller were implanted first. The native ventricles were then excised and the AbioCor thoracic unit was inserted in the orthotopic position and attached to atrial cuffs and outflow conduits via quick connectors. The Abiocor flow was adjusted to 4–8 L/min.

There was one intraoperative death caused by bleeding. There have been several morbid events. All six patients had prolonged intubation. Two had hepatic and renal failure. Other patients suffered recurrent gastrointestinal bleeding, acute cholecystitis requiring laparotomy, respiratory failure that required extracorporeal membrane oxygenization and malignant hyperthermia. There were two late deaths; one due to multiple organ failure (Day 56) and one due to bleeding and multiorgan failure (Day 151). There have been no mechanical failures and no device-related infections. Total days on support with the AbioCor are 369.

Although mechanical biventricular replacement remains a possibility for some patients with very advanced heart failure, few surgeons would envy the quality of life of these patients.

REFERENCES

Ankersmith, J., Tugulea, S., Spanier, T. *et al.* 1999: Activation-induced T-cell death and immune dysfunction after implantation of left ventricular assist device. *Lancet* **354**, 550–5.

Argenziano, M., Cantanese, K.A., Moazami, N. *et al.* 1997: The influence of infection on survival and successful transplantation in patients with left ventricular assist devices. *Journal of Heart and Lung Transplantation* **16**, 822–31.

Baldwin, R.T., Slogoff, S., Noon, G.P. *et al.* 1993: A model to predict survival at time of postcardiotomy intraaortic balloon pump insertion. *Annals of Thoracic Surgery* **55**, 908–13.

Buckley, M.J., Craver, J.M., Gold, H.K. *et al.* 1973: Intraaortic balloon pump assist for cardiogenic shock after cardiopulmonary bypass. *Circulation* **48** (Suppl. III), 90–4.

Busch, T., Sirbu, H., Zenker, D., Dalichau, H. 1997: Vascular complications related to intraaortic balloon counter pulsation: an analysis of ten years' experience. *Thoracic Cardiovascular Surgery* **45**, 55–9.

Christenson, J.T., Buswell, L., Velebit, V. *et al.* 1995: The intraaortic balloon pump for postcardiotomy heart failure. Experience with 169 intraaortic balloon pumps. *Thorac Cardiovasc Surg* **43**, 129–33.

DeBakey, M.E. 1971: Left ventricular bypass pump for cardiac assistance. Clinical experience. *American Journal of Cardiology* **27**, 685–92.

Dietl, C.A., Berkheimer, M.D., Woods, E.L. *et al.* 1996: Efficacy and cost effectiveness of preoperative intra-aortic balloon pump in patients with ejection fraction of 0.25 or less. *Annals of Thoracic Surgery* **62**, 401–8.

Dowling, R.D., Etoch, S.W., Stevens, K.A. *et al.* 2001: Current status of the AbioCor implantable replacement heart. *Annals of Thoracic Surgery* **71**, S147–9.

Dowling, R.D., Gray, L.A., Frazier, O.H. *et al.* 2002: Initital experience with the AbioCor implantable replacement heart. *American Association for Thoracic Surgery* **108**, abstract.

Farrar, D.J. 2000: The Thoratec ventricular assist device: a paracorporeal pump for treating acute and chronic heart failure. *Seminar Thoracic Cardiovascular Surgery* **12**, 243–50.

Frazier, O.H., Rose, E.A., MacMannus, Q. *et al.* 1992: Multicenter clinical evaluation of the Heartmate 1000 IP left ventricular assist device. *Annals of Thoracic Surgery* **53**, 1080–90.

Frazier, O.H., Rose, E.A., McCarthy, P. *et al.* 1995: Improved mortality and rehabilitation of transplant candidates treated with a long term implantable left ventricular assist system. *Annals of Thoracic Surgery* **222**, 327–8.

Frazier, O.H., Rose, E.A., Oz, M.C. *et al.* 2001a: Multicenter clinical evaluation of the Heart Mate vented electric left ventricular assist system in patients awaiting heart transplantation. *Journal of Thoracic and Cardiovascular Surgery* **122**, 1186–95.

Frazier, O.H., Myers, T.J., Jarvik, R.K. *et al.* 2001b: Research and development of an implantable axial flow left ventricular assist device: Jarvik 2000 Heart. *Annals of Thoracic Surgery* **71**, S125–32.

Goldstein, D.J., El-Amir, N.G., Ashton, R.C. *et al.* 1995: Fungal infection in left ventricular assist device recipients: incidence, prophylaxis and treatment. *ASAIO Journal* **41**, 873–5.

Griffith, B.P., Kormos, R.L., Borovetz, H.S. *et al.* 2001: HeartMate II left ventricular assist system: from concept to first clinical use. *Annals of Thoracic Surgery* **71**, S116–20.

Hall, C.W., Liotta, D., Henly, W.S. *et al.* 1964: Development of artificial intrathoracic circulatory pumps. *American Journal of Surgery* **108**, 685–92.

Hoerr, H.R. Jr, Kraemer, M.F., Williams, J.L. *et al.* 1987: *In vitro* comparison of the blood handling by the constrained vortex and twin roller blood pumps. *Journal Extracorporeal Technology* **19**, 316–21.

Jarvik, R.K., Westaby, S., Katsumata, T., Pigott, D., Evans, R.D. 1998: Left ventricular assist device power delivery: a percutaneous approach to avoid infection. *Annals of Thoracic Surgery* 65, 470–3.

Jett, G.K. 1996: ABIOMED BVS 5000: experience and potential advantages. *Annals of Thoracic Surgery* **61**, 301–4.

McCarthy, P.M., Schmitt, S.K., Vargo, R.L., Gordon, S., Keys, T.F., Hobbs, R.E. 1996: Implantable left ventricular assist device infections: implications for permanent use of the device. *Annals of Thoracic Surgery* **61**, 359–65.

Magovern, J.A., Sussman, M.J., Goldstein, A.H., Szydlowski, G.W., Savage, E.B., Westaby, S. 2001: Clinical results with the AB 180 left ventricular assist device. *Annals of Thoracic Surgery* **71**, S121–4.

Moazami, N., Roberts, K., Argenziano, M. *et al.* 1997: Asymptomatic microembolism in patients with long-term ventricular assist support. *ASAIO Journal* **43**, 177–80.

Moulopoulos, S.D., Topaz, O., Kolff, W.J. 1962: Diastolic balloon pumping (with carbon dioxide) in the aorta. A mechanical assistance to the failing circulation. *American Heart Journal* **63**, 669–75.

Noon, G.P., Morley, D.L., Irwin, S. *et al.* 2001: Clinical experience with the MicroMed DeBakey ventricular assist device. *Annals of Thoracic Surgery* **71**, 133–8.

Pagani, F.D., Aaroson, K.D., Swaniker, F., Bartlett, R.H. 2001: The use of extracorporeal life support in adult patient with primary cardiac failure as a bridge to implantable left ventricular assist device. *Annals of Thoracic Surgery* **71**, S77–81.

Pennington, D.G., McBride, L.R., Peigh, P.S., Miller, L.W., Swartz, M.T. 1994: Eight years experience with bridging to cardiac transplantation. *Journal of Thoracic and Cardiovascular Surgery* **107**, 472–80.

Portner, P.M., Jansen, P.G.M., Oyer, P.E., Wheeldon, D.R., Ramasamy, N. 2001: Improved outcome with an implantable left ventricular assist system: multicenter study. *Annals of Thoracic Surgery* **71**, 205–9.

Rose, E.A., Gelijins, A.C., Moskowitz, A.J. *et al.* 2001: Long-term mechanical left ventricular assistance for end stage heart failure. *New England Journal of Medicine* **345**, 1435–43.

Samuel, L.E., Holmes, E.C., Thomas, M.P. *et al.* 2001: Management of acute cardiac failure with mechanical assist: experience with the ABIOMED BVS 5000. *Annals of Thoracic Surgery* **71**, S67–72.

Schmid, C., Wyand, M., Navabi, D.G. *et al.* 1998a: Cerebral and systemic embolization during left ventricular support with the Novacor N100 device. *Annals of Thoracic Surgery* **65**, 1703–10.

Schmid, C., Weyand, M., Hammel, D., Deng, M.C., Nabavi, D., Scheld, H.H. 1998b: The effect of platelet inhibitors on thromboembolism after implantation of a Novacor N100 – preliminary results. *Thoracic Cardiovascular Surgery* **46**, 260–2.

Slater, J.P., Rose, E.A., Levin, H.R. *et al.* 1996: Low thromboembolic risk without anticoagulation using advanced design left ventricular assist devices. *Annals of Thoracic Surgery* **62**, 1321–7.

Spencer, F.C., Eiseman, B., Trinkle, J.K., Rodd, N.P. 1965: Assisted circulation for cardiac failure following intracardiac surgery with cardiorespiratory bypass. *Journal of Thoracic and Cardiovascular Surgery* **49**, 56–73.

Thomas, D.C., Buttler, K.C., Taylor, L.P. *et al.* 1997: Continued development of the Nimbus – University of Pittsburg (UOP) axial flow left ventricular assist system. *ASAIO Journal* **43**, M564–6.

Torchiana, D.F., Hirsch, G., Buckely, M.J. *et al.* 1997: Intra aortic balloon pumping for cardiac support: trends in practice and outcome, 1968 to 1995. *Journal of Thoracic and Cardiovascular Surgery* **27**, 140–2.

Vilacosta, I., Castillo, J.A., Peral, V. *et al.* 1995: Intramural aortic hematoma following intra-aortic balloon counterpulsation. Documentation by transesophageal echocardiography. *European Heart Journal* **16**, 2015–16.

Westaby, S. 1997: Mechanical circulatory support. In: Westaby, S., *Landmarks in Cardiac Surgery*. Oxford: Isis Medical Media, 279–307.

Westaby, S., Katsumata, T., Evans, R., Pigott, D.P., Jarvik, R.K. 1997: The Jarvik 2000 oxford system: increasing the scope of mechanical circulatory support. *Journal of Thoracic and Cardiovascular Surgery* **114**, 467–74.

Westaby, S., Katsumata, T., Howel, R. *et al.* 1998: Jarvik 2000 Heart: potential for bridge to myocyte recovery. *Circulation* **98**, 1568–74.

Westaby, S., Banning, A.P., Jarvik, R.K. *et al.* 2000: First permanent implant of the Jarvik 2000 heart. *Lancet* **356**, 900–3.

Westaby, S., Banning, A., Saito, S. *et al.* 2002: Circulatory support for long term treatment of heart failure. Experience with an intraventricular continuous flow pump. *Circulation* **105**, 2588–91.

Wieselthaler, G.M., Schima, H., Lassnigg, A.M. *et al.* 2001: Lessons learned from the first clinical implants of the DeBakey ventricular assist device axial pump: a single center report. *Annals of Thoracic Surgery* **71**, S139–43.

15

Extracorporeal membrane oxygenation

SCOTT K ALPARD, DAI H CHUNG AND JOSEPH B ZWISCHENBERGER

KEY POINTS

- Extracorporeal membrane oxygenation may be used to treat severe respiratory failure that is unresponsive to optimal conventional management, providing the patient is a newborn infant of more than 34 weeks' gestation, or an adult or child with treatable or reversible pulmonary disease of less than seven days' duration.
- Extracorporeal membrane oxygenation can be used to treat cardiac failure if it is likely that the cardiac condition will recover within a week, although severe left heart failure is probably better managed by left heart bypass.
- The beneficial effects of extracorporeal membrane oxygenation are related to decreasing the barotrauma and oxygen toxicity associated with mechanical ventilation, thus allowing the underlying lung pathology to resolve.
- Extracorporeal membrane oxygenation management requires a thorough understanding of oxygen delivery and consumption, CO_2 elimination and pulmonary pathophysiology.
- Complications of extracorporeal membrane oxygenation are common, and the success of

therapy is dependant on the recognition and management of complications, either mechanical or patient-related.
- Bleeding caused by combination of systemic anticoagulation and consumptive coagulopathy is the most common and one of the most difficult complications encountered.

INTRODUCTION

In the last two decades, two major developments in extracorporeal life support have occurred: technology has progressed to the point where injured lungs can be supported for several days to weeks in newborns, children, and adults; and specific patient populations with potentially reversible respiratory failure have been identified (Bartlett and Gazzaniga, 1978; Bartlett, 1990). Extracorporeal membrane oxygenation should be considered in the patient with severe respiratory failure unresponsive to optimal management if the patient is a newborn infant of greater than 34 weeks' gestational age, or a child or adult with treatable and reversible pulmonary disease of less than seven days' duration. However, extracorporeal membrane oxygenation should not be considered if the patient has extensive pulmonary fibrosis or other incurable disease, necrotizing pneumonitis, or has been treated with a ventilator with high pressure and high oxygen concentration for $\geq$1 week. Extracorporeal membrane oxygenation can also be used for cardiac failure in all age groups, but only if there is reason to believe that the patient will recover from their underlying cardiac condition within a week. Severe left ventricular failure may be better managed by left atrial–aortic extracorporeal life support or a total artificial heart, as a bridge to transplantation. Veno–arterial extracorporeal membrane oxygenation is reserved for patients with right ventricular or bi-ventricular failure, unresponsive to other modes of therapy, in which heart recovery or replacement is anticipated within five to seven days.

Extracorporeal membrane oxygenation is the term used to describe prolonged extracorporeal cardiopulmonary bypass achieved by extrathoracic vascular cannulation. A modified heart–lung machine is used, most often consisting of a distendible venous blood drainage reservoir, a servo-regulated roller pump, a membrane lung to exchange oxygen and carbon dioxide, and a countercurrent heat exchanger to maintain normal body temperature (Fig. 15.1, Fig. 15.2). The patient must be continuously anticoagulated with heparin to prevent thrombosis within the circuit and potential formation of thromboemboli. Various treatment modalities, such as nitric oxide, partial liquid ventilation, and extracorporeal membrane oxygenation, have shown isolated spectacular outcomes, but their application is limited by cost, complications, a labour-intensive nature and lack of validation by prospective randomized trials (Fig. 15.3). Even despite proposed or attempted randomized trials, the outcome may be biased because of a lack of strict blinded treatment arms. 'Protective' mechanical ventilation has become the standard supportive treatment for acute respiratory distress syndrome. Efforts continue to develop alternative ventilator management protocols and gas

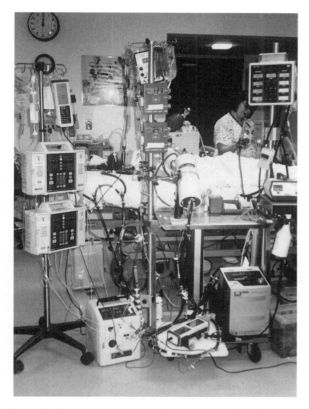

Figure 15.1 *Extracorporeal membrane oxygenation circuit.*

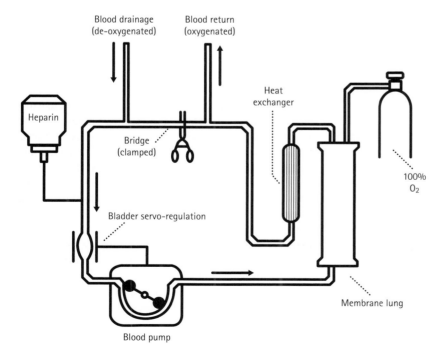

Figure 15.2 *Extracorporeal membrane oxygenation circuit.*

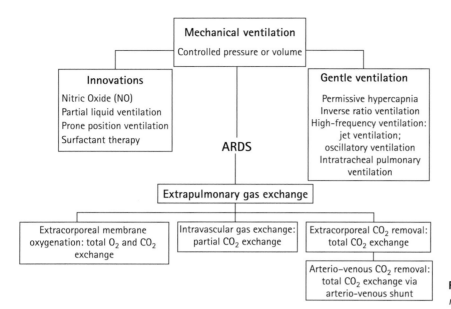

Figure 15.3 *Treatment options for acute respiratory distress syndrome (ARDS).*

exchange techniques to provide gentle ventilation, and to allow the lungs to recover from severe respiratory failure. Alternate treatment modalities for severe respiratory failure, including nitric oxide, high-frequency ventilation, surfactant, new ventilation techniques and management protocols, have affected the potential extracorporeal membrane oxygenation patient population.

HISTORY

John Gibbon Jr (Gibbon, 1937) and others developed the heart–lung machine in the 1930s and opened the era of cardiac surgery in the early 1950s. The use of an artificial pump and lung, however, was limited to one to two hours because of the inadequate oxygenator, which severely altered blood cells and proteins. The first membrane oxygenator was used clinically in 1956 (Clowes *et al.*, 1956). Early oxygenators exposed blood directly to gas mixtures to provide oxygenation and carbon dioxide removal. Cardiopulmonary bypass was provided by inserting cannulae directly into the heart or great vessels. The success of these devices resulted in the development of disposable, single-use, gas-interface oxygenators used for cardiac surgery. A time-dependent pathological response resulting in thrombocytopenia, haemolysis, coagulopathy, generalized oedema and multiorgan failure, appeared to result from direct exposure of blood to gaseous oxygen. The first attempts to separate the blood phase from the gas phase (similar to what occurs in the native lung) used semi-permeable membranes constructed of cellophane or polyethylene. These plastics were found to have low gas permeability and thus required very large surface areas to achieve adequate gas exchange (Clowes *et al.*, 1956;

Kolff and Effler, 1956). The membrane oxygenator became practical for long-term cardiopulmonary bypass with the introduction of silicone rubber as a membrane for gas transfer (Kolobow and Bowman, 1963). In the absence of direct gas exposure to blood, extracorporeal circulation could be carried out for weeks without haemolysis, significant capillary leak or organ deterioration.

Partial systemic anticoagulation was an important development in extracorporeal life support. Heparin anticoagulation sufficient to achieve an infinite clotting time had been used since the development of the first heart–lung machines. Bartlett *et al.* (1972) demonstrated that lower doses of systemic heparin could be safely used by carefully regulating the activated clotting time at the bedside within narrow ranges (activated clotting time 240–280 s). As a result, thrombosis in the extracorporeal circuit could be prevented, with reduced potential bleeding complications.

Concurrent with the development of open-heart surgery, the concept of intensive care units developed during the 1960s and early 1970s. Many patients, with various forms of respiratory failure, required mechanical ventilation to maintain adequate oxygenation and ventilation. Native lungs were frequently exposed to high pressures and volumes to provide adequate gas exchange (Kolobow, 1991). During this period, a new pathophysiological process, known as 'adult respiratory distress syndrome', came to be recognized. Failure of the lungs, either as primary pathology, or part of multiorgan failure, contributed to more than 50 per cent of all intensive care unit deaths. Extracorporeal membrane oxygenation with an 'artificial lung' was proposed as a possible solution to the problem of life-threatening respiratory failure, just as haemodialysis developed to support the failing kidney until organ recovery or renal transplant.

In 1975, investigators studying prolonged extracorporeal support met near Copenhagen to define goals and produce a benchmark publication (Zapol and Qvist, 1976). In addition, in the USA, the National Institutes of Health (NIH) ECMO study, which represented a multicentre, prospective, randomized study of extracorporeal membrane oxygenation in life-threatening respiratory failure, was begun. During this trial, many patients on extracorporeal membrane oxygenation remained on very high pressure mechanical ventilation, which may have contributed to ongoing lung injury. The study was terminated after enrolling 92 patients (less than a third of the projected study size) when survival rates of the extracorporeal membrane oxygenation and control groups were both less than 10 per cent. Death was frequently the result of technical complications, and autopsies uniformly revealed extensive pulmonary fibrosis (an irreversible injury). As a result of these findings, extracorporeal membrane oxygenation therapy for adults essentially stopped in the USA. From this study, several important conclusions were derived:

- application of extracorporeal membrane oxygenation to patients with irreversible pulmonary fibrosis is ineffective
- application to patients with reversible lung injury may work
- technical conduct of extracorporeal membrane oxygenation is critically important, and complications on extracorporeal membrane oxygenation are often life-threatening and must be reduced to a minimum if extracorporeal membrane oxygenation is to be 'successful'
- lungs will not heal when exposed to extremely high ventilator pressures.

Bartlett et al. (1976) persisted with application of the technique to a select population of patients with life-threatening, 'fatal' but reversible respiratory failure: neonates with respiratory failure characterized by pulmonary hypertension with right-to-left shunting. The technique of neonatal extracorporeal membrane oxygenation involved extrathoracic cannulation of the right internal jugular vein and right common carotid artery for partial veno–arterial cardiopulmonary bypass. Partial systemic anticoagulation with heparin was used to prevent circuit thrombosis and to minimize haemorrhagic complications. The most significant physiological concept to come from this experience was that of 'lung rest'. Early in the extracorporeal membrane oxygenation experience it became apparent that even profoundly injured lungs could recover if they were allowed to heal without the persistent application of high-pressure mechanical ventilation.

Although extracorporeal membrane oxygenation had been used since 1975, systematic collection of data did not begin until 1985. Since 1989, participating extracorporeal membrane oxygenation centres have voluntarily registered all patients with the Neonatal, Pediatric, and Adult ECMO Registry of the Extracorporeal Life Support Organization (ELSO). Information concerning patient demographics, pre-extracorporeal membrane oxygenation clinical features, indications, medical and technical complications, and outcomes on extracorporeal membrane oxygenation have been collected and updated continuously as new patients receive extracorporeal membrane oxygenation support. Key events in the history of extracorporeal membrane oxygenation are presented in Table 15.1.

NEONATE APPLICATION

Extracorporeal circulation for respiratory failure was first attempted in newborns in the 1960s (Rashkind et al., 1965). Bartlett et al. (1976) began clinical trials in 1972 and reported the first successful use of extracorporeal membrane oxygenation in newborn respiratory failure in 1976. During the initial experience in neonates, extracorporeal membrane oxygenation had an overall survival rate of 75–95 per cent (Bartlett et al., 1980, 1982a; Kirkpatrick et al., 1983). These results helped to establish the therapeutic effectiveness of extracorporeal membrane oxygenation in infants having met criteria predicting more than 80 per cent mortality. In 1986, Bartlett and colleagues (Bartlett et al., 1986) published their first 100 cases of extracorporeal membrane oxygenation for neonatal respiratory failure with an overall survival rate of 72 per cent. The collaborative UK ECMO trial (1998) concluded that extracorporeal membrane oxygenation support reduces the risk of death without a concomitant rise in severe disability. Comparing extracorporeal membrane oxygenation with conventional treatment, 61 per cent of the extracorporeal membrane oxygenation group ($n = 92$) were alive at one year versus 41 per cent of the conventionally treated group ($n = 93$). Extracorporeal membrane oxygenation has now become the standard treatment for severe respiratory failure in neonates based on successful phase I studies (Bartlett et al., 1976), two prospective randomized studies (Bartlett et al., 1985; O'Rourke et al., 1989) and worldwide application in over 28,163 patients with an overall 67 per cent survival rate (ECLS Organization, 2004).

Neonatal respiratory failure can be severe, progressive and rapidly fatal, yet is initially limited to a single organ. These characteristics make this disease state ideally suited for a treatment such as extracorporeal membrane oxygenation. Although there are a number of causes of respiratory failure in newborns (meconium aspiration, persistent pulmonary hypertension, congenital diaphragmatic hernia, sepsis), they share a common pathophysiological mechanism: pulmonary artery hypertension with persistent foetal circulation. Hypoxia, hypercarbia and acidosis cause pulmonary vasoconstriction that results in right-to-left shunting at the atrial, ductal and intrapulmonary

Table 15.1 *Key events in the history of extracorporeal membrane oxygenation for respiratory failure*

Date	Event
1965–1975	Unsuccessful attempts to support infants with both bubble and membrane oxygenators by Rashkind *et al.* (1965), Dorson *et al.* (1970), White *et al.* (1971) and Pyle *et al.* (1975)
1972	First successful treatment of adult respiratory distress syndrome with extracorporeal membrane oxygenation using partial veno–arterial bypass for three days by Hill *et al.* (1972)
1975	First neonatal extracorporeal membrane oxygenation survivor at University of California, Irvine, CA, by Bartlett *et al.* (1976)
1975–1979	US National Institutes of Health ECMO study of adults with respiratory failure shows 9% survival in both treatment and control groups (Zapol *et al.*, 1979)
1982	45 newborn cases with 23 survivors reported by Bartlett *et al.* (1982a) at University of Michigan, Ann Arbor, MI
1985, 1989	Randomized, prospective studies of extracorporeal membrane oxygenation for neonatal respiratory failure show superiority to conventional therapy (Bartlett *et al.*, 1985; O'Rourke *et al.*, 1989)
1986	Gattinoni *et al.* (1986) report 49% survival using extracorporeal CO_2 removal in adult respiratory distress syndrome
1988	Treatment of selected adult patients resumes in USA (Anderson *et al.*, 1992)
1988	ECMO Registry report: 715 neonatal cases at 18 centres with more than 80% survival (Toomasian *et al.*, 1988)
1989	Extracorporeal Life Support Organization (ECLS) study group formed
1989	Development (Zwischenberger *et al.*, 1985) and first successful treatment of neonates with single cannula double-lumen veno–venous extracorporeal membrane oxygenation (Anderson *et al.*, 1989)
1990	Overall survival rate of 83% in 3500 newborns with respiratory failure (Stolar *et al.*, 1991)
1992	ELSO Registry on extracorporeal membrane oxygenation for cardiac support with 46% in 553 cases after cardiac surgery (Zwischenberger and Cox, 1992)
1993	ELSO Registry on 285 paediatric cases at 52 centres with 49% survival (O'Rourke *et al.*, 1993)
1994	Double-lumen veno–venous extracorporeal membrane oxygenation has higher survival and lower complication rate (Zwischenberger *et al.*, 1994) (Note: probably biased by selection; later reports show veno–venous = veno–arterial)
1997	Percutaneous double-lumen veno–venous extracorporeal membrane oxygenation (Rich *et al.*, 1998b) Bartlett proposes 'best management' algorithm for adult severe respiratory failure (Rich *et al.*, 1998a)
1998	ELSO Registry report (ECLS, 1998): 13,138 neonatal cases with 80% survival; 1517 paediatric cases with 53% survival; 547 adult cases with 47% survival; 2297 paediatric cardiac cases with 42% survival
2004	ELSO Registry report (ECLS, 2004): 20,949 neonatal cases with 73% survival; 5713 paediatric cases with 48% survival; 1501 adult cases with 46% survival

levels. Shunting worsens the hypoxia, which in turn increases pulmonary vascular resistance, creating a downward cycle. Conventional methods for treating pulmonary artery hypertension have included mechanical ventilation with paralysis, induced respiratory alkalosis and inotropes to maintain adequate systemic vascular resistance. Up to five per cent of neonates will not respond to conventional treatment and may benefit from the 'lung rest' with normal gas exchange and circulatory support that can be achieved with extracorporeal membrane oxygenation (ECLS Organization, 1998).

PAEDIATRIC APPLICATION

Concurrent with the adult collaborative study, extracorporeal membrane oxygenation was evaluated in children.

Bartlett *et al.* (1980) as well as Kolobow *et al.* (1975) has reported an extracorporeal membrane oxygenation survival rate of 30 per cent in children and infants beyond the neonatal period with acute respiratory failure, whose predicted survival rate with conventional therapy was thought to be less than 10 per cent. Success was relatively infrequent and led to near abandonment of the technique. However, familiarity with extracorporeal membrane oxygenation use, and success in neonates, fostered confidence with the technique and an understanding of complications sufficient to re-initiate its use in children and adults. Paediatric clinical trials are subject to many of the same problems experienced in adult populations, notably diverse underlying disease processes and initiation of therapy after the onset of irreversible pulmonary changes. Green *et al.* (1996) reported the results from the Pediatric Critical Care Study Group multicentre analysis of extracorporeal membrane oxygenation for paediatric respiratory failure. Extracorporeal membrane oxygenation was associated with a significant reduction in mortality versus conventional or high-frequency ventilation (74 per cent survival with extracorporeal membrane oxygenation versus 53 per cent survival in control subjects). As of January 2004, extracorporeal membrane oxygenation had been used in over 2640 children with respiratory failure achieving an overall survival rate of 56 per cent (ECLS Organization, 2004). Extracorporeal membrane oxygenation has also been used for children needing cardiac support with a survival rate of 43 per cent (ECLS Organization, 2004). As currently applied to children and adults, extracorporeal membrane oxygenation is indicated in acute, potentially lethal respiratory failure that does not respond to conventional therapy when the underlying condition is potentially reversible.

ADULT APPLICATION

Hill et al. (1972) reported the first successful clinical use of extracorporeal membrane oxygenation in adults. A number of small patient series soon followed from the USA and Europe (Gille, 1975; Gille and Bagniewski, 1976). Initially, the overall survival rates were relatively low, but the successes were individually dramatic. In response to this early enthusiasm, the NIH sponsored a multi-institutional, prospective, randomized study of conventional mechanical ventilation versus extracorporeal membrane oxygenation in an adult population (Zapol et al., 1979). In this study of 90 adults with severe respiratory failure, the survival rate with extracorporeal membrane oxygenation was 9.5 per cent compared with 8.3 per cent using conventional treatment. The national experience at that time was only marginally better, with a reported pool survival rate of 15 per cent (Peirce, 1981). Extracorporeal membrane oxygenation did not change the outcome in a group of patients with severe respiratory failure, for whom therapy was begun after several days of mechanical ventilation with high-pressure and oxygen concentration. The cause of death in patients in both the extracorporeal membrane oxygenation and control groups was pulmonary fibrosis or necrotizing pneumonitis. However, extracorporeal membrane oxygenation provided safe and stable life support, and it seemed extracorporeal membrane oxygenation would be effective for high-risk patients if begun early, before pulmonary fibrosis or necrosis occurs. With the development of new equipment, a more clinically homogenous study group, earlier intervention, use of a lower fraction of inspired oxygen (FiO_2), and ventilation techniques that are less traumatic to the lung, survival rates with adult extracorporeal membrane oxygenation patients are improving (Kolobow, 1988a).

The first successful application of veno–arterial extracorporeal membrane oxygenation for status asthmaticus in an adult was reported in 1981 (MacDonnell et al., 1981). Status asthmaticus patients experience severe, reversible, reactive airway disease, with most deaths resulting from complications of mechanical ventilation (Conrad, 1995). Gattinoni and co-workers (Gattinoni et al., 1986), using a modified extracorporeal membrane oxygenation technique (low-frequency positive-pressure ventilation with extracorporeal carbon dioxide removal [LFPPV-ECCO$_2$R]) achieved 49 per cent survival in adult acute respiratory failure. Improvement in survival is also in part contributed to better patient selection, veno–venous perfusion, better regulation of anticoagulation and ventilator management directed towards 'lung rest'. With this information at hand, Morris et al. (1988) initiated a controlled trial of a three-step therapy for adult respiratory distress syndrome. Patients were randomly assigned to a control arm of protocol-controlled continuous positive-pressure ventilation or a new treatment arm of pressure-controlled inverse-ratio ventilation; if the patient failed to improve, LFPPV-ECCO$_2$R was used (Morris et al., 1988). The overall survival rate was 39 per cent in ECCO$_2$R and conventional therapy groups. Bartlett's experience, initially reported by Anderson et al. (1993a), demonstrated 47 per cent survival in adults with acute respiratory failure and 40 per cent survival with extracorporeal membrane oxygenation for cardiac support. Most recently, in a retrospective review of 100 adult patients with acute respiratory failure treated by Bartlett's group, Kolla et al. (1997a) reported a 54 per cent overall survival. Pre-extracorporeal membrane oxygenation variables found to be significant independent predictors of outcome included number of days of mechanical ventilation, P/F ratio and patient age. Rich et al. (1998a) also retrospectively evaluated Bartlett's standardized management protocol for acute respiratory failure utilizing 'lung protective' mechanical ventilation and extracorporeal membrane oxygenation in 141 patients. Forty-one patients showed improvement with the initial protocol of ventilator management (83 per cent survival), whereas 100 patients required extracorporeal membrane oxygenation support because of persistent respiratory failure (54 per cent survival). Overall, lung recovery occurred in 67 per cent of the acute respiratory failure patients, with a 62 per cent survival. Detailed and specific protocols for respiratory management to ensure consistent and uniform respiratory care may yield superior results to historical or non-protocol-controlled management and may decrease the need for extracorporeal membrane oxygenation. As of January 2004, 933 adults with severe respiratory failure treated with extracorporeal membrane oxygenation have been entered in the ELSO Registry with an overall survival rate of 53 per cent (ECLS Organization, 2004).

TRAUMA

Respiratory failure adds significant morbidity, mortality and cost to the care of patients with multiple trauma. High peak airway pressures, FiO_2 values and respiratory rates are often needed to achieve adequate oxygenation and ventilation, all of which are associated with barotrauma and oxygen toxicity (Kolobow et al., 1975). Extracorporeal membrane oxygenation has been safely used in adult and paediatric trauma patients with multiple injuries and severe respiratory failure (Fortenberry et al., 2003). It can provide cardiorespiratory support for trauma patients, allowing reduction of ventilatory support to less-damaging levels (Anderson et al., 1994). The primary risk with extracorporeal life support in trauma patients is severe bleeding because of the need for systemic heparinization. Anderson and colleagues (Anderson et al., 1994) published their experience with 24 moribund paediatric and adult patients who received extracorporeal membrane oxygenation support for respiratory failure from trauma. Fifteen patients (63 per cent) survived and were discharged from the hospital. Early intervention was found to be a key factor in their successful outcome. Michaels et al. (1999) reported that early institution of extracorporeal membrane oxygenation in adult trauma patients leads to improved oxygen delivery, diminished ventilator-induced lung injury and improved survival.

PATHOPHYSIOLOGY

The immediate beneficial effects of extracorporeal membrane oxygenation are related to decreasing the lung injury associated with mechanical ventilation. Gas exchange during extracorporeal membrane oxygenation takes place at ventilator settings that 'rest' the lungs in neonates, paediatric and adult populations. In general, extracorporeal membrane oxygenation provides pulmonary, cardiac or cardiopulmonary support for a period from days to several weeks to allow critical care management or primary therapy to resolve the underlying cause or primary injury.

Neonates

Persistent foetal circulation, also known as 'persistent pulmonary hypertension of the newborn', is a major pathophysiological mechanism of hypoxaemia in full-term infants, and represents a key clinical problem regardless of whether the primary condition is congenital diagphragmatic hernia, meconium aspiration or sepsis (Bartlett, 1986). In this condition, pulmonary arteriolar spasm results in high pulmonary vascular resistance and right-to-left shunting through the patent ductus arteriosus and foramen ovale. During extracorporeal membrane oxygenation, the lungs are exposed only to resting settings of low FiO_2, ventilator rate and airway pressures, allowing reversal of PFC and promoting recovery by minimizing the harmful effects of high-pressure mechanical ventilation.

Paediatric and adult patients

In children and adults, the challenge is to identify the causes of acute respiratory failure that may be reversible within the safe time limits (two to three weeks) of extracorporeal membrane oxygenation. Conditions treated successfully by extracorporeal membrane oxygenation include bacterial and viral pneumonias, fat and thrombotic pulmonary embolism, thoracic or extrathoracic trauma, shock, sepsis and near-drowning. As in neonates, lung rest from the harmful effects of excessive positive-pressure ventilation (high FiO_2, positive end-expiratory pressure, peak inspiratory pressure and minute ventilation) may be the universal benefit of extracorporeal membrane oxygenation in children and adults (Kolobow, 1988b).

Physiology of other organs during extracorporeal membrane oxygenation

Whereas red blood cell destruction occurs after several hours of bypass using a bubble oxygenator, there is minimal red cell loss attributable to the use of modern membrane lungs. Potential sources of red blood cell damage during long-term extracorporeal membrane oxygenation include mechanical injury from the roller pump and negative pressures within the circuit. Packed red blood cell transfusions are needed to maintain haematocrit, replace blood losses from wounds, blood sampling and the small amount of red cell destruction that occurs. Platelets adhere to the prosthetic surface where fibrinogen has been deposited within minutes of exposure. Adenosine diphosphate and serotonin release attracts additional platelets, causing platelet aggregates to form. These 'clumps' of platelets, including some white cells (and red cells in stagnant areas of the circuit), are released into the circulating blood and infused into the patient. They disaggregate and are eventually removed by the reticuloendothelial system (Hicks et al., 1973; Dutton et al., 1974). Platelets are continuously consumed during extracorporeal membrane oxygenation. If platelet consumption is balanced by increased platelet production, platelet counts stabilize; however, platelet transfusion is virtually always required in newborns and children. The effect of extracorporeal membrane oxygenation on white blood cells is less well known. Total and differential white blood cell counts are nearly normal during extracorporeal membrane oxygenation, ranging from 5000 to 15,000/mm^3 (DePalma et al., 1991; Hocker et al., 1991).

Bacterial infections generally resolve with antibiotic treatment, providing evidence that white cell function is adequate.

Fluid and electrolytes are managed as they would be in any critically ill patient. Increased capillary permeability usually occurs to some degree because of the patient's underlying disease as well as complement activation when extracorporeal membrane oxygenation is initiated (Westfall *et al.*, 1991). Both loop diuretics and osmotic agents can be used to treat hypervolaemic conditions. Pre-existing renal failure may be treated by dialysis using a haemofilter placed within the circuit. Although rarely a problem, significant amounts of free water are lost from the membrane lung. Cool and dry sweep gas exits the lung warmed and saturated with vapour. An infant can lose >150 mL/day of free water in this fashion. Serum-ionized calcium levels may fall when extracorporeal membrane oxygenation is started, resulting in cardiac dysfunction if not treated (Meliones *et al.*, 1991). This is significant when veno–venous extracorporeal membrane oxygenation is initiated, and can result in significant hypotension from low cardiac output. It is unclear whether this is caused by the citrate present in banked blood or a dilutional phenomenon.

Neonates are often kept on total parenteral nutrition, but enteral nutrition while on extracorporeal membrane oxygenation is gaining popularity. Hyperbilirubinaemia is common and may be severe. However, it typically resolves without sequelae and is probably related to haemolysis as well as cholestasis caused by lack of enteral nutrition on extracorporeal membrane oxygenation. Biliary calculi have been reported in two out of 121 patients in post-extracorporeal membrane oxygenation follow-up (Almond *et al.*, 1992). The haemolysis, total parenteral nutrition, diuretics and prolonged fasting associated with extracorporeal membrane oxygenation may predispose neonates to form early biliary stones. Although gastro-intestinal function may be normal, the majority of centres are reluctant to use enteral nutrition during extracorporeal membrane oxygenation. However, with the recent emphasis on the beneficial effects of enteral nutrition on the integrity of the intestinal gut barrier, this practice is changing. Piena *et al.* (1998) prospectively evaluated changes in small intestinal integrity in neonatal extracorporeal membrane oxygenation patients. Although intestinal integrity is compromised in neonates on extracorporeal membrane oxygenation, introducing enteral nutrition did not result in further deterioration. Pettignano *et al.* (1998) reported a higher percentage of extracorporeal membrane oxygenation patient survival in the enterally fed group compared with the total parenteral nutrition group (100 per cent versus 79 per cent). They concluded that enteral nutrition can be safely administered for nutritional support in paediatric patients undergoing veno–arterial or veno–venous extracorporeal membrane oxygenation.

Central nervous system function appears to be unaffected by extracorporeal membrane oxygenation. Infants may be awake and alert, and adults may be communicative during extracorporeal membrane oxygenation. The effect of microembolization from the extracorporeal circuit, although potentially harmful, seems to be of less practical importance. Mental function usually remains normal during prolonged extracorporeal membrane oxygenation. Tissue infarcts are rarely seen at autopsy, suggesting that microembolization during extracorporeal membrane oxygenation is not clinically significant. Veno–venous extracorporeal membrane oxygenation has a theoretical advantage over veno–arterial extracorporeal membrane oxygenation because of the concern of systemic effects of arterial embolization. Neurological and audiological sequelae have been reported in 10–20 per cent of veno–arterial extracorporeal membrane oxygenation survivors (Towne *et al.*, 1985; Glass *et al.*, 1989; Glass, 1993; Gleason, 1993; Graziani *et al.*, 1994; Wildin *et al.*, 1994; Glass *et al.*, 1995; Vaucher *et al.*, 1996; Graziani *et al.*, 1997a,b). Another 20–30 per cent with no evidence of severe handicap at one to three years of age have cognitive and visual–motor deficiencies at early school age, increasing the risk for future learning disabilities (Glass *et al.*, 1995). Graziani *et al.* (1997a) followed 271 infants treated with extracorporeal membrane oxygenation between 1985 and 1996. They concluded:

- hypotension before or during extracorporeal membrane oxygenation and the need for cardiopulmonary resuscitation before extracorporeal membrane oxygenation contribute to the pathogenesis of cerebral palsy
- profound hypocarbia before extracorporeal membrane oxygenation and delayed extracorporeal membrane oxygenation intervention are associated with a significant increased risk of hearing loss
- the type and severity of neurological and cognitive sequelae depends, in part, on the primary cause of the neonatal cardiorespiratory failure.

Physiology of the native lung during extracorporeal membrane oxygenation

During veno–arterial extracorporeal membrane oxygenation, left ventricular outflow falls proportionate to the extracorporeal blood flow, resulting in a decreased pulse pressure. Very high left atrial pressures will result if there is no left ventricular ejection, resulting in high pulmonary pressures and pulmonary oedema. During veno–arterial extracorporeal membrane oxygenation, a significant portion of the pulmonary blood flow is diverted through the extracorporeal circuit. There appear to be no major deleterious effects of reduced pulmonary blood flow unless normal ventilation is maintained. With normal ventilation of the native lungs during extracorporeal membrane oxygenation, pulmonary capillary pH can be as high as 8.0. Haemolysis and pulmonary haemorrhage can result even without marked systemic hypocarbia (Kolobow *et al.*, 1981; Foster and Kolobow, 1987). When extracorporeal membrane oxygenation is initiated, ventilatory settings are rapidly decreased to prevent further barotrauma from overdistention, as well as to prevent local tissue alkalosis. A low respiratory rate and normal inspiratory pressure or continuous positive end-expiratory pressure can be used during extracorporeal membrane oxygenation. A few sustained inflations above the alveolar opening pressure are provided periodically to prevent total lung collapse.

During veno–venous extracorporeal membrane oxygenation right ventricular output is normal and probably higher than before extracorporeal membrane oxygenation, since cardiac output increases after severe hypoxia is corrected. This exposes the pulmonary arterioles to blood with a relatively high pO_2, which may be beneficial in the treatment of pulmonary hypertension.

Oxygen delivery

Extracorporeal membrane oxygenation management requires a thorough understanding of oxygen delivery and oxygen consumption physiology. Oxygen consumption (VO_2) reflects the aerobic metabolic activity of tissues. Newborns use 5–8 mL/kg per minute of oxygen, children use 4–6 mL/kg per minute and adults use 3–5 mL/kg per minute. Oxygen consumption is decreased by hypothermia, sedation and complete paralysis. It is increased by exercise, shivering, catecholamines, hyperthermia and infection. Under normal steady-state conditions, the amount of oxygen taken up across the lungs into the pulmonary circulation equals the amount of oxygen consumed by the tissues. This concept, the Fick principle, is summarized by the following equation:

$$VO_2 = CO (CaO_2 - CVO_2)$$

where CaO_2 = arterial oxygen content and CVO_2 = mixed venous oxygen content. Oxygen consumption, under most circumstances, is independent of oxygen delivery. The amount of oxygen delivered to the tissues (DO_2) is the product of the cardiac output and CaO_2. Normally, DO_2 exceeds VO_2 by a factor of four to one. Saturated arterial blood corresponds to a mixed venous oxygen saturation of 75 per cent. When DO_2 is significantly reduced, VO_2 becomes supply-limited and falls, resulting in acidosis, hypotension, and a rise in blood lactate (that is, shock) (Bartlett, 1995).

During extracorporeal membrane oxygenation, DO_2 is controlled primarily by flow through the extracorporeal circuit as well as blood oxygenation in the membrane

lung and oxygen uptake through the native heart. Extracorporeal flow is set at the minimum amount that allows a 'normal' SVO_2, whereas pump flow is increased to treat falling PaO_2 and SVO_2. Pump flow may be decreased as PaO_2 rises when SVO_2 is normal, indicating lung recovery. Air–oxygen sweep gas mixtures can be used to reduce the pO_2 of the perfusate if significant arterial hyperoxia is present. Extracorporeal membrane oxygenation is most often applied to treat low DO_2 in the face of arterial hypoxia (hypoxic shock). During extracorporeal membrane oxygenation, systemic DO_2 is a combination of DO_2 from the extracorporeal circuit and across the native lung. This is most easily understood during veno–arterial extracorporeal membrane oxygenation. Total DO_2 is expressed as:

$$total\ DO_2 = (extracorporeal\ flow)\ (CaO_2\ post\text{-}membrane\ lung) + (CO)\ (CaO_2\ left\ ventricle)$$

This concept must be appreciated in order to interpret arterial blood gases sampled from the patient on veno–arterial extracorporeal membrane oxygenation.

Blood oxygenation in the membrane lung is a function of thickness of the blood film, membrane material and thickness, FiO_2, residence time of red cells in the gas exchange area, haemoglobin concentration, and the inlet saturation. All of these factors are included in a single descriptor of membrane lung function called 'rated flow' (Galletti *et al.*, 1972). Rated flow is the amount of normal venous blood that can be raised from 75 per cent to 95 per cent oxyhaemoglobin saturation in a given period. We use this information to plan which membrane lung to use, and to evaluate membrane lung performances during perfusion.

As long as extracorporeal blood flow is less than the rated flow of the membrane lung, the blood leaving the lung will be fully saturated. The amount of systemic DO_2 via the extracorporeal circuit is controlled by blood flow and the oxygen uptake capacity. If the haemoglobin concentration is low, or the venous blood saturation is high, the amount of oxygen that can be bound in the membrane lung is decreased. We can compensate for decreased oxygen binding capacity by increasing blood flow. Conversely, we can achieve DO_2 at low blood flow by increasing oxygen binding capacity. The resulting systemic pO_2 and systemic DO_2 are a function of DO_2 through the extracorporeal circuit and through the native heart and lung. In planning the size of the circuit and extracorporeal flow rate, it is assumed that there will be no gas exchange across the native lung. With this assumption, in veno–venous bypass, the PaO_2 and saturation will be identical to the values in the mixed right atrial blood. Because of the nature of veno–venous bypass, this saturation will not be higher than 95 per cent, and typically will be closer to 80 per cent saturation with a pO_2 of approximately 40 torr. Systemic oxygen delivery is perfectly adequate as long as there is a compensatory increase in cardiac output. A rise in systemic arterial pO_2 at constant extracorporeal flow may reflect very different physiological conditions. Improving lung function will result in greater oxygen saturation of left ventricular blood and correspondingly improving pO_2 in systemic arterial blood. However, decreased native lung blood flow will likewise result in a rising pO_2 as more of the systemic arterial blood is being contributed by the extracorporeal circuit. These patterns might be seen under conditions of pneumothorax, haemothorax or peri-cardial tamponade.

The best monitor of the adequacy of tissue oxygenation is mixed venous oxygen saturation. During veno–venous bypass, PaO_2 will be identical to the mixed right atrial pO_2, assuming there is no contribution from native lung gas exchange. Because some unsaturated blood is not captured by the venous drainage catheter, right atrial saturation is rarely more than 80–90 per cent. The resulting PaO_2 in arterial blood may be as low as 40 mmHg. The patient will therefore be relatively hypoxic and even cyanotic, but if the cardiac output is normal and haemoglobin level is adequate, oxygen delivery will be adequate and recovery can occur. Recovery is indicated by an increase in arterial pO_2 as the native lung contributes oxygen to pulmonary blood flow.

In veno–arterial bypass, the perfusate blood is typically 100 per cent saturated with a pO_2 of 500 torr. When the lung is not functioning, the left ventricular blood is identical to right atrial blood, typically with a saturation of 75 per cent and a pO_2 of 35 mmHg. Thus, during veno–arterial bypass, an increase in systemic pO_2 may signify improving lung function at constant flows, decreasing native cardiac output at constant extracorporeal flow, or increasing extracorporeal flow at constant native output. An interesting physiological property of the lung has been recognized with application of extracorporeal membrane oxygenation. Even the most severely injured lungs are capable of oxygen transfer if they are not required to provide any ventilatory function. This is the rationale behind $ECCO_2R$ and 'apnoeic oxygenation' as developed by Gattinoni et al. (1986). The lungs are inflated to moderate pressures (15–20 cmH$_2$O) and oxygen concentration is reduced, whereas CO_2 is removed by low-flow partial veno–venous bypass.

Carbon dioxide removal

Metabolic production of CO_2 approximates VO_2 (respiratory quotient = 1). Excretion of CO_2 across normal native lungs is exquisitely sensitive to alveolar ventilation with the rate and depth of breathing controlled to maintain $PaCO_2 \geqslant 40$ mmHg. The amount of CO_2 eliminated in extracorporeal circulation is a function of membrane lung geometry, material, surface area, blood pCO_2, blood flow and membrane lung ventilating gas flow. Usually the ventilating gas contains no CO_2 so the gradient for CO_2 transfer is the difference between the blood pCO_2 and zero (when gas flow rate is high). As pCO_2 drops during the passage of blood through the membrane lung, the gradient decreases and CO_2 excretion is less at the blood outlet than at the inlet end of the device. Consequently, the amount of CO_2 transfer is relatively independent of blood flow and only moderately dependent on inlet pCO_2, with the major determinant of CO_2 elimination being total surface area and flow rate of sweep gas. Characteristics of removal of CO_2 for a typical membrane lung at different levels of pCO_2 are shown over a range of blood flows. The capacity for CO_2 removal is considerably greater than the capacity for oxygen uptake at the rated flow. For any silicone rubber or microporous membrane oxygenator, CO_2 clearance will always be more efficient than oxygenation when the oxygenator is well ventilated and functioning properly.

The extracorporeal circuit is generally designed to supply total oxygen requirements. For this reason, the membrane lung will be capable of removing an excess of CO_2. Carbon dioxide transfer can be selectively increased by increasing sweep flow and the total surface area of the membrane lung in the extracorporeal circuit. Assuming there is no gas exchange across the native lung, the arterial pCO_2 will be the same as venous pCO_2 in veno–venous bypass; it will be a function of mixing perfusate and cardiac output blood in veno–arterial bypass. However, because of the efficiency of $ECCO_2R$, the systemic pCO_2 can be 'set' at any level by matching the membrane lung surface area and gas flow with the systemic production of CO_2.

During veno–venous bypass, oxygenated venous blood is returned to the venous circulation and mixed with systemic venous blood, raising its oxygen content. The final oxygen content depends on native lung function, oxygen saturation of blood from the extracorporeal membrane oxygenation circuit, and the amount of recirculation through the circuit. During veno–venous extracorporeal membrane oxygenation, if the native lung is not functioning, the PaO_2 can be no higher than the right atrial O_2, typically 85–90 per cent saturated (PaO_2 40–50 mmHg) and can be lower if there is more than 50 per cent recirculation through the extracorporeal membrane oxygenation circuit. Some of the mixed blood returns (recirculates) to the extracorporeal circuit while some enters the right ventricle and traverses the pulmonary vasculature and is shunted to the left heart and finally to the systemic arterial circulation. Veno–venous extracorporeal membrane oxygenation is limited by the amount of systemic venous return in the extracorporeal circuit. If systemic venous return is insufficient, adequate support may not be achieved. Veno–venous extracorporeal membrane oxygenation depends solely upon cardiac output to provide flow and is most useful in pure respiratory failure or when respiratory failure accompanies cardiac failure solely attributable to hypoxia or excessive intrathoracic pressures generated by mechanical ventilation.

PATIENT SELECTION

Patients selected for extracorporeal membrane oxygenation must have a potentially reversible underlying pathological process. Indications for extracorporeal membrane oxygenation support include acute reversible respiratory or cardiac failure unresponsive to optimal ventilator and pharmacological management, but from which recovery can be expected within a reasonable period (several days to three weeks) of extracorporeal support. The requirement for systemic heparinization limits the population for whom extracorporeal membrane oxygenation is appropriate to patients without bleeding complications, thereby relatively excluding premature infants (younger than 35 weeks' gestation) (Cilley et al., 1986) and patients with active bleeding. Other contraindications include those conditions incompatible with normal life after lung recovery (such as major brain injury), congenital or acquired immunodeficiency state, and mechanical ventilation for more than 7–10 days (as an indication of irreversible ventilator-induced lung injury).

Neonates

Extracorporeal membrane oxygenation has been applied to infants with a mortality risk of 80 per cent or greater by retrospective analysis of local patient populations. Included are neonates who, despite optimum medical management, demonstrated acute deterioration ($PaO_2 < 40$ mmHg or pH < 7.15 for two hours), failure to improve ($PaO_2 < 55$ mmHg and hypotension requiring inotropic support), uncontrolled air leak, pneumomediastinum or deterioration after congenital diaphragmatic hernia repair. Excessive alveolar-to-arterial oxygen gradients $P(A\text{-}a)O_2$ have been proposed as a qualification for extracorporeal membrane oxygenation. In a retrospective review by Krummel and associates (Krummel et al., 1984) a $P(A\text{-}a)O_2 > 620$ mmHg for 12 consecutive hours correlated with more than 90 per cent mortality. Many programmes currently use the oxygenation index as a criterion to determine the need to utilize extracorporeal membrane oxygenation support: mean airway pressure $\times$ FiO$_2$ $\times$ 100 divided by post-ductal PaO_2. Based on data generated before extracorporeal membrane oxygenation availability, after optimal conventional therapy, an oxygenation index consistently over 25 implies a 50 per cent mortality rate, and over 40 defines an 80 per cent mortality group.

Contraindications to neonatal extracorporeal membrane oxygenation include any evidence of intracerebral haemorrhage, other brain damage, multiple congenital anomalies and irreversible lung damage. In congenital diaphragmatic hernia, persistent fetal circulation (PFC) cannot be distinguished from pulmonary hypoplasia; therefore, in most centres all patients with diaphragmatic hernias are treated who otherwise meet local extracorporeal membrane oxygenation criteria (Zwischenberger and Bartlett, 1990). In some centres, a PaO_2 value >70 mmHg or a $PaCO_2 < 80$ mmHg is required at some time in the neonate's life as evidence of sufficient functional pulmonary parenchyma to avoid infants with fatal pulmonary hypoplasia. Potential extracorporeal membrane oxygenation candidates are evaluated with cranial ultrasound to rule out intraventricular haemorrhage and cardiac ultrasound to rule out congenital cardiac anomalies. Entry criteria should be evaluated at each hospital before extracorporeal membrane oxygenation therapy is begun because of regional differences in patient populations and treatment protocols.

Children and adults

Despite advances in ventilatory support, antibiotic therapy, and critical care, mortality from acute respiratory distress syndrome remains 50–80 per cent (Dal Nogare, 1989; Cunningham, 1991; Cox et al., 1992). The indication for extracorporeal membrane oxygenation in paediatric and adult patients is severe respiratory failure with a predicted mortality rate of $\geqslant$80 per cent. However, current techniques of ventilatory management are often associated with high inspiratory airway pressures (barotrauma), overdistending normal lung regions (volutrauma) and toxic levels of inspired oxygen, leading to exacerbated lung injury manifested by progressive deterioration in total lung compliance, functional residual capacity and arterial blood gases. High positive airway pressure also contributes to cardiovascular instability. Disappointing results with conventional management of acute respiratory distress syndrome patients have resulted in an increased urgency for developing alternative strategies that provide sufficient oxygenation, CO$_2$ removal and 'lung rest'. It has been recognized that the primary goal of respiratory support focuses on CO$_2$ removal and O$_2$ exchange with avoidance of high tidal volumes and airway pressures (Morris et al., 1994). Extracorporeal membrane oxygenation allows this goal to be maintained even when the lung is incapable of sufficient gas exchange.

Reversible acute respiratory failure in adults is difficult to define; therefore, adult criteria for extracorporeal membrane oxygenation are controversial (Zapol et al., 1979; Bone, 1986; Kolobow, 1988a). Selection criteria to identify patients with 90 per cent mortality risk are listed in Table 15.2. Most investigators use entry criteria from the NIH ECMO Study (Zapol et al., 1979). Many use a

P/F ratio < 100 and particular care must be taken to avoid therapy in patients with established pulmonary fibrosis. Lung biopsy may be necessary to determine the diagnosis and to measure the extent of irreversible lung damage. Patients with the potential for bleeding or those with major destruction of lung tissue are also not candidates for extracorporeal membrane oxygenation.

Table 15.2 *Extracorporeal circulation membrane oxygenation criteria for adults with ⩾90% mortality risk*

Indications	Contraindications
Failure of optimal conventional therapy	Age >60 years
Transpulmonary shunt >30%	Mechanical ventilation >5–7 days
Static lung compliance <0.5 mL/cmH$_2$O per kg	Incurable condition
Diffuse abnormal chest X-ray (four quadrants)	Severe bleeding potential
Cardiac failure or cardiac arrest	

TECHNIQUES AND MANAGEMENT

Extracorporeal membrane oxygenation has evolved into several formats, each with advantages and disadvantages depending upon the physiology to be corrected and the expertise of the extracorporeal membrane oxygenation team. A comparison of different extracorporeal treatment modalities is shown in Table 15.3.

Neonates

After the medical decision to initiate extracorporeal membrane oxygenation support is made, the informed consent for procedure is obtained while the circuit is prepared and primed with blood. Because the blood volume in the circuit is as much as twice the blood volume of the neonate, the appropriate haematocrit, pH and electrolyte concentration must be adjusted before cardiopulmonary bypass is instituted. Patients are cannulated with veno–arterial access if cardiac support is required for acute haemodynamic compromise (cardiac arrest) or for

Table 15.3 *Comparison of extracorporeal membrane oxygenation (ECMO), cardiopulmonary bypass (CPB), low-flow positive pressure ventilation with extracorporeal carbon dioxide removal (LFPPV–ECCO$_2$R), arterio–venous carbon dioxide removal (AVCO$_2$R) and artificial lung*

	ECMO	CPB	ECCO$_2$R	AVCO$_2$R	Artificial lung
Setting	Respiratory and/or cardiac failure	Cardiac surgery	Respiratory failure	Respiratory failure (investigational)	Respiratory failure (experimental)
Location	Extrathoracic	Intrathoracic	Extrathoracic	Extrathoracic	Extrathoracic
Type of support	VA (cardiac) VV (respiratory)	VA (total bypass)	VV (respiratory) (CO$_2$)	AV (respiratory) (CO$_2$)	PA–PA or PA–LA
Cannulation	VA: neck VV: neck and groin 1 cannula (VVDL)	Direct cardiac 2 cannulae (surgical)	Neck and groin 2 cannulae (surgical or percutaneous) 1 cannula (VVDL)	Groin 2 cannulae (percutaneous)	Transthoracic to major vessels
Blood flow	High (70–80% CO)	Total (100% CO)	Medium (30% CO)	Low (10–15% CO)	Total (100%)
Ventilatory support	Pressure-controlled ±high PEEP 10–12 breaths/min	None (anaesthesia)	High PEEP 2–4 breaths/min High FiO$_2$	Volume-controlled (algorithm-driven)	None necessary
Blood reservoir	Small (50 cc)	Yes (>1 L)	Small (50 cc)	No	No
Arterial filter	No	Yes	No	No	No
Blood pump	Roller or centrifugal	Roller or centrifugal	Roller or centrifugal	None	None
Heparinization	ACT 200–260	ACT > 400	ACT 200–260	ACT 200–260	ACT 200–260
Average length of extracorporeal support	Days to weeks	Hours	Days to weeks	Days to weeks	Days
Complications	Bleeding Organ failure	Intraoperative	Bleeding	Bleeding	Bleeding
Causes of death	Support terminated: PAP > 75% systemic; irreversible lung disease; cardiac dysrhythmias	Intraoperative Air embolism	Multiorgan failure Septic shock Haemorrhagic	Respiratory failure	Right heart failure

VA = veno–arterial; VV = veno–venous; AV = arterio–venous; PA = pulmonary artery; LA = left atrium; DL = direct line; ACT = activated clotting time.

transport on extracorporeal membrane oxygenation (Fig. 15.4). Veno–venous access is used in most cases without haemodynamic compromise and is the method of choice for patients with respiratory failure only (Fig. 15.5).

Dissection and cannulation are performed under local anaesthesia in the intensive care unit. The patient is heavily sedated with a combination of narcotics and sedatives, and is also paralysed for the procedure. An oblique incision in

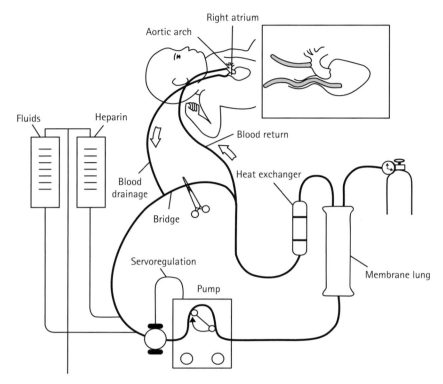

Figure 15.4 *Veno–arterial extracorporeal membrane oxygenation circuit.*

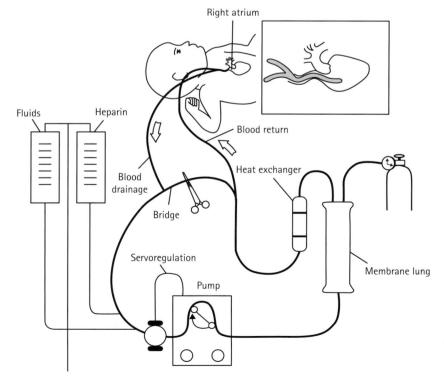

Figure 15.5 *Veno–venous extracorporeal membrane oxygenation circuit using the double-lumen catheter. Inset depicts cannulation of the right atrium by way of the right internal jugular vein. Side holes on the return lumen of the catheter direct oxygenated blood towards the tricuspid valve.*

the right side of the neck anterior to the sternocleidomastoid muscle exposes the internal jugular vein and common carotid artery. After dissection of vessels, the infant is given a 100-U/kg heparin bolus as a loading dose. The vessels are ligated distally, and cannulae are inserted in a proximal direction from the ligation site. The venous cannula is threaded through the right internal jugular vein into the right atrium and the arterial cannula is inserted into the common carotid artery so that its tip rests at the entrance to the aortic arch (Fig. 15.6). The right common carotid artery in a neonate can be successfully ligated with a relatively low complication rate, presumably because of abundant collateral flow (Campbell *et al.*, 1988). The largest catheters (8–14 F) that fit 'comfortably' inside the artery and vein are used. Catheter positions are confirmed by chest radiograph or ultrasonography.

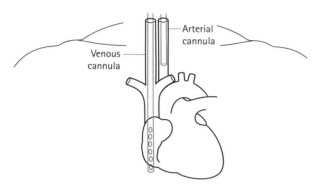

Figure 15.6 *The arterial catheter is positioned to reinfuse blood via the ascending aorta. The venous catheter aspirates blood from the atrium beneath the superior cavoatrial junction.*

Positioning and flow resistance of the venous drainage catheter determine the maximum blood flow; the catheter should be capable of delivering total cardiac support of 120 mL/kg per minute.

After cannulation is accomplished and bypass initiated, blood drains by gravity through the venous catheter to a servoregulated roller pump. The pump then perfuses the blood through a membrane lung (Avecor Cardiovascular, Minneapolis, MN) matched to the size of the patient (0.6, 0.8, 2.5, 3.5 or 4.5 m^2). Gas exchange occurs in the membrane lung as oxygen is added to the blood while water vapour and CO_2 are removed. Because CO_2 removal is much more efficient than oxygen transfer, exogenous CO_2 often must be added to the oxygen inflow to avoid hypocapnic alkalosis. The blood then passes through a heat exchanger and returns to the patient. Blood flow is gradually increased during the initial 15–20 minutes of bypass until approximately 80 per cent of the infant's cardiac output flows through the circuit (Fig. 15.7). Oxygenated blood from the circuit mixes in the aortic arch with poorly oxygenated blood from the left ventricle and ductus arteriosus to yield a mixed oxygen content adequate for the infant's metabolic requirements (Cilley *et al.*, 1987).

Once extracorporeal membrane oxygenation is established and appropriate pH, PaO_2 and $PaCO_2$ values are obtained, ventilator settings are reduced to minimize barotrauma and oxygen toxicity (peak inspiratory pressure, 15–20 cmH$_2$O; rate, 10 breaths/min; FiO$_2$, 0.3). The optimum positive end-expiratory pressure level is uncertain, but many programmes use high positive end-expiratory pressure (12–15 cmH$_2$O) with mean airway pressures of 13–16 cmH$_2$O, based on experimental studies in a neonatal lamb model of meconium aspiration (Kolobow

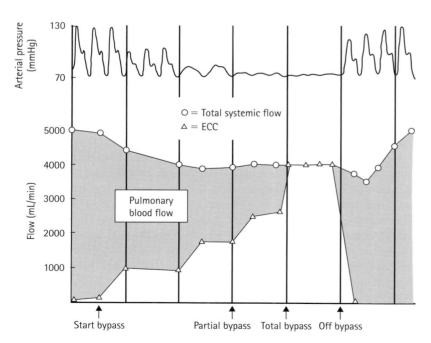

Figure 15.7 *Haemodynamic changes during veno–arterial bypass. Total flow and arterial blood pressure are shown during various levels of bypass. As blood is diverted from the right atrium to the extracorporeal circuit, pulmonary blood flow (and left ventricular flow) decreases to where there is no flow during total bypass. Pulse amplitude decreases, reaching nearly a non-pulsatile state during total bypass.*

et al., 1983) that showed decreased time of extracorporeal membrane oxygenation without increased barotrauma. A prospective, randomized study in neonates has also concluded that higher positive end-expiratory pressure safely prevents deterioration of pulmonary function during extracorporeal membrane oxygenation and results in more rapid lung recovery (Keszler et al., 1992).

Extracorporeal membrane oxygenation flow is maintained to achieve full respiratory support until lung improvement occurs. Pulmonary function is assessed by monitoring the saturation of venous drainage blood, pulmonary artery blood and arterial blood with a pulse oximeter. The usual flow for full support is 80–120 mL/kg per minute (average 300–400 mL/kg per minute) and is set to maintain PaO_2 between 70 mmHg and 90 mmHg. Adequate support is defined as the level of extracorporeal flow that results in normal arterial and mixed venous oxygenation, mean arterial pressure and organ function. During extracorporeal membrane oxygenation, chest physiotherapy, including suctioning through the endotracheal tube, is continued. Paralysing agents and vasoactive drugs are discontinued and patients are maintained alert and awake. Standard treatment for severe lung dysfunction is continued during extracorporeal membrane oxygenation, including bronchoscopy when necessary, and diuretics to eliminate excess volume. Although it is not necessary, monitoring native lung as well as membrane oxygenator VO_2 and VCO_2 can help to determine the total VO_2 (calculate the respiratory quotient) and assist in calculating indirect calorimetry for purposes of nutritional planning (Bartlett et al., 1982b). Identifying the fact that less than 25 per cent of total VO_2 is achieved through the native lung after the first week on support may represent dismal prognosis of lung recovery.

Anticoagulation must be maintained during the course of extracorporeal membrane oxygenation support. Heparin is administered into the circuit with a loading dose (100 U/kg) followed by a continuous infusion of approximately 30 U/kg per hour (20–70 U/kg per hour). Whole blood activated clotting time is measured each hour and maintained at two to three times normal values (220–260 s). Platelets, which may be destroyed by the membrane oxygenator, are administered when thrombocytopenia of $\geq$ 100,000–150,000 is observed. Haematocrit is maintained between 35 per cent and 45 per cent with packed red blood cell transfusions. Maintenance intravenous fluids, in the form of total parenteral nutrition, are delivered directly into the bypass circuit. Prophylactic antibiotics (ampicillin and gentamicin) are administered until extracorporeal membrane oxygenation cannulae are removed. A chest radiograph is obtained daily to monitor cannula positions as well as progress of lung recovery. Daily head ultrasound is recommended for the first week, and then on as-needed basis, depending on patients' clinical conditions.

When the lungs begin to recover, extracorporeal blood flow is reduced in a stepwise fashion until 10–20 per cent of the infant's cardiac output (usually 40–80 mL/min) is diverted through the circuit. Arterial pO_2 is maintained between 70 mmHg and 90 mmHg. The patient's ventilatory support is increased to moderate settings and then 'trial-off' is performed by clamping arterial and venous cannula tubings. A series of arterial blood gases is obtained to assess for adequacy of oxygenation and ventilation without the extracorporeal membrane oxygenation support. If blood gases represent adequate gas exchange via patient's lung, cannulae are removed and neck vessels are ligated proximally. The vessels can be repaired primarily, but this has resulted in high incidence of complications such as aneurysm, embolization, obstruction and bleeding. After decannulation, the infant is maintained with mechanical ventilation but is usually weaned to an oxygen hood within 48–72 hours. During the first three to four days off extracorporeal membrane oxygenation, the platelet count must be monitored closely for a precipitous drop while damaged platelets are removed from the circulation.

Termination of extracorporeal membrane oxygenation is indicated when the lungs have recovered or when signs of irreversible brain damage, uncontrollable bleeding or irreversible lung damage are present. Extracorporeal membrane oxygenation may be continued longer than three weeks if progressive improvement is seen or if open-lung biopsy demonstrates a reversible condition. In recent years, veno–venous extracorporeal membrane oxygenation, using a single cannula placed in the internal jugular vein, has been used to provide extracorporeal life support with excellent results in newborns (Anderson et al., 1989).

Paediatric and adult patients

For veno–arterial bypass, the same vessels used for neonatal extracorporeal membrane oxygenation are cannulated to deliver the oxygenated blood into the aortic arch. For veno–venous access, we prefer the right internal jugular vein for drainage and the right femoral vein for reinfusion (Figure 15.8). Rich et al. (1998b) recently compared atrial–femoral and femoral–atrial flow in adult veno–venous extracorporeal membrane oxygenation. Femoral–atrial bypass provided higher maximal extracorporeal flow, higher pulmonary arterial mixed venous oxygen saturation and required less flow to maintain equivalent mixed venous oxygen saturation than atrial–femoral bypass. In adults, 80–100 mL/kg per minute is an adequate blood flow rate. As in the neonate, the extracorporeal flow is increased until satisfactory gas exchange is achieved with low resting ventilator settings. Large membrane oxygenators (up to 4.5 m^2) are used, and if necessary, two oxygenators may be placed in parallel for increased gas exchange. The management and weaning of

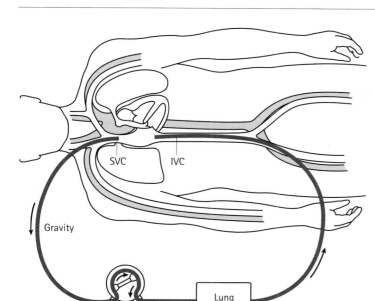

Figure 15.8 *Veno–venous bypass using the superior vena cava (SVC) as the venous outflow tract and the femoral vein as the arterial inflow tract. IVC = inferior vena cava.*

adults is similar to neonates, but survivors usually require a longer time on extracorporeal membrane oxygenation support. When pulmonary or cardiac function is sufficiently recovered to sustain acceptable haemodynamic and metabolic parameters off extracorporeal membrane oxygenation and on conventional management, the patient is taken off extracorporeal membrane oxygenation. Complications are primarily related to bleeding and circuit component failure.

Because the patient is on extracorporeal support and does not have to breathe, aspects of airway management unique to extracorporeal membrane oxygenation can be undertaken. For a large broncho-pleural fistula, selective ventilation of the opposite lung for a period of time, selective occlusion of the offending bronchus with a balloon catheter for one or two days, or cessation of ventilation altogether while the air leak seals are available management options. Once the air leak has been sealed for 48 hours, alveoli are recruited by hourly lung conditioning with application of continuous static airway pressure in the range of 20–30 cmH$_2$O. If the primary problems include excessive exudate or occlusion of the airways, flexible bronchoscopy with lavage can often help to clear the airway. The initial enthusiasm for perfluorocarbon liquid ventilation in these patients, to lavage the airways and improve alveolar recruitment and oxygenation, has dissipated for the paediatric patient population (Anderson *et al.*, 1989). Some centres favor early tracheostomy in respiratory failure patients in general because of the decreased incidence of nosocomial pneumonia from pharyngeal bacteria, easier airway access, as well as ventilator weaning (Bryant *et al.*, 1972; Rodriguez *et al.*, 1990). If tracheostomy has not been placed before extracorporeal membrane oxygenation, some undertake this procedure by percutaneous access on the first or second day of bypass

(Anderson and Bartlett, 1991). However, this involves the risk of bleeding at the tracheal stoma site, and if the patient may be weaned off bypass within a few days, tracheostomy should be postponed until the patient is off bypass.

Occasionally, extracorporeal membrane oxygenation can be used for the management of patients with severe airway obstruction secondary to status asthmaticus or airway occlusion caused by blood clots or other foreign material (Shapiro *et al.*, 1993). In these circumstances, oxygenation is usually more than adequate and the major problem is CO$_2$ retention, high intrathoracic pressures, cardiovascular collapse or barotrauma. Relatively low flow extracorporeal membrane oxygenation can be used for CO$_2$ removal and to permit lower ventilator settings to non-damaging settings (ECCO$_2$R). These patients usually recovery promptly and are ideally managed with extracorporeal membrane oxygenation.

Haemodynamics and cardiac status are monitored by pulse contour, pulmonary capillary wedge pressure, systemic blood pressure and signs of systemic perfusion. Mixed venous saturation is distorted in the veno–venous access patient because of recirculation. If there is any question about ventricular or valvular dysfunction, thrombi in the heart or peri-cardial tamponade, echocardiography should be performed. Frequently, inotropic support can be weaned off within a day or two on extracorporeal membrane oxygenation. If there is severe myocardial dysfunction unresponsive to inotropes, extracorporeal membrane oxygenation should be converted to veno–arterial support via the right common carotid artery to provide adequate haemodynamic support.

A progressive increase in pulmonary vascular resistance toward systemic levels is an ominous sign and usually represents progressive and irreversible fibrosis in the lung parenchyma. When mean pulmonary artery pressure is consistently greater than two-thirds of systemic pressure, the risk of right ventricular failure is high, and arrhythmias leading to ventricular tachycardia and fibrillation may occur. It is possible to support the circulation by converting to veno–arterial access at this point, but this situation has been uniformly fatal because of progressive lung injury. The right ventricular failure after prolonged veno–venous support may be considered a sign of irreversible lung injury. Conversely, if pulmonary artery pressure remains less than half systemic despite prolonged extracorporeal membrane oxygenation support for three of four weeks, extracorporeal membrane oxygenation support should be continued.

Patients who are considered for extracorporeal membrane oxygenation have usually been heavily sedated and frequently paralysed to facilitate ventilator management. As soon as stable extracorporeal membrane oxygenation is achieved, all sedative and paralytic drugs are discontinued until neurological functions are assessed. Most of these patients have had prolonged periods of hypoxia, usually associated with low blood flow and may not return to normal consciousness during the initial testing. Once the level of neurological function status has been verified, morphine and/or midazolam can be used to titrate to apparent patient comfort, allowing movement of all extremities, eyes, tongue and responses to simple commands. Patients are occasionally paralysed, in particular when the ventilator is set with a very long inspiratory phase and short expiratory phase. In addition, paralysis is necessary when patient agitation and activity increases VO_2 beyond the capability of the delivery system. Patients should be kept as awake and alert as possible during prolonged support. Even when the patient's condition requires paralysis, the paralytic agent is reversed daily to assess neurological functions. Any change in neurological function should prompt obtaining an immediate head CT scan to rule out diffuse swelling secondary to hypoxic ischaemic encephalopathy preceding the extracorporeal membrane oxygenation treatment, or localized intracranial bleeding or infarction. When it is apparent that severe brain damage has occurred, and does not rapidly improve within 24 hours, extracorporeal membrane oxygenation should be discontinued. On occasion, the diagnosis of cortical brain death can be made by physical examination after reversing pharmacological agents (lack of spontaneous movement, pupillary reflexes, and response to cold caloric stimulation of the ears). In such a case, clinical findings without head CT or EEG are adequate to confirm the diagnosis, although studies correlating clinical conditions may be reassuring to team or family members before discontinuing extracorporeal membrane oxygenation support.

When patients are managed at low activated clotting times and high platelet counts, either for procedures or to control bleeding, thrombosis may occur in the circuit. Monitoring the circuit carefully by examining directly for clots and determining pressure drops across the membrane oxygenators allow early recognition of clots in the circuit. The first sign of clotting in the circuit is an increase in pressure drop and loss of function in the membrane oxygenators. When clots in the circuit are localized to particular components, this component maybe replaced; however, the presence of clots throughout the circuit requires exchanging the entire circuit. A second identical circuit may be prepared and kept for rapid replacement (if necessary) when managing the patient with low heparin and high platelets to avoid significant delay between circuit exchange.

Occasionally, it is necessary to conduct surgical procedures while patients are on extracorporeal membrane oxygenation. Procedures such as evacuation of haemothorax, open lung biopsy or congenital diaphragmatic hernia repair have been performed during extracorporeal membrane oxygenation. Additionally, liver transplantation, lung transplantation, heart transplantation and evacuation of intracranial haematoma in patients on extracorporeal membrane oxygenation have also been performed. When undertaking elective or emergent operations on bypass, general guidelines such as lowering the activated clotting time parameters, increasing platelet counts or use of Amicar can be followed to minimize potential bleeding complications on extracorporeal membrane oxygenation.

Congenital diaphragmatic hernia

In 1981, the first cases of infants with congenital diaphragmatic hernia treated with extracorporeal membrane oxygenation were reported (Hardesty et al., 1981). The rationale for using extracorporeal membrane oxygenation in infants with congenital diaphragmatic hernia is to rest the lungs as pulmonary hypertension resolves without subjecting them to barotrauma. Since the introduction of extracorporeal membrane oxygenation as a treatment strategy for respiratory failure associated with congenital diaphragmatic hernia, improved survival rates have been reported (Redmond et al., 1987a; Weber et al., 1987; Bailey et al., 1989; Heiss et al., 1989; Van Meurs et al., 1990; Atkinson et al., 1991; Finer et al., 1992; Lessin et al., 1995; Mallik et al., 1995; van der Staak et al., 1995). The impact on mortality, however, has been institution-dependent, with survival rates varying from 34 per cent to 87 per cent (Lessin et al., 1995). Congenital diaphragmatic hernia has the lowest survival rate of all categories of neonatal respiratory failure for which extracorporeal membrane oxygenation is used. Current multicentre ELSO Registry data show infants with congenital diaphragmatic hernia treated with extracorporeal membrane oxygenation have a survival rate of 53 per cent (ECLS Organization, 2004). Despite the absence of reliable predictors to govern extracorporeal membrane oxygenation use, the technique remains the mainstay of congenital diaphragmatic hernia treatment. Veno–venous ECMO was compared to neoarterial ECMO in newborns with congenital diaphragmatic hernia and no significant difference in outcomes was reported (68 per cent vs 69 per cent) (Kugelman *et al.*, 2003). Although the role of extracorporeal membrane oxygenation as a treatment for congenital diaphragmatic hernia has been widely accepted, the timing of the surgical repair of the defect in relation to extracorporeal membrane oxygenation therapy remains controversial. It has been suggested that there is a survival advantage to congenital diaphragmatic hernia repair during the post-extracorporeal membrane oxygenation period; however, the timing of the congenital diaphragmatic hernia repair has been quite variable among extracorporeal membrane oxygenation centres.

Operative repair of the defect has been proposed while on extracorporeal membrane oxygenation (Connors *et al.*, 1990; Lally *et al.*, 1992; Wilson *et al.*, 1992, 1994; Stolar *et al.*, 1995). With this operative strategy, survival rates have been variable and as high as 80 per cent (Connors *et al.*, 1990; West *et al.*, 1992; Wilson *et al.*, 1994). Congenital diaphragmatic hernia patients have a higher risk of complications than other extracorporeal membrane oxygenation patients. They have longer runs and are generally kept less anticoagulated, leading to more mechanical complications. Since they undergo a major operation (congenital diaphragmatic hernia repair) either just before or during extracorporeal membrane oxygenation, these patients also experience more haemorrhagic complications. In a review of 483 cases of congenital diaphragmatic hernia, the overall incidence of haemorrhage was 43 per cent, with fatal haemorrhage occurring in 4.8 per cent of cases (Vazquez and Cheu, 1994). The locations of bleeding in descending order were surgical site (24 per cent), intracranial (11 per cent), cannulation site (7.5 per cent), gastrointestinal (5 per cent), pleural cavity (3.5 per cent), abdominal (2.8 per cent) and pulmonary (1.9 per cent).

Criteria for determining extracorporeal membrane oxygenation use in infants with congenital diaphragmatic hernia has been based on variable institutional factors predicting ⩾80 per cent mortality for all cases of neonatal respiratory failure treated with conventional mechanical ventilation. Indications for extracorporeal membrane oxygenation in neonates with congenital diaphragmatic hernia are inadequate oxygen delivery despite adequate volume resuscitation, pharmacological support and ventilation. If infants experience respiratory failure after congenital diaphragmatic hernia repair, they are placed on extracorporeal membrane oxygenation postoperatively. As delayed repair became more common, congenital diaphragmatic hernia repair has been performed during extracorporeal membrane oxygenation support at many institutions. Delaying repair until the infant is off extracorporeal membrane oxygenation is

another option in which favourable results have been reported (Adolph *et al.*, 1995; Sigalet *et al.*, 1995).

The overall survival rate for neonates with congenital diaphragmatic hernia is unknown. Previous studies have suggested that the mortality rate has remained approximately 50 per cent even with the increased use of extracorporeal membrane oxygenation support (Adzick *et al.*, 1985; Wilson *et al.*, 1991; Sharland *et al.*, 1992; Harrison *et al.*, 1994; Lessin *et al.*, 1995). Variation in published survival rates is quite high, and represents institutional differences in management strategies and perhaps patient accrual. Evolution of mechanical ventilation techniques, extracorporeal support, use of surfactant, nitric oxide and different timing of surgical intervention have all contributed to variable survival rates from different institutions.

Clinically, chronic lung disease has been reported in congenital diaphragmatic hernia survivors requiring extracorporeal membrane oxygenation (Lund *et al.*, 1994; D'Agostino *et al.*, 1995); however, it is unclear whether this represents apparent pathophysiology of congenital diaphragmatic hernia or sequelae of iatrogenic barotauma. Studies have identified a number of non-pulmonary morbidities in congenital diaphragmatic hernia survivors, in particular in infants requiring aggressive management of severe respiratory failure: neurological abnormalities have been the most common problems found in a number of series. Abnormalities in both motor and cognitive skills have been identified (D'Agostino *et al.*, 1995; Stolar *et al.*, 1995). Other neurological problems reported have included visual disturbances, hearing loss, seizures, abnormal cranial CT and MRI scans, and abnormal electroencephalogram (EEG) studies (Lund *et al.*, 1994; D'Agostino *et al.*, 1995).

VENO–VENOUS EXTRACORPOREAL MEMBRANE OXYGENATION

Development of veno–venous extracorporeal membrane oxygenation and clinical experience

The most widely used strategy for long-term perfusion support has been veno–arterial extracorporeal membrane oxygenation. Of the 18,703 neonatal extracorporeal membrane oxygenation cases reported to the ELSO Registry as of January 2004, 13,080 have been supported with veno–arterial perfusion and only 3968 cases with veno–venous extracorporeal membrane oxygenation (ECLS Organization, 2004). However, the veno–venous approach is not new; its use in animals was first described in 1969 (Kolobow *et al.*, 1969). Hanson and colleagues (Hanson *et al.*, 1973) showed that veno–venous perfusion could be used to support adequate gas exchange in lambs breathing nitrogen. Lamy and colleagues (Lamy et al., 1975) investigated the effects of various cannulation routes, including veno–venous support, on the pulmonary circulation; and, in 1979, Delaney and co-workers (Delaney et al., 1979) studied the effects of veno–venous as compared with veno–arterial flow on lung transvascular fluid dynamics. The technique of veno–venous extracorporeal membrane oxygenation, as performed by Gattinoni et al. (1986) and Kolobow (1988a), is different from veno–arterial extracorporeal membrane oxygenation (Table 15.4) (Klein et al., 1985). This technique prevents damage to diseased lungs by reducing their motion (pulmonary rest), although three to five 'sighs' with low-frequency positive-pressure ventilation (LFPPV) are provided each minute to preserve the functional residual capacity. With this method, oxygen uptake and CO_2 removal are dissociated: oxygenation is accomplished primarily through the lungs, whereas CO_2 is cleared through extracorporeal removal ($ECCO_2R$). $LFPPV$-$ECCO_2R$ is performed at an extracorporeal blood flow of 20–30 per cent of cardiac output. Vascular access is achieved via combinations of jugular–femoral, femoral–femoral or saphenous–saphenous veins. Veno–venous access, emphasizing CO_2 removal, is promising, although most infants and children go through a phase of diminished lung function requiring oxygenation support. It is possible to supply all O_2 requirements during veno–venous bypass by increasing the flow to 100–120 per cent of cardiac output. The efficiency of oxygen transfer is decreased because of the elevated saturation of the venous blood

(recirculation); however, this can be offset by increasing extracorporeal blood flow. In a recent retrospective review of 94 patients, Bartlett's group (Pranikoff et al., 1999) concluded that percutaneous cannulation can be used for veno–venous extracorporeal membrane oxygenation in adults.

Advantages

If the lungs are not functioning, all gas exchange requirements can be achieved during veno–venous bypass by increasing the flow to 100–120 per cent of cardiac output. Veno–venous extracorporeal membrane oxygenation has the advantage of maintaining normal pulmonary blood flow and avoiding arterial cannulation with its risk of systemic microemboli. Total support of gas exchange with veno–venous perfusion, returning the perfusate blood into the venous circulation through the femoral vein or a modified jugular venous drainage catheter, also has the advantage of avoiding carotid artery ligation (Zwischenberger et al., 1985).

Bartlett's group developed a polyurethane double-lumen catheter for single-site cannulation of the internal jugular vein (Anderson et al., 1989, 1993a). A tidal flow veno–venous system with a single-lumen catheter (Zwischenberger et al., 1985) has been developed to aid venous gas exchange. Efficient wire-wound cannulae, which are capable of sufficient flow for total gas exchange, can be inserted in large children (>15 kg) and adults by

Table 15.4 *Comparison of veno–arterial and veno–venous extracorporeal membrane oxygenation*

	Veno–arterial	Veno–venous
Cannulation sites	Internal jugular vein, right atrium or femoral vein plus right common carotid, axillary or femoral artery or aorta (directly)	Internal jugular vein alone (double-lumen or single-lumen tidal flow) Jugular–femoral Femoro–femoral Sapheno–saphenous Right atrium (directly)
Organ support	Gas exchange and cardiac output	Gas exchange only
Systemic perfusion	Circuit flow and cardiac output	Cardiac output only
Pulse contour	Reduced pulsatility	Normal pulsatility
Central venous pressure	Unreliable	Accurate guide to volume status
Pulmonary artery pressure	Unreliable	Reliable
Effect of R–L shunt	Mixed venous into perfusate blood	None
Effect of L–R shunt (PDA)	Pulmonary hyperperfusion may shunt	No effect on flow Require increased flow usual PDA physiology
Blood flow for full gas exchange	80–100 cc/kg per h	100–120 cc/kg per h
Circuit SVO_2	Reliable	Unreliable
Circuit recirculation	None	15–30%
Arterial pO_2s	60–150 torr	45–80 torr
Arterial oxygen saturation	≥95%	80–95%
Indicators of O_2 insufficiency	Mixed venous saturation or pO_2 Calculated oxygen consumption	Cerebral venous saturation Da-VO_2 across the membrane Patient PaO_2 Pre-membrane saturation trend

percutaneous insertion (Seldinger technique). Although jugulo–femoral veno–venous bypass is feasible in neonates, the advantages do not outweigh the disadvantages (Klein et al., 1985). The occasional need for better cardiopulmonary support, and the additional complexity of two-vein veno–venous bypass favours veno–arterial bypass for haemodynamically unstable neonates.

Outcome

Since the 14-French veno–venous direct line catheter became commercially available in 1989, more than 3428 neonates have been treated, with an 86 per cent overall survival (ECLS Organization, 2004). A multicentre retrospective comparison of veno–arterial access to veno–venous direct line for newborns with respiratory failure undergoing extracorporeal membrane oxygenation was undertaken (Anderson et al., 1993b). Overall survival in patients undergoing veno–arterial bypass was 87 per cent, whereas survival in patients undergoing veno–venous direct line was 95 per cent. Eleven patients required conversion from veno–venous direct line to veno–arterial because of insufficient support, with 10 survivors. Average bypass time for newborns on veno–arterial bypass was 132 ($\pm$7.4) hours versus 100 ($\pm$5.1) hours on veno–venous direct line bypass, and neurological complications were more common in veno–arterial bypass. Haemorrhagic, cardiopulmonary and mechanical complications, other than kinking of the veno–venous direct line catheter, occurred with equal frequency in each group.

When the entire ELSO Registry experience of veno–arterial versus veno–venous direct line was compared, the survival for veno–arterial (1990–1992, $n = 3146$) was 81 per cent, whereas that for veno–venous direct line (1990–1992, $n = 576$) was 91 per cent (Zwischenberger et al., 1994). The average duration of veno–arterial extracorporeal membrane oxygenation was 141 ($\pm$89) hours and of veno–venous direct line was 120 ($\pm$64) hours. Comparison of specific mechanical complications demonstrated that veno–venous direct line had a significantly higher prevalence of restrictive sutures and kinking in the cannulae. When comparing the specific patient complication rates between techniques, veno–venous direct line had a much lower rate of major neurological complications. The prevalence and survival rates with seizures or cerebral infarction were significantly lower with veno–venous direct line and seemed to have a substantial effect on overall survival. Therefore, during the initial experience, veno–venous direct line extracorporeal membrane oxygenation had a higher survival rate and a lower rate of major neurological complications (Zwischenberger et al., 1994). As of January 2004, veno–arterial versus veno–venous direct line survival is 75 per cent versus 86 per cent, respectively (ECLS Organization, 2004).

Although patients in which this technique was used may have been more carefully selected and 'more stable' than veno–arterial extracorporeal membrane oxygenation patients, early success may lead to an important conceptual change in the use of extracorporeal membrane oxygenation technology. The current practice of waiting until the natural lungs become severely dysfunctional and then having to support cardiopulmonary function almost completely, as with veno–arterial extracorporeal membrane oxygenation, may give way to the concept of early lung assistance. Single-site cannulation has already become the ideal method of choice for most newborns with respiratory failure without haemodynamic compromise. Similarly, continued catheter development will allow percutaneous access for veno–venous direct line extracorporeal membrane oxygenation. A single-cannula tidal flow veno–venous extracorporeal membrane oxygenation system has been developed which allows percutaneous access (Chevalier et al., 1993; Kolla et al., 1997b).

COMPLICATIONS DURING EXTRACORPOREAL MEMBRANE OXYGENATION, AND THEIR MANAGEMENT

The success or failure of a course of therapy including extracorporeal membrane oxygenation is completely dependent upon the prompt recognition and management of related complications as they emerge. Complications during extracorporeal membrane oxygenation are the rule, not the exception (Upp et al., 1994; Zwischenberger et al., 1994). Unfortunately, it is the nature of long-term heart–lung bypass that potentially catastrophic complications arise unexpectedly and progress rapidly. An understanding of the physiology relevant to extracorporeal membrane oxygenation, familiarity with the extracorporeal membrane oxygenation circuit and the attainment of a certain level of confidence in managing patients on extracorporeal membrane oxygenation prepare us to deal with most of the problems routinely encountered with this technique. The complications encountered in extracorporeal membrane oxygenation can be classified as mechanical or patient complications. Any mechanical component of the extracorporeal membrane oxygenation apparatus may fail, and constant system checks and monitoring prevent most complications from becoming management disasters. Although patient complications span the entire field of critical care, they are often related to systemic heparinization, such as intracranial haemorrhage, gastrointestinal haemorrhage and cannula site bleeding.

Mechanical complications

The collective experience of complications during extracorporeal membrane oxygenation from the ELSO Registry

Table 15.5 *Mechanical complications*

Neonatal	Percentage incidence	Paediatric/cardiac/adult	Percentage incidence
Clots in circuit	62	Other	46.2
Cannula problems	14	Oxygenator failure	22.3
Other	12.8	Cannula problems	18.2
Air in circuit	7.5	Tubing rupture	7.2
Oxygenator failure	7.2	Pump malfunction	4.6
Cracks in connectors	4.7	Heat exchanger	1.6
Pump malfunction	2.1		
Cannula kinking	2.2		
Heat exchanger	1.3		
Haemofilter malfunction	1.8		
Other tubing rupture	1.1		
Restrictive sutures	0.6		

has been reviewed (ECLS Organization, 2000). There were 13,417 mechanical complications reported in 19,750 extracorporeal membrane oxygenation cases, or an average of 0.68 mechanical complications per case. Mechanical complications, in descending order of frequency, are listed in Table 15.5. Revealingly, the most common mechanical complication for the paediatric, cardiac and adult groups listed in the ELSO Registry is that of 'other'. This reflects the fact that, in addition to the identifiable components listed above, the entire circuit is subject to failure, including the bladder box, connectors, electrical components, power sources, plugs, oxygen sources, carbogen tanks, blenders and circuit monitoring equipment.

Clots in the circuit are the single most common mechanical complication, representing well over half (62 per cent) of the mechanical complications reported (ECLS Organization, 2000). Major clots can lead to oxygenator failure or a consumption coagulopathy as well as the potential for pulmonary or systemic emboli. The extracorporeal circuit presents a large foreign surface for activation of neutrophils, lymphocytes and platelets, releasing inflammatory mediators and causing free-radical activity (Cavarocchi *et al.*, 1986; De Puydt *et al.*, 1993; Eberhart, 1993; Robinson *et al.*, 1993; Bergman *et al.*, 1994). Despite initial encouraging reports of heparin-coated Carmeda® extracorporeal membrane oxygenation in decreasing bleeding complications (Nagaraj *et al.*, 1992; Rais-Bahrami *et al.*, 1993; Bergman *et al.*, 1994), the significant bleeding complications on extracorporeal membrane oxygenation remain problematic.

Cannulae are inserted with great care to avoid vascular damage during insertion, since loss of control of the

internal jugular vein can result in massive mediastinal bleeding, and dissection of the carotid artery intima can progress to a lethal aortic dissection. The venous cannula, however, can be advanced too little or too much, either of which can cause cannula obstruction. Similarly, the venous catheter can enter the subclavian vein or cross the foramen ovale. Anatomic variations of the right atrium (aneurysmal atrial septum or redundant eustachian valve) can also interfere with venous return. The use of echocardiography to confirm cannula position has been recommended because routine radiography of the chest can fail to demonstrate cannula malposition (Nagaraj *et al.*, 1992; Rais-Bahrami *et al.*, 1993). Problems with arterial cannulation malposition can affect patients' haemodynamic status. Insertion too far into the ascending aorta can cause increased after-load to left ventricular outflow, and may contribute to left ventricular failure. In addition, the cannula can cross the aortic valve, causing aortic insufficiency. Insertion too far down the descending aorta can compromise coronary and cerebral oxygenated blood flow as well as 'streaming' of hyperoxygenated blood from the extracorporeal membrane oxygenation circuit without adequate mixing. The distance from the orifice of the innominate artery to the take-off of the right subclavian artery can be a remarkably short 1.0–1.5 cm. If the arterial cannula is pulled out to the point at which the arterial infusion selectively enters the right subclavian artery, the right upper extremity can be infused with the entire post-oxygenator blood flow while the rest of the body becomes hypoxic and cyanotic. Cannula-induced vertebral steal while on veno–arterial extracorporeal membrane oxygenation can occur with decreased blood flow to the right arm and retrograde flow in the right vertebral artery (Alexander *et al.*, 1992).

Oxygenator failure has decreased in frequency to 7.2 per cent. Any failing membrane should be changed immediately upon recognition to prevent an air or blood leak. A double diamond tubing arrangement with dual connectors located at both pre- and post-oxygenator, allows in-line replacement of the oxygenator without interrupting extracorporeal membrane oxygenation flow. Air in the circuit (7.5 per cent) can represent from small bubbles seen in the bladder to a complete venous air lock. Venous air lock usually results from dislodgment of the venous cannula so that one or more of the sideholes is outside the vessel (Faulkner *et al.*, 1993). Massive airlock requires the patient to come off extracorporeal membrane oxygenation support with either removal of the air or replacement of an entire extracorporeal membrane oxygenation circuit. For small amounts of air in the venous line, the air can be moved to the venous reservoir by sequentially raising the venous line to aspirate the air out of the venous reservoirs.

The extracorporeal membrane oxygenation circuit is designed to pump blood safely and efficiently, but a large bolus of air can develop and circulate rapidly, and is commonly fatal. There are several potential sources of such an embolus. When the partial pressure of oxygen in the blood is very high as seen post-oxygenator, oxygen can easily be forced out of solution. Hitting the membrane or operating the circuit in a low ambient pressure environment (such as in-flight in a non-pressurized cabin) may produce foam in the top of the oxygenator. Operating the pump with a clamp on the venous side of the circuit, with the bladder in the 'prime' mode or with the outlet arm of the bladder kinked can generate a markedly negative pressure in the blood path and pull large amounts of gas out of solution, resulting in cavitation. This is the problem the bladder box system is designed to avoid.

Probably the most dramatic air embolus occurs when a small tear develops in the membrane, allowing blood to leak into the gas path of the oxygenator. The blood gradually moves down to the gas exhalation port where it may either be blown out in small drops onto the floor, or accumulate and form a clot. If this clot obstructs the egress of gas, back pressure will develop inside the gas path of the oxygenator. When the gas pressure exceeds that of the blood, a large bolus of gas crosses the membrane and appears in the blood path. As it surges out the membrane to the heat exchanger (and the arterial line filter, if it is used), the gas trapping capacity of these two devices (on the order of 45 mL for each) may rapidly be exceeded, and the embolus will push into the arterial line toward the aorta.

The solution to these problems rests on prevention and a rapid response when air embolism is recognized. Keeping the pO_2 in the membrane blood at 600 mmHg or less, carefully monitoring the bladder box, strictly prohibiting placement of extraneous clamps on the circuit and adherence to precautions with regard to the procedure for 'walking the raceway' will eliminate most problems. Lightly touching the gas exhalation port of the membrane with your finger as a part of the hourly circuit check will alert the practitioner when there is blood other than just water being expelled. However, occluding the gas exhalation port even briefly can cause a precipitous rise in the gas phase pressure across the membrane, risking membrane rupture and/or formation of air embolus.

If air is headed toward the arterial cannula, a clamp is immediately placed on the arterial tubing close to the patient. The pump is immediately turned off, the main bridge is unclamped, and the venous line is clamped. The patient should be hand bagged or the ventilator should be returned to its pre-extracorporeal membrane oxygenation settings, and the problem in the circuit identified and corrected. Once the patient is 'off bypass', lower the head relative to the body as much as possible in order to move any air pockets away from the cerebral circulation. Using a sterile catheter-tipped syringe, aspirate any accessible air back out of the arterial cannula. If a hyperbaric chamber is available and the patient is stable, its immediate use should also be considered.

Tubing rupture has become much less frequent with the introduction of Super Tygon (S65HL) (Norton Performances Plastics, Inc., Akron, OH, USA) raceway tubing (Toomasian *et al.*, 1987). Previously, polyvinyl chloride (PVC) tubing required advancing the raceway every 24 hours to prevent tube fatigue and rupture. With prolonged extracorporeal membrane oxygenation, the raceway should be advanced approximately every 36 hours for neonates with 1/4-inch Super Tygon tubing and every 96–120 hours in older patients with 3/8-inch Super Tygon tubing. Pump failure, similarly, has become more rare as direct and belt drive pumps have been manufactured specifically with long-term extracorporeal support in mind. Occasionally, the pump 'cuts' out and stops pumping blood. This is a manifestation of inadequate venous return to the pump and may simply be a response to hypovolaemia that can be corrected easily with intravascular volume expansion. Although heat exchanger malfunction occurs in only one per cent of cases, it may cause severe hypothermia or haemodilution in the infant. Additionally, defective heat exchangers have been responsible for aluminum particle emboli (Vogler *et al.*, 1988); however, redesign has eliminated this problem.

Patient complications

The management of the patient on extracorporeal membrane oxygenation, including patient-related complications, spans the entire field of critical care. In July 1999, ELSO Registry reports of patient complications during extracorporeal membrane oxygenation were 34,641 patient complications or an average of 1.75 complications per case (ECLS Organization, 1999). The incidence of patient-related complications is nearly three times that of the mechanical circuit-related events. Bleeding is one of the most devastating and difficult problems encountered. Patient complications, in descending order of frequency, include intracranial haemorrhage, seizures, surgical site haemorrhage, haemofiltration or dialysis, abnormal creatinine, hypertension, cardiac dysfunction, haemolysis, electrolyte abnormalities, pneumothorax, positive blood culture (sepsis), gastrointestinal haemorrhage and arrhythmias (Table 15.6).

Moderate bleeding (more than 10 cc/h in neonates) is frequently seen at the neck cannulation site. This problem is minimized by use of electrocautery at the time of surgical exposure, cannulation, and the liberal use of a topical haemostatic agent, such as Gelfoam thrombin. At many centres, neck wounds are packed with a topical haemostatic agent before closure, which decreases the incidence of bleeding for the duration of the extracorporeal membrane oxygenation course and is easily removed at decannulation.

Table 15.6 *Patient complications*

Complication	Percentage
Haemofiltration or dialysis	8.4
Intracerebral haemorrhage	6.2
Abnormal creatinine	5.8
Seizures	5.3
Inotropes on extracorporeal membrane oxygenation	5.2
Hypertensive	4.9
Surgical site bleeding	4.9
Haemolysis	4.8
Other haemorrhage	3.9
Sepsis (culture positive)	3.9
Abnormal potassium	3.9
Other cardiovascular	3.5
Acid-base abnormalities	3.4
Hyperbilirubinaemia	3.2
Arrhythmias	3.2
Abnormal glucose	2.9
Pneumothorax	2.8
Other pulmonary	2.6
Abnormal sodium	2.3
Myocardial stun	2.2
Other neurological	1.9
Cannula site bleeding	1.8
Abnormal calcium	1.4
Cardiopulmonary resuscitation required	1.4
Symptomatic PDA	1.3

When bleeding from the neck incision is observed, local pressure, topical placement of haemostatic agents (Gelfoam thrombin, Oxycel, topical thrombin) and injection of cryoprecipitate fibrin glue into the wound have all been successful. If topical treatment methods are unsuccessful, consider decreasing the heparin infusion rate to keep the activated clotting time between 180 s and 220 s, and maintaining the platelet count > 100,000. Any time the neck incision bleeds more than 10 cc/h for two hours despite the treatment strategies outlined above the wound should be explored. Once haemostasis is achieved with electrocautery, the wound should be packed with a topical haemostatic agent and reclosed.

Bleeding into the site of a previous invasive procedure is a frequent complication. Intracranial, gastrointestinal, intrathoracic, abdominal and retroperitoneal bleeding have all been observed in neonates on extracorporeal membrane oxygenation. Bleeding from other sites occurs in approximately 10.8 per cent of cases. Significant bleeding that is not attributable to the neck incision is not routine and must be dealt with aggressively. A decreasing haematocrit, a rising heart rate, a fall in the blood pressure or a progressive rise in the PaO_2 on veno–arterial extracorporeal membrane oxygenation disproportionate to observed improvements in the patient's pulmonary status all suggest bleeding. In addition, neurological changes, the development of seizures, intrathoracic tamponade or abdominal distention all raise suspicions of the presence of bleeding into these respective areas. Although plain chest radiographs can suggest bleeding, such findings should be aggressively evaluated by ultrasound exam of the respective organ space, or even CT scan evaluation, if necessary.

Minor surgical procedures may be required during extracorporeal membrane oxygenation; however, they should not be taken lightly. Bleeding complications have occurred after seemingly trivial procedures. Arterial cutdown may be needed if appropriate access can not be obtained before the initiation of extracorporeal membrane oxygenation, or if access is lost. Tube thoracostomy may be required to drain haemothorax or pneumothorax. At the time of these minor invasive procedures, skin incisions can be made with the cutting mode of an electrocautery. Muscles should be cauterized and not torn. Fibrin glue (cryoprecipitate, calcium and thrombin solution) applied to wounds will help to decrease bleeding complications. Although bleeding may be a significant problem, liberal use of cautery, application of fibrin glue, and a low threshold for re-exploration permit nearly any procedure to be performed.

The development of safe and reliable heparin-bonded, non-thrombogenic surfaces potentially ushers in an entirely new era in extracorporeal membrane oxygenation (Shanley et al., 1992; Lazzara et al., 1993; Tsuno et al., 1993), allowing safer application of extracorporeal membrane oxygenation to patients with conditions currently considered contraindicated. The use of heparin-bonded circuits also appears to decrease platelet, leukocytes, complement and kinin system activation (Plotz et al., 1993). Despite early enthusiasm for its potential benefits, the initial experiences with heparin-bonded tubings have not been successful.

Aminocaproic acid and aprotinin have been recommended to decrease bleeding and intracerebral haemorrhage complications during extracorporeal membrane oxygenation (van Oeveren et al., 1987; Dietrich et al., 1989; Fraedrich et al., 1989; Brunet et al., 1992; Feindt et al., 1993; Wachtfogel et al., 1993; Wilson et al., 1993; Spannagl et al., 1994, Wilson et al., 1994). Wilson and colleagues (Wilson et al., 1993, 1994) reported that aminocaproic acid, an inhibitor of fibrinolysis, administered just before or after cannulation (100 mg/kg bolus, then 30 mg/kg per hour infusion), significantly decreased bleeding in high-risk neonates. The incidence of intracerebral haemorrhage was also reduced. In 298 patients, Downard and colleagues (Downard et al., 2003) reported a significant reduction in the incidence of surgical site bleeding with the use of aminocaproic acid; however, the rate of intracranial hemorrhage was not significantly affected. Presently, a randomized prospective study is ongoing. Brunet and colleagues (Brunet et al., 1992) reported that aprotinin infusion (2×10^6 kIU loading dose, then 5×10^5 kIU/h) resulted in resolution of life-threatening bleeding in two adult patients during prolonged ECCO$_2$R. Further clinical trials will be required to determine its safety and efficiency during prolonged extracorporeal membrane oxygenation.

The subject of intracerebral haemorrhage in neonates has been reviewed extensively (Tarby and Volpe, 1982). As a rule, the appearance of a new intracerebral haemorrhage or enlargement of a pre-existing bleed are indications to discontinue extracorporeal membrane oxygenation support if possible. Factors that increase the pressure gradient between the blood vessel lumen in the germinal matrix and the surrounding brain tissue increase the likelihood of small-vessel rupture and haemorrhage. Factors contributing to intracerebral haemorrhage in all critically ill neonates include hypoxia, hypercapnia, acidosis, ischaemia, hypotension, sepsis, coagulopathy, thrombocytopenia, venous hypertension, seizures, birth trauma and rapid infusions of colloid or hypertonic solution. Mechanical ventilation has also been associated with an increased rate of intracerebral haemorrhage in premature infants with respiratory distress syndrome.

During extracorporeal membrane oxygenation, infants are exposed to a number of conditions that may increase the risk of intracerebral haemorrhage, including ligation of the right common carotid artery and internal jugular vein, systemic heparinization, thrombocytopenia, coagulopathy and hypertension (Cilley et al., 1986; Gleason, 1993, Schumacher, 1993). In a retrospective analysis of neonates undergoing extracorporeal membrane oxygenation therapy, birthweight and gestational age were the most significant factors correlating with the incidence of intracranial haemorrhage during extracorporeal membrane oxygenation (Cilley et al., 1986). Cranial ultrasound can aid in the diagnosis of intracerebral haemorrhage (von Allmen et al., 1992; Lazar et al., 1994).

Patients in whom veno–arterial extracorporeal membrane oxygenation is used commonly have ligation of the right common carotid artery and internal jugular veins. Decreased cerebral blood flow and increased cerebral venous hypertension have been considered as a source of intracerebral haemorrhage (Alexander et al., 1992; Taylor and Walker, 1992; Gleason, 1993; Schumacher, 1993). Schumacher et al. (1988) reported right-sided central nervous system lesions in eight of 69 extracorporeal membrane oxygenation patients; however, these patients were also profoundly hypoxic and hypotensive upon initiation of extracorporeal membrane oxygenation. Others have shown no evidence of a higher incidence of right-sided central nervous system lesions (Campbell et al., 1988). Blood flow to the right cerebral hemisphere is preserved after right carotid artery ligation by collateral circulation via the external carotid artery and the anterior communicating artery of the Circle of Willis. Non-invasive vascular studies have demonstrated that adequate cerebral blood

flow occurs during extracorporeal membrane oxygenation as well as early after decannulation (Raju et al., 1989; Lohrer et al., 1992) and in the late follow-up period (Towne et al., 1985; Taylor et al., 1989). Ten infants also underwent digital intravenous angiography; in each case, there was prompt bilateral filling of both middle cerebral arteries (Lohrer et al., 1992). No consistently lateralized EEG abnormalities were observed during or after extracorporeal membrane oxygenation when compared with tracings obtained before cannulation of the right common carotid artery (Streletz et al., 1992). These studies suggest that collateral circulation is readily established in neonates despite the ligation of the common carotid artery. Because of continued concerns about long-term effects of common carotid artery ligation, a few centres reconstruct the artery at decannulation (Spector et al., 1991; Moulton et al., 1991; Baumgart et al., 1994). Carotid reconstruction, however, introduces the potential for carotid dissection, aneurysm, thrombosis, emboli or late stenosis. Desai et al. (1999) prospectively evaluated serial Doppler ultrasonography and long-term neurodevelopmental outcomes in neonates whose right common carotid artery was reconstructed after extracorporeal membrane oxygenation. Reconstructions were successful (<50 per cent right common carotid artery stenosis by Doppler ultrasonography) 76 per cent, and no significant differences were seen between reconstructed and ligated groups in neonatal complications or extracorporeal membrane oxygenation courses. Compared with a historical control group, patients with right common carotid artery reconstruction had fewer brain scan abnormalities and tended to be less likely to have cerebral palsy. Therefore, right common carotid artery reconstruction after veno–arterial extracorporeal membrane oxygenation may improve outcome.

During extracorporeal membrane oxygenation, infants are anticoagulated with heparin infusions of 30–60 U/kg per hour to maintain activated clotting times of two to three times normal. Although heparinization may not cause intracerebral haemorrhage, it may allow rapid progression of haemorrhage with atypical sonographic characteristics of intracerebral haemorrhage (von Allmen et al., 1992; Lazar et al., 1994). The extracorporeal circuit also exposes the infant's blood to a large surface area of foreign material, creating the setting for ongoing blood surface interactions. Heparin infusion rates must be carefully adjusted to prevent large variations in the degree of anticoagulation. Adequate oxygenation must be maintained and rapid changes in systemic blood pressure avoided. Hypertension must be avoided and rapidly treated when present. Before extracorporeal membrane oxygenation treatment, cranial ultrasound is mandatory to identify patients with pre-existing intracerebral haemorrhage.

Instability of previously well-controlled coagulation parameters (activated clotting time, platelet count, fibrinogen) may represent an early predictor of an intracranial event (Hirthler *et al.*, 1992; Stallion *et al.*, 1994). Haemolysis is a complication often related to the extracorporeal membrane oxygenation membrane and/or circuit (Steinhorn *et al.*, 1989). Clots in the circuit or membrane may promote a coagulopathy by activation of complement, white blood cells, platelets or coagulation factors to cause erythrocytes to adhere and lyse on the fibrin strands (Eberhart, 1993).

Thrombocytopenia during extracorporeal membrane oxygenation may result from several factors:

- decreased production
- increased consumption
- sequestration in, or removal to, extravascular sites
- dilution.

Thrombocytopenia is expected during the use of extracorporeal membrane oxygenation as platelets are altered and as platelet aggregates in the extracorporeal circuit are preferentially sequestered in the lung, liver and spleen (Anderson *et al.*, 1986; De Puydt *et al.*, 1993; Robinson *et al.*, 1993). Thrombocytopenia in the neonate is significant in that existing bleeding may be exacerbated or bleeding may occur spontaneously. A platelet count <100,000/mm^3 is considered abnormal. Hypoxia has been shown to be a factor in the inhibition of platelet production by blood forming organs. Thrombocytopenia can occur up to four days after the termination of extracorporeal membrane oxygenation for the treatment of neonatal respiratory failure; therefore, platelet counts need to be measured frequently during this critical period (Anderson *et al.*, 1986). Thrombocytopenia must be avoided by using platelet transfusion as often as necessary to maintain adequate platelet counts during, as well as after extracorporeal membrane oxygenation when thrombocytopenia may occur.

Ultrasound of the kidneys to exclude major anatomic anomalies is mandatory in the presence of any elevated creatinine or persistently poor response to intravenous furosemide (1–2 mg/kg). Oliguria during extracorporeal membrane oxygenation is common, especially during the first 24–48 hours. Sell *et al.* (1987a) report the use of continuous haemofiltration for renal failure during extracorporeal membrane oxygenation. Continuous haemofiltration removes plasma water and dissolved solutes while retaining proteins and cellular components of the intravascular space. The classic indications for dialysis hold true with continuous haemofiltration on extracorporeal membrane oxygenation: hypervolaemia, hyperkalaemia and azotaemia. Hyperkalaemia and hypervolaemia are easily managed with continuous haemofiltration, but azotaemia is more difficult to manage because of chronic haemolysis during extracorporeal membrane oxygenation. The continuous haemofiltration apparatus is easily added in-line to the extracorporeal membrane oxygenation circuit, and allows removal of up to 10 mL/kg per hour.

Systolic hypertension is a dangerous side effect of extracorporeal membrane oxygenation. Sell *et al.* (1987b) reported that 38 of 41 newborns treated with extracorporeal membrane oxygenation developed systolic blood pressures >90 mmHg. Forty-four per cent of patients with persistent hypertension developed detectable intracerebral haemorrhage and 27 per cent developed clinically significant intracerebral haemorrhage. The development of a medical management protocol using hydralazine, nitroglycerin and captopril has decreased the incidence of clinically significant intracerebral haemorrhage associated with hypertensive episodes. We currently use hydralazine 0.1 mg/kg IV for systolic hypertension >90 mmHg.

It is unusual to have catastrophic haemodynamic deterioration while a patient is on veno–arterial extracorporeal membrane oxygenation. The factors that deserve immediate evaluation when this occurs include venous catheter displacement, inadequate systemic volume status, and the possibility of extracorporeal membrane oxygenation circuit failure. Major cardiac dysfunction is usually not appreciated during veno–arterial extracorporeal membrane oxygenation when full supportive flow (120 mL/kg per minute) can be provided.

Ionized hypocalcaemia is a frequent occurrence after initiation of extracorporeal membrane oxygenation and can contribute to hypotension on extracorporeal membrane oxygenation (Meliones *et al.*, 1991). 'Stunned myocardium' after extracorporeal membrane oxygenation is defined as left ventricular shortening fraction decrease by ⩾25 per cent with initiation of extracorporeal membrane oxygenation and returning to normal after 48 hours on extracorporeal membrane oxygenation (Martin *et al.*, 1991; Hirschl *et al.*, 1992; Holley *et al.*, 1994). This syndrome can occur despite relief of hypoxia. Underlying congenital heart disease can be 'masked' by respiratory failure in two per cent of cases requiring extracorporeal membrane oxygenation (Palmisano *et al.*, 1992). Veno–arterial extracorporeal membrane oxygenation is preferred over veno–venous support in these cases.

If cardiac arrest, dysrhythmia, or a drop in cardiac output secondary to severe myocardial dysfunction occurs, the initial treatment of choice while on veno–arterial extracorporeal membrane oxygenation is simply to increase the pump flow. This may require the addition of blood volume to the circuit. Continued extracorporeal membrane oxygenation or circulatory support is likely to be one of the most effective therapeutic measures. Treatment may include the administration of standard 'arrest' medications, correction of the electrolyte abnormalities, addition of antiarrhythmic agents, treatment with sympathomimetic agents or inotropes, or even countershock. If pump flow cannot be increased sufficiently to compensate for the fall in intrinsic cardiac output, or if the patient is on veno–venous extracorporeal membrane oxygenation, the episode must be handled much the same as a cardiac arrest in any other patient. Most importantly, the most common cause of cardiac dysfunction in ventilated neonates is hypoxia from respiratory, not cardiac failure. Assess the infant for inadvertent extubation or the development of a tension pneumothorax. The reason why one cannot achieve the desired extracorporeal membrane oxygenation flows may be that venous return to the patient's heart is being impeded by the accumulation of blood or air in the chest or pericardium (Zwischenberger and Bartlett, 1990).

Extreme acid-base imbalance caused by the addition of too much or too little CO_2 to the sweep gas, hypoxia caused by removal (or absence) of the tubing to the gas inlet port of the oxygenator, or hypovolaemia from failure to clamp the main bridge are just a few examples of the numerous ways in which circuit problems can precipitate such an event. The goal is to restore normal cardiac and respiratory function in the fastest and least traumatic manner possible. Once the potential problems outlined above have been eliminated, one should consider intrathoracic complications within the patient that can cause immediate haemodynamic deterioration on extracorporeal membrane oxygenation: pericardial tamponade and tension haemothorax or pneumothorax (Zwischenberger et al., 1988, 1989).

Pericardial tamponade and tension haemothorax and/ or pneumothorax show a similar pathophysiology of increasing intrapericardial pressure and decreasing venous return. Perfusion is initially maintained by the non-pulsatile flow of the extracorporeal membrane oxygenation flow and progressive haemodynamic deterioration. With decreased venous return to the heart, pulmonary blood flow as well as the native cardiac output are decreased. Therefore, the relative contribution of the extracorporeal circuit to peripheral perfusion is increased, and peripheral perfusion is initially maintained by the non-pulsatile flow of the extracorporeal membrane oxygenation circuit (post-oxygenator $pO_2 > 300$ torr). The PaO_2 will increase while the patient actually has decreased peripheral perfusion with a decreased pulse pressure and decreased SvO_2. Decreased SvO_2 confirms the decreased DO_2 achieved by the extracorporeal membrane oxygenation flow, and further haemodynamic deterioration of the patient. The triad of increased PaO_2, decreased peripheral perfusion (as evidenced by decreased pulse pressure and decreased SvO_2) followed by decreased extracorporeal membrane oxygenation flow with progressive haemodynamic deterioration is consistently associated with tension pneumothorax (Zwischenberger and Bartlett, 1990).

The diagnosis of tension haemothorax and pneumothorax is best confirmed by chest X-ray. Extracorporeal membrane oxygenation does not affect the classic appearance of tension haemothorax or pneumothorax on chest X-ray. Similarly, pericardial tamponade may be suggested on chest X-ray by enlargement of the cardiac silhouette. The most helpful tool, however, is an echocardiogram,

which will demonstrate a pericardial effusion and may also identify a haemothorax.

For emergency treatment of both tension haemothorax, pneumothorax and pericardial tamponade, a percutaneous drainage catheter should be placed to reverse the pathophysiology. For pericardial tamponade, placement of an angiocatheter into the pericardium using ultrasound guidance seems most safe and reliable. Once partial drainage using the angiocatheter has relieved the tamponade, a guide wire may be passed using a modified Seldinger technique to place a drainage tube with multiple holes (for example No. 5 Fr. paediatric feeding tube). For tension haemothorax and/or pneumothorax, a needle, angiocatheter and chest tube are all acceptable options for emergent decompression.

Sepsis is both an indication for and a complication of extracorporeal membrane oxygenation. However, according to the ELSO Registry, only five per cent of all patients requiring extracorporeal membrane oxygenation demonstrate positive blood cultures. This is a remarkably low incidence given the duration of cannulation, the large surface area involved and frequency of access to the circuit.

The pathophysiology of PFC is a right-to-left shunt and a patent ductus arteriosus during severe respiratory failure in the newborn. Therefore, when extracorporeal membrane oxygenation is initiated, a patent ductus arteriosus is always present. When pulmonary hypertension resolves, flow through the ductus reverses (becomes left-to-right shunting). A persistent left-to-right shunt across the ductus arteriosus may lead to pulmonary oedema. Decreased systemic oxygenation may result both from pulmonary oedema and decreased systemic blood flow. Both of these conditions will require increasing the extracorporeal membrane oxygenation flow to maintain adequate gas exchange and perfusion. Similarly, if renal failure occurs and a previous hypoxic or ischaemic insult cannot be identified, the possibility of decreased renal perfusion during extracorporeal membrane oxygenation as a result of a patent ductus arteriosus must be considered. Therefore, a patent ductus arteriosus on extracorporeal membrane oxygenation may present with various signs:

- a decreased $PaCO_2$
- decreased peripheral perfusion
- decreased urine output
- acidosis
- rising extracorporeal membrane oxygenation flow and volume requirements.

The clinical diagnosis may be confirmed as with other neonatal patients by use of Doppler echocardiography or angiography. Some centres have tried using intravenous indomethacin to treat patent ductus arteriosus while on extracorporeal membrane oxygenation; however, this may increase the risks of bleeding in patients on extracorporeal membrane oxygenation because of its effects on platelet function. Once the diagnosis is established, most pro-grammes will 'run the patient relatively dry' while main-taining supportive extracorporeal membrane oxygenation flow until the patent ductus arteriosus closes. Although this often means a few additional days on extracorporeal mem-brane oxygenation, surgical ligation is rarely necessary.

Occasionally, a patient's respiratory status does not improve despite two to three weeks of extracorporeal membrane oxygenation support. An echocardiogram is repeated to ensure an absence of patent ductus arteriosus with predominant left-to-right shunt as well as congenital heart defect such as total anomalous venous return. We then attempt to trial-off extracorporeal membrane oxy-genation with increased ventilator settings. If the patient fails repeated trial-off extracorporeal membrane oxygena-tion with increased ventilator settings, cardiac catheteri-zation and/or open lung biopsy must be considered to rule out a potentially irreversible disease process, such as congenital pulmonary lymphangiectasis. If no correctable lesions are found, a decision must be made to discon-tinue extracorporeal membrane oxygenation support or to continue indefinitely if there are objective signs of improvement without any complications.

CARDIAC SUPPORT

The pioneering usage of extracorporeal membrane oxy-genation in patients with severe cardiac failure was first reported in the 1950s but it was not commonly used until the 1980s (Bartlett et al., 1977). Although prior experience had shown success in infants with severe respiratory fail-ure, early results in post-operative cardiac failure were disappointing. Later experience demonstrated the effec-tiveness of extracorporeal membrane oxygenation in some post-cardiotomy patients. Considerations for extracor-poreal membrane oxygenation include the complexity of the heart defects, the need for continued heparinization to prevent clotting in the circuit and the incidence of infection related to the surgical implantation of the system (Zapol et al., 1979; Weinhaus et al., 1989; Anderson et al., 1990; Klein et al., 1990; Raithel et al., 1991).

Since then, the use of extracorporeal membrane oxy-genation has been extended to cardiac and pulmonary support after cardiac surgery in children and infants (Kanter et al., 1987; Bavaria et al., 1988). The first suc-cessful application of extracorporeal membrane oxy-genation in post-cardiotomy failure was reported by Soeter and colleagues in 1973 (Soeter et al., 1973). The effect of extracorporeal membrane oxygenation on the heart includes a decrease in pre-load, a slight increase in afterload and a concomitant elevation in left ventricular wall stress. Advantages include support of both right and left ventricles, improvement of systemic oxygenation and ease of placement. Extracorporeal membrane oxygenation support in post-cardiotomy patients may be provided

with either veno–arterial or veno–venous cannulation. Veno–arterial cannulation provides the optimal cardiac support when ventricular dysfunction is the predomi-nate clinical problem. However, studies have also shown that veno–venous bypass, primarily by improving venous oxygenation, may improve myocardial oxygenation and decrease pulmonary vascular resistance in selected patients, thus providing adequate cardiac recovery and support (Miyamura et al., 1996).

Cannulation

Veno–arterial extracorporeal membrane oxygenation may be performed by extrathoracic cannulation (carotid artery and jugular vein, or femoral artery and vein), or more commonly transthoracic cannulation through the median sternotomy incision (the aorta and the right atrium). Carotid–jugular cannulation may best be used in patients who are weaned from cardiopulmonary bypass in the operating room and develop myocardial dysfunc-tion with cardiogenic shock after operation. Advantages of this approach are a separate incision site remote from the median sternotomy wound and a lower incidence of bleeding from the mediastinal wound. Both of these factors may contribute to a decreased risk of mediastinal infection (Karl et al., 1990).

In patients with a cavopulmonary connection (Glenn or Fontan circulation), direct access from the jugular vein to the right atrium is not feasible; therefore, a trans-thoracic approach is required in these cases. Femoral arterio–venous cannulation can be used in certain older children, with placement of intravascular catheters into the inferior vena cava or right atrium through the femoral vein and into the common femoral or iliac artery for arterial return. The venous return with this type of cannulation may be restrictive unless a centrifugal type pump which provides active venous drainage is used. The advantage of this peripheral technique includes the noninvasive surgical approach and more secure cannula fixation.

Transthoracic cannulation is preferable in patients who cannot be weaned from cardiopulmonary bypass in the operating room or in those circumstances where the chest was opened for the purpose of resuscitation in the post-operative period. The major disadvantage of the transthoracic approach includes the potential risks of mediastinal haemorrhage, infection and cannula dislodg-ment during repositioning or transport. Anticoagulation with heparin is maintained with activated clotting times of approximately 200 s. If bleeding persists, the activated clot-ting time parameters can be lowered. The platelet count should be maintained >100,000/mm^3 with transfusions given as needed. The leukocyte-filtered and/or irradiated blood product should be used if transplantation is likely to occur. This avoids further pre-sensitization and antibody development that might promote allograft rejection, and also restricts cytomegalovirus exposure. The development of heparin-bonded circuits may help to reduce the need for significant anticoagulation, with its attendant risks (Fosse *et al.*, 1994). The standard cannulae for bypass can be converted to the extracorporeal membrane oxygenation circuit and brought out through or below the median sternotomy incision. Whenever possible, the sternum should be closed unless prevented by oedema of the myocardium. Closure will help to decrease the incidence of infection and bleeding during this period. The goal of extracorporeal membrane oxygenation support in patients after cardiac surgery differs from that in neonates with hypoxaemia resulting from pulmonary dysfunction. Maintenance of adequate tissue perfusion while providing complete or nearly complete cardiac bypass is the primary goal.

The prevention of cardiac distention and minimization of myocardial energy expenditure are vital to potential myocardial recovery. Flows as high as 150 mL/kg per minute are frequently needed to reduce both right and left atrial pressure. When left atrial pressures remain elevated despite optimal flow, it is critical to vent the left atrium to the venous drainage system. This scenario is frequently found in patients with multiple aortopulmonary collaterals. High flows should be maintained for 48–72 hours before attempting to wean from extracorporeal membrane oxygenation.

During extracorporeal membrane oxygenation support it is important to maintain adequate pulmonary ventilation to prevent atelectasis while recognizing that this may also create hypocarbia and excessive PaO_2. This should be controlled by reducing ventilatory rate (not tidal volume) and adjusting the O_2 and CO_2 flow to the membrane. Adequate tidal volume and extracorporeal flow rates should never be altered to manage PaO_2 or PCO_2. Veno–venous cannulation provides oxygenation support to venous blood. When myocardial dysfunction is primarily caused by inadequate oxygenation or elevated pulmonary vascular resistance, significant improvement may be accomplished by increasing the saturation of the venous blood. Such situations are uncommon in paediatric cardiac patients and thus veno–venous extracorporeal membrane oxygenation has infrequently been used in this patient population.

The pre-operative use of extracorporeal membrane oxygenation in infants with congenital heart disease is controversial (Table 15.7). In patients with cyanotic heart disease and cardiopulmonary collapse associated with hypercyanotic spells, pulmonary hypertension or sepsis, indications for extracorporeal membrane oxygenation includes arterial oxygen saturation <60 per cent on maximal medical therapy, with hypotension and metabolic acidosis (Karl *et al.*, 1990). The duration of extracorporeal membrane oxygenation support ranged from one to 38 days. Seven of eight patients underwent corrective or palliative surgery while on extracorporeal membrane oxygenation or within 48 hours after decannulation. The survival rate was 62 per cent, and survivors

Table 15.7 *Indications for extracorporeal membrane oxygenation support*

Pre-operative

Arterial O_2 saturation <60% on 100% FiO_2, maximal medical therapy support with inotropes, vasodilators and pharmacological paralysis and sedation, associated with hypotension and metabolic acidosis

Peri-operative

Inability to wean from cardiopulmonary bypass despite maximal inotropic therapy and/or intra-aortic balloon pump

Post-operative

Low cardiac output as defined by progressive decrease in urine output, elevated right atrial and left atrial filling pressures despite maximal inotropic support, widened atrio-ventricular O_2 difference

had normal growth and development. Other groups have also described the successful use of extracorporeal membrane oxygenation as a bridge to transplant in paediatric patients (Jurmann *et al.*, 1991) and as a lifesaving therapy after lung transplantation (Zenati *et al.*, 1996).

Intraoperative extracorporeal membrane oxygenation is used when a child cannot be weaned from cardiopulmonary bypass despite maximal inotropic therapy and optimal operative repair. Decisions about venting of the left ventricle at the time of initiation of extracorporeal membrane oxygenation in the operating room depend on the measurement of left atrial pressure on full extracorporeal membrane oxygenation support. If the left ventricle distends or left atrial pressure rises above 10 mmHg despite adequate flow rates, the left atrium should be vented. In the majority of patients placed on extracorporeal membrane oxygenation for inability to wean from cardiopulmonary bypass, extracorporeal membrane oxygenation is maintained via the original bypass cannulae. To improve and simplify venous return, bi-caval cannulation should be converted to a single venous cannula. The patient is then converted to a closed extracorporeal membrane oxygenation system with brief clamping of the cannulae and connection of sterile lines on the operative field. In patients with systemic-to-pulmonary shunts, pulmonary blood flow can be limited by partial occlusion of the shunt. This may be opened gradually to provide pulmonary blood flow and possible pulmonary parenchymal nutrition before weaning from extracorporeal membrane oxygenation.

The development of postoperative low cardiac output requiring extracorporeal membrane oxygenation support represents a unique group of patients. These patients usually present with decreased urine output (<1 mL/kg per hour), poor peripheral perfusion, low systemic venous saturation (wide AVO_2 difference) and elevated filling pressures despite maximal inotropic and diuretic support. Myocardial injury in these patients is usually less than in those who cannot be weaned from cardiopulmonary bypass. The interval between surgery and initiation of extracorporeal membrane oxygenation may provide sufficient time for recovery of normal coagulation, an important factor which may positively affect the outcome of these infants and children (Weinhaus *et al.*, 1989).

Weaning

The ability to decrease inotropic support along with improvement in renal function and diuresis of retained fluid are initial indicators of myocardial recovery. After a period of time in which myocardial contractility is permitted to improve, an attempt is made to wean from extracorporeal membrane oxygenation. With reasonable inotropic support, extracorporeal membrane oxygenation flow is gradually lowered to 100–200 mL/min. If myocardial contractility remains satisfactory, and the filling pressures are low, decannulation may be accomplished.

Complications

As previously discussed, mechanical support of infants and children with extracorporeal membrane oxygenation results in several possible complications. The major complication of post-cardiotomy extracorporeal membrane oxygenation in paediatric patients is haemorrhage. Approximately 40–50 per cent of children require re-exploration for haemorrhage during the time of support. To minimize the magnitude of bleeding, the activated clotting time is maintained at approximately 200 s and the platelet count is kept >100,000/mm^3. The primary determinant of significant haemorrhage is the duration of extracorporeal membrane oxygenation (Sell *et al.*, 1986). Keeping the chest open is sometimes necessary to facilitate re-exploration and to prevent periods of cardiac tamponade. The use of heparin-coated circuits and oxygenators presents promising possibilities, with improved biocompatibility and less complement activation (Karl, 1994). Another important complication of prolonged extracorporeal membrane oxygenation is mediastinal infection and sepsis. This is a result of continued bleeding from mediastinal structures, multiple cannulae and catheters in the mediastinal cavity, exiting through the skin, low cardiac and renal output, and multiple transfusions. To decrease the incidence of infection, broad-spectrum coverage with antibiotics and aseptic technique, with attempts to minimize the time on extracorporeal membrane oxygenation are encouraged.

Clinical results

The results of extracorporeal membrane oxygenation for paediatric cardiac support, reported by numerous investigators, are summarized in Table 15.8. Early survival was 40–44 per cent, with somewhat better survival

Table 15.8 *Extracorporeal membrane oxygenation for cardiac support*

Author	Year	No. of patients	Survival (%)
Bartlett *et al.*	1977	4	25
Pennington *et al.*	1984	4	75
Redmond *et al.*	1987	9	55.6
Kanter *et al.*	1987	13	26
Rogers *et al.*	1989	10	70
Weinhaus *et al.*	1989	14	35.7
Klein *et al.*	1990	36	61
Delius *et al.*	1990	6	33.3
Galantowicz and Stolar	1991	20	20
Ziomek *et al.*	1992	24	54
Raithel *et al.*	1992	65	35
Hunkeler *et al.*	1992	8	62.5
del Nido *et al.*	1992	11	64
del Nido *et al.*	1994	14	50
Walters *et al.*	1995	73	57.5
Black *et al.*	1995	31	45
del Nido	1996	68 (14 bridge-to-transplant; resuscitation post-arrest)	38
Wang *et al.*	1996	18	33.3
Kulik *et al.*	1996	64	33
Ishino *et al.*	1996	6	33.3
Doski *et al.*	1997	839	60.8
Peek and Firmin	1997	–	43–61
Ko *et al.*	1997	3	100
Saker *et al.*	1997	1	100
Goldman *et al.*	1997	12	66
Trittenwein *et al.*	1997	3	100
Langley *et al.*	1998	9	22
Duncan *et al.*	1998	11	64
Delius	1998	22	50
Younger *et al.*	1999	21	36
Magovern and Simpson	1999	55	36
Hopper *et al.*	1999	32	56
Pagani *et al.*	1999	14	43
Jaski *et al.*	1999	10	40
Ibrahim *et al.*	2000	26	96
Duncan *et al.*	2001	12	83
Aharon *et al.*	2001	50	50
Kirshborn *et al.*	2002	31	39 (ECMO pre-tx)
		12	33 (ECMO post-tx)

(43–54 per cent) when the lesion was tetralogy of Fallot, truncus arteriosus, atrio–ventricular canal or total anomalous pulmonary venous return. Lower survival rates (14 per cent) have been reported for single ventricle, hypoplastic left heart syndrome, and other malformations requiring a Fontan procedure. Difference in survival rates suggests that the improved survival is associated with a complete bi-ventricular operative repair while an operation with shunt dependent pulmonary blood flow is associated with lower overall recovery rates. A decreased survival rate of 0–27 per cent is found when the patient is unable to be weaned from cardiopulmonary bypass, suggesting a greater degree of myocardial damage in these patients.

THE FUTURE

The future of extracorporeal support depends on the development of techniques and devices to make the technique less invasive, safer and simpler in management. The use of percutaneous catheters without surgical exploration can reduce potential bleeding wounds. Most extracorporeal membrane oxygenation for respiratory support will be carried out in the veno–venous mode using a single catheter with two lumens or a single-lumen tidal flow system. Percutaneous access has become the favourable approach for patients over the age of two. The use of the Seldinger wire-guided technique with sequential dilators and placement of large catheters directly, or with peel-away sheaths, has had an impact on decreasing the incidence of bleeding complications from cannulation sites. Cannulation can be accomplished quickly and easily under a variety of circumstances, including on-extracorporeal membrane oxygenation transport and emergency access.

The future of extracorporeal membrane oxygenation also includes laminar flow oxygenators; safe, simple automatic pumps; non-thrombogenic surfaces to eliminate bleeding complications; advances in respiratory and cardiac care; and new approaches to clinical trials. A system for long-term extracorporeal membrane oxygenation with reduced heparinization and minimal plasma leakage has been reported (Kitano et al., 1997). Although the initial intravenacaval gas exchange device (IVOX®) trials identified problems of inadequate gas exchange and technical placement difficulties, they also showed that non-thrombogenic coating and a totally implantable prosthetic lung is possible (Conrad et al., 1994). Temporary or permanent implantable devices may have a major role in the future of mechanical support for respiratory failure. The servo-regulated roller pump will be replaced by simpler, safer pumps including electronically servo-regulated centrifugal pumps, mechanically servo-regulated peristaltic pumps or ventricle pumps.

Heparin-bonded oxygenators, pump chambers and extracorporeal circuits may allow extracorporeal membrane oxygenation for days without bleeding, complications or formation of clots. Systemic heparinization is still required, primarily because if extracorporeal membrane oxygenation must be interrupted for any reason, blood in the circuit will clot very quickly. Unfortunately, the thrombocytopenia and platelet dysfunction that

accompanies extracorporeal membrane oxygenation has not been eliminated by the availability of heparin-bonded circuits. Heparin-bonded circuits have been used for extracorporeal membrane oxygenation in patients with major coagulopathies who are bleeding significantly at the time extracorporeal membrane oxygenation is instituted. This advance makes it possible to use extracorporeal membrane oxygenation for patients who cannot come off conventional cardiopulmonary bypass in the operating room, patients with major trauma and active bleeding, and patients after major operations, such as thoracotomy for lung transplantation.

Once the extracorporeal circuit has been exposed to blood, even a conventional plastic circuit without heparin bonding can be used for hours or days without clotting as long as high-flow extracorporeal membrane oxygenation is maintained. In the future, combinations of surface coatings including heparin and modifications to minimize platelet adherence with low-level anticoagulation, will further extend the use of extracorporeal membrane oxygenation. Various groups have tested heparin-coated circuits and reported reduced thrombogenicity and reductions in required systemic heparinization for prolonged support (Nojiri et al., 1995; Palmer et al., 1995; Moen et al., 1996; Weerwind et al., 1998). Recently, the use of nitric oxide in the sweep gas to decrease platelet adhesion has been proposed (Mellgren et al., 1996).

With improvement in technique, and simplification of extracorporeal membrane oxygenation, the indications may be expanded. With improved circuit safety, single-vein access and minimal anticoagulation, indications for extracorporeal membrane oxygenation will change from moribund patients to patients with moderate respiratory and cardiac failure. Extracorporeal membrane oxygenation will become an adjunct therapy option to conventional ventilation and pharmacological management rather than something to try when standard ventilation and pharmacology is failing. At the same time, simpler methods of treatment of acute pulmonary and cardiac failure may significantly decrease the need for extracorporeal membrane oxygenation. Extracorporeal membrane oxygenation will continue to gain wider application as temporary mechanical support of the circulation in children and adults with cardiac failure. New applications of extracorporeal membrane oxygenation will include emergency room and cath lab resuscitation in cardiac failure, resuscitation in trauma and haemorrhagic shock, and use as an adjunct to perfusion and temperature control. Many of the lessons learnt in extracorporeal membrane oxygenation have already been applied to bypass for cardiac surgery (servo-regulation, mixed venous saturation monitoring, membrane lungs, standardized descriptors of vascular access catheters).

Extracorporeal membrane oxygenation has led to better understanding of pulmonary pathophysiology. It has changed the management of congenital diaphragmatic hernia from a rush to the operating room to intensive care unit management until the relief of pulmonary hypertension with elective repair of the defect days or even weeks after birth. Extracorporeal membrane oxygenation permits the evaluation of innovative approaches to lung hypoplasia in the newborn, and earlier and more extensive use of extracorporeal membrane oxygenation will lead to the study of pharmacological agents to reverse fibrosis and growth factors to enhance lung growth. The study of extracorporeal membrane oxygenation has brought the proper emphasis to the separation of oxygenation from CO_2 removal and the realization that high peak airway pressure during attempted hyperventilation for CO_2 clearance is the major culprit in ventilator-induced injury. A return to pressure limited mechanical ventilation has occurred, with extracorporeal membrane oxygenation acting as an adjunct when low pressure mechanical ventilation does not achieve adequate CO_2 clearance.

Different techniques (nitric oxide, pressure controlled inverse ratio ventilation and permissive hypercapnia, intravenous oxygenation (IVOX), arterio–venous carbon dioxide removal ($AVCO_2R$) (Zwischenberger et al., 1999; Conrad et al., 2001), liquid ventilation, and a paracorporeal artificial lung (PAL) (Lynch et al., 2000; Haft et al., 2001; Lick et al., 2001; Zwischenberger et al., 2002)) highlight the fact that the tools used to sustain gas exchange in the patient with respiratory failure in the near future may be very different from now. The availability of extracorporeal membrane oxygenation has made it possible to study these innovative and numerous methods of lung management. Currently, acute respiratory distress syndrome is primarily treated with mechanical ventilation, aimed at restoring normal blood gases by manipulating minute ventilation and oxygen concentration while the lungs recover from the initial injury or disease process.

The array of alternative ventilator management strategies that can be used in the management of acute respiratory distress syndrome is impressive. Despite the religious zeal with which many such strategies are defended, few prospective clinical trials can confirm the effectiveness in terms of improving survival. 'Cousins' of extracorporeal membrane oxygenation, intravascular (intravenacaval or IVOX) gas exchange devices and $AVCO_2R$ are designed to supply supplemental gas exchange with the potential for percutaneous access and 'routine' intensive care management. Despite spectacular results in reported individuals, the multicentre trials on IVOX, NO and partial liquid ventilation have all been disappointing.

Clinical experiments comparing extracorporeal membrane oxygenation to other treatments are difficult because blinding is impossible and 'standard therapy' is not standardized and changes frequently. Furthermore, an extensive learning curve is required for many of the newer techniques before definitive study, and randomization may be refused. The best way to evaluate new methods in life

support technology will continue to be the approach used by Timmons and Green in the Pediatric Respiratory Failure evaluation (Philips, 1990; Green et al., 1995). Data were pooled into a common database and evaluated by multivariate analysis to determine which factors were associated with death or survival. Data were further analysed by a matched-pairs analysis. This approach to evaluation of life support techniques when applied in a prospective fashion has significant advantages over randomized studies and is the best method of analysis for the future.

REFERENCES

Adolph, V., Flageole, H., Perreault, T. et al. 1995: Repair of congenital diaphragmatic hernia after weaning from extracorporeal membrane oxygenation. Journal of Pediatric Surgery 30, 349–52.

Adzick, N.S., Harrison, M.R., Glick, P.L., Nakayama, D.K., Manning, F.A., deLorimier, A.A. 1985: Diaphragmatic hernia in the fetus: prenatal diagnosis and outcome in 94 cases. Journal of Pediatric Surgery 20, 357–61.

Aharon, A.S., Drinkwater, D.C. Jr., Churchwell, K.B. et al. 2001: Extracorporeal membrane oxygenation in children after repair of congenital cardiac lesions. Annals of Thoracic Surgery 72, 2095–102.

Alexander, A.A., Mitchell, D.G., Merton, D.A. et al. 1992: Cannula-induced vertebral steal in neonates during extracorporeal membrane oxygenation: detection with color Doppler US. Radiology 182, 527–30.

von Allmen, D., Babcock, D., Matsumoto, J. et al. 1992: The predictive value of head ultrasound in the ECMO candidate. Journal of Pediatric Surgery 27, 36–9.

Almond, P.S., Adolph, V.R., Steiner, R., Hill, C.B., Falterman, K.W., Arensman, R.M. 1992: Calculous disease of the biliary tract in infants after neonatal extracorporeal membrane oxygenation. Journal of Perinatology 12, 18–20.

Anderson, H.L., Bartlett, R.H. 1991: Elective tracheostomy for mechanical ventilation by the percutaneous technique. In: Jeffer, J.D., ed. Clinic in chest medicine. Philadelphia, PA: WB Saunders: 555–60.

Anderson, H.L. III, Cilley, R.E., Zwischenberger, J.B., Bartlett, R.H. 1986: Thrombocytopenia in neonates after extracorporeal membrane oxygenation. ASAIO Trans 32, 534–7.

Anderson, H.L., Attorri, R.J., Custer, J.R. 1990: Extracorporeal membrane oxygenation for pediatric cardiopulmonary failure. Journal of Thoracic and Cardiovascular Surgery 99, 1011–21.

Anderson, H.L. III, Otsu, T., Chapman, R.A., Bartlett, R.H. 1989: Venovenous extracorporeal life support in neonates using a double lumen catheter. ASAIO Trans 35, 650–3.

Anderson, H.L. III, Delius, R.E., Sinard, J.M. et al. 1992: Early experience with adult extracorporeal membrane oxygenation in the modern era. Annals of Thoracic Surgery 53, 553–63.

Anderson, H. III, Steimle, C., Shapiro, M. et al. 1993a: Extracorporeal life support for adult cardiorespiratory failure. Surgery 114, 161–73.

Anderson, H.L. III, Snedecor, S.M., Otsu, T., Bartlett, R.H. 1993b: Multicenter comparison of conventional venoarterial access versus venovenous double-lumen catheter access in newborn infants undergoing extracorporeal membrane oxygenation. *Journal of Pediatric Surgery* **28**, 530–4.

Anderson, H.L., Shapiro, M.B., Delius, R.E. 1994: Extracorporeal life support for respiratory failure after multiple trauma. *Journal of Trauma* **37**, 266–72.

Atkinson, J.B., Ford, E.G., Humphries, B. *et al.* 1991: The impact of extracorporeal membrane support in the treatment of congenital diaphragmatic hernia. *Journal of Pediatric Surgery* **26**, 791–3.

Bailey, P.V., Connors, R.H., Tracy, T.F. Jr, Stephens, C., Pennington, D.G., Weber, T.R. 1989: A critical analysis of extracorporeal membrane oxygenation for congenital diaphragmatic hernia. *Surgery* **106**, 611–15.

Bartlett, R.H. 1986: Respiratory support with extracorporeal membrane oxygenation in newborn respiratory failure. In: Welch, K., Randolph, J., Ravitch, M., eds. *Pediatric surgery* (fourth edition). Chicago, IL: Year Book Medical Publishers: 74–7.

Bartlett, R.H. 1990: Extracorporeal life support for cardiopulmonary failure. *Current Problems Surgery* **27**, 621–705.

Bartlett, R.H. 1995: Physiology of extracorporeal life support. In: Zwischenberger, J.B., Bartlett, R.H., eds. *ECMO. Extracorporeal cardiopulmonary support in critical care.* Ann Arbor, MI: Extracorporeal Life Support Organization: 27–52.

Bartlett, R.H., Gazzaniga, A.B. 1978: Extracorporeal circulation for cardiopulmonary failure. *Current Problems in Surgery* **15**, 1–96.

Bartlett, R.H., Drinker, P.A., Burns, N.E., Fong, S.W., Hyans, T. 1972: The toroidal membrane oxygenator: design, performance, and prolonged bypass testing of a clinical model. *Transactions of the American Society for Artificial Internal Organs* **18**, 369–74.

Bartlett, R.H., Gazzaniga, A.B., Jefferies, M.R. *et al.* 1976: Extracorporeal membrane oxygenation (ECMO) cardiopulmonary support in infancy. *Transactions of the American Society for Artificial Internal Organs* **22**, 80–93.

Bartlett, R.H., Gazzaniga, A.B., Fong, S.W., Jefferies, M.R., Roohk, H.V., Haiduc, N. 1977: Extracorporeal membrane oxygenator support for cardiopulmonary failure. Experience in 28 cases. *Journal of Thoracic and Cardiovascular Surgery* **73**, 375–86.

Bartlett, R.H., Gazzaniga, A.B., Wetmore, N.E., Rucker, R., Huxtable, R.F. 1980: Extracorporeal membrane oxygenation (ECMO) in the treatment of cardiac and respiratory failure in children. *Transactions of the American Society for Artificial Internal Organs* **26**, 578–81.

Bartlett, R.H., Andrews, A.F., Toomasian, J.M., Haiduc, N.J., Gazzaniga, A.B. 1982a: Extracorporeal membrane oxygenation for newborn respiratory failure: forty-five cases. *Surgery* **92**, 425–33.

Bartlett, R.H., Dechert, R.E., Mault, J., Ferguson, S., Kaiser, A.M., Erlandson, E.E. 1982b: Measurement of metabolism in multiple organ failure. *Surgery* **92**, 771–8.

Bartlett, R.H., Roloff, D.W., Cornell, R.G., Andrews, A.F., Dillon, P.W., Zwischenberger, J.B. 1985: Extracorporeal circulation in neonatal respiratory failure: a prospective randomized study. *Pediatrics* **76**, 479–87.

Bartlett, R.H., Gazzaniga, A.B., Toomasian, J., Coran, A.G., Roloff, D., Rucker, R. 1986: Extracorporeal membrane oxygenation (ECMO) in neonatal respiratory failure: 100 cases. *Annals of Surgery* **204**, 236–45.

Baumgart, S., Streletz, L.J., Needleman, L. *et al.* 1994: Right common carotid artery reconstruction after extracorporeal membrane oxygenation: vascular imaging, cerebral circulation, electroencephalographic, and neurodevelopmental correlates to recovery. *Journal of Pediatrics* **125**, 295–304.

Bavaria, J.E., Ratcliff, M.B., Gupta, K.B. 1988: Changes in left ventricular systolic wall stress during biventricular circulatory assistance. *Annals of Thoracic Surgery* **45**, 526–32.

Bergman, P., Belboul, A., Friberg, L.G., Al-Khaja, N., Mellgren, G., Roberts, D. 1994: The effect of prolonged perfusion with a membrane oxygenator (PPMO) on white blood cells. *Perfusion* **9**, 35–40.

Black, M.D., Coles, J.G., Williams, W.G. *et al.* 1995: Determinants of success in pediatric cardiac patients undergoing extracorporeal membrane oxygenation. *Annals of Thoracic Surgery* **60**, 133–8.

Bone, R.C. 1986: Extracorporeal membrane oxygenation for acute respiratory failure. *Journal of the American Medical Association* **256**, 910.

Brunet, F., Mira, J.P., Belghith, M. *et al.* 1992: Effects of aprotinin on haemorrhagic complications in acute respiratory distress syndrome patients during prolonged extracorporeal CO_2 removal. *Intensive Care Medicine* **18**, 364–7.

Bryant, L.R., Trinkle, J.K., Mobin-Uddin, K. 1972: Bacterial colonization profile with tracheal intubation and mechanical ventilation. *Archives of Surgery* **104**, 647–51.

Campbell, L.R., Bunyapen, C., Holmes, G.L., Howell, C.G. Jr, Kanto, W.P. Jr. 1988: Right common carotid artery ligation in extracorporeal membrane oxygenation. *Journal of Pediatrics* **113**, 110–13.

Cavarocchi, N.C., England, M.D., Schaff, H.V. *et al.* 1986: Oxygen free radical generation during cardiopulmonary bypass: correlation with complement activation. *Circulation* **74**, III130–3.

Chevalier, J.Y., Couprie, C., Larroquet, M. *et al.* 1993: Venovenous single lumen cannula extracorporeal lung support in neonates. A five year experience. *ASAIO Journal* **39**, M654–8.

Cilley, R.E., Zwischenberger, J.B., Andrews, A.F., Bowerman, R.A., Roloff, D.W., Bartlett, R.H. 1986: Intracranial haemorrhage during extracorporeal membrane oxygenation in neonates. *Pediatrics* **78**, 699–704.

Cilley, R.E., Wesley, J.R., Zwischenberger, J.B. 1987: Metabolic rates of newborn infants with severe respiratory failure treated with extracorporeal membrane oxygenation. *Curr Surg* **44**, 48–51.

Clowes, J. Jr, Hopkins, A.L., Nevill, W.E. 1956: An artificial lung dependent upon diffusion of oxygen and carbon dioxide through plastic membranes. *Journal of Thoracic and Cardiovascular Surgery* **32**, 630–7.

Collaborative UK ECMO (extracorporeal membrane oxygenation) Trial. 1998: Follow-up to 1 year of age. *Pediatrics* **101**, E1.

Connors, R.H., Tracy, T. Jr, Bailey, P.V., Kountzman, B., Weber, T.R. 1990: Congenital diaphragmatic hernia repair on extracorporeal membrane oxygenation. *Journal of Pediatrics Surgery* **25**, 1043–6.

Conrad, S.A. 1995: Selection criteria for use of extracorporeal membrane oxygenation in adults. In: Zwischenberger, J.B., Bartlett, R.H., eds. *ECMO. Extracorporeal cardiopulmonary support in critical care.* Ann Arbor, MI: Extracorporeal Life Support Organization: 385–400.

Conrad, S.A., Zwischenberger, J.B., Eggerstedt, J.M., Bidani, A. 1994: In vivo gas transfer performance of the intravascular oxygenator in acute respiratory failure. *Artificial Organs* **18**, 840–5.

Conrad, S.A., Zwischenberger, J.B., Grier, L.R., Alpard, S.K., Bidani, A. 2001: Total extracorporeal arteriovenous carbon dioxide removal in acute respiratory failure: a phase I clinical study. *Intensive Care Medicine* **27**, 1340–51.

Cox, C.S., Zwischenberger, J.B., Graves, D., Raymond, G. 1992: Mortality from acute respiratory distress syndrome remains unchanged. *American Review of Respiratory Disease* **145**, A83.

Cunningham, A.J. 1991: Acute respiratory distress syndrome – two decades later. *Yale Journal of Biology and Medicine* **64**, 387–402.

D'Agostino, J.A., Bernbaum, J.C., Gerdes, M. *et al.* 1995: Outcome for infants with congenital diaphragmatic hernia requiring extracorporeal membrane oxygenation: the first year. *Journal of Pediatric Surgery* **30**, 10–15.

Dal Nogare, A.R. 1989: Adult respiratory distress syndrome. *American Journal of Medical Science* **298**, 413–30.

Delaney, A.G., Zapol, W.M., Erdmann, A.J. III. 1979: Lung transvascular fluid dynamics with extracorporeal membrane oxygenation in unanesthetized lambs. *Journal of Thoracic and Cardiovascular Surgery* **77**, 252–8.

Delius, R.E. 1998: As originally published in 1990: Prolonged extracorporeal life support of pediatric and adolescent cardiac transplant patients. Updated in 1998. *Annals of Thoracic Surgery* **65**, 877–8.

Delius, R.E., Zwischenberger, J.B., Cilley, R. *et al.* 1990: Prolonged extracorporeal life support of pediatric and adolescent cardiac transplant patients. *Annals of Thoracic Surgery* **50**, 791–5.

DePalma, L., Short, B.L., Van Meurs, K., Luban, N.L. 1991: A flow cytometric analysis of lymphocyte subpopulations in neonates undergoing extracorporeal membrane oxygenation. *Journal of Pediatrics* **118**, 117–20.

De Puydt, L.E., Schuit, K.E., Smith, S.D. 1993: Effect of extracorporeal membrane oxygenation on neutrophil function in neonates. *Critical Care Medicine* **21**, 1324–7.

Desai, S.A., Stanley, C., Gringlas, M. *et al.* 1999: Five-year follow-up of neonates with reconstructed right common carotid arteries after extracorporeal membrane oxygenation. *Journal of Pediatrics* **134**, 428–33.

Dietrich, W., Barankay, A., Dilthey, G. *et al.* 1989: Reduction of homologous blood requirement in cardiac surgery by intraoperative aprotinin application – clinical experience in 152 cardiac surgical patients. *Thoracic Cardiovascular Surgery* **37**, 92–8.

Dorson, W. Jr, Meyer, B., Baker, E. *et al.* 1970: Response of distressed infants to partial bypass lung assist. *Transactions of the American Society for Artificial Internal Organs* **16**, 345–51.

Doski, J.J., Butler, T.J., Louder, D.S., Dickey, L.A., Cheu, H.W. 1997: Outcome of infants requiring cardiopulmonary resuscitation before extracorporeal membrane oxygenation. *Journal of Pediatric Surgery* **32**, 1318–21.

Downard, C.D., Betit, P., Chang, R.W., Garza, J.J., Arnold, J.H., Wilson, J.M. 2003: Impact of AMICAR on hemorrhagic complications of ECMO: a ten-year review. *Journal of Pediatric Surgery* **38**, 1212–16.

Duncan, B.W., Ibrahim, A.E., Hraska, V. *et al.* 1998: Use of rapid-deployment extracorporeal membrane oxygenation for the resuscitation of pediatric patients with heart disease after cardiac arrest. *Journal of Thoracic and Cardiovascular Surgery* **116**, 305–11.

Duncan, B.W., Bohn, D.J., Atz, A.M., French, J.W., Laussen, P.C., Wessel, D.L. 2001: Mechanical circulatory support for the treatment of children with acute fulminant myocarditis. *Journal of Thoracic and Cardiovascular Surgery* **122**, 440–8.

Dutton, R.C., Edmunds, L.H. Jr, Hutchinson, J.C., Roe, B.B. 1974: Platelet aggregate emboli produced in patients during cardiopulmonary bypass with membrane and bubble oxygenators and blood filters. *Journal of Thoracic and Cardiovascular Surgery* **67**, 258–65.

Eberhart, R.C. 1993: Interactions of blood and artificial surfaces: in search of 'heparin-free' cardiopulmonary bypass. In: Arensman, R.M., Cornish, J.D., eds. *Extracorporeal life support.* Boston, MA: Blackwell Scientific:105–25.

Extracorporeal Life Support (ECLS) Organization. 1998: *ECMO Registry report.* Ann Arbor, MI: Extracorporeal Life Support Organization.

Extracorporeal Life Support (ECLS) Organization. 1999: *ECMO Registry report.* Ann Arbor, MI: Extracorporeal Life Support Organization.

Extracorporeal Life Support (ECLS) Organization. 2000: *Registry report.* Ann Arbor: MI: Extracorporeal Life Support Organization.

Extracorporeal Life Support (ECLS) Organization. January 2004: *Registry report.* Ann Arbor: MI: Extracorporeal Life Support Organization.

Faulkner, S.C., Chipman, C.W., Baker, L.L. 1993: Trouble shooting the extracorporeal membrane oxygenator circuit and patient. *Journal of Extracorporeal Technology* **24**, 120–9.

Feindt, P., Volkmer, I., Seyfert, U., Huwer, H., Kalweit, G., Gams, E. 1993: Activated clotting time, anticoagulation, use of heparin, and thrombin activation during extracorporeal circulation: changes under aprotinin therapy. *Thoracic Cardiovascular Surgery* **41**, 9–15.

Finer, N.N., Tierney, A.J., Hallgren, R., Hayashi, A., Peliowski, A., Etches, P.C. 1992: Neonatal congenital diaphragmatic hernia and extracorporeal membrane oxygenation. *CMAJ* **146**, 501–8.

Fortenberry, J.D., Meier, A.H., Pettignano, R., Heard, M., Chambliss, C.R., Wulkam, M., 2003: Extracorporeal life support for posttraumatic acute respiratory distress syndrome at a children's medical center. *Journal of Pediatric Surgery* **38**, 1221–6.

Fosse, E., Moen, O., Johnson, E. 1994: Reduced complement and granulocyte activation with heparin-coated cardiopulmonary bypass. *Annals of Thoracic Surgery* **58**, 472–4.

Foster, A.H., Kolobow, T. 1987: A potential hazard of ventilation during early separation from total cardiopulmonary bypass. *Journal of Thoracic and Cardiovascular Surgery* **93**, 150–1.

Fraedrich, G., Weber, C., Bernard, C., Hettwer, A., Schlosser, V. 1989: Reduction of blood transfusion requirement in open heart surgery by administration of high doses of aprotinin – preliminary results. *Thoracic Cardiovascular Surgery* **37**, 89–91.

Galantowicz, M.E., Stolar, C.J. 1991: Extracorporeal membrane oxygenation for perioperative support in pediatric heart transplantation. *Journal of Thoracic and Cardiovascular Surgery* **102**, 148–52.

Galletti, P.M., Richardson, P.D., Snider, M.T. 1972: A standardized method for defining the overall gas transfer performance of artificial lungs. *Transactions of the American Society for Artificial Internal Organs* **18**, 359–68.

Gattinoni, L., Pesenti, A., Mascheroni, D. *et al.* 1986: Low-frequency positive-pressure ventilation with extracorporeal CO_2 removal in severe acute respiratory failure. *Journal of the American Medical Association* **256**, 881–6.

Gibbon, J.H. Jr. 1937: Artificial maintenance of circulation during experimental occlusion of the pulmonary artery. *Archives of Surgery* **34**, 1105–31.

Gille, J.P. 1975: World census on long-term perfusion for respiratory support. In: Zapol, W.M., Qvist, J., eds. *First International Conference on Membrane Technology.* Copenhagen.

Gille, J.P., Bagniewski, A.M. 1976: Ten years of use of extracorporeal membrane oxygenation (ECMO) in the treatment of acute respiratory insufficiency (ARI). *Transactions of the American Society for Artificial Internal Organs* **22**, 102–9.

Glass, P. 1993: Patient neurodevelopmental outcomes after neonatal extracorporeal membrane oxygenation. In: Arensman, R.M., Cornish, J.D., eds. *Extracorporeal life support.* Boston, MA: Blackwell Scientific Publications: 241–51.

Glass, P., Miller, M.K., Short, B.L. 1989: Morbidity for survivors of extracorporeal membrane oxygenation: neurodevelopmental outcome at 1 year of age. *Pediatrics* **83**, 72–8.

Glass, P., Wagner, A.E., Papero, P.H. 1995: Neurodevelopmental status at age five years of neonates treated with extracorporeal membrane oxygenation. *Journal of Pediatrics* **127**, 447–57.

Gleason, L.A. 1993: ECMO and the brain. In: Arensman, R.M., Cornish, J.D., eds. *Extracorporeal life support.* Boston, MA: Blackwell Scientific: 138–55.

Goldman, A.P., Kerr, S.J., Butt, W. *et al.* 1997: Extracorporeal support for intractable cardiorespiratory failure due to meningococcal disease. *Lancet* **349**, 466–9.

Graziani, L.J., Streletz, L.J., Baumgart, S. 1994: The predictive value of neonatal electroencephalograms before and during extracorporeal membrane oxygenation. *Journal of Pediatrics* **125**, 969–75.

Graziani, L.J., Baumgart, S., Desai, S., Stanley, C., Gringlas, M., Spitzer, A.R. 1997a: Clinical antecedents of neurologic and audiologic abnormalities in survivors of neonatal ECMO. *Journal of Child Neurology* **12**, 415–22.

Graziani, L.J., Gringlas, M., Baumgart, S. 1997b: Cerebrovascular complications and neurodevelopmental sequelae of neonatal ECMO. *Clin Perinatol* **24**, 655–75.

Green, T.P., Moler, F.W., Goodman, D.M. 1995: Probability of survival after prolonged extracorporeal membrane oxygenation in pediatric patients with acute respiratory failure. *Critical Care Medicine* **23**, 1132–9.

Green, T.P., Timmons, O.D., Fackler, J.C., Moler, F.W., Thompson, A.E., Sweeney, M.F. 1996: The impact of extracorporeal membrane oxygenation on survival in pediatric patients with acute respiratory failure. Pediatric Critical Care Study Group. *Critical Care Medicine* **24**, 323–9.

Haft, J.W., Montoya, P., Alnajjar, D. *et al.* 2001: An artificial lung reduces pulmonary impedence and improves right ventricular efficiency in pulmonary hypertension. *Journal of Thoracic and Cardiovascular Surgery* **122**, 1094–100.

Hanson, E.L., Bartlett, R.H., Burns, N.E. *et al.* 1973: Prolonged use of a membrane oxygenator in air-breathing and hypoxic lambs. *Surgery* **73**, 284–98.

Hardesty, R.L., Griffith, B.P., Debski, R.F., Jeffries, M.R., Borovetz, H.S. 1981: Extracorporeal membrane oxygenation. Successful treatment of persistent fetal circulation following repair of congenital diaphragmatic hernia. *Journal of Thoracic and Cardiovascular Surgery* **81**, 556–63.

Harrison, M.R., Adzick, N.S., Estes, J.M., Howell, L.J. 1994: A prospective study of the outcome for fetuses with diaphragmatic hernia. *Journal of the American Medical Association* **271**, 382–4.

Heiss, K., Manning, P., Oldham, K.T. *et al.* 1989: Reversal of mortality for congenital diaphragmatic hernia with ECMO. *Annals of Surgery* **209**, 225–30.

Hicks, R.E., Dutton, R.C., Ries, C.A., Price, D.C., Edmunds, L.H. Jr. 1973: Production and fate of platelet aggregate emboli during venovenous perfusion. *Surgery Forum* **24**, 250–2.

Hill, J.D., O'Brien, T.G., Murray, J.J. *et al.* 1972: Prolonged extracorporeal oxygenation for acute post-traumatic respiratory failure (shock-lung syndrome). Use of the Bramson membrane lung. *New England Journal of Medicine* **286**, 629–34.

Hirschl, R.B., Heiss, K.F., Bartlett, R.H. 1992: Severe myocardial dysfunction during extracorporeal membrane oxygenation. *Journal of Pediatric Surgery* **27**, 48–53.

Hirthler, M.A., Blackwell, E., Abbe, D. *et al.* 1992: Coagulation parameter instability as an early predictor of intracranial hemorrhage during extracorporeal membrane oxygenation. *Journal of Pediatric Surgery* **27**, 40–3.

Hocker, J.R., Wellhausen, S.R., Ward, R.A., Simpson, P.M., Cook, L.N. 1991: Effect of extracorporeal membrane oxygenation on leukocyte function in neonates. *Artificial Organs* **15**, 23–8.

Holley, D.G., Short, B.L., Karr, S.S., Martin, G.R. 1994: Mechanisms of change in cardiac performance in infants undergoing extracorporeal membrane oxygenation. *Critical Care Medicine* **22**,1865–70.

Hopper, A.O., Pageau, J., Job, L., Heart, J., Deming, D.D., Peverini, R.L. 1999: Extracorporeal membrane oxygenation for perioperative support in neonatal and pediatric cardiac transplantation. *Artificial Organs* **23**, 1006–9.

Hunkeler, N.M., Canter, C.E., Donze, A., Spray, T.L. 1992: Extracorporeal life support in cyanotic congenital heart disease before cardiovascular operation. *American Journal of Cardiology* **69**, 790–3.

Ibrahim, A.E., Duncan, B.W., Blume, E.D., Jonas, R.A. 2000: Long-term follow-up of pediatric cardiac patients requiring mechanical circulatory support. *Annals of Thoracic Surgery* **69**, 186–92.

Ishino, K., Weng, Y., Alexi-Meskishvili, V. *et al.* 1996: Extracorporeal membrane oxygenation as a bridge to cardiac transplantation in children. *Artificial Organs* **20**, 728–32.

Jaski, B.E., Lingle, R.J., Overlie, P. *et al.* 1999: Long-term survival with use of percutaneous extracorporeal life support in patients presenting with acute myocardial infarction and cardiovascular collapse. *ASAIO Journal* **45**, 615–18.

Jurmann, M.J., Haverich, A., Demertzis, S. 1991: Extracorporeal membrane oxygenation as a bridge to lung transplantation. *European Journal of Cardiothoracic Surgery* **5**, 94–8.

Kanter, K.R., Pennington, G., Weber, T.R., Zambie, M.A., Braun, P., Martychenko, V. 1987: Extracorporeal membrane oxygenation for postoperative cardiac support in children. *Journal of Thoracic and Cardiovascular Surgery* **93**, 27–35.

Karl, T.R. 1994: Extracorporeal circulatory support in infants and children. *Seminar of Thoracic and Cardiovascular Surgery* **6**, 154–60.

Karl, T.R., Lyer, K.S., Mee, R.B. 1990: Infant extracorporeal membrane oxygenation cannulation technique allowing preservation of carotid and jugular vessels. *Annals of Thoracic Surgery* **50**, 488–9.

Keszler, M., Ryckman, F.C., McDonald, J.V. 1992: A prospective multicenter randomized study of high vs low positive end-expiratory pressure during extracorporeal membrane oxygenation. *Journal of Pediatrics* **120**, 107–13.

Kirkpatrick, B.V., Krummel, T.M., Mueller, D.G., Ormazabal, M.A., Greenfield, L.J., Salzberg, A.M. 1983: Use of extracorporeal membrane oxygenation for respiratory failure in term infants. *Pediatrics* **72**, 872–6.

Kirshborn, P.M., Bridges, N.D., Myung, R.J., Gaynor, J.W., Clark, B.J., Spray, T.L. 2002: Use of extracorporeal membrane oxygenation in pediatric thoracic organ transplantation. *Journal of Thoracic and Cardiovascular Surgery* **123**, 130–6.

Kitano, Y., Takata, M., Miyasaka, K. *et al.* 1997: Evaluation of an extracorporeal membrane oxygenation system using a nonporous membrane oxygenator and a new method for heparin coating. *Journal of Pediatric Surgery* **32**, 691–7.

Klein, M.D., Andrews, A.F., Wesley, J.R. *et al.* 1985: Venovenous perfusion in extracorporeal membrane oxygenation for newborn respiratory insufficiency. A clinical comparison with venoarterial perfusion. *Annals of Surgery* **201**, 520–6.

Klein, M.D., Shaheen, K.W., Whittlesey, G.C., Pinsky, W.W., Arciniegas, E. 1990: Extracorporeal membrane oxygenation for the circulatory support of children after repair of congenital heart disease. *Journal of Thoracic and Cardiovascular Surgery* **100**, 498–505.

Ko, W.J., Chen, Y.S., Chou, N.K., Wang, S.S., Chu, S.H. 1997: Extracorporeal membrane oxygenation in the perioperative period of heart transplantation. *Journal of Formosan Medical Association* **96**, 83–90.

Kolff, W.J., Effler, D.B. 1956: Disposable membrane oxygenator (heart–lung machine) and its use in experimental and clinical surgery while the heart is arrested with potassium citrate according to the Melrose technique. *Transactions of the American Society for Artificial Internal Organs* **2**, 13–21.

Kolla, S., Awad, S.S., Rich, P.B., Schreiner, R.J., Hirschl, R.B., Bartlett, R.H. 1997a: Extracorporeal life support for 100 adult patients with severe respiratory failure. *Annals of Surgery* **226**, 544–66.

Kolla, S., Crotti, S., Lee, W.A. *et al.* 1997b: Total respiratory support with tidal flow extracorporeal circulation in adult sheep. *ASAIO Journal* **43**, M811–16.

Kolobow, T. 1988a: An update on adult extracorporeal membrane oxygenation – extracorporeal CO_2 removal. *ASAIO Trans* **34**, 1004–5.

Kolobow, T. 1988b: Acute respiratory failure. On how to injure healthy lungs (and prevent sick lungs from recovering). *ASAIO Trans* **34**, 31–4.

Kolobow, T. 1991: Extracorporeal respiratory gas exchange: a look into the future. *ASAIO Trans* **37**, 2–3.

Kolobow, T., Bowman, R.L. 1963: Construction and evaluation of an alveolar membrane artificial heart lung. *Transactions of the American Society for Artificial Internal Organs* **9**, 238–43.

Kolobow, T., Zapol, W., Pierce, J. 1969: High survival and minimal blood damage in lambs exposed to long term (1 week) veno-venous pumping with a polyurethane chamber roller pump with and without a membrane blood oxygenator. *Transactions of the American Society for Artificial Internal Organs* **15**, 172–7.

Kolobow, T., Stool, E.W., Sacks, K.L. 1975: Acute respiratory failure, survival following ten days' support with a membrane lung. *Journal of Thoracic and Cardiovascular Surgery* **69**, 947–53.

Kolobow, T., Spragg, R.G., Pierce, J.E. 1981: Massive pulmonary infarction during total cardiopulmonary bypass in unanesthetized spontaneously breathing lambs. *International Journal of Artificial Organs* **4**, 76–81.

Kolobow, T., Moretti, M.P., Mascheroni, D. *et al.* 1983: Experimental meconium aspiration syndrome in the preterm fetal lamb: successful treatment using the extracorporeal artificial lung. *Transactions of the American Society for Artificial Internal Organs* **29**, 221–6.

Krummel, T.M., Greenfield, L.J., Kirkpatrick, B.V. 1984: Alveolar–arterial oxygen gradients versus the neonatal pulmonary insufficiency index for prediction of mortality in ECMO candidates. *Journal of Pediatric Surgery* **19**, 380–4.

Kugelman, A., Gangitano, E., Pincros, J., Tantivit, P., Taschuk, R., Durand, M. 2003: Venovenous versus venoarterial extracorporeal membrane oxygenation in congenital diaphragmatic hernia. *Journal of Pediatric Surgery*, **38**, 1131–6.

Kulik, T.J., Moler, F.W., Palmisano, J.M. *et al.* 1996: Outcome-associated factors in pediatric patients treated with extracorporeal membrane oxygenator after cardiac surgery. *Circulation* **94**, II63–8.

Lally, K.P., Paranka, M.S., Roden, J. *et al.* 1992: Congenital diaphragmatic hernia. Stabilization and repair on ECMO. *Annals of Surgery* **216**, 569–73.

Lamy, M., Eberhart, R.C., Fallat, R.J., Dietrich, H.P., Ratliff, J., Hill, J.D. 1975: Effects of extracorporeal membrane oxygenation (ECMO) on pulmonary haemodynamics, gas exchange and prognosis. *Transactions of the American Society for Artificial Internal Organs* **21**, 188–98.

Langley, S.M., Sheppard, S.V., Tsang, V.T., Monro, J.L., Lamb, R.K. 1998: When is extracorporeal life support worthwhile following repair of congenital heart disease in children? *European Journal of Cardiothoracic Surgery* **13**, 520–5.

Lazar, E.L., Abramson, S.J., Weinstein, S., Stolar, C.J.H. 1994: Neuroimaging of brain injury in neonates treated with extracorporeal membrane oxygenation: lessons learned from serial examinations. *Journal of Pediatric Surgery* **29**, 186–91.

Lazzara, R.R., Magovern, J.A., Benckart, D.H., Maher, T.D. Jr, Sakert, T., Magovern, G.J. Jr. 1993: Extracorporeal membrane oxygenation for adult post cardiotomy cardiogenic shock using a heparin bonded system. *ASAIO Journal* **39**, M444–7.

Lessin, M.S., Thompson, I.M., Deprez, M.F., Cullen, M.L., Whittlesey, G.C., Klein, M.D. 1995: Congenital diaphragmatic hernia with or without extracorporeal membrane oxygenation: are we making progress? *Journal Am Coll Surg* **181**, 65–71.

Lick, S.D., Zwischenberger, J.B., Wang, D., Deyo, D.J., Alpard, S.K., Chambers, S.D. 2001: Improved right heart function with a compliant inflow artificial lung in series with the pulmonary circulation. *Annals of Thoracic Surgery* **72**, 899–904.

Lohrer, R.M., Bejar, R.F., Simko, A.J., Moulton, S.L., Cornish, J.D. 1992: Internal carotid artery blood flow velocities before, during, and after extracorporeal membrane oxygenation. *American Journal of Diseases of Children* **146**, 201–7.

Lund, D.P., Mitchell, J., Kharasch, V., Quigley, S., Kuehn, M., Wilson, J.M. 1994: Congenital diaphragmatic hernia: the hidden morbidity. *Journal of Pediatric Surgery* **29**, 258–62.

Lynch, W.R., Montoya, J.P., Brant, D.O., Schreiner, R.J., Iannettoni, M.D., Bartlett, R.H. 2000: Hemodynamic effect of a low-resistance artificial lung in series with the native lungs of sheep. *Annals of Thoracic Surgery* **69**, 351–6.

MacDonnell, K.F., Moon, H.S., Sekar, T.S., Ahluwalia, M.P. 1981: Extracorporeal membrane oxygenator support in a case of severe status asthmaticus. *Annals of Thoracic Surgery* **31**, 171–5.

Magovern, G.J.J., Simpson, K.A. 1999: Extracorporeal membrane oxygenation for adult cardiac support: the Allegheny experience. *Annals of Thoracic Surgery* **68**, 655–61.

Mallik, K., Rodgers, B.M., McGahren, E.D. 1995: Congenital diaphragmatic hernia: experience in a single institution from 1978 through 1994. *Annals of Thoracic Surgery* **60**, 1331–5.

Martin, G.R., Short, B.L., Abbott, C. 1991: Cardiac stun in infants undergoing extracorporeal membrane oxygenation. *Journal of Thoracic and Cardiovascular Surgery* **101**, 607–11.

Meliones, J.N., Moler, F.W., Custer, J.R. et al. 1991: Hemodynamic instability after the initiation of extracorporeal membrane oxygenation: role of ionized calcium. Critical Care Medicine 19, 1247–51.

Mellgren, K., Friberg, L.G., Mellgren, G., Hedner, T., Wennmalm, A., Wadenvik, H. 1996: Nitric oxide in the oxygenator sweep gas reduces platelet activation during experimental perfusion. Annals of Thoracic Surgery 61, 1194–8.

Michaels, A.J., Schriener, R.J., Kolla, S. et al. 1999: Extracorporeal life support in pulmonary failure after trauma. Journal of Trauma 46, 638–45.

Miyamura, H., Sugawara, M.A., Watanabe, H., Eguchi, S. 1996: Blalock–Taussig operation with an assist of venovenous extracorporeal membrane oxygenation. Annals of Thoracic Surgery 62, 565–6.

Moen, O., Fosse, E., Braten, J. et al. 1996: Differences in blood activation related to roller/centrifugal pumps and heparin-coated/uncoated surfaces in a cardiopulmonary bypass model circuit. Perfusion 11, 113–23.

Morris, A.H., Menlove, R.L., Rollins, R.J. 1988: A controlled clinical trial of a new 3-step therapy that includes extracorporeal CO_2 removal for acute respiratory distress syndrome. Transactions of the American Society for Artificial Internal Organs 34, 48–53.

Morris, A.H., Wallace, C.J., Menlove, R.L. et al. 1994: Randomized clinical trial of pressure-controlled inverse ratio ventilation and extracorporeal CO_2 removal for adult respiratory distress syndrome. American Journal of Respiratory and Critical Care Medicine 149, 295–305.

Moulton, S.L., Lynch, F.P., Cornish, J.D., Bejar, R.F., Simko, A.J., Krous, H.F. 1991: Carotid artery reconstruction following neonatal extracorporeal membrane oxygenation. Journal of Pediatric Surgery 26, 794–9.

Nagaraj, H.S., Mitchell, K.A., Fallat, M.E., Groff, D.B., Cook, L.N. 1992: Surgical complications and procedures in neonates on extracorporeal membrane oxygenation. Journal of Pediatric Surgery 27, 1106–9.

del Nido, P.J., Dalton, H.J., Thompson, A.E., Siewers, R.D. 1992: Extracorporeal membrane oxygenator rescue in children during cardiac arrest after cardiac surgery. Circulation 86, II300–4.

del Nido, P.J., Armitage, J.M., Fricker, F.J. et al. 1994: Extracorporeal membrane oxygenation support as a bridge to pediatric heart transplantation. Circulation 90, II66–9.

del Nido, P.J. 1996: Extracorporeal membrane oxygenation for cardiac support in children. Annals of Thoracic Surgery 61, 336–9.

Nojiri, C., Hagiwara, K., Yokoyama, K. et al. 1995: Evaluation of a new heparin bonding process in prolonged extracorporeal membrane oxygenation. ASAIO Journal 41, M561–7.

O'Rourke, P.P., Crone, R.K., Vacanti, J.P. et al. 1989: Extracorporeal membrane oxygenation and conventional medical therapy in neonates with persistent pulmonary hypertension of the newborn: a prospective randomized study. Pediatrics 84, 957–63.

O'Rourke, P.P., Stolar, C.J., Zwischenberger, J.B., Snedecor, S.M., Bartlett, R.H. 1993: Extracorporeal membrane oxygenation: support for overwhelming pulmonary failure in the pediatric population. Collective experience from the extracorporeal life support organization. Journal of Pediatric Surgery 28, 523–8.

van Oeveren, W., Jansen, N.J., Bidstrup, B.P. et al. 1987: Effects of aprotinin on hemostatic mechanisms during cardiopulmonary bypass. Annals of Thoracic Surgery 44, 640–5.

Pagani, F.D., Lynch, W., Swaniker, F. et al. 1999: Extracorporeal life support to left ventricular assist device bridge to heart transplant: a strategy to optimize survival and resource utilization. Circulation 100, II206–10.

Palmer, K., Ehren, H., Benz, R., Frenckner, B. 1995: Carmeda surface heparinization in neonatal extracorporeal membrane oxygenation systems: long-term experiments in a sheep model. Perfusion 10, 307–13.

Palmisano, J.M., Moler, F.W., Custer, J.R., Meliones, J.N., Snedecor, S., Revesz, S.M. 1992: Unsuspected congenital heart disease in neonates receiving extracorporeal life support: a review of ninety-five cases from the Extracorporeal Life Support Organization Registry. Journal of Pediatrics 121, 115–17.

Peek, G.J., Firmin, R.K. 1997: Extracorporeal membrane oxygenation for cardiac support. Coronary Artery Disease 8, 371–88.

Peirce, E.C. II. 1981: Is extracorporeal membrane oxygenation a viable technique. Annals of Thoracic Surgery 31, 102–4.

Pennington, D.G., Merjavy, J.P., Codd, J.E., Swartz, M.T., Miller, L.L., Williams, G.A. 1984: Extracorporeal membrane oxygenation for patients with cardiogenic shock. Circulation 70, I130–7.

Pettignano, R., Heard, M., Davis, R., Labuz, M., Hart, M. 1998: Total enteral nutrition versus total parenteral nutrition during pediatric extracorporeal membrane oxygenation. Critical Care Medicine 26, 358–63.

Philips, J.B. 1990: Treatment of PPHNS. In: Long, W.A., ed. Fetal and neonatal cardiology. Philadelphia, PA: Saunders: 691–701.

Piena, M., Albers, M.J., Van Haard, P.M., Gischler, S., Tibboel, D. 1998: Introduction of enteral feeding in neonates on extracorporeal membrane oxygenation after evaluation of intestinal permeability changes. Journal of Pediatric Surgery 33, 30–4.

Plotz, F.B., van Oeveren, W., Bartlett, R.H., Wildevuur, C.R. 1993: Blood activation during neonatal extracorporeal life support. Journal of Thoracic and Cardiovascular Surgery 105, 823–32.

Pranikoff, T., Hirschl, R.B., Remenapp, R., Swaniker, F., Bartlett, R.H. 1999: Venovenous extracorporeal life support via percutaneous cannulation in 94 patients. Chest 115, 818–22.

Pyle, R.B., Helton, W.C., Johnson, F.W. et al. 1975: Clinical use of the membrane oxygenator. Archives Surgery 110, 966–70.

Rais-Bahrami, K., Martin, G.R., Schnitzer, J.J., Short, B.L. 1993: Malposition of extracorporeal membrane oxygenation cannulas in patients with congenital diaphragmatic hernia. Journal of Pediatrics 122, 794–7.

Raithel, S.C., Boegner, E., Fiore, A. 1991: Extracorporeal membrane oxygenation in children following cardiac surgery. Circulation 84, 240.

Raithel, S.C., Pennington, D.G., Boegner, E., Fiore, A., Weber, T.R. 1992: Extracorporeal membrane oxygenation in children after cardiac surgery. Circulation 86, II305–10.

Raju, T.N., Kim, S.Y., Meller, J.L., Srinivasan, G., Ghai, V., Reyes, H. 1989: Circle of Willis blood velocity and flow direction after common carotid artery ligation for neonatal extracorporeal membrane oxygenation. Pediatrics 83, 343–7.

Rashkind, W.J.K., Freeman, A., Klein, D. 1965: Evaluation of a disposable plastic, low-volume, pumpless oxygenator as a lung substitute. Jornal de Pediatrica 66, 94–102.

Redmond, C., Heaton, J., Calix, J. et al. 1987a: A correlation of pulmonary hypoplasia, mean airway pressure, and survival in congenital diaphragmatic hernia treated with extracorporeal membrane oxygenation. Journal of Pediatric Surgery 22, 1143–9.

Redmond, C.R., Graves, E.D., Falterman, K.W., Ochsner, J.L., Arensman, R.M. 1987: Extracorporeal membrane oxygenation for respiratory and cardiac failure in infants and children. *Journal of Thoracic and Cardiovascular Surgery* **93**, 199–204.

Rich, P.B., Awad, S.S., Kolla, S. *et al.* 1998a: An approach to the treatment of severe adult respiratory failure. *Journal of Critical Care* **13**, 26–36.

Rich, P.B., Awad, S.S., Crotti, S., Hirschl, R.B., Bartlett, R.H., Schreiner, R.J. 1998b: A prospective comparison of atrio–femoral and femoro–atrial flow in adult venovenous extracorporeal life support. *Journal of Thoracic and Cardiovascular Surgery* **116**, 628–32.

Robinson, T.M., Kickler, T.S., Waler, L.K., Ness, P., Bell, W. 1993: Effect of extracorporeal membrane oxygenation on platelets in newborns. *Critical Care Medicine* **21**, 1029–34.

Rodriguez, J.L., Steinberg, S.M., Luchetti, F.A. 1990: Early tracheostomy for primary airway management in the surgical critical care setting. *Surgery* **108**, 655–9.

Rogers, A.J., Trento, A., Siewers, R.D. 1989: Extracorporeal membrane oxygenation for postcardiotomy shock in children. *Annals of Thoracic Surgery* **47**, 903–6.

Saker, D.M., Walsh-Sukys, M., Spector, M., Zahka, K.G. 1997: Cardiac recovery and survival after neonatal myocardial infarction. *Pediatr Card* **18**, 139–42.

Schumacher, R.E. 1993: Risks of neonatal ECMO. In: Arensman, R.M., Cornish, J.D., eds. *Extracorporeal life support.* Boston, MA: Blackwell Scientific: 226–40.

Schumacher, R.E., Barks, J.D., Johnston, M.V. *et al.* 1988: Right-sided brain lesions in infants following extracorporeal membrane oxygenation. *Pediatrics* **82**, 155–61.

Sell, L.L., Cullen, M.L., Lerner, G.R. 1986: Hemorrhagic complications during extracorporeal membrane oxygenation. Prevention and treatment. *Journal of Pediatric Surgery* **21**, 1087–8.

Sell, L.L., Cullen, M.L., Whittlesey, G.C., Lerner, G.R., Klein, M.D. 1987a: Experience with renal failure during extracorporeal membrane oxygenation: treatment with continuous hemofiltration. *Journal of Pediatric Surgery* **22**, 600–2.

Sell, L.L., Cullen, M.L., Lerner, G.R., Whittlesey, G.C., Shanley, C.J., Klein, M.D. 1987b: Hypertension during extracorporeal membrane oxygenation: cause, effect, and management. *Surgery* **102**, 724–30.

Shanley, C.J., Hultquist, K.A., Rosenberg, D.M., McKenzie, J.M., Shah, N.L., Bartlett, R.H. 1992: Prolonged extracorporeal circulation without heparin. Evaluation of the Medtronic Minimax oxygenator. *ASAIO Journal* **38**, M311–16.

Shapiro, M.B., Kleaveland, A.C., Bartlett, R.H. 1993: Extracorporeal life support for status asthmaticus. *Chest* **103**, 1651–4.

Sharland, G.K., Lockhart, S.M., Heward, A.J., Allan, L.D. 1992: Prognosis in fetal diaphragmatic hernia. *American Journal of Obstetrics and Gynecology* **166**, 9–13.

Sigalet, D.L., Tierney, A., Adolph, V. *et al.* 1995: Timing of repair of congenital diaphragmatic hernia requiring extracorporeal membrane oxygenation support. *Journal of Pediatric Surgery* **30**, 1183–7.

Soeter, J.R., Mamiya, R.T., Sprague, A.Y. 1973: Prolonged extracorporeal oxygenation for cardiorespiratory failure after tetralogy correction. *Journal of Thoracic and Cardiovascular Surgery* **66**, 214–18.

Spannagl, M., Dietrich, W., Beck, A., Schramm, W. 1994: High dose aprotinin reduces prothrombin and fibrinogen conversion in patients undergoing extracorporeal circulation for myocardial revascularization. *Thrombosis Haemostasis* **72**, 159–60.

Spector, M.L., Wiznitzer, M., Walsh-Sukys, M.C., Stork, E.K. 1991: Carotid reconstruction in the neonate following ECMO. *Journal of Pediatric Surgery* **26**, 357–9.

Stallion, A., Cofer, B.R., Rafferty, J.A., Ziegler, M.M., Ryckman, F.C. 1994: The significant relationship between platelet count and hemorrhagic complications on ECMO. *Perfusion* **9**, 265–9.

van der Staak, F.H., de Haan, A.F., Geven, W.B., Doesburg, W.H., Festen, C. 1995: Improving survival for patients with high-risk congenital diaphragmatic hernia by using extracorporeal membrane oxygenation. *Journal of Pediatric Surgery* **30**, 1463–7.

Steinhorn, R.H., Isham-Schopf, B., Smith, C., Green, T.P. 1989: Hemolysis during long-term extracorporeal membrane oxygenation. *Journal of Pediatrics* **115**, 625–30.

Stolar, C.J., Snedecor, S.M., Bartlett, R.H. 1991: Extracorporeal membrane oxygenation and neonatal respiratory failure: experience from the extracorporeal life support organization. *Journal of Pediatric Surgery* **26**, 563–71.

Stolar, C.J., Crisafi, C.A., Driscoll, Y.T. 1995: Neurocognitive outcome for neonates treated with extracorporeal membrane oxygenation: are infants with congenital diaphragmatic hernia different? *Journal of Pediatric Surgery* **30**, 366–71.

Streletz, L.J., Bej, M.D., Graziani, L.J. *et al.* 1992: Utility of serial EEGs in neonates during extracorporeal membrane oxygenation. *Pediatr Neurol* **8**, 190–6.

Tarby, T.J., Volpe, J.J. 1982: Intraventricular hemorrhage in the premature infant. *Pediatr Clin North Am* **29**, 1077–104.

Taylor, G.A., Walker, L.K. 1992: Intracranial venous system in newborns treated with extracorporeal membrane oxygenation: Doppler US evaluation after ligation of the right jugular vein. *Radiology* **183**, 453–6.

Taylor, G.A., Short, B.L., Fitz, C.R. 1989: Imaging of cerebrovascular injury in infants treated with extracorporeal membrane oxygenation. *Journal of Pediatrics* **114**, 635–9.

Toomasian, J.M., Kerby, K.A., Chapman, R.A., Heiss, K.F., Hirschl, R.B., Bartlett, R.H. 1987: Performance of a rupture-resistant polyvinyl chloride tubing. *Proc Am Acad Cardiovasc Perfusion* **8**, 56–9.

Toomasian, J.M., Snedecor, S.M., Cornell, R.G., Cilley, R.E., Bartlett, R.H. 1988: National experience with extracorporeal membrane oxygenation for newborn respiratory failure. Data from 715 cases. *ASAIO Trans* **34**, 140–7.

Towne, B.H., Lott, I.T., Hicks, D.A., Healey, T. 1985: Long-term follow-up of infants and children treated with extracorporeal membrane oxygenation (ECMO): a preliminary report. *Journal of Pediatric Surgery* **20**, 410–14.

Trittenwein, G., Furst, G., Golej, J. *et al.* 1997: Preoperative extracorporeal membrane oxygenation in congenital cyanotic heart disease using the AREC system. *Annals of Thoracic Surgery* **63**, 1298–302.

Tsuno, K., Terasaki, H., Otsu, T., Okamoto, T., Sakanashi, Y., Morioka, T. 1993: Newborn extracorporeal lung assist using a novel double lumen catheter and a heparin-bonded membrane lung. *Intensive Care Med* **19**, 70–2.

Upp, J.R. Jr, Bush, P.E., Zwischenberger, J.B. 1994: Complications of neonatal extracorporeal membrane oxygenation. *Perfusion* **9**, 241–56.

Van Meurs, K.P., Newman, K.D., Anderson, K.D., Short, B.L. 1990: Effect of extracorporeal membrane oxygenation on survival of infants with congenital diaphragmatic hernia. *Journal of Pediatrics* **117**, 954–60.

Vaucher, Y.E., Dudell, G.G., Bejar, R. 1996: Predictors of early childhood outcome in candidates for extracorporeal membrane oxygenation. *Journal of Pediatrics* **128**, 109–17.

Vazquez, W.D., Cheu, H.W. 1994: Hemorrhagic complications and repair of congenital diaphragmatic hernias: does timing of the repair make a difference? Data from the Extracorporeal Life Support Organization. *Journal of Pediatric Surgery* **29**, 1002–5.

Vogler, C., Sotelo-Avila, C., Lagunoff, D., Braun, P., Schreifels, J.A., Weber, T. 1988: Aluminum-containing emboli in infants treated with extracorporeal membrane oxygenation. *New England Journal of Medicine* **319**, 75–9.

Wachtfogel, Y.T., Kucich, U., Hack, C.E. *et al.* 1993: Aprotinin inhibits the contact, neutrophil, and platelet activation systems during simulated extracorporeal perfusion. *Journal of Thoracic and Cardiovascular Surgery* **106**, 1–9.

Walters, H.L. III, Hakimi, M., Rice, M.D., Lyons, J.M., Whittlesey, G.C., Klein, M.D. 1995: Pediatric cardiac surgical extracorporeal membrane oxygenation: multivariate analysis of risk factors for hospital death. *Annals of Thoracic Surgery* **60**, 329–36.

Wang, S.S., Chen, Y.S., Ko, W.J., Chu, S.H. 1996: Extracorporeal membrane oxygenation support for postcardiotomy cardiogenic shock. *Artificial Organs* **20**, 1287–91.

Weber, T.R., Connors, R.H., Pennington, D.G. *et al.* 1987: Neonatal diaphragmatic hernia. An improving outlook with extracorporeal membrane oxygenation. *Archives Surgery* **122**, 615–18.

Weerwind, P.W., van der Veen, F.H., Lindhout, T., de Jong, D.S., Cahalan, P.T. 1998: *Ex vivo* testing of heparin-coated extracorporeal circuits: bovine experiments. *International Journal of Artificial Organs* **21**, 291–8.

Weinhaus, L., Canter, C., Noetzel, M., McAlister, W., Spray, T.L. 1989: Extracorporeal membrane oxygenation for circulatory support after repair of congenital heart defects. *Annals of Thoracic Surgery* **48**, 206–12.

West, K.W., Bengtson, K., Rescorla, F.J., Engle, W.A., Grosfeld, J.L. 1992: Delayed surgical repair and ECMO improves survival in congenital diaphragmatic hernia. *Annals of Surgery* **216**, 454–60.

Westfall, S.H., Stephens, C., Kesler, K., Connors, R.C., Tracy, T.F. Jr, Weber, T.R. 1991: Complement activation during prolonged extracorporeal membrane oxygenation. *Surgery* **110**, 887–91.

White, J.J., Andrews, H.G., Risemberg, H., Mazur, D., Haller, J.A. Jr. 1971: Prolonged respiratory support in newborn infants with a membrane oxygenator. *Surgery* **70**, 288–96.

Wildin, S.R., Landry, S.H., Zwischenberger, J.B. 1994: Prospective, controlled study of developmental outcome in survivors of extracorporeal membrane oxygenation: the first 24 months. *Pediatrics* **93**, 404–8.

Wilson, J.M., Lund, D.P., Lillehei, C.W., Vacanti, J.P. 1991: Congenital diaphragmatic hernia: predictors of severity in the ECMO era. *Journal of Pediatric Surgery* **26**, 1028–33.

Wilson, J.M., Lund, D.P., Lillehei, C.W., O'Rourke, P.P., Vacanti, J.P. 1992: Delayed repair and preoperative ECMO does not improve survival in high-risk congenital diaphragmatic hernia. *Journal of Pediatric Surgery* **27**, 368–72.

Wilson, J.M., Bower, L.K., Fackler, J.C., Beals, D.A., Bergus, B.O., Kevy, S.V. 1993: Aminocaproic acid decreases the incidence of intracranial haemorrhage and other hemorrhagic complications of ECMO. *Journal of Pediatric Surgery* **28**, 536–40.

Wilson, J.M., Bower, L.K., Lund, D.P. 1994: Evolution of the technique of congenital diaphragmatic hernia repair on ECMO. *Journal of Pediatric Surgery* **29**, 1109–12.

Younger, J.G., Schreiner, R.J., Swaniker, F., Hirschl, R.B., Chapman, R.A., Bartlett, R.H. 1999: Extracorporeal resuscitation of cardiac arrest. *Academic Emergency Medicine* **6**, 700–7.

Zapol, W.M., Qvist, J. 1976: *Artificial lungs for acute respiratory failure.* New York, NY: Academic Press.

Zapol, W.M., Snider, M.T., Hill, J.D. *et al.* 1979: Extracorporeal membrane oxygenation in severe acute respiratory failure. A randomized prospective study. *Journal of the American Medical Association* **242**, 2193–6.

Zenati, M., Pham, S.M., Keenan, R.J., Griffith, B.P. 1996: Extracorporeal membrane oxygenation for lung transplant recipients with primary severe donor lung dysfunction. *Transplant International* **9**, 227–30.

Ziomek, S., Harrell, J.E. Jr, Fasules, J.W. *et al.* 1992: Extracorporeal membrane oxygenation for cardiac failure after congenital heart operation. *Annals of Thoracic Surgery* **54**, 861–78.

Zwischenberger, J.B., Bartlett, R.H. 1990: Extracorporeal circulation for respiratory or cardiac failure. *Seminar of Thoracic and Cardiovascular Surgery* **2**, 320–31.

Zwischenberger, J.B., Cox, C.S. Jr. 1992: ECMO in the management of cardiac failure. *ASAIO Journal* **38**, 751–3.

Zwischenberger, J.B., Cilley, R.E., Hirschl, R.B., Heiss, K.F., Conti, V.R., Bartlett, R.H. 1988: Life-threatening intrathoracic complications during treatment with extracorporeal membrane oxygenation. *Journal of Pediatric Surgery* **23**, 599–604.

Zwischenberger, J.B., Bowers, R.M., Pickens, G.J. 1989: Tension pneumothorax during extracorporeal membrane oxygenation. *Annals of Thoracic Surgery* **47**, 868–71.

Zwischenberger, J.B., Toomasian, J.M., Drake, K., Andrews, A.F., Kolobow, T., Bartlett, R.H. 1985: Total respiratory support with single cannula venovenous ECMO: double lumen continuous flow vs. single lumen tidal flow. *Transactions of the American Society for Artificial Internal Organs* **31**, 610–15.

Zwischenberger, J.B., Nguyen, T.T., Upp, J.R. Jr *et al.* 1994: Complications of neonatal extracorporeal membrane oxygenation. Collective experience from the Extracorporeal Life Support Organization. *Journal of Thoracic and Cardiovascular Surgery* **107**, 838–49.

Zwischenberger, J.B., Conrad, S.A., Alpard, S.K., Grier, L.R., Bidani, A. 1999: Percutaneous extracorporeal arteriovenous CO_2 removal for severe respiratory failure. *Annals of Thoracic Surgery* **68**, 181–7.

Zwischenberger, J.B., Wang, D., Lick, S.D., Deyo, D.J., Alpard, S.K., Chambers, S.D. 2002: The paracorporeal artificial lung improves 5-day outcomes from lethal smoke/burn-induced acute respiratory distress syndrome in sheep. *Annals of Thoracic Surgery* **74**, 1011–8.

16

The extended use of the extracorporeal circuit

PHILIP H KAY, ANIL KUMAR MULPUR, DUMBOR NGAAGE, SAMIR SHAH, KIERAN HORGAN, JOHN POLLITT AND STEPHEN D HANSBRO

KEY POINTS

- Cardiopulmonary bypass can be used to improve operating conditions on other organs, both inside and outside the thorax.
- Cardiopulmonary bypass with deep hypothermic circulatory arrest provides excellent operating conditions for radical nephrectomy, combined with removal of tumour thrombus, extending along the inferior vena cava and into the right atrium.
- Femoro–femoral bypass with profound hypothermia and circulatory arrest facilitates surgery on arterio–venous malformations and intracranial aneurysms in the brain stem. However, this technique is now largely replaced by selective embolization.
- Cardiopulmonary bypass is the most efficient and physiological method of rewarming hypothermic patients who have suffered a cardiac arrest. It is most successful in patients who have not suffered concomitant asphyxia (avalanche or drowning).
- The cytotoxic agent, melphalan, is effective in treating recurrent melanoma using the technique of isolated hypothermic limb perfusion.

INTRODUCTION

The introduction of the extracorporeal oxygenator system by Gibbon (1954) laid the foundation for the dramatic development that has occurred in open-heart surgery during the last half-century. During this period other surgical disciplines have also appreciated the benefits of circulatory control. The first group of surgeons to take advantage of these techniques were the cardiothoracic and cardiovascular surgeons operating in their non-cardiac discipline. The role of cardiopulmonary bypass in supporting surgery to the descending thoracic aorta and the carina of the trachea is well described. It is not the purpose of this chapter to review these surgical techniques, but to explore the more peripheral roles for the extracorporeal circuit.

UROLOGY

Renal cell carcinoma extending along the ipsilateral renal vein, inferior vena cava and into the right atrium presents a complex surgical problem. Radical nephrectomy and inferior vena cavotomy, with removal of the tumour thrombus, represents the best hope for long-term survival. We have adopted a multidisciplinary approach to this problem, involving combined teams of urologists and cardiac surgeons. The role of the cardiac surgeon is to utilize the techniques of extracorporeal circulation and deep hypothermic arrest to provide easy and safe operating conditions, particularly when the tumour thrombus is being delivered from the inferior vena cava.

We have now used this technique in nine patients, the majority (eight) with right-sided hypernephroma. At the start of the procedure the urologist opens the abdomen via a chevron, sub-costal incision. A final assessment of the operability of the tumour is made. The kidney is dissected along with the sub-hepatic section of the inferior vena cava. This is a difficult and haemorrhagic procedure owing to the engorged intra-abdominal veins secondary to the inferior vena cava obstruction. Access to the engorged kidney is improved by the median sternotomy incision. The venous engorgement is reduced after the establishment of cardiopulmonary bypass. We insert two venous cannulae, one low down in the right atrium, the second into the superior vena cava via the right atrial appendage. The return is to the ascending aorta. The patient is cooled to 15°C and the aorta left unclamped.

Once the temperature has cooled to 15°C the kidney and renal vein are removed. The circulation is arrested and retrograde cerebral perfusion through the snared cannula in the superior vena cava is commenced at a rate of 300 mL/min, with a passive return to a vent in the aortic root (Ngaage et al., 2001).

The inferior vena cava is opened at the level of the excised renal vein. The tumour is densely adherent to the caval wall and may also extend into the hepatic veins. A finger is used to establish a plane between the tumour and caval wall, rather like performing an endarterectomy. Concurrently, the cardiac surgeon removes the cannula from the right atrium and inserts his finger through the purse string into the atrium. Working from above a similar plane between the tumour and caval wall is established until the finger of the cardiac surgeon and that of the urologist working from below meet within the liver. The tumour is then delivered from the infra-hepatic vena cava. It is this safe delivery of the tumour from the inferior vena cava in a bloodless field that is the hallmark of this technique. The inferior vena cava is then repaired. Sometimes it is possible to close the incision directly, though on other occasions the renal tumour has been so densely adherent to the wall of the inferior vena cava, particularly at the junction with the subtending renal vein, that a patch repair using autologous pericardium is required. The mean circulatory arrest time has been 27 minutes (range 10–36 minutes). The additional benefit of retrograde cerebral perfusion, particularly with such relatively short circulatory arrest times, remains a matter for debate (Reich et al., 2001).

Eight patients survived this radical surgery. All suffered a deterioration in renal function with a mean doubling of the pre-operative serum creatinine. Two patients required temporary post-operative renal support. All patients who were anaemic at the start of the procedure required modest blood transfusion (mean four units, range two to eight units). This demonstrates good circulatory control in a potentially extremely haemorrhagic situation.

Such surgery must be regarded as being palliative. There have been two late deaths, one 30 months after surgery because of extensive recurrent tumour, the second patient died of unconnected causes. The remaining six patients are alive eight to 37 (mean 18) months after radical nephrectomy. Each of the surviving patients has evidence of residual or recurrent tumour.

NEUROSURGERY

Arterio–venous malformations and intracranial aneurysms, particularly in the brain stem, can present a severe technical challenge to the neurosurgeon. Williams et al. (1991) reported the use of cardiopulmonary bypass with profound hypothermia and circulatory arrest to facilitate this complex surgery.

Our experience in this field is limited to five cases. Initially, cardiopulmonary bypass via a formal median sternotomy incision was used with a pulmonary artery vent to prevent cardiac distension.

More recently we have used femoro–femoral bypass with monitoring of the pulmonary artery pressures by Swan–Ganz catheter and left ventricular dimensions with transoesophageal echocardiography. If the aortic valve is competent and the venous drainage adequate then left ventricular distension should not occur. In the event of such distension a left ventricular vent can be inserted directly into the apex of the left ventricle via a small anterior thoracotomy.

In each of these cases the cardiopulmonary bypass circuit has provided excellent operating conditions, enabling successful neurosurgery to be performed. This technique is now largely being replaced by selective embolization.

RESUSCITATION OF VICTIMS OF HYPOTHERMIC CARDIAC ARREST

The human body has three thermal zones:

1 A superficial zone formed by the skin and subcutaneous tissue with a normal temperature of 34°C.
2 An intermediate zone composed of the skeletal muscles with a normal temperature of 35°C.
3 A deep zone comprising the body cavities with a normal core temperature of 37°C.

Acute hypothermia is a life-threatening condition that occurs when the core temperature drops below 35°C. It is classified into mild (32–35°C), moderate (28–32°C) and severe (below 28°C). Patients with severe hypothermia may suffer a cardiac arrest and present comatose, pulseless and with fixed, dilated pupils yet still be salvageable. Althaus and colleagues (Althaus et al., 1982) reported that 80 per cent of patients with core temperatures between 24°C and 35°C would not survive without active therapeutic measures.

In 1967 two groups, working independently, reported the first successful use of cardiopulmonary bypass in rewarming hypothermic patients. Davies and Millar (1967) used femoro–femoral bypass to successfully resuscitate an 82-year-old woman with a rectal temperature of 33.3°C. In the same year Kugelberg and colleagues (Kugelberg *et al.*, 1967) used femoro–femoral bypass to revive a 59-year-old man with a core temperature of 21.4°C.

Following this early experience, Gregory and colleagues (Gregory *et al.*, 1991) showed that cardiopulmonary bypass is the most efficient and physiological method of rewarming hypothermic patients. With a blood or core temperature gradient of 6°C and a flow of 4 L/min, the core temperature can rise by up to 10°C per hour, depending on the size of the patient.

Cardiopulmonary bypass has several advantages over other methods of rewarming. The deep thermal zone is rewarmed rapidly. This in turn expedites the recovery of cardiopulmonary, metabolic, hormonal and enzymatic homeostasis. In addition there is a decreased incidence of 'rewarming collapses' (Webb, 1986). In a recent review Walpoth and colleagues (Walpoth *et al.*, 1997) reported a 64 per cent survival in a series of 11 patients with severe hypothermia (rectal temperatures between 17°C and 26°C), rewarmed using cardiopulmonary bypass. All patients had suffered a cardiac arrest and had been in coma for 1.5–3.7 hours with dilated, non-reacting pupils at the commencement of cardiopulmonary bypass.

We have successfully used femoro–femoral bypass to re-warm a young drug addict who became hypothermic with subsequent cardiac arrest, following an overdose. However, this technique is less successful in patients who have suffered concomitant asphyxia in addition to their hypothermia, as in the case of victims of avalanche or drowning. Two young children who fell through the ice and presented with cardiac arrest of two hours' duration and rectal temperatures of 24°C could not be resuscitated. In these cases massive endothelial leakage and gross elevation of serum potassium levels (12 mmol/L) signalled widespread cell death.

ISOLATED HYPERTHERMIC CYTOTOXIC LIMB PERFUSION

Isolated hyperthermic limb perfusion is a technique that is used to deliver high-dose chemotherapy to a tumour-bearing region of the body, without subjecting the patient to the systemic toxicity and side-effects associated with chemotherapy. It was first described by Creech *et al.* (1958) as an alternative to amputation. The patient had developed approximately 80 satellite metastases on the leg two years after wide excision of a melanoma. The limb was perfused with melphalan (L-Phenylalanine mustard) and a complete

remission achieved. The patient died 16 years later at the age of 92, free of recurrent tumour.

Isolated hyperthermic limb perfusion is particularly applicable to tumours with a high propensity for regional recurrent metastases and without the tendency to haematogenous spread. It can be delivered in either the therapeutic or adjuvant setting. The most common indication is the management of advanced melanoma of the leg with multiple fungating, ulcerating and bleeding metastases. Occasionally isolated hyperthermic cytotoxic limb perfusion is used in locally advanced soft tissue sarcoma that is surgically inoperable. Melphalan is the cytotoxic drug of choice for isolated hyperthermic cytotoxic limb perfusion. It is equally effective alone as when used in combination with other cytotoxic agents. Melphalan was initially selected for metastatic melanoma as phenylalanine is a metabolite of melanin, which should facilitate drug entry into the melanin-producing malignant cells. It is a long-acting alkylating agent that causes alkylation of cellular DNA, disrupting the tumour cells. It also interferes with cell replication by forming cross-links between the strands of the double helix.

The dose of melphalan can be calculated with reference either to the total patient body weight or the limb volume. At this hospital we use the 'Rule of Nines' method to calculate the weight of the limb. This method lists the leg as 18 per cent body surface area while the arm is listed as nine per cent.

Weight of lower limb = Total body weight × 0.18.
Weight of upper limb = Total body weight × 0.09.

Melphalan is then prescribed at a dose of 1.5–2.0 mg/kg for the lower limb and 1.0–1.5 mg/kg for the upper limb.

More recently recombinant human tumour necrosis factor alpha has been added to the perfusate. This is one of the central cytokines that mediates the systemic inflammatory response to injury. The maximum tolerated dose is limited to 400 mg/m^2 (Selby *et al.*, 1987). Tumour necrosis factor activates and selectively destroys the tumour-associated microvasculature (Eggermont *et al.*, 1997) and also enhances tumour-selective drug uptake (Eggermont and ten Hagen 2001). Toxicity includes systemic septic shock with hypotension, tachycardia, decreased systemic vascular resistance and increased cardiac output. Results show a markedly elevated response rate, particularly for previously unresponsive tumours such as soft tissue sarcomas, which may subsequently be rendered operable.

Hyperthermia appears to have a synergistic role with the cytotoxic agents. Nineteenth-century observations on patients with malignancy revealed that those who experienced fevers related to bacterial septicaemia occasionally had a reduction in tumour size. Formal experiments by Criel in the 1960s showed that hyperthermia increased response rates to radiation therapy, particularly with

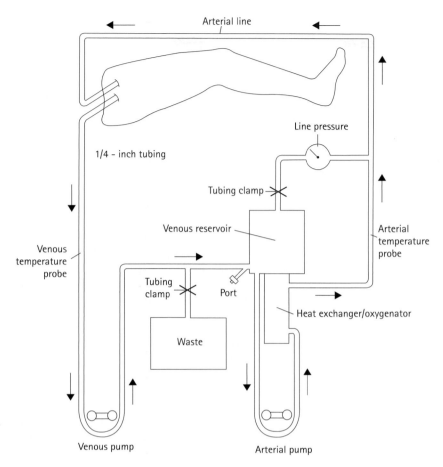

Figure 16.1 *Isolated limb perfusion circuit.*

temperatures above 40°C. Cavaliere and colleagues (Cavaliere *et al.*, 1967) found that hyperthermic perfusion at between 40°C and 41°C for four hours, without any chemotheraputic drugs caused tumour size to decrease. The precise mechanism of this thermal potentiation is not clear. There is little information about the optimal limb perfusion temperature, but it is now generally accepted that a limb temperature of 40°C should be maintained. This is classified as mild hyperthermia. Elevation of limb temperature above this level requires careful monitoring to avoid neural and muscular damage.

Most patients will be fit for isolated hyperthermic cytotoxic limb perfusion, but care should be taken in the selection of patients with proven cardio, respiratory or peripheral vascular disease. The procedure demands close interaction between anaesthetic, surgical, perfusion and nursing staff. It is performed under general anaesthetic with invasive monitoring of central venous and arterial pressures. Cannulation of the vascular pedicle to the lower limb is achieved by exposing the iliac vessels through an extra peritoneal approach. Any enlarged nodes are removed. An 18 French, right-angled cannula is inserted into the artery and a 20 French, right-angled cannula into the vein. Any vascular side branches are occluded to minimize systemic leakage. A tourniquet is applied at the transitional zone between the trunk and the lower limb to prevent systemic leak of perfusate. A Steinmann pin secured to the anterior superior iliac spine serves as a suitable pivot for the tourniquet. A sterile latex Esmarch bandage is used as the tourniquet.

The extracorporeal circuit is shown in Figure 16.1. We use a paediatric membrane oxygenator and tubing pack. This reduces the priming volume and therefore the potential for haemodilution. The circuit is primed with 300 mL Hartmann solution and 300 mL Geloflex; 25 mmol of 8.4 per cent sodium bicarbonate is added to the prime to make the solution less acidic. Heparin, 5000 U is also added to the prime. The oxygen demand of the limb is increased because of hyperthermia, therefore, it is essential to maintain the haematocrit of the limb above 15 per cent to ensure adequate oxygen delivery.

The dilutional effects of the prime can be calculated as follows:

$$\text{Total body blood volume} = \text{weight in kg} \times 70 = y\,\text{mL}$$

$$\text{Total body red cell volume} = y\,\text{mL} \times \text{haematocrit}$$

$$\text{Blood volume in limb} = y\,\text{mL} \times 0.18\ \text{(lower limb)}$$

$$\text{Total red cell in limb} = \text{Total body red cell volume} \times 0.18$$

$$\text{Perfusion volume of limb} = \text{Blood volume in limb} + \text{prime volume}$$

$$\text{Haematocrit of perfusion limb} = \frac{\text{Total red cells in limb}}{\text{perfusion volume of limb}}$$

If the calculated haematocrit of the perfusion limb falls below 15 per cent packed red cells can be added to the prime of the circuit. The volume of packed red cells required can be calculated as follows.

$$\text{Red blood cells required} = \text{Perfusion volume of limb} \times \text{required haematocrit.}$$

$$\text{Red cells to add} = \text{Red cells required} - \text{total red cells in limb.}$$

$$\text{Additional packed cells to add} = \frac{\text{Red cells to add}}{0.70 \, (\text{haematocrit of packed cells})}$$

The patient is fully heparinized (300 IU/kg) before cannulation and adequate activated clotting times are established before initiating bypass. The isolated limb perfusion is initiated by adjusting the roller pumps on the arterial and venous sides of the circuit whilst maintaining the volume of blood in the venous reservoir at a constant level, gradually increasing perfusion flow rate up to 1200 mL/min. The tourniquet is then applied to the root of the limb. Observing both the central venous pressure and the venous reservoir level will identify any blood losses from the perfusion circuit to the systemic circulation.

Oxygen partial pressures are kept above 30 kPa, with a normal base excess and CO_2 partial pressure between 5.3 kPa and 6.0 kPa. Local vasodilation within the limb is facilitated by the supplementation of isoflurane at one 1–2 per cent. This results in improved delivery of the cytotoxic agents to the limb tissues.

When the limb temperature reaches the required range (40°C at the calf probe) the perfusion flow rate is reduced to approximately 350 mL/min, again maintaining a constant volume in the venous reservoir. The 60-minute perfusion with cytotoxic agents is then commenced. The melphalan dose is administered at two time points; 0 minutes and 30 minutes into the infusion port on the venous arm of the circuit. This provides two peaks in drug concentration with satisfactory background levels. After 60 minutes' circulation with the cytotoxic agent, and before the release of the tourniquet, the blood from the limb is washed out with 2 L of colloid and 1 L of 0.9 per cent sodium chloride. The returning blood from the limb is diverted to a waste container by clamping at the venous reservoir inlet and opening the waste washout line. The washout takes about 10 minutes to perform, after which the pump is stopped and the venous line clamped. Heparinization is reversed by administration of protamine. Decannulation is performed in standard fashion.

Radioactive tracers have been used to continuously monitor the rate of leakage during a perfusion. Radio-labelled albumen (I^{131}) can be introduced into the perfusate and leaks detected via a scintillation scanner placed over the heart. However, with the use of a relatively low perfusion rate (350 mL/min) leakage does not appear to be a significant problem.

Upper limb perfusion is performed via the axillary vessels. An infraclavicular approach has the advantage of allowing a more proximal cannulation of the vessels, combined with access to the apical group of the axillary lymph nodes for staging.

In our experience isolated hyperthermic cytotoxic limb perfusion is most successful for patients who present with a limited number of small cutaneous melanotic nodules more than two years after surgical excision of the primary melanoma. In these circumstances it is frequent to achieve complete response rates in approximately 80 per cent of patients with a median duration of 18–24 months. Where such a response is achieved, further success may be obtained by a second perfusion at the time of the later recurrence. In situations where patients present with larger nodules, in particular subcutaneous lesions more than 2 cm in diameter, it is more difficult to achieve a complete response. A partial response or even stasis of the disease may be beneficial in terms of palliation for these patients. The median duration of response for this latter patient group is shorter, with further progression of disease usually evident within nine months of treatment. However, the clinical behaviour of melanoma is so variable that even some patients with obvious melanoma recurrences on the limb, and no detectable systemic disease, can achieve complete response rates for many years. When the initial response to isolated hyperthermic cytotoxic limb perfusion has been either shortlived or absent we have found no advantage in repeating isolated hyperthermic cytotoxic limb perfusion.

Although isolated hyperthermic cytotoxic limb perfusion is now a recognized technique in the armamentarium of surgical oncologists, it is not without mortality and morbidity. Mortality is normally caused by bone marrow suppression from systemic cytotoxic drug leakage. The most common form of morbidity is acute regional toxicity. It is characterized by localized oedema, erythema and pain. Other manifestations may include temporary loss of nails, dryness or blistering of skin, alopecia and neuralgia. Most of these factors are treated conservatively. More sinister complications include muscle damage and acute renal failure secondary to rhabomyolysis. Limb swelling and lymph oedema is common and often recalcitrant to treatment as many patients have undergone regional lymphadenectomy. All these complications relate directly to the operative technique. Meticulous attention to detail and multidisciplinary team working is the key to successful outcomes.

REFERENCES

Althaus, U., Aeberhard, P., Schupback, P., Nachbur, B.H., Muhlemann, W. 1982: Management of profound accidental hypothermia with cardiorespiratory arrest. *Annals of Surgery* **195**, 492–5.

Cavaliere, R., Ciocatto, E.C., Giovanella, B.C. *et al.* 1967: Selective heat sensitivity of cancer cells. Biochemical and clinical studies. *Cancer* **20**, 1351–67.

Creech, O.J., Krementz, E.T., Ryan, R.F. 1958: Regional perfusion utilizing an extracorporeal circuit. *Annals of Surgery* **148**, 616–32.

Davies, D.M., Millar, I.A. 1967: Accidental hypothermia treated by extracorporeal blood rewarming. *Lancet* **1**, 1036–7.

Eggermont, A.M.M., Schraffordt Koops, H., Klausner, J.M., Lienard, D., Kroon, B.B., Schlag, P.M., Ben-Ari, G., Lejeune, F.J. 1997: Isolated limb perfusion with tumour necrosis factor alpha and chemotherapy for advanced extremity soft tissue sarcomas. *Seminars in Oncology* **24**, 547–55.

Eggermont, A.M.M., ten Hagen, T.L. 2001: Isolated limb perfusion for extremity soft tissue sarcomas, in-transit metastases and other unresectable tumours: credits, debits and future perspectives. *Current Oncology Reports* **3**, 359–67.

Gibbon, J.H. 1954: Application of a mechanical heart and lung apparatus to cardiac surgery. *Minnesota Medicine* **37**, 171–80.

Gregory, J.S., Bergstein, J.M., Aprahamian, C., Witmann, D.H. 1991: Comparison of three methods of rewarming from hypothermia: advantages of extracorporeal blood rewarming. *Journal of Trauma* **13**, 1247–52.

Kugelberg, J., Schuller, H., Berg, B., Kallum, B. 1967: Treatment of accidental hypothermia. *Scandinavian Journal of Thoracic and Cardiovascular Surgery* **1**, 142–6.

Ngaage, D.L., Sharpe, D.A.C., Prescott, S., Kay, P.H. 2001: Safe techniques for removal of extensive renal tumours. *Annals of Thoracic Surgery* **71**, 1679–81.

Reich, D.L., Uysal, S., Ergin, A., Griepp, R.B. 2001: Retrograde cerebral perfusion as a method of neuroprotection during thoracic aortic surgery. *Annals of Thoracic Surgery* **72**, 1774–82.

Selby, P., Hobbs, S., Viner, C. *et al.* 1987: Tumour necrosis factor in man: clinical and biological observations. *British Journal of Cancer* **56**, 803–8.

Walpoth, B.H., Walpoth-Aslan, B.N., Mattle, H.P. *et al.* 1997: Outcome of survivors of accidental deep hypothermia and circulatory arrest treated with extracorporeal blood warming. *New England Journal of Medicine* **337**, 1500–5.

Webb, P. 1986: Afterdrop of body temperature during rewarming: an alternative explanation. *Journal of Applied Physiology* **60**, 385–90.

Williams, M.D., Rainer, W.C., Fieger, H.G. Jr. 1991: Cardiopulmonary bypass, profound hypothermia and circulatory arrest for neurosurgery. *Annals of Thoracic Surgery* **52**, 1069–74.

17

Cardiopulmonary bypass during Port-access™ and robotic surgery

ALAN P KYPSON AND W RANDOLPH CHITWOOD Jr

KEY POINTS

- Recent advances in perfusion technology, visualization, instrumentation and robotics mean that effective, safe minimally invasive cardiac surgery is now becoming a practical reality.
- Endovascular bypass requires a purpose-built catheter system, with appropriate manipulation of venous drainage, aortic occlusion and cardioplegia delivery.
- Perfusion management during endovascular bypass is more complex and requires a high level of vigilance and expertise from the perfusionist.
- The development of minimally invasive surgery may be considered to progress in a stepwise fashion (levels 1–4) with each level of technical complexity being mastered before progress to the next level.
- Preliminary data suggest that, although operative times are longer, minimally invasive operations can be done in a safe manner, using appropriate modifications of bypass technology.
- Clearly, further study is needed to determine whether endovascular bypass and minimal access surgery have advantages in terms of outcomes such as long-term results, recovery times and cost-effectiveness.

INTRODUCTION

Conventional cardiac surgery has been performed traditionally through a median sternotomy, which provides generous exposure of the operative field and allows ample access to cardiac structures for cannulation and institution of cardiopulmonary bypass. During the past decade, improvements in endoscopic equipment and techniques have resulted in an explosion of minimally invasive general, urological, gynaecological and thoracic surgical procedures. Because of their more complex nature, most cardiovascular procedures require a median sternotomy and cardiopulmonary bypass. Thus, minimally invasive cardiac techniques have only been attempted recently. It is only after modifications in cardiopulmonary bypass, reductions in the size of incisions and alternate incision site usage that the possibilities of minimally invasive cardiac surgery have been realized. Advances in cardiopulmonary perfusion, intracardiac visualization, instrumentation and robotic telemanipulation have hastened a shift toward efficient and safe minimally invasive cardiac surgery. Today, cardiac surgery done through small incisions has become standard practice for many surgeons, and patients are becoming more aware of its increasing availability.

Minimally invasive cardiovascular surgery can be performed using the Port-access™ system, which is based on closed-chest cardiopulmonary bypass (Cardiovations Inc., Ethicon, Somerville, NJ). Introduced in 1996 (Pompili et al., 1996; Stevens et al., 1996), Port-access™ cardiac surgery combines a minimal surgical approach with avoidance of a median sternotomy, total cardiopulmonary bypass and an arrested heart. The system provides extrathoracic cardiopulmonary bypass by use of a special set of endovascular catheters that provide either or both antegrade and retrograde cardioplegic arrest, as well as ventricular decompression. Aortic clamping, cardioplegic arrest and ventricular decompression are achieved by means of a multipurpose endovascular balloon catheter that is usually placed through femoral vessel access into the ascending aorta. When integrated into a modified cardiopulmonary bypass circuit, this system creates a platform that facilitates both epicardial and intracardiac procedures done through a mini-thoracotomy. Ultimately, this method should facilitate the performance of operations in a closed-chest environment using robotic assistance.

Robotic cardiac surgery has evolved as the next level of 'minimal invasiveness', as assisted vision and advanced instrumentation have developed. New robotic methods now offer near endoscopic possibilities for cardiac surgeons. In 1998, Carpentier and colleagues (Carpentier et al., 1998) performed the first true robotic mitral valve operation using the da Vinci™ surgical system (Intuitive Surgical Inc., Sunnyvale, CA). Subsequently, our group performed the first da Vinci™ mitral repair in the USA (Chitwood et al., 2000). This system provides both tele- and micro-manipulation of tissues in confined spaces. The surgeon operates from a console and becomes immersed in a three-dimensional view of the operative field. Through a computer, the surgeon's motions are reproduced in scaled proportion through 'micro-wrist' instruments that are mounted on robotic arms inserted through the chest wall. These instruments emulate human X–Y–Z axis wrist activity throughout seven degrees of motion. Here, too, access to the heart is limited, and traditional cannulation techniques have been abandoned to make this new technology clinically applicable. A combination of new and more traditional cardiopulmonary bypass approaches now can be used in minimally invasive approaches to heart surgery. As direct control of cannula placement and surveillance becomes more removed from the surgeon, the role of the anesthesiology and perfusion team becomes even more critical as compared with standard cardiac procedures.

Since 1996, more than 3210 procedures have been performed worldwide using the Port-access™ system (Port-access International Registry, 2000). Cardiac surgeons and their teams have performed a broad array of operations, including coronary artery bypass grafting (CABG) (Galloway et al., 1999; Grossi et al., 1999; Gulielmos et al., 1999); heart valve replacement or repair (Reichenspurner et al., 1998; Vanermen et al., 1999; Kort et al., 2001; Kypson et al., 2002a); atrial septal defect repair (Kappert et al., 1999; Yozu et al., 2001); multivalve

procedures (Colvin et al., 2000; Kypson and Glower, 2002b; Tripp et al., 2002); valve or coronary combination procedures (Tabry et al., 2000); re-operative procedures on patients with a prior median sternotomy (Onnasch et al., 2002; Trehan et al., 2002) and robotic-assisted cardiac operations (Loulmet et al., 1999; Reichenspurner et al., 1999; Mohr et al., 2001).

ENDOVASCULAR CATHETER SYSTEM

The endovascular cardiopulmonary bypass system (ENDOCPB™) (Cardiovations Inc., Ethicon, Somerville, NJ) is a cannula or catheter-based system that enables cardiopulmonary bypass and cardioplegic cardiac arrest without requiring a median sternotomy (Table 17.1). The essential components of the ENDOCPB™ system are:

- an endovascular venous cannula (Quickdraw™), which drains the inferior vena cava or right atrium
- a femoral arterial cannula (Endoreturn™)
- a direct aortic perfusion cannula, placed through a thoracic trocar or small incision (Endodirect™)
- an endo-aortic occlusion clamp (Endoclamp™)
- a percutaneous coronary sinus cardioplegia catheter (Endoplege™)
- a percutaneous pulmonary artery vent (Endovent™) for cardiac decompression during cardiopulmonary bypass.

The Endoreturn™ arterial cannula delivers oxygenated blood during cardiopulmonary bypass. It is thin-walled and has a wire-wound section for flexibility and kink resistance, an atraumatic tip, and a hydrophilic coating to facilitate insertion. After exposing the femoral artery, the cannula is placed over guidewire directed coaxial dilators using the Seldinger technique. This device comes in 21 French (F) [0.275 (OD)] or 23F [0.301 (OD)]. This cannula has a Y connection site for arterial inflow and a separate haemostatic valve for endo-aortic balloon clamp passage (Fig. 17.1). The Endodirect™ cannula is another arterial cannula variant and permits direct cannulation of the ascending aorta through a small incision or trocar site. It has a bevelled tip with an end hole, side perfusion

Table 17.1 *Components of the ENDOCPB™ system*

Quickdraw	Venous cannual
Endoreturn	Femoral arterial cannula
Endodirect	Aortic perfusion cannula
Autoincisor	Blade-tipped introducer for Endodirect
Endoclamp	Endo-aortic balloon clamp
Endoplege	Percutaneous coronary sinus catheter
Endovent	Percutaneous pulmonary artery vent

™Cardiovations Inc., Ethicon, Somerville, NJ, USA.

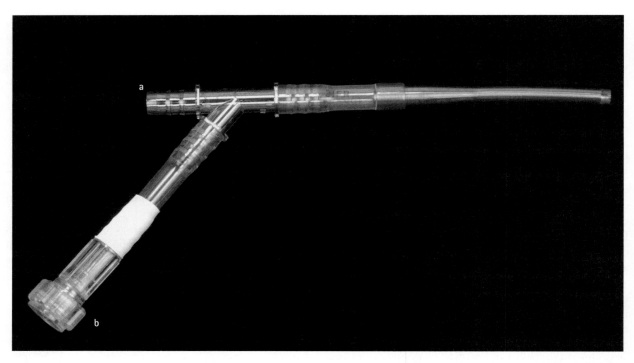

Figure 17.1 *Endoreturn™ arterial cannula (21F) with: (a) 3/8-inch barbed connector for arterial inflow tubing; (b) haemostatic valve that allows passage of the Endoclamp™.*

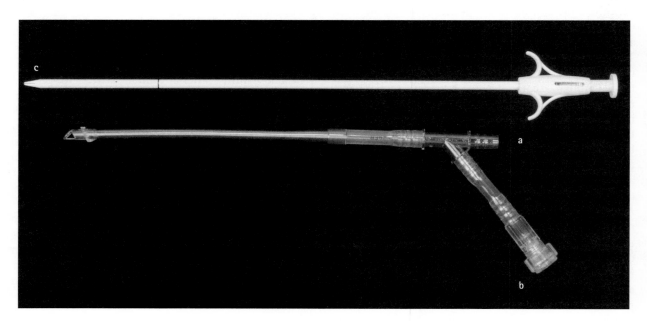

Figure 17.2 *Endodirect™ arterial cannula (24F) with the Autoincisor™. Note: (a) the 3/8-inch barbed connector for arterial inflow tubing; (b) haemostatic valve that allows for passage of the Endoclamp™; (c) the tip of the blade is at the end of the Autoincisor™.*

holes and a suture slot ring with tourniquet tubing posts for immobilization. The dilator accompanying the Endo-direct™ cannula contains a spring-loaded blade tip that incises the aorta for introduction (Fig. 17.2). Both arterial cannulae are available without a side arm if an external or transthoracic cross-clamp is to be used.

The thin-walled Quickdraw™ venous cannula couples directly to the venous tubing of the heart–lung machine. This soft tip cannula contains multiple side holes with both wire-wound and plain tubing segments for clamping (Fig. 17.3). This cannula comes in 22F and 25F sizes, either of which can be inserted by femoral venous cutdown or

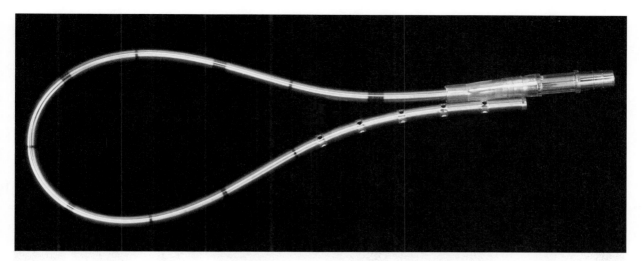

Figure 17.3 *Quickdraw™ venous drainage cannula (25F) with a 3/8-inch barbed connector for venous outflow tubing. Note the multiple side holes at the tip.*

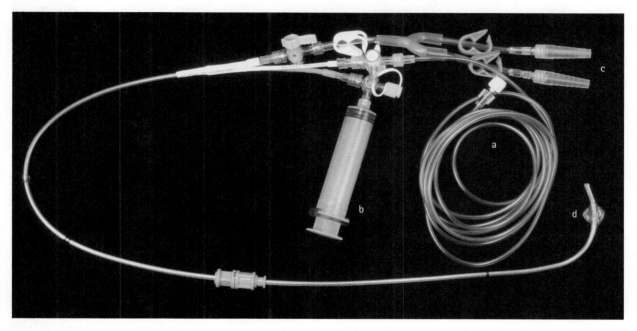

Figure 17.4 *Endoclamp™ catheter. Note: (a) the aortic root pressure monitoring line; (b) the 35 mL syringe for balloon inflation; (c) a Y-connector for aortic root cardioplegia and venting; (d) balloon.*

percutaneously via the Seldinger technique. Optimally, this cannula is positioned in the right atrium under intra-operative transoesophageal echocardiographic guidance.

The Endoclamp™ is a 10.5F, wire-wound, triple-lumen catheter with an elastomeric balloon near the tip. When inflated, it concentrically occludes the ascending aorta. Furthermore, the large central lumen enables both delivery of aortic root cardioplegia and venting. The two remaining lumens serve as conduits for balloon and aortic root pressure monitoring (Fig. 17.4). The aortic root vent line contains a negative pressure relief valve that allows venting while avoiding excessive negative pressure. This balloon clamp is passed through the side arm of the arterial cannula and positioned above the tubulosinus ridge using transoesophageal echocardiography. A securing hub provided on the introducer tubing allows the balloon catheter to be locked in place. The catheter comes in 65 cm and 100 cm lengths, depending on whether it is placed from the peripheral or central approach.

Retrograde cardioplegia delivery is possible using the jugular vein-placed Endoplege™ catheter. This endovascular coronary sinus catheter is a 9F triple-lumen catheter

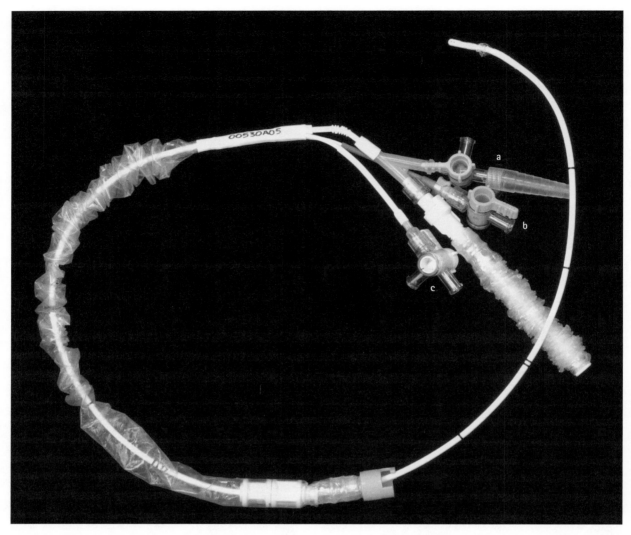

Figure 17.5 *Endoplege™ catheter. Note: (a) the cardioplegia delivery line; (b) the balloon inflation lumen; (c) the coronary sinus pressure monitoring lumen.*

with an elastomeric balloon near its tip (Fig. 17.5). It is inserted into the right internal jugular vein percutaneously through an 11F introducer sheath. This catheter can occlude the coronary sinus, deliver retrograde cardioplegia and monitor coronary sinus pressures simultaneously. A shaft torque device allows catheter steering for ideal positioning in the coronary sinus, which must be confirmed by transoesophageal echocardiography.

The Endovent™ returns to the cardiopulmonary bypass circuit pulmonary blood not drained by the venous cannula. It has a single-lumen pre-shaped catheter (8.3F) that is inserted percutaneously via the internal jugular or subclavian veins. It has a small, integrated balloon, much like a Swan–Ganz catheter, that allows flow-directed positioning in the main pulmonary artery. Figure 17.6 illustrates the final position of all cannulae and catheters used in the ENDOCPB™ system.

Modification of the cardiopulmonary bypass circuit

In traditional median sternotomy-based cardiac surgery, gravity venous drainage has been the mainstay of cardiopulmonary perfusion for many years. This technique has proved safe and inexpensive. Varying the difference in height between the patient's right atrium and the venous reservoir usually creates an adequate negative pressure head to achieve optimal venous return to the pump. However, large-diameter cannulae are generally necessary to achieve adequate flow rates. In minimally invasive cardiac surgery, there is no median sternotomy and access for direct insertion of large-bore cannulae is not feasible. As mentioned, new ultra-thin catheter designs with multiple side holes optimize flow rates and provide maximum drainage. Despite these improved catheters for minimally

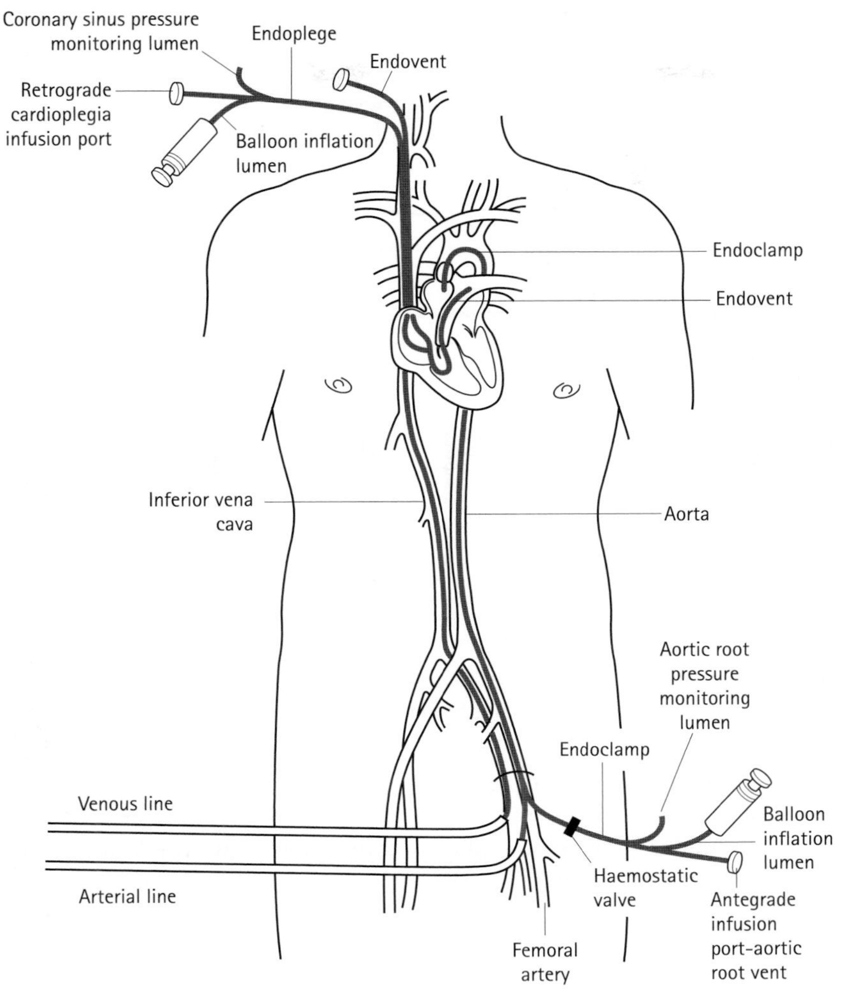

Figure 17.6 *Final position of all cannulae and catheters in the ENDOCPB™ system allowing closed-chest cardiopulmonary bypass and cardiac arrest.*

invasive cardiac surgery, gravity-assisted venous drainage is often inadequate because of cannula length and relatively small diameter. Under optimal conditions these cannulae drain only 75–80 per cent of venous return using gravity. Unless the left ventricle is decompressed completely, the heart continues to eject blood and after arrest the intracardiac operative field remains flooded. Therefore, most surgeons now use augmented venous return to provide total cardiopulmonary support with adequate cardiac decompression.

Assisted drainage improves siphoning of venous blood that increases blood return flow to the cardiopulmonary bypass machine. A variety of methods can be used to implement assisted venous drainage but, most commonly, kinetically assisted and vacuum-assisted venous drainage are used.

Kinetically assisted venous drainage utilizes a centrifugal pump, placed between the venous cannula and the venous reservoir. This kinetic pump generates negative pressure siphoning that enhances venous return. This method improves venous drainage by 20–40 per cent in

comparison to gravity circuits (Toomasian *et al.*, 1998). With kinetically assisted venous drainage, venous blood is pumped actively into either an open or closed venous reservoir. Centrifugal pump inertia regulates siphoning of venous blood and, as the pump speed is increased, more central suction is generated. Pressure in the venous conduit is monitored proximal to the pump inlet, allowing the perfusionist to regulate the amount of blood returned. Excessive negative pressure can cause haemolysis and/or right atrial collapse around the venous cannula, impeding venous return. Unfortunately, kinetically assisted venous drainage has two drawbacks: the cost that the pump adds to the cardiopulmonary bypass circuit, and depriming of the centrifugal pump if air is introduced from the cannulation site. In a series of experiments, LaPietra *et al.* (2000) found that kinetically assisted venous drainage was unable to handle gaseous microemboli from a small continuous air leak. System air leaks require constant manual clearing of both pump and reservoir, which may result in frequent interruptions of cardiopulmonary bypass (Ogella, 1999). In contrast, vacuum-assisted venous drainage handles

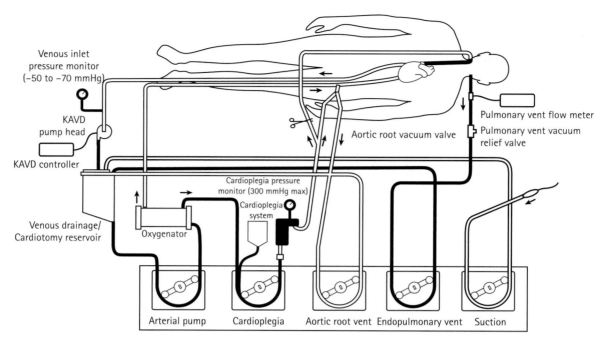

Figure 17.7 *A typical cardiopulmonary bypass circuit for Port-access™ and robotic cardiac surgery. Note the capability of both antegrade and retrograde cardioplegia administration. Assisted venous drainage is also in use.*

macroscopic air entrapment more efficiently with less depriming. Moreover, the cost is much less than kinetically assisted venous drainage as no centrifugal pump head is required.

Vacuum-assisted venous drainage utilizes a standard vacuum suction source connected to an open or hard-shell venous reservoir, which creates suction in the entire drainage system and increases venous return. Vacuum-assisted venous drainage requires close regulation of the vacuum source to avoid negative pressure variations found in most hospital wall suction units. Excessive vacuum-assisted venous drainage can also cause trauma to the blood components in addition to cracking or imploding of the venous reservoir. Regulators must be used to maintain precise vacuum pressures. Also, positive and negative pressure relief valves must be incorporated into the reservoir to prevent both over- and underpressure and to ensure consistent extracorporeal flow rates (Almany and Sistino, 2002). Vacuum-assisted venous drainage cannot be applied to closed systems using a venous reservoir bag or collapse occurs.

Unfortunately, it has been shown that both techniques of augmented venous return introduce gaseous microemboli while on cardiopulmonary bypass (Willcox *et al.*, 1999). The application of any negative pressure in the venous line can facilitate entrapment of air (Willcox, 2002). This is a matter for concern as these gaseous emboli seem to contribute to patient neurocognitive deficits after cardiopulmonary bypass. Figure 17.7 illustrates a typical cardiopulmonary bypass circuit for Port-access™ surgery.

Perfusion management

Perfusion using the Port-access™ extracorporeal system is managed through standard protocols for the flow rate, heparinization, hypothermia, myocardial protection and acid-base status. After heparinization (300 U/kg), the femoral vein is cannulated using the Seldinger method. Next, the arterial circulation is accessed (femoral or direct), and the balloon clamp is prepared. The aortic root and balloon pressure monitoring lines are passed off the field and flushed. Simultaneously, the cardioplegia line is flushed with cold cardioplegia. Partial cardiopulmonary bypass is initiated using gravity drainage. Then, assisted drainage is begun and venous return augmented by applying monitored negative pressures between 50 mmHg and 80 mmHg. Pressures greater than 100 mmHg can collapse atrial tissue around the venous cannula, diminishing the venous blood flow. Blood incompletely drained by the venous cannula can be returned by suctioning the pulmonary artery vent, which has a pressure relief valve that prevents excessive negative pressures. The amount of blood aspirated through this vent is an indicator of optimal venous cannula positioning with flows of less than 100 mL/min indicating complete cardiopulmonary bypass support.

The Endoclamp™ is then positioned in the ascending aorta above the tubulosinus ridge and proximal to the innominate artery. Transoesophageal echocardiography should be used to monitor balloon inflation and occlusion of the ascending aorta. The balloon is inflated with diluted contrast solution, in case fluoroscopic conformation is needed. To seal the balloon optimally, it is important to keep the heart empty and prevent left ventricular ejection, which can cause dislodgement. This is done by decreasing pump inflow flow and initiating aortic root venting. Alternatively, asystole can be obtained briefly from an adenosine infusion, which allows the balloon to seal firmly and ensures stabilization of the balloon clamp (Farhat *et al.*, 2002). The balloon pressure is monitored continuously after inflation and maintained between 250 mmHg and 350 mmHg. After transoesophageal echocardiography or fluoroscopic confirmation of ideal balloon position, the extracorporeal flow rate is re-established at normal levels. During balloon inflation, the perfusionist monitors right radial artery pressure to determine distal balloon dislodgment and occlusion of the innominate artery. Conversely, a sudden drop in the balloon pressure suggests migration of the balloon across the aortic valve and into the left ventricle.

Once the intra-aortic balloon is positioned properly, antegrade cardioplegia can be infused. During antegrade delivery, the distal pressure must be verified to assure delivery and inadvertent recirculation through the aortic root vent suction line. The cardioplegia infusion pressure is measured continuously and should not exceed 350 mmHg at maximal flow rates between 250 mL/min and 300 mL/min. As cardioplegia infusion continues, aortic root pressure rises to 60–80 mmHg. Failure of this rise may indicate an incompetent aortic valve or malpositioned balloon clamp. Retrograde cardioplegia infusion can be delivered via the endo-coronary sinus balloon catheter. Infusions begin at low flow rates (50 mL/min) and slowly increase to 150–200 mL/min. Simultaneously, coronary sinus pressure must be monitored and should not exceed 40 mmHg. As with antegrade cardioplegia infusions, the aortic root can be vented through the Endoclamp™ aortic root lumen.

After completion of the procedure, the balloon clamp is deflated and the aortic root vented simultaneously. As the patient is being rewarmed, ventilation is re-established, aortic and pulmonary root venting is discontinued, and the clamp is withdrawn during a brief suspension of pump flow. As vacuum assist is diminished, the left ventricle is allowed to eject. Weaning from cardiopulmonary bypass is done according to the standard perfusion protocol. After administration of protamine sulfate, all Port-access™ cannulae are removed.

Perfusion management during Port-access™ surgery requires the perfusionist to monitor more parameters as surges in systemic or cardioplegia flow can dislodge the endovascular balloon clamp, causing disruptions of operations. Changes in cardiopulmonary bypass parameters are often subtle, and more vigilance is required of the perfusionist. Moreover, anesthesiologists must monitor the position of the endoclamp continuously during the occlusion phase. Table 17.2 lists recommended pressures and

Table 17.2 *Normal flows, pressure and volume measurements during Port-access™ cardiac surgery*

Aortic root pressure during:	
delivery of antegrade cardioplegia	60–80 mmHg
delivery of retrograde cardioplegia	0–20 mmHg
venting	0–10 mmHg
Cardioplegia line pressure	<350 mmHg
Coronary sinus pressure during cardioplegia delivery	20–40 mmHg
Endoplege™ balloon inflation volume	0.2–0.5 mL
Endoclamp™ balloon pressure	250–350 mmHg
Endoclamp™ balloon volume	20–40 mL
Endoreturn™ cannula line pressure	<350 mmHg
Endodirect™ cannula line pressure	<350 mmHg
Endovent™ flow:	
initial flow	Up to 250 mL/min
maintainenance phase	<40 mL/min
Venous inlet pressure	−40 to −80 mmHg

flow levels for Port-access™ minimally invasive cardiac surgery.

Patient contraindications

In patients with severe peripheral vascular disease or atheromatous aortas, insertion of ENDOCPB™ system cannulas can be dangerous. These patients are predisposed to retrograde visceral and cerebral atherosclerotic embolization as well as retrograde arterial dissections. As inflation of the Endoclamp™ results in intra-aortic balloon pressures of 250–350 mmHg, patients with aortic aneurysms or significant ectasia should not be considered for this approach.

In the presence of severe aortic insufficiency, positioning the balloon clamp can be very difficult. Moreover, aortic insufficiency can impede antegrade cardioplegia administration, resulting in inadequate myocardial preservation and left ventricular distension. Furthermore, conditions precluding transoesophageal echocardiographic probe insertion contraindicate usage of this system, as its use is vital to positioning and monitoring of all catheters.

EVOLUTION OF MINIMALLY INVASIVE CARDIAC SURGERY

Traditionally, cardiac surgery has been done most often through a median sternotomy, which provides generous access to the heart and great vessels. Traditional cannulation for cardiopulmonary bypass has required direct, manual access to the heart and its surrounding topography. To perform the ideal cardiac operation, surgeons will need to operate in restricted spaces through tiny incisions, which require modified perfusion, assisted vision and advanced instrumentation. Although the ideal cardiac operation has not been achieved widely, minimally invasive cardiac surgery has continued to evolve toward video-assisted or video-directed operations. Moreover, new robotic methods now offer near-endoscopic possibilities for cardiac surgeons (Fig. 17.8). Both video-assisted and direct-vision Port-access™ surgery is now within the reach of most cardiac surgeons. In the future, coronary artery bypass surgery may be performed through multiple small port sites on a beating heart, obviating the need for cardiopulmonary bypass. Nevertheless, in order to perform intra-cardiac surgery and complex myocardial revascularization, the heart will still need to be arrested and isolated from the systemic circulation with a cross-clamp. This is where the evolution of perfusion technology has become so important in providing the opportunity to perform these minimally invasive operations.

Modified perfusion technology has facilitated minimally invasive cardiac surgery greatly. As discussed, current developments for minimal access surgery include smaller arterial and venous cannulae, transthoracic cannulation methods, balloon endo-aortic clamping devices, percutaneous coronary sinus cardioplegia catheters and assisted or suction venous drainage. Assisted venous drainage has been a major advance in facilitating minimally invasive cardiac surgery making the selection of smaller cannula sizes possible. This technology in now being used for minimally invasive aortic and mitral valve surgery, as well as the endoscopic coronary operations.

The development of minimally invasive heart surgery may be considered analogous to an Everest ascent, embarking from a conventional or 'base camp' operation and advancing progressively toward less invasiveness through experience and acclimatization. A nomenclature that parallels this 'mountaineering' analogy is shown in Table 17.3. In this scheme, entry levels of technical complexity are mastered before advancing past small incision, direct-vision approaches (Level I), toward more complex video-assisted procedures (Level II or Level III) and, lastly, to robotic surgery (Level IV). With the constant evolution of new technology and surgical expertise, many established surgeons have already attained serial 'comfort zones' along this trek.

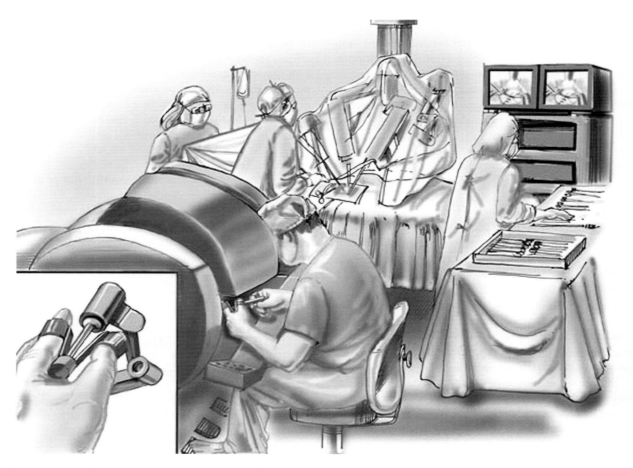

Figure 17.8 *da Vinci™ robotic manipulation system (Intuitive Surgical Inc., Sunnyvale, CA, USA). Note the surgeon seated at the operative console manipulating the robotic instruments (see inset) and instrument cart positioned over the patient. There is a patient-side surgeon, and video monitors allow the operative team to view the surgery.*

Table 17.3 *Minimally invasive cardiac surgery*

Level 1
direct vision
mini (10–12 cm) incisions

Level 2
video-assisted
micro (4–6 cm) incisions

Level 3
video-directed and robot-assisted
micro or port incisions (1 cm)

Level 4
robotic tele-manipulation
port incisions (1 cm)

Level 1: direct vision minimally invasive cardiac surgery

Early on, minimally invasive cardiac surgery was based solely on modifications of traditional incisions, and nearly all operations were done under direct vision. In 1996, the first truly minimally invasive aortic valve operations were reported. Using either mini-sternal or para-sternal incisions, Cosgrove and Sabik (1996), Cohn *et al.* (1997) and Gundry *et al.* (1998) showed encouraging results with low surgical mortality (one to three per cent) and morbidity. At the Brigham and Women's Hospital, the right atrium is cannulated directly through the parasternal incision. A separate lower skin incision is used for the inferior caval cannula. In early cases, Cosgrove and Gillinvov (1998) used this method; however, they now introduce a small 23F cannula directly into the right atrium through the mini-sternotomy. We have used a single 19F internal jugular cannula introduced percutaneously. Our group has also established percutaneous femoral-to-right atrial access using a 23F Bio-Medicus™ cannula (Medtronic Inc., Minneapolis, MN) introduced by the Seldinger technique (Chitwood, 1999). Augmented venous drainage has been excellent using a Bio-Medicus™ vortex pump. We currently extend sternal incisions for aortic surgery only to

the third interspace. Loulmet *et al.* (1998) use a percutaneously introduced femoral venous cannula that has dual-stage drainage ports (Fig. 17.9a). This catheter can be used with caval snares to perform atrial septal and tricuspid surgery as well. We have used this cannula for mitral operations and atrial septal defect closures with great success. After the operation, both the jugular and femoral percutaneous venous cannulae can be removed, applying local pressure alone for haemostasis. We have not experienced any complications using either the percutaneous jugular or femoral method.

For most mini-sternotomies and parasternal incisions, central arterial cannulation is used most frequently. Gundry *et al.* (1998) use a flexible cannula that can be introduced with or without a guide wire (see Fig. 17.9b). We cannulate the transverse aortic arch for aortic surgery using a non-kinking Bio-Medicus™ cannula. However, many minimally invasive cardiac operations still employ retrograde femoral arterial perfusion, especially for mitral surgery.

By early 1997, the Port-access™ surgical system became used more widely. This technique, developed mainly for coronary and mitral valve surgery, requires retrograde femoral arterial perfusion, femoral–atrial venous drainage and an intraluminal aortic balloon Endoclamp™ for occlusion. For both central and peripheral arterial cannulation (with retrograde arterial perfusion), our group uses the Bio-Medicus™ wire-wound arterial cannula. For both regions, we introduce either a 17F or 19F cannula through a purse-string suture using the Seldinger technique. Using these cannulas, excellent flow rates with acceptable perfusion pressures have been obtained. In patients with peripheral atherosclerosis, we cannulate the aorta through a mini-thoracotomy with video assistance. Direct aortic occlusion using a standard cross-clamp can be used for minimally invasive valve surgery. Specialized flexible-handle clamps have been developed to increase exposure and prevent inadvertent dislodgement. Gundry *et al.* (1998) use a right-angled cross-clamp with the tip placed slightly toward the transverse arch. For mitral operations, done through a mini-thoracotomy, we developed a percutaneous transthoracic aortic cross-clamp

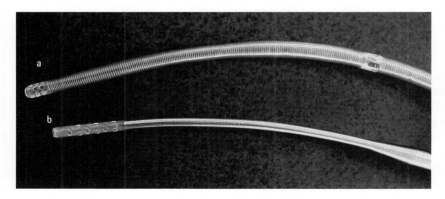

Figure 17.9 *(a) Percutaneous femoral vein two-stage venous return cannula designed by Carpentier. This cannula can be used to isolated superior and inferior caval venous drainage from the right atrium. It can be used for mitral, tricuspid and interarterial surgery; (b) thin-walled (19F) flexible arterial perfusion cannula (Bio-Medicus™, Medtronic Inc., Minneapolis, MN, USA).*

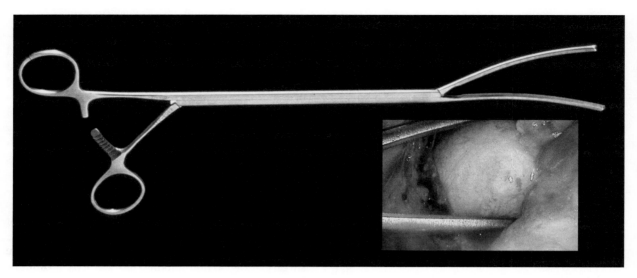

Figure 17.10 *The Chitwood transthoracic aortic cross-clamp (Scanlan International Inc., Minneapolis, MN, USA). The shaft is 4 mm in diameter and is passed through the third intercostal space. (Inset) The posterior or fixed prong of the clamp is passed through the transverse sinus, under direct or video visualization to avoid injury to either the right pulmonary artery, left atrial appendage or left main coronary artery. The mobile prong is passed ventral to the aorta as far as the main pulmonary artery.*

(Fig. 17.10). This clamp is inserted percutaneously through a 4-mm incision in the right lateral third intercostal space. The posterior, or immobile, 'fork' of the clamp is positioned carefully through the transverse sinus. We prefer camera-directed placement for maximal safety.

In contrast, the balloon clamp is introduced through a channel in either the peripheral or central arterial perfusion cannula. The occlusive balloon is positioned, under echocardiographic control, just above the tubulosinus ridge in the ascending aorta. Balloon pressures must be continuously monitored and antegrade cardioplegia is given via a central catheter lumen. Continuous echocardiographic monitoring is important to detect balloon migration.

Myocardial preservation in minimally invasive cardiac surgery has been similar to sternotomy-based operations. Many surgeons prefer to use antegrade cardioplegia. Limited exposure makes retrograde coronary sinus catheter insertion more difficult and less easy to control should complications arise. Generally, for aortic and mitral surgery, an initial dose of arresting cardioplegia is given via the occluded aortic root. For supplemental cardioplegia, doses are administered either into the coronary ostia for aortic surgery or aorta for mitral operations. With our 'micromitral' mini-thoracotomy, we insert the cardioplegia needle directly into the ascending aorta through the incision, under videoscopic control.

Air removal is particularly difficult in minimally invasive cardiac surgery. The cardiac apex cannot be elevated, and difficulty exists in manipulating the heart. Air is often sequestered in pulmonary veins and along the interventricular septum. Carbon dioxide infusions have been particularly helpful for air removal (Webb *et al.*, 1997). This gas is much more soluble in blood than air and displaces it. Near the end of the operation, we infuse carbon dioxide (1–2 L/min) into both the left atrium and ventricle and then ventilate both lungs to draw the gas deep into the pulmonary veins. Constant carbon dioxide infusion into the chest cavity can elevate the patient's $PaCO_2$ level if the pump suckers are continuously maintained open. After atriotomy closure, we suction vent the aortic root and compress the right coronary artery upon cross-clamp release. As the heart beats, we gently reclamp the aorta to expel the residual air into the vent suction. With the Endoclamp™, similar maneuvers should be applied to remove residual cardiac air. Constant transoesophageal echocardiographic monitoring should assure adequate air removal before weaning the patient from cardiopulmonary bypass.

Level 2: micro-incision and video-assisted operations

Cardiac surgery is the last specialty to utilize the benefits afforded by video assistance. Cardiac surgeons have lagged behind other surgical specialists in using assisted vision for complex operations. Micro-incisions are considered as 4–6-cm skin incisions, and video assistance indicates that 50–70 per cent of the operation is done while viewing the operative field from a screen. Similarly, port incisions connote incisions ≤3–4 cm, and video direction implies that most of the operation is done via secondary or assisted vision.

Video assistance was used first for closed chest internal mammary artery harvests and congenital heart operations (Burke *et al.*, 1995; Acuff *et al.*, 1996; Nataf *et al.*, 1996). Although Kaneko *et al.* (1996) first described the use of video assistance for mitral valve surgery done through a sternotomy, it was Carpentier who, in February 1996, performed the first video-assisted mitral valve repair via a mini-thoracotomy using ventricular fibrillation (Carpentier *et al.*, 1996). Three months later, our group performed a mitral valve replacement using a micro-incision, videoscopic vision, percutaneous transthoracic aortic clamp and retrograde cardioplegia (Chitwood *et al.*, 1997a,b,c). In 1998, Mohr (Mohr *et al.*, 1998) reported the Leipzig experience of 51 minimally invasive mitral operations using Port-access™ technology, a 4-cm incision and three-dimensional videoscopy. Video technology was helpful for replacement and simple repair operations; however, complex reconstructions were still approached under direct vision. Simultaneously, our group reported 31 patients using video-assistance with a two-dimensional 5-mm camera. Complex repairs were possible and included quadrangular resections, sliding valvuloplasties and chordal replacements with no major complications and mortality less than one per cent (Chitwood *et al.*, 1997c).

Levels 3–4: micro- or port incisions, video-directed and robotic operations

Level 3 video-directed and Level 4 robotic or computer-assisted operations may be the future of cardiac surgery. Certainly, as our experience has grown, mitral valve surgery certainly seems to be heading in that direction. With the assistance of a voice-activated robot-driven camera, AESOP™3000 (Computer Motion, Inc., Santa Barbara, CA) cardiac surgery entered the robotic age. With this device, a voice-controlled robotic arm allows hands-free camera manipulation. The surgeon commands camera movements verbally, providing a direct eye–brain action. This technology has enabled use of even smaller incisions with better valve and sub-valvular visualization. Our Level 3 operations have been done completely under video direction, without direct vision of the valve. In Europe, Reichenspurner *et al.* (2000) and Mohr (Falk *et al.*, 1998) have used three-dimensional systems successfully and now control image position using an AESOP™3000 robotic arm. In June of 1998, our group performed the first video-directed mitral operation in the USA using a voice-activated robotically controlled Vista™ camera (Vista Cardiothoracic Systems Inc., Westborough, MA) and the AESOP™3000 system (Chitwood *et al.*, 1997a,b). Visual accuracy was improved by camera voice manipulation by the operating surgeon. We now use the robotic arm routinely and have done over 250 videoscopic mitral

operations successfully using this device. Image stability during complex surgical manoeuvres remains crucial. The addition of three-dimensional visualization, robotic camera control and instrument tip articulation seems the next essential step toward a totally endoscopic mitral operation where wrist-like instruments and three-dimensional vision could transpose surgical manipulations from outside the chest wall to deep within cardiac chambers.

Innovations in computer-assisted, robotic mitral surgery are rapidly increasing. Within a week in May 1998, Carpentier in Paris and Mohr in Leipzig performed the first mitral valve repairs and coronary grafts using the da Vinci™ articulated intracardiac 'wrist' robotic device (Carpentier *et al.*, 1999; Loulmet *et al.*, 1999; Mohr *et al.*, 1999a,b). The 'micro-wrist' permits intra-atrial instrument articulation with the seven full degrees of freedom offered by the human wrist (Chitwood *et al.*, 2000). The surgeon operates from a master console using three-dimensional vision to affect simultaneous, filtered and scaled movements in a robotic slave that drives intracardiac articulated instruments. The operator essentially becomes transported to the valvular topography affecting 'tele-presence' at all levels of vision, dexterity, access and proprioception. Recently, Grossi of New York University partially repaired a mitral valve using Zeus™ (Computer Motion Inc., Santa Barbara, CA) (Grossi *et al.*, 2000). In May 2000 (Chitwood *et al.*, 2000), using the da Vinci™ system, our group performed the complete repair of a mitral valve in North America. Using the articulated wrist instruments, a trapezoidal resection of a large P2 was performed with the defect closed using multiple interrupted sutures, followed by implantation of a No. 28 Cosgrove annuloplasty band (Figs 17.11 and 17.12). Subsequently, we have performed 20 mitral repairs as part of a Food and Drug Administration (FDA)-approved trial designed to determine the safety and efficacy of da Vinci™ and a total of 50 have been carried out to date. Recently, an FDA-approved, multi-centre trial involving 112 patients has concluded. As of September 2002, more than 100 mitral operations have been done between the Leipzig, Frankfurt, Broussais and East Carolina University groups using da Vinci™. This technology represents the final step in the evolution toward a truly endoscopic mitral operation. Future refinements in these devices are needed to apply this new technology more widely.

Results

A number of studies have assessed the use of the Port-access™ platform in mitral valve surgery. Grossi *et al.* (2001) used the Port-access™ system in 100 patients undergoing mitral valve repair and compared them with a cohort of 100 conventional median sternotomy mitral operations. These workers reported a peri-operative

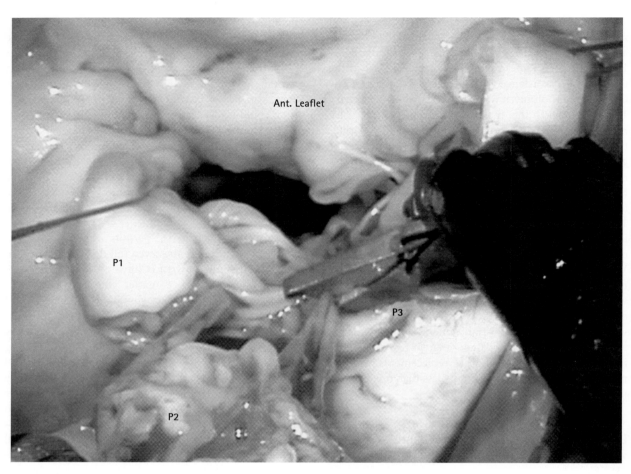

Figure 17.11 *da Vinci™ mitral valve repair: the P2 segment of the posterior leaflet is being resected by robotic micro-scissors. The annulus is reduced and both P1 and P3 approximated.*

mortality of one per cent for the former group. These results indicate that Port-access™ mitral valve surgery can be done safely with results similar to those for conventional median sternotomy. Both echocardiographic and NYHA functional improvements were compatible with results from median sternotomy patients. Glower *et al.* (1998) investigated retrospectively the advantages and disadvantages of the Port-access™ system versus median sternotomy in 41 patients undergoing mitral valve surgery. Overall operative times were longer and the overall complication rate was similar with the hospital length of stay trending downward, although not reaching statistical significance. The major difference was return to normal activity, which was significantly less in the Port-access™ group as compared with the median sternotomy group (4 (±2) weeks versus 9 (±1) weeks). In an early report on Port-access™ mitral valve surgery by Mohr *et al.* (1998), the mortality rate was 9.8 per cent with two retrograde aortic dissections, leading to conversion to median sternotomy and demonstrating clearly a learning curve with this new technology. Furthermore, four of the

51 patients (7.8 per cent) had a transient neurological event. In contradistinction, Galloway *et al.* (1999) analysed the outcome of New York University patients undergoing Port-access™ mitral valve repair and replacement. Ninety-three per cent of 321 patients were completed with Port-access™ techniques. Operative mortality for Port-access™ mitral repair was 1.5 per cent in 137 patients and 3.3 per cent in 184 patients undergoing mitral valve replacement. Galloway *et al.* (1999) concluded that morbidity and mortality rates were similar to those associated with open-chest operations. In addition to mitral valve surgery, Port-access™ has been successfully applied to patients undergoing tricuspid valve surgery. Kypson and Glower (2002a) reported 33 patients with one conversion to median sternotomy secondary to a left ventricular tear that resulted from adhesions to a prior left thoracotomy.

Coronary artery bypass grafting (CABG) using Level 3 and Level 4 techniques has been more difficult to adapt because of the greater complexity of the procedure in a closed-chest environment. Steps such as identifying the proper distal coronary target, opening the artery and using

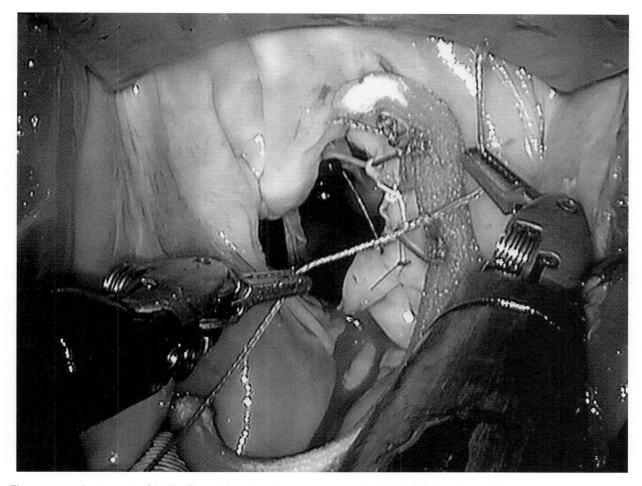

Figure 17.12 *Instruments of da Vinci™ are tying sutures to secure an annuloplasty band along the posterior annulus.*

fine suture (7-0 or 8-0 monofilament) to create a vascular anastomosis are technically challenging with current technology. Nevertheless, there is moderate experience with Port-access™ and robotically assisted CABG.

The two largest single-centre series reported include 31 patients from the New York University group (Ribakove *et al.*, 1998). Fifteen of the 31 patients (48.4 per cent) underwent single-vessel CABG, whereas 38.7 per cent underwent double-bypass and 12.9 per cent underwent triple-bypass. There were no documented peri-operative infarctions, mortality or aortic dissection. There were no conversions. Overall anastomotic patency before discharge was 98 per cent. Reichenspurner *et al.* (1998) reported 60 patients, 92 per cent of whom received single-vessel CABG. The peri-operative mortality was 1.6 per cent with a one per cent incidence of aortic dissection. More recently, the first report of the Port Access™ International Registry (Galloway *et al.*, 1999) documented the results of 555 bypass procedures performed worldwide. Forty-eight per cent were single-vessel grafts. Peri-operative complications included 2.2 per cent strokes and one per cent myocardial infarctions, with a one per cent mortality of

patients with no re-operations. The median hospital stay was four days. Grossi *et al.* (1999) compared 302 Port-access™ CABG patients with patients undergoing conventional bypass grafting in the Society of Thoracic Surgery national database. The hospital mortality for Port-access™ was 0.99 per cent versus 1.2 per cent in the conventional group. Ventilatory support greater than one day was 1.7 per cent in the Port-access™ group versus 3.8 per cent in the conventional access group. The rate of stroke was 1.7 per cent versus 1.2 per cent in the conventional group.

COMPLICATIONS OF MINIMALLY INVASIVE CARDIAC SURGERY

Port-access™ does not eliminate some of the patho-physiological consequences of cardiopulmonary bypass. Furthermore, certain complications may result from the unique technological aspects of the system, such as vascular access via the femoral vessels, placement of a large balloon clamp in the ascending aorta, migration of the endo-aortic balloon, and percutaneous cannulation and occlusion of the coronary sinus.

Complications at the site of femoral arterial cannulation include damage and stenosis after removing the cannulae, as well as acute limb ischaemia, thrombosis, lymphocele and local groin infections. Cannulation of the femoral vein can also lead to deep venous thrombosis with potential secondary pulmonary embolism. Arterial dissections related to cannulation or to the balloon clamp placement are the most-feared complication. This can result from a ruptured or traumatized atheromatous plaque or from vascular trauma related to the passage and/or inflation of the Endoclamp™. Mohr *et al.* (1998) reported two dissections in 51 patients. These results prompted some changes in the cannula and guidewire design. The overall incidence of dissections has decreased to 0.18 per cent. Another unusual complication relating to catheters of the Port-access™ system is the entrapment of the pulmonary artery vent by atriotomy closure sutures. To eliminate this complication, the anesthesiologist should check the mobility of this vent immediately after atriotomy closure while the patient is still on cardiopulmonary bypass.

Another substantial complication related to cardiopulmonary bypass is that of adverse central nervous system events. Some aspects of the Port-access™ system may affect these complications in a very unique way – in particular, retrograde arterial and aortic blood flow, and limited access to the cardiac chambers for proper 'de-airing' manoeuvres. Retrograde aortic blood flow associated with femoral artery cannulation has been recognized as a potential risk factor for adverse neurological outcomes, presumably because reversal of flow tends to disrupt atheromatous debris and direct it toward the brain. Furthermore, passage of the cannulae and catheters can dislodge atheromatous plaques as well. The balloon clamp, on the other hand, eliminates the need for an external cross-clamp with the resultant mural crush injury. Inflation of a soft balloon may result in less fracturing of atheromatous plaques with a reduction in potentiating embolic material. Unfortunately, balloon dislodgment with migration can occlude the innominate artery, and this has been implicated in some post-operative neurological events.

SUMMARY

Port-access™ and robotic cardiac surgery allow the surgeon to perform operations that traditionally called for a median sternotomy through much smaller incisions. Modifications in cardiopulmonary perfusion have become necessary as the surgeon is now removed from the operative field. At present, operative times are longer, demonstrating the increased complexity of the entire operation. Minimally invasive cardiac surgery requires transoesophageal echocardiographic expertise and a team approach with the anesthesiologist and the perfusionist playing a role as critical as that of the surgeon. Preliminary data suggest that these minimally invasive operations can be done in a safe manner with appropriate modifications of the cardiopulmonary bypass circuit (Siegel *et al.*, 1997; Toomasian *et al.*, 1997; Gooris *et al.*, 1998; Groh and Fallen, 1998; Ceriana *et al.*, 2000). Further study is needed to analyse the outcomes, long-term efficacy, recovery times and cost-effectiveness of Port-access™ and robotic cardiac surgery.

REFERENCES

Acuff, T.E., Landrenau, R.J., Griffith, B.P., Mack, M.J. 1996: Minimally invasive coronary artery bypass grafting. *Annals of Thoracic Surgery* **61**, 135–7.

Almany, D.K., Sistino, J.J. 2002: Laboratory evaluation of the limitations of positive pressure safety valves on hard-shell venous reservoirs. *Journal of Extra-Corporeal Technology* **34**, 115–17.

Burke, R.P., Wernovsky, G., van der Velde, M., Hansen, D., Castaneda, A.R. 1995: Video-assisted thoracoscopic surgery for congenital heart disease. *Journal of Thoracic and Cardiovascular Surgery* **109**, 499–507.

Carpentier, A., Loulmet, D., LeBret, E., Haugades, B., Dassier, P., Guibourt, P. 1996: Chirurgie à coeur ouvert par video-chirurgie et mini-thoracotomie-primer cas (valvuloplastie mitrale) opéré avec succès. *Comptes Rendus De L'Academie des Sciences: Sciences de la vie* **319**, 219–23.

Carpentier, A., Loulmet, D., Aupecle, B. *et al.* 1998: Computer assisted open heart surgery. First case operated on with success. *Comptes Rendus De L Academic Des Science Serie III* **321**, 437–42.

Carpentier, A., Loulmet, D., Aupecle, B., Berrebi, A., Relland, J. 1999: Computer-assisted cardiac surgery. *Lancet* **353**, 379–80.

Ceriana, P., Pagnin, A., Locatelli, A. *et al.* 2000: Monitoring aspects during port-access cardiac surgery. *Journal of Cardiovascular Surgery* **41**, 579–83.

Chitwood, W.R. Jr. 1999: Minimally invasive cardiac valve surgery. In: Franco, K.L., Verrier, E.D. (eds)., *Advanced therapy in cardiac surgery.* Hamilton, Ontario, BC Decker Inc. 145–58.

Chitwood, W.R., Elbeery, J.R., Chapman, W.H.H. *et al.* 1997a: Video-assisted minimally invasive mitral valve surgery: the 'micro-mitral' operation. *Journal of Thoracic and Cardiovascular Surgery* **113**, 413–14.

Chitwood, W.R., Elbeery, J.R., Moran, J.M. 1997b: Minimally invasive mitral valve repair: using a mini-thoracotomy and trans-thoracic aortic occlusion. *Annals of Thoracic Surgery* **63**, 1477–9.

Chitwood, W.R. Jr, Wixon, C.L., Elbeery, J.R., Moran, J.M., Chapman, W.H., Lust, R.M. 1997c: Video-assisted minimally invasive mitral valve surgery. *Journal of Thoracic and Cardiovascular Surgery* **114**, 773–80.

Chitwood, W.R. Jr, Nifong, L.W., Elbeery, J.E. *et al.* 2000: Robotic mitral valve repair: trapezoidal resection and prosthetic annuloplasty with the da Vinci surgical system. *Journal of Thoracic and Cardiovascular Surgery* **120**, 1171–2.

Cohn, L.H., Adams, D.H., Couper, G.S., Bichell, D.P. 1997: Minimally invasive aortic valve replacement. *Seminar of Thoracic and Cardiovascular Surgery* **9**, 331–6.

Colvin, S.B., Grossi, E.A., Ribakove, G., Galloway, A.C. 2000: Minimally invasive aortic and mitral operation. *Oper Tech Card Thorac Surg* **5**, 212–20.

Cosgrove, D.M., Sabik, J.F. 1996: Minimally invasive approach for aortic valve operations. *Annals of Thoracic Surgery* **62**, 596–7.

Cosgrove, D.M., Gillinvov, A.M. 1998: Partial sternotomy for mitral valve operations. *Oper Tech Card Thorac Surg* **1**, 62–72.

Falk, V., Walther, T., Autschbach, R., Diegeler, A., Battelini, R., Mohr, F.W. 1998: Robot-assisted minimally invasive solo mitral valve operation. *Journal of Thoracic and Cardiovascular Surgery* **115**, 470–1.

Farhat, F., Coddens, J., Vanermen, H., Mikaeloff, P., Jegaden, O. 2002: Adenosine in port access surgery: a means for stabilizing the endoaortic clamp. *Heart Surgery Forum* **5**, E9–10.

Galloway, A.C., Shemin, R.J., Glower, D.D. 1999: First report of the port access international registry. *Annals of Thoracic Surgery* **67**, 51–8.

Glower, D.D., Landolfo, K.P., Clements, F. *et al.* 1998: Mitral valve operation via port access versus median sternotomy. *European Journal of Cardiothoracular Surgery* **14**, S143–7.

Gooris, T., van Vaerenbergh, G., Coddens, J., Bouchez, S., Vanermen, H. 1998: Perfusion techniques for port-access surgery. *Perfusion* **13**, 243–7.

Groh, M.A., Fallen, D.M. 1998: Alteration of the traditional extracorporeal bypass circuit to accommodate port-access minimally invasive cardiac procedures using endovascular based cardiopulmonary bypass. *Artificial Organs* **22**, 775–80.

Grossi, E.A., Groh, M.A., Lefrak, E.A. 1999: Results of a prospective multicentre study on port-access coronary bypass grafting. *Annals of Thoracic Surgery* **68**, 1475–7.

Grossi, E.A., LaPietra, A., Applebaum, R.M. *et al.* 2000: Case report of robotic instrument-enhanced mitral valve surgery. *Journal of Thoracic and Cardiovascular Surgery* **120**, 1169–71.

Grossi, E.A., LaPietra, A., Ribakove, G.H. *et al.* 2001: Minimally invasive versus sternotomy approaches for mitral reconstruction: comparison of intermediate-term results. *Journal of Thoracic and Cardiovascular Surgery* **121**, 708–13.

Gulielmos, V., Wagner, F.M., Waetzig, B. 1999: Clinical experience with minimally invasive coronary artery and mitral valve surgery with the advantage of cardiopulmonary bypass and cardioplegic arrest using the port access technique. *World Journal of Surgery* **23**, 480–5.

Gundry, S.R., Shattuck, O.H., Razzouk, A.J., del Rio, M.J., Sardari, F.F., Bailey, L.L. 1998: Facile minimally invasive cardiac surgery via ministernotomy. *Annals of Thoracic Surgery* **65**, 1100–4.

Kaneko, Y., Kohno, T., Ohtsuka, T., Ohbuchi, T., Furuse, A., Konishi, T. 1996: Video-assisted observation in mitral valve surgery. *Journal of Thoracic and Cardiovascular Surgery* **111**, 279–80.

Kappert, U., Wagner, F.M., Gulielmos, V., Taha, M., Schneider, J., Schueler, S. 1999: Port access surgery for congenital heart disease. *European Journal of Cardiothoracic Surgery* **16**, S86–8.

Kort, S., Applebaum, R.M., Grossi, E.A. *et al.* 2001: Minimally invasive aortic valve replacement: echocardiographic and clinical results. *American Heart Journal* **142**, 476–81.

Kypson, A.P., Glower, D.D. 2002a: Minimally invasive tricuspid operation using port access. *Annals of Thoracic Surgery* **74**, 43–5.

Kypson, A.P., Glower, D.D. 2002b: Port-access approach for combined aortic and mitral valve surgery. *Annals of Thoracic Surgery* **73**, 1657–8.

LaPietra, A., Grossi, E.A., Pua, B.B. *et al.* 2000: Assisted venous drainage presents the risk of undetected air microembolism. *Journal of Thoracic and Cardiovascular Surgery* **120**, 856–63.

Loulmet, D.F., Carpentier, A., Cho, P.W. *et al.* 1998: Less invasive techniques for mitral valve surgery. *Journal of Thoracic and Cardiovascular Surgery* **115**, 772–9.

Loulmet, D., Carpentier, A., d'Attellis, N. *et al.* 1999: Endoscopic coronary artery bypass grafting with the aid of robotic assisted instruments. *Journal of Thoracic and Cardiovascular Surgery* **118**, 4–10.

Mohr, F.W., Falk, V., Diegler, A., Walther, T., van Son, J.A., Autschbach, R. 1998: Minimally invasive port-access mitral valve surgery. *Journal of Thoracic and Cardiovascular Surgery* **115**, 567–76.

Mohr, F.W., Falk, V., Diegeler, A., Autschback, R. 1999a: Computer-enhanced coronary artery bypass surgery. *Journal of Thoracic and Cardiovascular Surgery* **117**, 1212–14.

Mohr, F.W., Onnasch, J.F., Falk, V. *et al.* 1999b: The evolution of minimally invasive mitral valve surgery – 2 year experience. *European Journal of Cardiothoracic Surgery* **15**, 233–9.

Mohr, F.W., Falk, V., Diegeler, A. *et al.* 2001: Computer-enhanced 'robotic' cardiac surgery: experience in 148 patients. *Journal of Thoracic and Cardiovascular Surgery* **121**, 842–53.

Nataf, P., Lima, L., Regan, M. *et al.* 1996: Minimally invasive coronary surgery with thoracoscopic internal mammary dissection: surgical technique. *Journal of Cardiac Surgery* **11**, 288–92.

Ogella, D.A. 1999: Advances in perfusion technology – an overview. *Journal of Indian Medical Association* **97**, 436–7, 441.

Onnasch, J.F., Schneider, F., Falk, V., Walther, T., Gummert, J., Mohr, F.W. 2002: Minimally invasive approach for redo mitral valve surgery: a true benefit for the patient. *Journal of Cardiac Surgery* **17**, 14–19.

Pompili, M.F., Stevens, J.H., Burdon, T.A. *et al.* 1996: Port-access mitral valve replacement in dogs. *Journal of Thoracic and Cardiovascular Surgery* **112**, 1268–74.

Port-Access International Registry. *Clinical report.* 2000.

Reichenspurner, H., Welz, A., Gulielmos, V., Boehm, D., Reichart, B. 1998: Port-access cardiac surgery using endovascular cardiopulmonary bypass: theory, practice, and results. *Journal of Cardiac Surgery* **13**, 275–80.

Reichenspurner, H., Damiano, R.J., Mack, M. *et al.* 1999: Use of the voice-controlled and computer-assisted surgical system Zeus for endoscopic coronary artery bypass grafting. *Journal of Thoracic and Cardiovascular Surgery* **118**, 11–16.

Reichenspurner, H., Boehm, D.H., Gulbins, H. *et al.* 2000: Three-dimensional video and robot-assisted port-access mitral valve surgery. *Annals of Thoracic Surgery* **69**, 1176–81.

Ribakove, G.H., Miller, J.S., Anderson, R.V. *et al.* 1998: Minimally invasive port-access coronary artery bypass grafting with early angiographic follow-up: initial clinical experience. *Journal of Thoracic and Cardiovascular Surgery* **115**, 1101–10.

Siegel, L.C., St Goar, F.G., Stevens, J.H. 1997: Monitoring considerations for port-access cardiac surgery. *Circulation* **96**, 562–8.

Stevens, J.H., Burdon, T.A., Peters, W.S. *et al.* 1996: Port-access coronary artery bypass grafting: a proposed surgical method. *Journal of Thoracic and Cardiovascular Surgery* **111**, 567–73.

Tabry, I., Costantini, E., Reyes, E. 2000: Left sided heartport approach for combined mitral valve and coronary bypass surgery. *Heart Surgery Forum* **3**, 334–6.

Toomasian, J.M., Williams, D.L., Colvin, S.B., Reitz, B.A. 1997: Perfusion during coronary and mitral valve surgery utilizing minimally invasive port-access technology. *Journal of Extra-Corporeal Technology* **29**, 66–72.

Toomasian, J.M., McCarthy, J.P. 1998: Total extrathoracic cardiopulmonary support with kinetic assisted venous drainage: experience in 50 patients. *Perfusion* **13**, 137–43.

Trehan, N., Mishra, Y.K., Mathew, S.G., Sharma, K.K., Shrivastava, S., Mehta, Y. 2002: Redo mitral valve surgery using the port-access system. *Asian Cardiovasc Thorac Ann* **10**, 215–18.

Tripp, H.F., Glower, D.D., Lowe, J.E., Wolfe, W.G. 2002: Comparison of port access to sternotomy in tricuspid or mitral/tricuspid operations. *Heart Surgery Forum* **5**, 136–40.

Vanermen, H., Wellens, F., De Geest, R., Degrieck, I., Van Praet, F. 1999: Video-assisted port-access mitral valve surgery: from debut to routine surgery. Will trocar-port-access cardiac surgery ultimately lead to robotic cardiac surgery? *Seminar of Thoracic and Cardiovascular Surgery* **11**, 223–4.

Webb, W.R., Harrison, L.H. Jr, Helmcke, F.R. 1997: Carbon dioxide field flooding minimizes residual intracardiac air after open heart operations. *Annals of Thoracic Surgery* **64**, 1489–91.

Willcox, T.W. 2002: Vacuum-assisted venous drainage: to air or not to air, that is the question. Has the bubble burst? *Journal of Extra-Corporeal Technology* **34**, 24–8.

Willcox, T.W., Mitchell, S.J., Gorman, D.F. 1999: Venous air in the bypass circuit: a source of arterial line emboli exacerbated by vacuum-assisted drainage. *Annals of Thoracic Surgery* **68**, 1285–9.

Yozu, R., Shin, H., Maehara, T., Iino, Y., Mitsumaru, A., Kawada, S. 2001: Port-access cardiac surgery. Experience with 34 cases at Keio University Hospital. *Jpn Journal of Thoracic and Cardiovascular Surgery* **49**, 360–4.

18

Cardiac surgery without cardiopulmonary bypass

JOSEPH P McGOLDRICK

KEY POINTS

- Surgeons focusing on avoiding cardiopulmonary bypass rather than avoiding the sternotomy *per se*.
- 'Beating heart' surgery must not prevent complete coronary revascularization.
- Median sternotomy combined with traction sutures and appropriate patient positioning has afforded safer access to all the coronary arteries.
- The widespread use of 'stabilizing' devices combined with intracoronary 'shunting' has largely obviated the need for pharmacologically induced bradycardia, and greatly facilitates an improved coronary anastomosis.
- 'Off-pump' surgery is a proven viable alternative to conventional coronary artery bypass grafting (CABG) in those with poor left ventricular function, or with other co-existing risk factors.
- As technology has evolved, we are now seeing, in some centres, more than 90 per cent of CABG being performed by off-pump CABG techniques.

INTRODUCTION

During recent years an increasing number of cardiac surgeons have resurrected the practice of unsupported 'beating heart' coronary operations for selected groups of patients. Kolosov (1967) popularized such techniques in the 1960s, whereas the technique has regained surgeons' attention as a less invasive and alternative approach to conventional coronary artery bypass grafting (CABG). Long considered by surgeons as the gold standard, cardiopulmonary bypass-supported coronary procedures are now being closely questioned, as such procedures remain characterized by a number of significant side effects.

Even the choice of access to the heart has received renewed attention. In avoiding sternotomy in favour of a small anterior thoracotomy, minimally invasive direct CABG (MIDCAB) attracts interest as an alternative technique – albeit largely limited to single-vessel coronary procedures. For some, the issue of access was of secondary importance; the focus of some surgeons devoted to minimally invasive approaches rapidly shifted towards the avoidance of cardiopulmonary bypass rather than avoiding the sternotomy itself. Such surgery currently receives the illustrious working title of 'Off-pump coronary artery bypass grafting' (OP-CABG). This change in emphasis away from MIDCAB offered greater opportunities to treat the significantly larger number of patients affected with multi-vessel disease.

How readily did the cardiac surgical community adopt such 'new' procedures? Initially, the beating heart operative technique was deemed to be more technically demanding; however, the introduction and continuous refinement in mechanical coronary stabilizers considerably improved the feasibility and outcome of these procedures. The surgical 'comfort zone' was expanded for many practitioners of surgery without cardiopulmonary bypass. Although the beating heart procedure was shown to be a suitable alternative to conventional cardiopulmonary bypass operations in select patients carrying high surgical risk, it is still not yet considered on a systematic basis for a majority of patients.

Clearly then, to gain credibility as a robust alternative to conventional procedures, beating heart operations must respond to all anatomies, use similar vascular conduits and achieve both equivalent technical results and comparable mortality and morbidity rates. It must certainly maintain a low conversion rate to cardiopulmonary bypass. Additionally, the beating heart operation must not prevent the patient from receiving complete coronary revascularization. This review traces the re-emergence of beating heart surgery and seeks to address some of its controversies. The indications, complications and results of coronary artery surgery without bypass are discussed.

Minimally invasive cardiac surgery – emerging strategies

Most patient concerns and demands for less invasive surgery are focused on comfort, cosmetic appearance, and rehabilitation that are all related to the degree of invasiveness. Conceptually, the degree of invasiveness of cardiac surgery depends on two factors:

- the surgical approach – the length of the skin incision, the degree of retraction and aggression to the tissue, the loss of blood
- the use of cardiopulmonary bypass.

Regarding specific definitive surgical strategies, four categories of less invasive cardiac surgery can be distinguished:

- direct coronary artery surgery on the beating heart *via sternotomy* without cardiopulmonary bypass (OP-CABG)
- MIDCAB on the beating heart *via a parasternal or left anterior small thoracotomy*
- limited or modified approaches using conventional techniques and instruments with either conventional cardiopulmonary bypass or the endovascular Endocardiopulmonary bypass system
- true port-access surgery in which all surgical acts are performed through ports and the heart is arrested with the endo-aortic clamp catheter.

These options offer different advantages in terms of reducing invasiveness and also have different learning curves. Although minimally invasive cardiac surgery is undergoing explosive evolution, the indications for the different surgical categories above are yet to be determined. The remainder of this review will address principally coronary revascularization procedures that take place without the use of cardiopulmonary bypass, namely MIDCAB and OP-CABG procedures.

It is interesting to reflect on the important advances that led to the widespread development of cardiac surgery:

- the description of the median sternotomy incision
- the development of cardiopulmonary bypass by Gibbon, and its clinical application in 1953
- improving techniques of myocardial protection.

It is certainly ironic that the current goals of less invasive CABG are the avoidance of cardiopulmonary bypass and the minimization of the access by avoiding median sternotomy (antero-lateral mini-thoracotomy, full endoscopic approach). The median sternotomy has always provided excellent simultaneous exposure to all of the cardiac valves and the epicardial coronary arteries. Good exposure has always been a necessity for the extensive corrections needed to treat the complex heart disease of most patients requiring surgery. Not all cardiac surgeons have embraced the sense of change in coronary revascularization!

Despite all the recent advancements, many surgeons feel that a cardioplegic-arrested heart is still to be considered the 'gold standard' in coronary artery surgery as it enables optimal exposure for even the most difficult coronary revascularization.

These concepts in less invasive surgery (optimistically 'minimally invasive' surgery) are not confined to cardiac surgery – they have dramatically affected many surgical sub-specialities. Advances in port access and video instrumentation have made laparoscopic and thorocoscopic surgery possible, whereas the desire to lessen incisional pain and hospital stay has made less invasive surgery an ever expanding field. Traditionally, minimally invasive surgical strategies have not been a major factor in adult cardiac surgery. That situation is changing each day.

Minimally invasive cardiac surgery: a need for change?

Cardiopulmonary bypass and cardioplegic arrest are, of themselves, non-physiological and inflict a total-body invasion. Pathophysiological changes occur from systemic inflammatory, coagulopathic, high vascular resistance, low output states, neuropsychiatric phenomena and cerebrovascular accident (Baumgartner *et al.*, 1999).

Although the majority of patients undergoing CABG tolerate cardiopulmonary bypass well, certain patient sub-groups have a higher incidence of adverse outcomes from the procedure, including the elderly and patients with profound ventricular dysfunction, prior cardiovascular accident, and pulmonary and renal dysfunction. It is these types of high-risk patients who may benefit the most from OP-CABG compared with standard cardiopulmonary bypass.

The cause of renal dysfunction after a cardiac operation is multifactorial and usually attributed to several issues, such as the use of cardiopulmonary bypass, perioperative cardiovascular compromise or toxic insults to the kidneys (Ascione *et al.*, 1999). Free plasma haemoglobin, elastase and endothelin, and free radicals including superoxide, hydrogen peroxide and the hydroxyl radicals can be generated during cardiopulmonary bypass and can induce injury in the renal brush-border membrane (Regragui *et al.*, 1995). Non-pulsatile flow, renal hypoperfusion, hypothermia and duration of cardiopulmonary bypass are also thought to have adverse affects on renal function. The benefit to the kidneys of the avoidance of cardiopulmonary bypass in the performance of OP-CABG is discussed later in this chapter.

Historical perspective

Although most 'off-pump' cardiac surgery is confined to coronary revascularization, it was in the area of valve surgery that the first beating heart procedure was performed. Henry Souttar is credited with the first successful procedure in 'beating heart' surgery when, in 1925, he performed 'finger' dilatation on a stenosed Mitral valve (Westaby and Benetti, 1996). His first attempt was sadly his last. Such was the adverse tide of opinion against him (and others whose attempts were not successful) that he could not find another suitable case thereafter.

Longmire (unreported) performed the first direct anastomosis between the left internal thoracic artery and the left anterior descending coronary artery in 1958 after failed endarterectomy. Sabiston performed a right coronary artery saphenous vein graft in 1962 and DeBakey succeeded with a vein bypass of the left coronary artery without cardiopulmonary bypass in 1964 (Sabiston, 1974). In 1967, Kolosov reported his success in performing left internal thoracic artery grafting to the left anterior descending artery and grafting of a lateral circumflex vessel on a beating heart – through a left thoracotomy (Kolosov, 1967). Favaloro (1968), Garrett and colleagues (Garrett *et al.*, 1973), Trapp and Bisarya (1975) and Ankeney (1975) also performed CABG without cardiopulmonary bypass between 1968 and 1975. Later they abandoned the procedure.

After 1968, widespread adoption of cardiopulmonary bypass and cardioplegia greatly facilitated CABG, and stimulated an exponential rise in both the number and complexity of cases performed. This was enough to stifle further efforts to operate on the beating heart at a time when vascular surgical techniques and myocardial protection were relatively primitive.

A few surgeons persisted, although largely for economic reasons. In Argentina and Brazil, Benetti and colleagues (Benetti *et al.*, 1991) and Buffolo *et al.* (1996) independently reported large series of operations performed via median sternotomy with simple interruption of coronary flow. Pfister and colleagues (Pfister *et al.*, 1992) also reported successful 'coronary bypass without cardiopulmonary bypass'. These workers reported 220 off-bypass operations, comparing the outcome with 220 conventional operations matched for number of grafts, left ventricular function and date of operation. They concluded that selected patients with left anterior descending artery and right coronary disease could safely undergo non-pump coronary surgery and that left ventricular function was better preserved than after cardioplegic arrest.

Akins (1994), too, compared coronary operations performed with and without cardiopulmonary bypass, and documented better preservation of left ventricular function despite extended periods of unprotected regional ischaemia. Benetti *et al.* (1991) took intraoperative left ventricular biopsies and demonstrated superior preservation of the mitochondria in the non-bypass patients.

Myocardial reperfusion injury plays a central role in the pathophysiology of myocardial stunning, but is unimportant in non-pump patients, despite individual coronary occlusion times of 15–30 minutes. Cardiopulmonary bypass activates neutrophils, which contribute to reperfusion injury. Temporary obstruction of a stenosed artery in a non-bypass case does not cause the same degree of injury as global ischaemia followed by reperfusion with activated neutrophils (Westaby, 1995). Collectively, the data from these groups suggest that non-pump coronary bypass is safe, cost-effective and beneficial, notably for patients with impaired ventricles. For those who do not accept blood transfusion, avoiding haemodilution virtually guarantees this.

Benetti and colleagues some years later (Benetti and Sani, 1994) seem to be the first surgeons who suggested that CABG could be performed through a small left thoracotomy with the aid of a thoracoscope. Benetti presented his ideas at the International Symposium on Myocardial Protection in Chicago in October 1994 (Benetti, 1994). At the International workshop on Arterial Conduits for Myocardial Revascularisation held in Rome in November 1994, Benetti and Sani (1994) and Subramanian *et al.* (1995) demonstrated the clinical use of minimally invasive coronary artery bypass grafting (MICAB).

Spence (1994) also presented MICAB experimental studies on dogs. In 1995, Benetti and co-workers reported the technique (Benetti and Ballester, 1995). It fell to Calafiore *et al.* (1996) to popularize MICAB through a small left anterior thoracotomy and report the world's largest series of operations, extending the indications to patients with multi-vessel coronary artery disease.

Aims of less invasive coronary surgery

A coronary artery bypass operation, whether conventional or less invasive, is a major life event to the patient. Conventional coronary operations with cardiopulmonary bypass are both relatively safe and effective. The pump oxygenator provides continuous systemic circulation, whereas cardioplegic arrest ensures myocardial protection. Based on the results of conventional coronary surgery, the patient expects long-term relief of angina, improved quality of life, and often to live longer. Any drive towards cost containment must not influence this goal. The aims of less invasive coronary surgery are to reduce peri-operative morbidity and ultimately to promote earlier hospital discharge (Westaby and Benetti, 1996).

In thoracic, abdominal and pelvic surgery a less invasive operation equates with a smaller incision, if not more of them! However, surgical invasiveness depends on the severity of post-operative physiological derangement and its effect on recovery. When the surgical wound discomfort has settled, the single most important comorbidity is cerebral injury. Viewed a different way, less invasive coronary surgery depends primarily on the avoidance of the damaging effects of cardiopulmonary bypass and only secondarily on access through smaller incisions.

The incision

Since the beginning of cardiac surgery, median sternotomy represented the standard approach to most cardiac procedures and the initial focus of surgeons was appropriately on survival as opposed to aesthetics. As the results improved, the cosmetic and psychological implications of surgery become more important in the evaluation of these procedures.

There are many surgeons who perform 'off-pump' CABG through a median sternotomy while shying away from mini-thoracotomy. Median sternotomy provides unparalleled access to the left anterior descending artery and right coronary arteries, which can be grafted while the heart supports the circulation. In good hands, with a short procedure, the morbidity of sternotomy is very low, even in patients undergoing bilateral internal thoracic artery grafts.

Sternotomy allows easy access to both internal thoracic arteries and allows vein or radial arterial grafts to be anastomosed to the aorta with a side clamp. Sternotomy allows early or immediate extubation and early discharge from hospital. There have been many varieties of partial sternotomy described. Partial lower sternotomy keeps the manubrium intact, and provides sufficient access for left internal thoracic artery to left anterior descending artery or right internal thoracic artery to right coronary artery anastomoses.

Alternatives to median sternotomy have been refined (Hanlon et al., 1969; Laks and Hammonds, 1980; Brutel de la Riviere et al., 1981; Bedard et al., 1986). Brutel de la Riviere et al. (1981) were the first to describe a bilateral sub-mammarian incision combined with a vertical sternotomy, after development of a superior flap to expose the suprasternal notch and an inferior flap extending beyond the xyphoid process (Hanlon et al., 1969).

Dubois (1989) described the first laparoscopic cholecystectomy. By 1991 technology had permitted a miniaturized video camera to be placed at the end of a thoracoscope. This stimulated an explosion in thoracic video-assisted surgery. There is now an irresistible drive towards minimal access coronary revascularization and a large and rapidly developing support industry. Future comparative studies will show whether these small incisions have an actual advantage in recovery or morbidity or whether their interest is entirely aesthetic. The use of minimally invasive techniques in valvular surgery is certainly based on aesthetic interest.

The minimal access approach began with the left internal thoracic artery to the left anterior descending artery through a 10 cm transverse incision over the fourth costal cartilage (Subramanian et al., 1997). Although patients were able to leave hospital 48–72 hours post-operatively, many complained bitterly of wound pain. Other less invasive approaches have followed, including the sub-xiphoid approach for anastomoses of the right gastro-epiploic artery to the posterior descending coronary artery.

PATIENT SELECTION FOR LESS INVASIVE OPERATIONS

MIDCAB

Most clinicians in the field refer to CABG without cardiopulmonary bypass through an anterolateral minithoracotomy incision as minimally invasive direct coronary artery bypass (MIDCAB). The incision has often been term a 'LAST' procedure – 'Limited Anterior Short Thoracotomy'. This surgical technique is appropriate for patients with left anterior descending artery or right coronary artery disease. A pedicled left internal thoracic artery graft of good calibre is required, and T-grafts, using radial artery can be used for the principal diagonal artery. Right coronary artery MIDCAB has not been as successful as left anterior descending artery grafts.

Limiting angina after left anterior descending artery restenosis is an indication for patients with isolated left anterior descending artery disease and possibly some patients with multi-vessel disease where other lesions are not surgically significant. Elderly patients with comorbidities or organ impairment and those with malignancy may be good candidates if adequate revascularization can be achieved with a single graft.

Patients with a small left anterior descending artery, a calcified vessel or a deep intra-myocardial left anterior descending artery are not good candidates for MIDCAB. Obesity, chronic obstructive airways disease (COAD) and a history of irradiation to the chest wall may contraindicate the method. Some surgeons, including the author, have found MIDCAB to be an ideal solution to re-operation on the left anterior descending artery in the presence of functioning grafts to the circumflex and right coronary arteries.

MIDCAB initially required one-lung ventilation and induced bradycardia to improve operating conditions. The difficult anastomotic exposure encountered with MIDCAB surgery has prompted some institutions to require immediate post-operative validation of graft patency through Doppler flow, thermoimaging or radiographic means.

Sternotomy without bypass: OP–CABG

Because of the difficulties described above, an alternative approach to MIDCAB surgery has emerged as the more preferential operation at many institutions. Referred to in this article as 'off-pump CABG' (OP-CABG), this technique is practised through a full sternotomy incision. When compared with the anterior thoracotomy access approach used in the MIDCAB procedure, the median sternotomy optimizes surgical exposure whilst minimizing post-operative pain. Additionally, the number of grafts and their locations limit the MIDCAB approach.

The technology currently available has allowed the OP-CABG procedure to reach multiple, targeted coronary locations and in many ways obviates the need for a so-called 'hybrid' procedure (combined MIDCAB and PTCA). The transition from MIDCAB to OP-CABG surgery has allowed cardiac surgeons to obtain improved anastomotic conditions while eliminating the need for both one-lung ventilation and induced bradycardia. Single or multiple bypasses are performed through a variety of graft conduits. These conduits include the internal thoracic arteries, saphenous vein and radial arteries.

Partial lower sternotomy

This approach has been used to offer good access to both internal thoracic arteries, and to give excellent exposure to the left and right coronary arteries. Selection criteria are the same as for a MIDCAB procedure.

Sub–xiphoid gastro–epiploic graft

This is a technique sometimes employed where access is sought to the posterior descending branch of the right coronary artery in re-operations where the graft conduit is the right gastro-epiploic artery. Adhesions from previous cardiac surgery can actually facilitate this procedure.

The method is indicated where patent grafts to the left coronary system exist. Naturally, previous gastric surgery or upper abdominal procedures are a relative contraindication. The gastro-epiploic artery should only be used for grafting the posterior descending coronary artery when a high grade stenosis exists. In the event of a less significant coronary stenosis where the gastro-epiploic artery competes with low flow, the graft will immediately adapt to its situation, reducing its size (O'Neil *et al.*, 1991). If the native coronary flow is brisk, the gastro-epiploic artery can even be perfused retrogradely, causing steal and hypoperfusion with ischaemia in the coronary artery territory (Spence *et al.*, 1995).

TECHNICAL CONSIDERATIONS IN OFF–PUMP SURGERY

Trauma

Both cardiopulmonary bypass and sternotomy provide a trauma stimulus to the patient that can be alleviated. Carrying out OP-CABG with perfusion assist devices in the left or right ventricles can reduce the effects of cardiopulmonary bypass, but it seems to many that it is the trauma of cardiopulmonary bypass itself that is to be avoided in 'beating heart' surgery. Musculoskeletal trauma can be minimized by reducing incision length, the amount of muscle divided and the amount of bone or rib divided or removed.

Access

As previously mentioned, MIDCAB requires the accurate placement of the incision to access the relevant coronary artery, usually the left anterior descending artery, and the harvesting of a good calibre high-quality length of internal thoracic artery. Usually only the left anterior descending artery is grafted, though sequential 'jump' grafts to the diagonal vessels can also be performed. The incision for the mini-thoracotomy is placed transversely or obliquely along the fifth intercostal space starting from the mid-clavicular line and spreading medially for 5–6 cm. Although the initial access appears limited, it allows for a clear dissection of the internal thoracic artery directly or thoracoscopically.

Parasternal incisions have been employed though the resulting rib excision is more traumatic even though the internal thoracic artery is well visualized. In mini-thoracotomy, after locating the internal thoracic artery, the use of a specially constructed spreader allows good mobilization of the internal thoracic artery by direct open dissection to above the first rib (Boonstra *et al.*, 1997; Qaqish *et al.*, 1997). There are several retractors of this type available, most elevate the upper ribs while pressing down on the lower one. These retractors can also be used in reverse to improve distal dissection below the fourth or fifth intercostal space. Video assistance has also been employed – this helps mostly by illumination and provides an alternative to a headlight.

The internal thoracic arteries can also be harvested videoscopically in either thorax. The actual port placements are critical to access the length of the internal thoracic artery and to prevent 'fencing' of the instruments. Both diathermy and harmonic scalpel techniques have been described (Nataf et al., 1996; Mack et al., 1997; Ohtsuka et al., 1997).

Pericardial access

Although a full sternotomy may not be considered by some as minimally invasive, it facilitates the performance of multiple CABG without bypass. Whilst hemi-sternotomy has been mentioned, a full sternotomy is the incision of choice for circumflex grafting off-bypass (Arom et al., 1996). To expose the posterior vessels the following manoeuvres are important.

1 Placing very deep pericardial sutures on the left side of the pericardium just above the pulmonary veins and at the diaphragm. Pulling up on even one of these sutures will elevate and rotate the heart to present the left anterior descending artery and left ventricular apex.
2 Mobilization of the right pleura or pericardium and dividing the connections between them and the diaphragm allows a space for the elevated heart to lie in. This space can be further increased by elevating the right sternal border and/or by widely opening the pleura. The heart can then be rotated over to access the circumflex vessels.

3 Rotation of the patient to the right and in a steep Trendelenberg head-down position. This improves right ventricular filling, which has been shown experimentally and clinically to be a manoeuvre that maintains cardiac output during elevation of the heart (Garrett et al., 1973; Grundeman et al., 1997; Jansen et al., 1998). The mechanism of action is debated, although it undoubtedly overcomes partial kinking and restriction of inflow of blood to the right ventricle rather than any aid to the left ventricle. Steep, down Trendelenberg positioning may also assist displacement of the apex out of the pericardium to allow easier access to the posterior vessels. Rotation to the right also helps by preventing the weight of the elevated heart compressing posteriorly down onto the right atrium, vena cavae and ventricular input.

Stabilization

Early experience with minimally invasive cardiac surgery (MIDCAB) did not involve the use of stabilizers. Traction sutures or adenosine and other pharmacological agents were used to steady the motion of the heart (Robinson et al., 1998). The wider introduction of different types of stabilizers into clinical practice has made it far easier to operate on a beating heart.

Although there is an expanding array of devices made available to surgeons, there are two essential types:

• the suction device known as the 'octopus'
• the footplate device (see Figs 18.1–18.3).

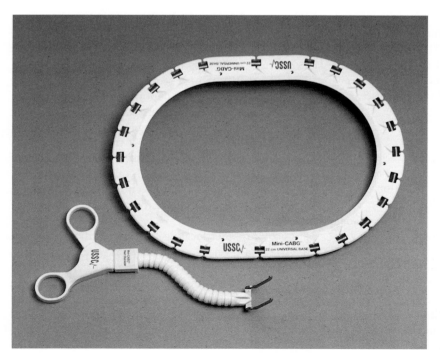

Figure 18.1 *USSC stabilizer ring with attachable or detachable footplate stabilizer for MIDCAB or OP-CABG.*

The suction device has two roles in that it can steady the heart by lifting and thereby reducing pressure on the ventricle, and it may also be used in part to rotate or present the heart. The foot devices are much simpler to attach: they fit onto or are a part of the chest spreader and are much less bulky and less surgically obtrusive – an advantage with the use of small incisions. They do cause pressure on the ventricle, which may adversely affect ventricular function, and they have only limited value in a presentation function.

The literature is quite clear on the significant contribution that the stabilizer has made to improved outcomes in beating heart surgery compared with no stabilizer. Poirier *et al.* (1999) published the Montreal Heart Institute's quantitative assessment of coronary anastomoses performed off bypass and also concluded that, in their experience, patients who underwent CABG with a stabilizer had a greater number of CABGs than did a 'non-stabilized' group.

Some authors have reported early post-operative angiographic results after revascularization of the beating heart with or without a mechanical restraining device. Buffalo and colleagues (Buffolo *et al.*, 1996) compared, in a non-randomized study, early angiographic results of the left internal thoracic artery graft to the left anterior descending artery in 60 patients performed with or without cardiopulmonary bypass. Ninety-three per cent of coronary anastomoses were patent in both groups. Benetti and colleagues

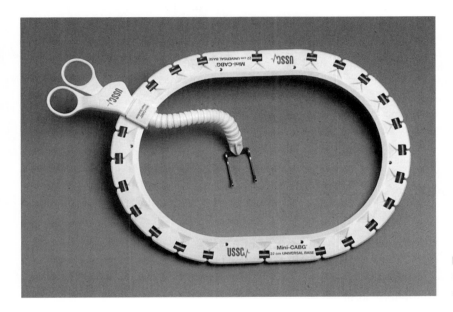

Figure 18.2 *USSC stabilizer ring with footplate stabilizer for MIDCAB or OP-CABG.*

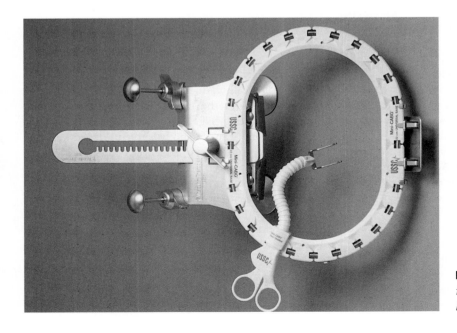

Figure 18.3 *USSC stabilizer ring with footplate stabilizer and thoralift for MIDCAB.*

(Benetti *et al.*, 1991) also studied a similar group of 54 patients (72 saphenous vein grafts and 24 internal thoracic artery grafts) with angiograms obtained during the first four weeks after surgery. They reported patency rates of 93 per cent with saphenous vein grafts and 88 per cent with internal thoracic artery grafts. Such reports documented patients early in the experience of these groups.

Conclusions from these and other investigators show that CABG on the beating heart performed with a mechanical myocardial wall restraining device results in lesser residual luminal stenosis at the anastomotic site, and better anastomotic coronary blood flow, than does the same procedure performed without stabilization.

Suturing technique

Before the widespread use of stabilizers, surgeons performed newer methods of suture orientation and placement to accommodate their new method of performing the anastomosis. With good stabilization there is virtually no need to alter one's tried and tested suturing style. A single circular suture (parachute) technique affords excellent vision of the entire suture circumference, and enables the occluder to remain *in situ* until the last suture is placed. The occluder is then removed after haemostasis is ensured. It is the author's view that a 'heel-and-toe-first' technique effectively fixes either end of the anastomosis and allows more potential for tearing of a coronary if the stabilization is less than ideal.

Ischaemia

Off-pump and MIDCAB surgery will produce local ischaemia from temporary occlusion of the native coronary vessel. Surgeons practising such techniques are acutely aware that resultant ischaemia may induce arrhythmias such as ventricular fibrillation or marked bradycardia, impaired ventricular performance or frank myocardial infarction. Operative ischaemia can result in ST-changes on the ECG or significant cardiac enzyme rise may be seen post-operatively. It is important to note that measurements of cardiac enzymes, especially of troponin (Hadjinikolaou *et al.*, 1997; Babatasi *et al.*, 1998; Bonatti *et al.*, 1998; Spooner *et al.*, 1998) all show very low levels of troponin rise in OP-CABG surgery compared with on-pump surgery, with the usual levels of troponin rise being 0.3 mcg/L compared with on-pump levels of about 1–2 mcg/L. Data acquired during the early experience of MIDCAB (Stanbridge *et al.*, 1997) showed that the ECG-ST change monitored by the anaesthetist rarely showed ST elevation above 1 mm.

The predictability of ECG-ST was shown to relate to the degree of native stenosis of the vessel being grafted

Table 18.1 *Relationship between degree of stenosis and ischaemic changes during MIDCAB surgery**

Percentage proximal stenosis	100	90	70	50
ST elevation (mm)	0.27	0.63	1.83	5.85

*ST elevation and percentage of native proximal stenosis in 50 patients (Stanbridge and Hadjinikolaou, 1999).

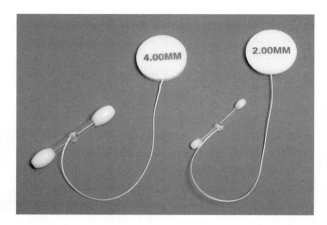

Figure 18.4 *Intracoronary shunts.*

(Hadjinikolaou *et al.*, 1997). Table 18.1 shows correlation of ECG-ST changes with native stenosis so that if the percentage native stenosis is 75 per cent or less then some ECG change may be expected. Additionally, it has been observed by the author and by other experienced off-pump surgeons that large right native coronary arteries have a disturbing habit of demonstrating arrhythmia on occlusion. Local ischaemia is rarely clinically significant, unless there is a mild proximal native stenosis or a large dominant right coronary artery.

Techniques to avoid regional myocardial ischaemia

Methods currently employed to combat ischaemia include pharmacologically induced bradycardia, ischaemic 'preconditioning' and the rapidly increased use of intracoronary shunting (Fig. 18.4). The practice of ischaemic pre-conditioning appears to be surgeon-dependant, and there remains controversy as to how necessary or beneficial it is to perform a pre-conditioning manoeuvre before completing an anastomosis (Malkowski *et al.*, 1998).

Intracoronary shunting has proved an invaluable adjunct in performing off-pump anastomoses safely and under good vision (Rivetti *et al.*, 1997). Shunting can prevent ischaemic phenomena, and can control bleeding through the vessel during the anastomoses. Excess blood loss through an arteriotomy may in theory also be a cause of ischaemia, especially if the vessel is not clamped

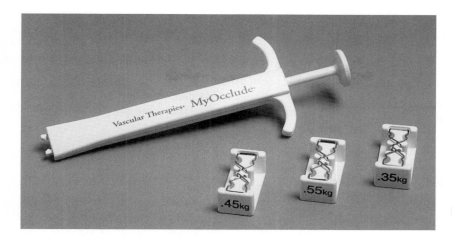

Figure 18.5 *Occluder clips, Vascular Therapies.*

proximally. It must also be noted that shunting can be a cumbersome technique at times, and can certainly damage the native vessel endothelium.

In summary, the main indications for shunting are:

- mild proximal native vessel stenosis (<75 per cent)
- a large dominant right coronary being grafted in its distal main part before the posterior descending bifurcation
- elevation of the ECG-ST segment by 2 mm or more
- any situation in which good haemostasis cannot be obtained (Stanbridge and Hadjinikolaou, 1999).

Haemostasis and vessel occlusion

Whilst making the operative field secure and the vessel stable is the most important prerequisite for reducing the risk of anastomotic stenosis or occlusion, it is fair to conclude that effective operative haemostasis is the second most important requirement for a good anastomosis. Vessel occlusion and irrigation are the two most common adjuncts to assuring a clear and precise surgical field. Before vessel occlusion, some preliminary dissection is required around the target vessel. This may lead to troublesome bleeding of a kind not normally encountered when grafting a vessel on a heart arrested by cardioplegia.

Three main techniques are employed to temporarily occlude a coronary artery before an OP-CABG procedure.

1 *Suture technique.* Usually a single silastic suture is employed to pass under the native coronary, which is then crossed and pulled up to give soft 'atraumatic' occlusion with haemostasis. This technique is particularly suited to grafting of the main right coronary artery. This vessel is often diseased and may fail to accept snugging or clipping.

2 *Snugging sutures.* These sutures are used with a snugger often over a pledget of felt or rubber and pressed down

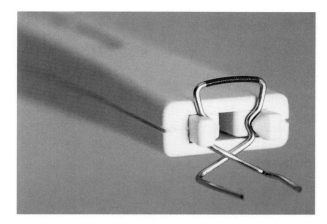

Figure 18.6 *Occluder clips, Vascular Therapies.*

to occlude the target vessel. This technique has received criticism, perhaps harshly, as damage to the vessel has been proposed as the cause of proximal or distal vessel stenosis with suture occlusion (Gundry, 1992; Pagni *et al.*, 1997), although there are experimental data offering evidence to the contrary (Perrault *et al.*, 1997), especially if the snaring is performed gently! Clearly, if the occlusion suture is also used to position the artery, damage is more likely.

3 *Clips.* Many types of soft metal clips are available and have been effective in occluding the native vessel. A degree of dissection is often required before their operative placement to prevent them 'flying off' (Figs 18.5 and 18.6).

Despite all the above techniques, vessel occlusion may still be inadequate because of collateral flow. For this reason the author and others have placed their faith in additional irrigation techniques. The author favours a technique that employs a combination of intracoronary shunting or vessel occluder and a blower technique of a CO_2 or saline 'mist' blown at the coronary artery – obviating the need for cumbersome occluding sutures or any form of clipping.

Blowers and irrigation

If a blower is to be used, safety factors will dictate that CO_2, and not air or oxygen, is used as the gas mixed with saline. Carbon dioxide is very soluble in blood and will be much less likely to cause gas embolism, whereas nitrogen in air can. The CO_2 is humidified, as dry gas blowing over the coronary artery anastomosis will cause the endothelium to dry out quickly and produce desiccation changes.

Anaesthetic implications of minimally invasive cardiac surgery

Minimally invasive approaches to myocardial revascularization provide several challenges to the cardiac anaesthetist. The key areas for consideration include pre-operative assessment and preparation, and safe induction and maintenance of anaesthesia, leading to smooth, early, pain-free emergence. Several workers have shown that early extubation can be achieved in the majority of these patients (Subramanian et al., 1997; Wasnick and Acuff, 1997; Heres et al., 1998).

PRE-OPERATIVE ASSESSMENT

In addition to standard cardiac evaluation, careful review of the coronary anatomy and pathology and discussions between surgeon and anaesthetist are essential. This will help identify specific needs, such as 'unconventional' positioning for different approaches, and the possibility of intraoperative complications, including dysrhythmias, hypotension and a need for conversion to cardiopulmonary bypass.

Light pre-medication will facilitate early emergence and extubation. Facilities for transthoracic defibrillation and pacing should be available, as should arrangements for maintaining body temperature.

INTRA-OPERATIVE CONSIDERATIONS

The aims during induction and maintenance of anaesthesia are to provide cardiac stability whilst facilitating early emergence and extubation. Tachycardia and extremes of blood pressure should be avoided. Appropriate volume loading is useful in this regard. The quoted improvements in surgical retractors and heart stabilizers have reduced the need for pharmacological interventions to provide a quiet surgical field (Heres et al., 1998; Lampa and Ramsey, 1999).

Monitoring should include ECG with continuous sinus tachycardia analysis, intra-arterial blood pressure and central venous access. The use of pulmonary artery catheters and/or transoesophageal echocardiography can be useful in patients with reduced ventricular function having multiple grafts (Lampa and Ramsey, 1999).

The use of a double-lumen endotracheal tube and one lung anaesthesia will facilitate surgery performed through a mini-thoracotomy and thoracoscopic procedures.

POST-OPERATIVE CONSIDERATIONS

The majority of these patients are suitable for 'fast-tracking'. Good analgesia is essential for early emergence and extubation and a smooth post-operative course. Various techniques, including combinations of systemic and intrathecal opioids, neural blockade via intercostal and intrapleural blocks, and thoracic epidurals and non-steroidal anti-inflammatory drugs have been described (Heres et al., 1998; Lampa and Ramsey, 1999).

RESULTS

Stanbridge and Hadjinikolaou (1999) reviewed the valuable experience of many centres when publishing a meta-analysis comparing MIDCAB surgery with OP-CABG through a sternotomy. Although this analysis contrasts the experience in two differing types of MICAS, there were valuable conclusions and valid inferences in comparing off-pump surgery with procedures performed with cardiopulmonary bypass. The analysis was presented to an International Symposium addressing the 'Present State of Minimally Invasive Cardiac Surgery – Meet the Experts', in Dresden, Germany in December 1998.

The analysis was based on 63 centres reporting 3304 cases of MIDCAB surgery, and 21 centres reporting over 3060 cases of off-pump surgery through a sternotomy. Several centres reported on both MIDCAB and sternotomy. Death was reported in 66 per cent of MIDCAB and 90 per cent of off-pump sternotomy reports. Myocardial infarction was less well reported, with some 30 per cent of reports mentioning this. There was no difference in early or late deaths between the two groups (1.6 per cent MIDCAB:2.2 per cent sternotomy). There was a higher infarction rate with MIDCAB that did not quite achieve statistical significance (2.9 per cent MIDCAB:1.45 per cent sternotomy; $p < 0.03$) (Table 18.2).

Graft patency and vessel stenosis were extracted and back-calculated to give exact numbers and proportions compared with angiography. Sixty per cent of reports mentioned occlusion rates in MIDCAB after investigation with angiography or non-invasive means, such as Doppler scanning, and 35 per cent commented on stenoses. Forty-three of 63 centres reported with angiography, and this accounted for reports in nearly 50 per cent of cases.

Table 18.2 *Mortality and myocardial infarction**

	N	Percentage available	Increase (%)
MIDCAB surgery (3304 patients from 63 centres)			
death early	31/1836	60	1.6
death late	6/599	18	1.0
myocardial infarction	32/1106	33	2.9[a]
Off-pump sternotomy surgery (3060 patients from 21 centres)			
death early	62/2819	92	2.2
death late	0/110	4	0.0
myocardial infarction	13/899	29	1.45[b]

*Stanbridge and Hadjinikolaou, 1999.
[a] $p \leqslant 0.05$.
[b] $p \leqslant 0.03$.

Table 18.3 *Patency and stenosis in MIDCAB surgery**

	N	Increase (%)
By invasive/non-invasive (3304 patients)		
occlusion early	86/2208	3.9
stenosis early	17/1698	1.0
total anastomatic problems	137/1343	10.2
By angiography (1727 patients from 43 centres)		
occlusion early	50/1281	3.9
stenosis early	64/977	6.6
total anastomatic problems	114/1281	8.9

*Stanbridge and Hadjinikolaou, 1999.

Table 18.4 *Patency and stenosis**

	Data	Percentage (%)
Off-pump sternotomy by invasive or non-invasive techniques (3060 patients)		
occlusion early	21/436	4.9
stenosis early	4/239	1.6
total anastomotic problems	13/239	5.4

	Off-pump (%)	MIDCAB (%)	p value
MIDCAB compared with off-pump sternotomy surgery by angiography			
occlusion early	4.7	3.9	NS
stenosis early	1.4	6.6	0.001
total anastomotic problems	6.4	10.5	0.08

*Stanbridge and Hadjinikolaou, 1999.
NS = not significant.

The use of angiography in sternotomy off-pump series was small, with only 432 cases of 3060 being analysed (14 per cent). The results are summarized in Tables 18.3, 18.4 and 18.5.

Table 18.5 *MIDCAB surgery**

	No stabilizer	Stabilizer	p value
Patency and stenosis with and without stabilizers			
n	575	898	1473
occlusion early	5.4	3.6	NS
stenosis early	9.6	3.7	0.002
total anastomotic problems	6	5.4	0.0001
late graft stenosis	3.3	1.9	NS
Mortality and myocardial infarction			
n	575	898	NS
early mortality	1.6 (4/251)	2.0 (11/560)	NS
late mortality	5.4 (2/205)	3.6 (2/199)	NS
peri-operative myocardial infarction	2.4 (4/169)	3.2 (16/493)	NS
conversions	5.3 (9/169)	5.2 (26/503)	NS

*Stanbridge and Hadjinikolaou, 1999.
NS = not significant.

The occlusion rates did not vary between those detected by angiography alone and those in which either angiography or non-invasive means were used (Table 18.3). The occlusion rate for MIDCAB was 3.9 per cent, and for sternotomy off-pump 4.9 per cent. Stenoses were reported angiographically at the anastomosis site or in the native left anterior descending artery vessel whether proximal or distal, or in the LIMA graft. The incidence of stenosis in MIDCAB was 6.6 per cent and for sternotomy off-pump was 1.4 per cent. This difference was significant at the $p < 0.001$ level (Table 18.4). A combination total for occlusion or stenosis showed a high incidence in the MIDCAB group (10.5 per cent), which was significantly higher than the sternotomy group (6.4 per cent) at angiography ($p < 0.08$).

The role of stabilization in the high MIDCAB occlusion or stenosis group was found to be critical. Four major series showed comparative data for the period before stabilizers were used against that after their introduction. These data are summarized in Table 18.5. After the introduction of stabilizers the combined occlusion and stenosis rate altered significantly – it was halved in each series! Stenosis rates on these four comparative MIDCAB reports showed a high incidence (9.6 per cent), which was significantly reduced with stabilization to 3.7 per cent ($p < 0.002$). The combined occlusion and stenosis rate was very high at 16 per cent and was reduced significantly to five per cent ($p < 0.0001$).

Stabilization did not produce any change in the incidence of early or late death, of myocardial infarction or of conversion to sternotomy (constant at five per cent) in these series.

In the total series there was no significant difference in length of stay (4.6 days), incidence of atrial fibrillation (nine per cent), or between conversion to sternotomy (MIDCAB group) or to bypass (sternotomy group) (five per cent). Interestingly, grafting the right coronary artery by MIDCAB produced worse results than the left anterior descending artery, whether alone or as a combined operation.

There was a startling uniformity in Stanbridge's meta-analysis with respect to comparison of occlusion rates. When angiography was compared with other non-invasive techniques there was little difference between the diagnostic modalities, suggesting there may be little difference between Doppler analysis and angiography in detecting occlusions, though not stenoses. An important finding was that while MIDCAB carried a non-significant higher occlusion rate than off-pump sternotomy, this became identical (3.6 per cent) as soon as stabilizers were introduced.

Many centres in this meta-analysis showed real and important improvements in results as soon as they adopted a practice incorporating the use of stabilizers. It is interesting to observe that not all MIDCAB reports were bad when stabilization was not routinely practised; however, the results overall are good enough to suggest that stabilization is a critical step in beating-heart surgery. Stanbridge and Hadjinikolaou (1999) concluded that the evidence strongly supports the view that stabilizers should always be used in MIDCAB surgery. In addition, and logically, stabilizers should always be used in off-pump sternotomy beating heart surgery. Left anterior descending artery occlusion rates with stabilization (3.6 per cent) compare favourably with those recorded by conventional surgery (4.9 per cent) (Mack et al., 1998). The fate of the LIMA graft with stabilization performed by MIDCAB or off-pump sternotomy appears as good as with conventional surgery.

The large series of both MIDCAB and sternotomy CABG show that stenosis in the graft vessel or its host is a significant finding. This finding is perhaps overlooked in conventional CABG when not many post-operative angiograms have been done, but we are all aware of late findings of stenosis in the host or graft vessel. This finding focuses surgeons on the quality of their anastamoses as well as the quality of their grafts and how they treat the native vessel either side of the anastamosis.

It is to be noted in the reports to the International Symposium on MICAS in Dresden 1998 that no particular or consistent definition was set for myocardial infarction – that merely being set by the reporting groups. It was thought perhaps this fact alone accounted for the apparent lower incidence of myocardial infarction with sternotomy off-pump than with MIDCAB.

Right internal mammary artery anastomosis to right coronary artery had a poorer result than left anterior descending artery grafts in both MIDCAB and off-pump sternotomy. This could be explained by the different characteristics of the right coronary artery, its position for anastamosis and the higher incidence of poor target finding.

The incidence of atrial fibrillation is much reduced (nine per cent) compared with often-quoted statistics (15–30 per cent) and this is widely taken to reflect less interference to the atrium or pericardium in CABG without bypass, and is particularly true of MIDCAB.

In summary, it is clear from many reviews that there is a higher early stenosis rate and total anastomotic problem rate with MIDCAB compared with off-pump CABG, but this rate equalizes with the use of stabilizers. Moreover, there is an unexplained low and lower rate of myocardial infarction in sternotomy off-pump compared with MIDCAB. The overall success of both these modalities of surgery off bypass using stabilizers has encouraged more centres in their endeavours to perform revascularization surgery without extracorporeal circulation.

PRIMARY CABG OFF-PUMP IN SITUATIONS OF IMPAIRED LEFT VENTRICULAR FUNCTION

Moshkovitz et al. (1997) and other groups have reported excellent operative results of conventional CABG performed in patients with severely impaired left ventricular function using different cardioplegic and left ventricular preservation techniques. He puts forward an argument that, as these results are similar to their own group's results for OP-CABG in poor left ventricular patients, CABG without cardiopulmonary bypass should rightly be regarded as a legitimate myocardial protection technique. This is especially true, they state, for patients with extreme left ventricular dysfunction, or for those with significant co-existing risk factors for conventional CABG, such as acute myocardial infarction and cardiogenic shock.

The report from the Chaim Sheba Medical Centre (Moshkovitz et al., 1997) details outcomes of 75 patients with left ventricular ejection fraction of ⩽0.35, who underwent primary CABG without cardiopulmonary bypass. Thirty-two (43 per cent) patients had congestive heart failure, 11 (15 per cent) were referred within 24 hours of an evolving infarct and 21 (28 per cent) up to one week after acute myocardial infarction. Eighteen patients (24 per cent), six of whom were in cardiogenic shock, underwent emergency operations. The mean number of grafts was 1.9 (range one to four) and IMA usage was 85 per cent. Only 23 per cent of patients had a graft to the circumflex artery. Two patients (2.7 per cent) died perioperatively and one sustained a stroke. At a mean follow-up of 28 months, 13 patients had died and angina had returned in seven (10.5 per cent). One- and four-year actuarial survival was 96 per cent and 73 per cent, respectively. It is clear that off-pump surgery is at least a viable alternative to conventional CABG, in particular for patients with extreme left ventricular dysfunction or with other co-existing risk factors, such as acute myocardial infarction and cardiogenic shock.

ALTERNATIVE APPROACHES TO CORONARY DISEASE WITH INTEGRATED CORONARY REVASCULARIZATION

Integrated coronary revascularization combines minimally invasive CABG with left internal mammary artery–left anterior descending artery grafting and percutaneous coronary intervention. The rationale for the emergence of such combination strategies lies in the attempts to glean the benefits of both forms of revascularization at the same time in the ischaemic patient. As the rapid expansion in available options of myocardial revascularization has occurred both in the interventional cardiology and in the surgical field then it was obvious that the 'gap' between percutaneous and surgical coronary revascularization would narrow. One can see that, as percutaneous techniques move from 'plain old angioplasty' to more invasive and costly techniques, surgery is moving towards less invasive and less expensive approaches (Table 18.6).

The successful and cost-effective application of MICABG has created the basis for a new approach to multi-vessel coronary artery disease by combining the minimally invasive surgical revascularization of the left anterior descending artery using the left internal mammary artery with percutaneous coronary intervention of the circumflex or right coronary artery. The aim was to offer a safe and efficacious treatment with the best possible short- and long-term results at low cost and short hospital stay.

Zenati *et al.* (1999) reported that, for their series of patients, integrated coronary revascularization (left internal mammary artery–left anterior descending artery

and PTCA or stenting of other vessels in patients with multi-vessel disease) was a safe and effective treatment. Even patients at high risk, with left main stem disease, low ejection fraction, advanced age and significant comorbidities, were successfully treated with no mortality and minimal morbidity. The elimination of cardiopulmonary bypass in these patients with particularly high risk may avoid the significant incidence of neurological sequelae reported with routine CABG (Roach *et al.*, 1996).

Zenati *et al.* (1999), in an attempt to offer the best revascularization strategy to patients with multi-vessel coronary artery disease, hypothesized that integrated revascularization could provide 'the best of two possible worlds', promoting a complementary role of minimally invasive surgery and interventional cardiology.

In their series of 31 consecutive patients undergoing interventional coronary revascularization, the acute procedural rate was 100 per cent. Freedom from repeat revascularization at 10.8 months' follow-up was 90.4 per cent; one case of sub-acute thrombosis owing to non-compliance with aspirin–ticlopidine regimen occurred and two cases of recurrence of coronary artery disease proximal to the site of stent placement were noted. No clinical restenosis was observed. Patency of the left internal mammary artery–left anterior descending artery anastomosis was 100 per cent. Survival was 100 per cent at 10.8 months. Unlike others, these workers did not observe increased bleeding caused by the more intense anticoagulation required for stents.

Zenati *et al.* (1999) concluded, as many including the author have, that it is reasonable for the future to envision the formation of a practical 'partnership' between interventional cardiology and coronary bypass surgery, with the development of revascularization centres in which different procedures are performed by a closely co-ordinated team of operators with different backgrounds.

BEATING HEART SURGERY SUPPORTED BY ASSIST DEVICES

Ventricular assist devices have been successfully used to support patients during CABG. These techniques avoid the risk of cardiopulmonary bypass and an artificial oxygenator because the patients' own lungs are functioning. Sweeney and Frazier (1992) reported good results when using ventricular assist device-supported CABG in high-risk patients. They used the β-blocking agent, esmolol, as an adjunct to make the heart flaccid. The technique, using both left- and right-sided assist with Bio-Medicus pumps, is cumbersome with the risk of device-related complications.

In a few cases Sweeney and Frazier (1992) used an intracorporeal axial blood flow pump for left ventricular

Table 18.6 *Myocardial revascularization strategies*

Percutaneous coronary intervention:
   percutaneous transluminal coronary angioplasty
   stenting
   atherectomy
   laser angioplasty
   percutaneous transmyocardial laser revascularization
   combination of the above
Surgical revascularization:
   CABG
   MICABG
   transmyocardial laser revascularization
   integrated coronary revascularization (MICABG + PTCA or stent)

support with encouraging results. This method has the potential to become an alternative to the MIDCAB procedure as it provides the surgeon with an approach by which he can reach more than one vessel, while avoiding the negative effects of cardiopulmonary bypass. It can also provide a less dramatic way of using the MIDCAB approach, operating on the beating heart but with the convenience of a sternotomy giving better control over the surgical field.

In 1994 Lönn reported their clinical experience using an axial blood flow pump (hemopump). The hemopump was inserted into the left ventricle through a graft sutured to the aorta 5–6 cm distal to the aortic valve. Transoesophageal echo was occasionally used to confirm the position of the pump. Esmolol was given as a bolus followed by an infusion to ensure flaccidity. Thirty-two patients were randomizd prospectively. The study group was operated on using the hemopump as circulatory support. Operations were performed on the beating heart. The control group was operated on using cardiopulmonary bypass, aortic cross-clamping and cardioplegic arrest.

The results showed that all patients went through the procedure without major complications and were discharged from the hospital. No statistical differences were observed between the groups for time on support (hemopump, 60.5 min; cardiopulmonary bypass, 70.5 min) or total operating time (hemopump, 178 min; cardiopulmonary bypass 162 min). The number of grafts was greater in the cardiopulmonary bypass group (hemopump, 1.8; range 1–3; cardiopulmonary bypass, 2.5; range, 1–4). Statistical differences were found for intraoperative bleeding (hemopump mean, 312 mL; cardiopulmonary bypass mean, 582 mL) and myocardial trauma, as measured by post-operative troponin-T values (hemopump, 0.23 μg/L; cardiopulmonary bypass, 1.17 μg/L). These researchers concluded that they had delivered the benefits of safe surgery with reduced bleeding and myocardial damage without prolonging intraoperative support or total operating time. The author will let the reader decide how 'minimally invasive' such a procedure is, and if it offers a simpler alternative to conventional coronary surgery performed with cardiopulmonary bypass.

CONCLUSIONS

Robert Kennedy stated, 'Progress is a nice word, but change is its motivator, and change has its enemies.' Many surgeons (including the author) have asked themselves, 'Why change a good operation?' My own feeling is that the question, 'Is there a future for minimally invasive cardiac surgery?' should, more appropriately, be 'Is there a future for cardiac surgery without minimally invasive cardiac surgery?'

In an editorial responding to critics of minimally invasive cardiac surgery, entitled 'Cardiac Surgery of the 1990's: the "Inertia of success"', Mack *et al.* (1999) stated that although conventional CABG has been a good operation for the past 30 years, and had contributed to the health of millions of patients, innovation for the most part had stopped. Although there were some advances, including better myocardial protection, safer oxygenators and greater use of arterial conduits to prolong longevity, these were merely upgrades of basically a speciality that was not re-inventing itself.

As evidence of this we can look at the frequency of procedures being performed for coronary revascularization. Catheter-based procedures, which were initiated in 1979, took a mere 10 years to surpass cardiac surgical procedures in the number of procedures performed. The figures compiled from industry sales data in 1998 of worldwide case volumes showed that twice the number of catheter-based procedures are performed worldwide (1,500,000) compared with coronary bypass procedures (750,000). Mack *et al.* (1999) concluded that surgeons must have the courage to embrace change and continually re-invent themselves and their practices. The editorial concluded, 'we must not become stagnant by the inertia of our past success and fail to grasp the opportunity for change.'

At present, the MIDCAB procedure has found its niche in revascularization. In 1998, it is estimated that approximately seven per cent of all coronary bypass operations performed worldwide were performed by a beating-heart approach. Of these beating-heart procedures, approximately 10 per cent (44,000) appear to be MIDCAB procedures. The MIDCAB procedure seems to have found a niche for a number of reasons:

1 It is applicable, mostly, to only single-vessel disease on the anterior surface of the heart.
2 Wider use of improved catheter-based techniques and stents limits its application.
3 The ability to perform a beating-heart anastomosis through a limited access incision has proved a formidable challenge for many surgeons.

For all the above reasons, minimally invasive cardiac surgery appears to have evolved to off-pump beating-heart surgery performed through a median sternotomy approach or OP-CABG. The reasons for the wider acceptance of OP-CABG compared with MIDCAB procedures include:

- the ability to address multi-vessel disease
- 'surgeon-friendly' wider access approaches with much less concern if conversion to cardiopulmonary bypass is necessary
- improved technology, including second-generation stabilizers
- new techniques that allow access to the posterior arterial circulation of the heart without significant haemodynamic compromise.

In many centres in Europe and the USA, more than 90 per cent of all CABG is performed by OP-CABG techniques. Although the literature does not document on a randomized basis the benefits of OP-CABG versus conventional coronary bypass techniques, with the rapid evolution of these techniques, those results should be forthcoming.

Technology continues to evolve, and will continue to expand the application of minimally invasive cardiac surgery, but it also improves conventional surgical techniques. Indeed, one of the more significant contributions of minimally invasive surgery may be the 'coat-tail effect' that is conveyed to conventional bypass surgery. There is a plethora of new technology that attempts to eliminate the undesirable effects of conventional bypass surgery. Some of these developments include newer oxygenators, arterial aortic filters to trap and eliminate atherosclerotic emboli and, very significantly, newer methods of providing circulatory assistance for off-pump beating-heart surgery. This chapter has already referred to a number of axial flow micropumps that have been developed, which allow univentricular and biventricular support without the need for artificial oxygenation.

The ability to perform coronary bypass surgery by a totally endoscopic approach is a formidable challenge that is being addressed in many centres, with varying technologies. There has been intense interest in the field of robotics to facilitate endoscopic coronary bypass surgery. The principal underlying role of robotics for coronary bypass surgery is that the introduction of 'computer assistance' with robotics allows the enhanced precision necessary for an endoscopic vascular anastomosis to be performed. There have been at least 250 robotically assisted operations performed worldwide of which 80 have been cardiac procedures (Mack *et al.*, 1999). The cardiac procedures performed using robotic or computer assistance include internal mammary artery harvest, atrial septal defect repair, mitral valve repair and CABG.

For all this innovation, the introduction of new technology has to comply with safety standards and match the good results that are currently offered with conventional surgery. Surgeons have taken account that coronary bypass surgery on the beating heart is a microsurgical procedure on a moving target and technically somewhat demanding when the procedure is performed through a limited access. To minimize this risk, appropriate indication and patient selection is crucial.

Future generations of cardiac surgeons, especially those in training, will have to become familiar with minimally invasive techniques. As catheter-based therapy becomes more complex with the use of multiple stents per procedure and with the use of expensive 2b/3a agents and the need for repeat target vessel revascularization, cardiac surgery, especially when performed by a minimally invasive approach, may become the most cost-effective treatment for coronary artery disease.

As cardiac surgery becomes less invasive, and cardiology becomes more invasive, it is possible that both specialities will evolve into one in which a 'cardiac interventionalist' will have the ability to perform catheter-based techniques along with surgical intervention. This delivery of multi-modality cardiac interventional therapy may define the cardiac revascularization specialist of the next decade.

To exist is to change, to change is to mature, to mature is to go on creating one's self endlessly.

Henri Bergson

REFERENCES

Ankeney, J.L. 1975: To use or not to use the pump oxygenator in coronary bypass operations. *Annals of Thoracic Surgery* **19**, 108–9.

Arom, K.V., Emery, R.W., Nicoloff, D.M. 1996: Mini-sternotomy for coronary artery bypass grafting via left anterior small thoracotomy without cardiopulmonary bypass. *Annals of Thoracic Surgery* **62**, 1271–2.

Ascione, R., Lloyd, C.T., Underwood, M.J., Gomes, W.J., Angelini, G.D. 1999: On-pump versus off-pump coronary revascularization: evaluation of renal function. *Annals of Thoracic Surgery* **68**, 493–8.

Akins, C.W. 1994: Controversies in myocardial revascularization: coronary artery surgery for single vessel disease. *Semin Thorac Cardiovasc Surg* **6**, 109–15.

Babatasi, G., Massetti, M., Nataf, P., Fradin, S., Khayat, A. 1998: Safety of beating heart anastomosis during video assisted coronary surgery attested by cardiac troponin. *Artifical Organs* **22**, 508–13.

Baumgartner, F.J., Gheissari, A., Capouya, E.R., Panagiotides, G.P., Katouzian, A., Yokoyama, T. 1999: Technical aspects of total revascularization in off-pump coronary bypass via sternotomy approach. *Annals of Thoracic Surgery* **67**, 1653–8.

Bedard, P., Keon, W.J., Brais, M.P., Goldstein, W. 1986: Submammary skin incision as a cosmetic approach to median sternotomy. *Annals of Thoracic Surgery* **41**, 339–41.

Benetti, F.J. 1994: Symposium on myocardial protection: looking towards the 21st century. Chicago, IL, October.

Benetti, F.J., Ballester, C. 1995: Use of thoracoscopy and a minimal thoracotomy in mammary-coronary bypass to left anterior descending artery without extra corporeal circulation. Experience in two cases. *Journal Cardiovascular Surgery* **36**, 159–61.

Benetti, F.J., Sani, G. 1994: International workshop on arterial conduits for myocardial revascularization. Universita Cattolica del Sacro Cuore, Rome, Italy, November.

Benetti, F.J., Naselli, G., Wood, M., Geffner, L. 1991: Direct myocardial revascularization without extra-corporeal circulation. Experience in 700 patients. *Chest* **100**, 312–16.

Bonatti, J., Hangler, H., Hormann, C., Mair, J., Falkensammer, J., Mair, P. 1998: Myocardial damage after minimally invasive coronary artery bypass grafting on the beating heart. *Annals of Thoracic Surgery* **66**, 1093–6.

Boonstra, P.W., Grandjean, J.G., Mariani, M.A. 1997: Local immobilization of the left anterior descending artery for minimally invasive coronary bypass grafting. *Annals of Thoracic Surgery* **63** (Suppl, 6), S76–8.

Brutel de la Riviere, A., Brom, G.H.M., Brom, A.G. 1981: Horizontal submammary skin incision for median sternotomy. *Annals of Thoracic Surgery* **32**, 101–4.

Buffolo, E., de Andrade, C.S., Branco, J.N., Teles, C.A., Anuiar, L.F., Gomes, W.J. 1996: Coronary artery bypass grafting without cardiopulmonary bypass. *Annals of Thoracic Surgery* **61**, 63–6.

Calafiore, A.M., Giamarco, G.D., Teodori, G. *et al.* 1996: Left anterior coronary artery grafting via left anterior small thoracotomy without cardiopulmonary bypass. *Annals of Thoracic Surgery* **61**, 1659–65.

Dubois, F., Berthelot, G., Levard, H. 1989: Cholocystectomy by coelioscopy [French]. *Presse Med* **18**(19), 980–2.

Favaloro, R.G. 1968: Saphenous vein autograft replacement of severe segmental coronary occlusion. *Annals of Thoracic Surgery* **5**, 334–9.

Garrett, H.E., Dennid, E.W., DeBakey, M.E. 1973: Aorto-coronary bypass with saphenous vein graft. Seven year follow-up. *Journal of the American Medical Association* **223**, 792–4.

Grundeman, P.F., Borst, C., van Herwaarden, J.A., Mansvelt-Beck, H.J., Jansen, E.W.L. 1997: Haemodynamic changes during displacement of the beating heart by the Utrecht 'Octopus' method. *Annals of Thoracic Surgery* **67**, S88–92.

Gundry, S.R. 1992: Discussion of Pfister J.A., Salah Z.M., Garcia J.M. Coronary artery bypass without cardiopulmonary bypass. *Annals of Thoracic Surgery* **54**, 1085–92.

Hadjinikolaou, L.N., Cohen, A.S., Aitkenhead, H., Richmond, W., Stanbridge, R.D. 1997: Troponin-T in minimal invasive coronary operations. *Annals of Thoracic Surgery* **63**, 1511–12.

Hanlon, C.R., Barner, H.B., Wilman, V.L., Mudd, J.G., Kaiser, G.C. 1969: Atrial septal defect results of repair in adults. *Archives of Surgery* **99**, 275–81.

Heres, E.K., Marquez, J., Malkowski, M.J., Magovern, J.A., Gravlee, G.P. 1998: Minimally invasive direct coronary artery bypass: anesthetic, monitoring and pain control considerations. *Journal of Cardiothoracic and Vascular Anesthesiology* **4**, 385–9.

Jansen, E.W., Borst, C., Lahpor, J.R. *et al.* 1998: Coronary artery bypass grafting without cardiopulmonary bypass using the Octopus method: results in the first one hundred patients. *Journal of Cardiothoracic and Vascular Anesthesiology* **116**, 60–7.

Kolosov, V. 1967: Mammary artery–coronary artery anastomosis as a method for treating angina pectoris. *Journal of Cardiothoracic and Vascular Anesthesiology* **54**, 535–44.

Laks, H., Hammonds, G.M. 1980: A cosmetically acceptable incision for the median sternotomy. *Journal of Cardiothoracic and Vascular Anesthesiology* **79**, 146–9.

Lampa, M., Ramsay, J. 1999: Anesthetic implications of new surgical approaches to myocardial revascularization. *Curr Opin Anesth* **12**, 3–8.

Lonn, L., Peterzen, B., Granfeld, H. (1994): Coronary artery operation with support of the Haemopump Cardiac Assist System. *Annals of Thoracic Surgery* **58**, 519–23.

Mack, M., Acuff, T., Yong, P., Jett, G.K., Carter, D. 1997: Minimally invasive thoracoscopically assisted coronary artery bypass surgery. *European Journal of Cardiothoracic Surgery* **12**, 20–4.

Mack, M.J., Osbourne, J.A., Shennib, H. 1998: Arterial graft patency in coronary artery bypass grafting: what do we really know? *Annals of Thoracic Surgery* **66**, 1055–9.

Mack, M.J., Damiano, R., Matheny, R., Reichenspurner, H., Carpentier, A. 1999: 'The inertia of success' a response to

minimally invasive coronary bypass, a dissenting opinion. *Circulation* **99**, 1404–6.

Malkowski, M.J., Kramer, C.M., Parvizi, S.T. *et al.* 1998: Transient ischemia does not limit regional dysfunction in humans: a transesophageal echocardiographic study during minimally invasive coronary artery bypass surgery. *J Am Coll Cardiol* **31**, 1035–9.

Moshkovitz, Y., Sternik, L., Paz, Y. *et al.* 1997: Primary coronary artery bypass grafting in impaired left ventricular dysfunction. *Annals of Thoracic Surgery* **63**, S44–7.

Nataf, P., Lima, L., Regan, M. *et al.* 1996: Minimally invasive coronary surgery with thorascopic internal mammary dissection: surgical technique. *Journal of Thoracic and Cardiovascular Surgery* **11**, 288–97.

Ohtsuka, T., Wolf, R.K., Hiratzka, L.F., Wurnig, P., Flege, J.B. 1997: Thoracoscopic IMA harvest for MICABG using the harmonic scalpel. *Annals of Thoracic Surgery* **63** (Suppl. 6), S107–9.

O'Neil, G.S., Chester, A.H., Allen, S.P. *et al.* 1991: Endothelial function of human gastroepiploic artery. Implications for its use as a bypass graft. *Journal of Thoracic and Cardiovascular Surgery* **102**, 561–5.

Pagni, S., Qagish, N.K., Senior, D.G., Spence, P.A. 1997: Anastomotic complications in minimally invasive coronary bypass grafting. *Annals of Thoracic Surgery* **63** (Suppl. 6), S64–7.

Perrault, L.P., Menasche, P., Bidouard, J.P. *et al.* 1997: Snaring of the target vessel in less invasive bypass operations does not cause endothelial dysfunction. *Annals of Thoracic Surgery* **63**, 751–5.

Pfister, A.J., Zaki, M.S., Garcia, J.M. *et al.* 1992: Coronary artery bypass without cardiopulmonary bypass. *Annals of Thoracic Surgery* **54**, 1085–91.

Poirier, N.C., Carrier, M., Lesperance, J. *et al.* 1999: Quantitative angiographic assessment of coronary anastomoses performed without cardiopulmonary bypass. *Journal of Thoracic and Cardiovascular Surgery* **117**, 292–7.

Qaqish, N.K., Pagni, S., Spence, P.A. 1997: Instrumentation for minimally invasive internal thoracic harvest. *Annals of Thoracic Surgery* **63** (Suppl. 6), S97–9.

Regragui, I.A., Izzat, M.B., Birdi, I., Lapsley, M., Bryan, A.J., Angelini, G.D. 1995: Cardiopulmonary bypass perfusion temperature does not influence perioperative renal function. *Annals of Thoracic Surgery* **60**, 160–4.

Rivetti, L.A., Gandra, S.M. 1997: Initial experience using an intraluminal shunt during revascularization of the beating heart. *Annals of Thoracic Surgery* **63**, 1742–7.

Roach, G.W., Kangchuger, M., Mangano, C.M. *et al.* 1996: Adverse cerebral outcomes after coronary bypass surgery. *New England Journal of Medicine* **335**, 1857–63.

Robinson, M.C., Thielmeier, K.A., Hill, B.B. 1998: Transient ventricular asystole using adenosine during minimally invasive and open sternotomy coronary artery bypass grafting. *Annals of Thoracic Surgery* **66**, 30–4.

Sabiston, D.C. 1974: The coronary circulation. *Johns Hopkins Med J* **134**, 314–29.

Spence, P. 1994: International workshop on arterial conduits for myocardial revascularization. Universita Cattolica del Sacro Cuore, Rome, Italy, November.

Spence, P.A., Montgomery, W.D., Stantamore, W.P. 1995: High flow demand on small arterial coronary bypass conduits promotes graft spasm. *Journal of Thoracic and Cardiovascular Surgery* **110**, 952–62.

Spooner, T.H., Dyrud, P.E., Monson, B.K., Dixon, G.E., Robinson, L.D. 1998: Coronary artery bypass on the beating heart with the octopus; a North American experience. *Annals of Thoracic Surgery* **66**, 1032–5.

Stanbridge, R. De L., Hadjinikolaou, L.K., Cohen, A.S., Foale, R.A., Davies, W.D., Al Kutoubi, A. 1997: Minimally invasive coronary revascularization through parasternal incisions without cardiopulmonary bypass. *Annals of Thoracic Surgery* **63** (Suppl. 6), S53–6.

Stanbridge, R.D., Hadjinikolaou, L.K. 1999: Technical adjuncts in beating heart surgery. Comparison of MIDCAB to off-pump sternotomy: a meta-analysis. *European Journal of Cardiothoracic Surgery* **16**(Suppl. 2) S24–33.

Stanbridge, R., De L, Symons, G.V., Banwell, P.E. 1995: Minimal access surgery for coronary artery revascularization. *Lancet* **346**, 837.

Subramanian, V.A., Sani, G., Bennetti, F.J., Calafiore, A.M. 1995: Minimally invasive coronary bypass surgery: a multicentre report of preliminary clinical experience. *Circulation* **92**(Suppl. 1) 645 (abstract).

Subramanian, V.A., McCabe, J.C., Geller, C.M. 1997: Minimally invasive direct coronary artery bypass grafting: two-year clinical experience. *Annals of Thoracic Surgery* **64**, 1648–55.

Sweeney, M.S., Frazier, O.H. 1992: Device supported revascularization: safe help for sick hearts. *Annals of Thoracic Surgery* **54**, 1065–70.

Trapp, W.G., Bisarya, R. 1975: Placement of coronary artery bypass graft without pump oxygenator. *Annals of Thoracic Surgery* **19**, 1–9.

Wasnick, J.D., Acuff, T. 1997: Anesthesia and minimally invasive thoracoscopically assisted coronary artery bypass: a brief clinical report. *Journal of Cardiothoracic and Vascular Anesthesia* **5**, 552–5.

Westaby, S. 1995: Coronary surgery without cardiopulmonary bypass. *British Heart Journal* **73**, 203–5.

Westaby, S., Benetti, F.J. 1996: Less invasive coronary surgery: consensus from the Oxford meeting. *Annals of Thoracic Surgery* **62**, 924–31.

Zenati, M., Chen, H.A., Griffith, B.P. 1999: Alternative approach to multivessel coronary disease with integrated coronary revascularization. *Journal of Thoracic and Cardiovascular Surgery* **117**, 439–46.

The development of clinical perfusion education and standards in the UK and Ireland

MICHAEL WHITEHORNE

INTRODUCTION

Kirklin (1990), during his analysis of the development of cardiac surgery, described three distinct eras:

- innovation 1954–1970
- consolidation 1970–1985
- scientific development 1985–2000.

Interestingly, the same analysis can be applied to the development of the science of clinical perfusion.

INNOVATION

The decade between the mid-1950s and mid-1960s spawned a new era in cardiac surgery in the United Kingdom. During this decade, Cleland, Melrose and Bentall (Cleland *et al.*, 1968) assisted by an immensely dedicated team of enthusiastic nurses and technicians, performed the first procedures utilising cardiopulmonary bypass in the UK. The heart and lung equipment used and prototypes had been developed by Dr Dennis Melrose at the Hammersmith Hospital Royal Postgraduate Medical School and manufactured by New Electronic Products Ltd. As a result of the innovative work of Melrose, New Electronic Products manufactured and released the first-generation pump oxygenators into the UK market. Figure 19A.1 illustrates the first of these models used and modified at King's College Hospital, London in 1964.

Initially, this equipment was operated by anaesthetists and physiologists assisted by interested personnel from varied backgrounds, including electricians, instrument curators, engineers and laboratory technicians.

Many of these assistants would become significantly involved in the design and function of pumping and oxygenating equipment, and were soon to become totally responsible for their operation during cardiac surgical procedures. These early innovators, without knowing, had given birth to a new allied medical profession, which we now know as 'clinical perfusion science'. This was an era rich in experimentation and research, leading to tremendous advancements in surgical techniques, instrumentation and medical equipment. Figure 19A.2 gives us an example of how equipment and its components were designed, custom built and assembled 'in-house'. The custom-designed pump oxygenator shown here was used at King's College Hospital to investigate the preservation of organs such as kidneys, livers and hearts. It was also used in 250 heart and lung transplant procedures on pigs in 1967.

CONSOLIDATION

The years between 1970 and 1985 witnessed momentous scientific and technological advances in cardiac surgery. It became increasingly apparent that this new profession, in order to stay abreast of rapidly changing technology, would need to supplement its newly found practical skills with some medical and scientific academic knowledge. Strongly encouraged by eminent surgeons and

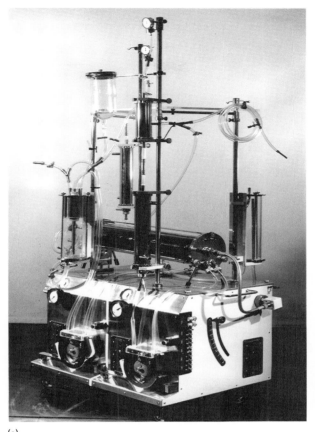

(a)

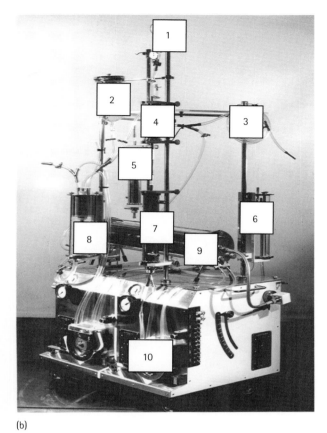

(b)

Figure 19 A.1 *(a) First-generation pump oxygenator used at King's College Hospital, London, 1964; (b) key to components: (1) Tygos pressure gauge; (2) blood reservoir; (3) femoral line with femoral cannulae; (4) New Electronic Products filter and bubble trap (arterial); (5) New Electronic Products heat exchanger (arterial); (6) New Electronic Products blood reservoir with high pressure suction; (7) New Electronic Products large heat exchanger; (8) New Electronic Products cardiotomy reservoir with low pressure suction; (9) New Electronic Products 'K CROSS' disk oxygenator; (10) New Electronics DeBakey twin roller pump console (modified by King's College Hospital, London). (Reproduced courtesy of Mr Andreas Patellopoulos ACP MBE, Chief Clinical Perfusionist, King's College Hospital 1963–1999.)*

anaesthetists at the time, many clinical perfusionists from the UK and Ireland joined together and, in 1974, the Society of Perfusionists of Great Britain and Ireland was formed, whose motto was aptly 'education, education, education'. The primary objective of the Society at this time was the education of clinical perfusionists.

At this time many perfusionists subscribed to and supported the Society's aim of improving education. Many attended colleges around the UK and Ireland in pursuit of qualifications relating to medical physics and physiological measurement at ordinary national diploma (OND) and higher national diploma (HND) levels. These qualifications became the basic requirement for clinical perfusionists entering the profession at that time. The Society, now well-established, grew in size and confidence, and in 1981 staged the first World Congress on Perfusion.

With a rapidly growing profession, the Society recognized that a uniform standard in perfusion science was required urgently across the UK and Ireland.

The accreditation process

In 1988 the Society introduced an accreditation system. This ensured that all clinical perfusionists would follow a uniform education programme. The accreditation system was made up of several components:

1 Theoretical examination comprising six written papers: (i) anatomy; (ii) physiology; (iii) pharmacology; (iv) pathology; (v) perfusion management; (vi) perfusion services.
2 Practical examination. This part of the programme requires that two senior clinical perfusionists with at

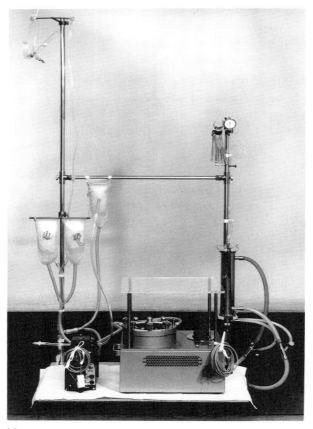

(a)

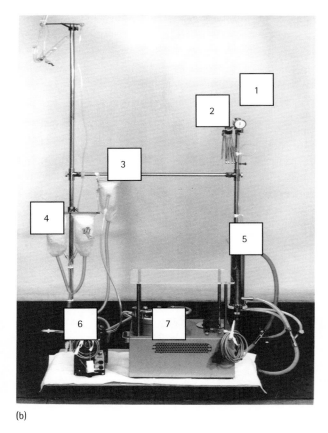

(b)

Figure 19 A.2 *(a) Custom-designed pump oxygenator designed and used at King's College Hospital, London for animal research, 1967; (b) key to components: (1) Tygos pressure gauge; (2) tubing clamps; (3) Polystan cardiotomy reservoir with low pressure suction; (4) Polystan cardiotomy reservoirs with King's College Hospital-designed bubble oxygenator; (5) New Electronic Products heat exchanger; (6) Watson Marlow pump for low pressure suction; (7) Associated Engineering Industries (AEI) roller pump. (Reproduced courtesy of Mr Andreas Patellopoulos ACP MBE, Chief Clinical Perfusionist, King's College Hospital 1963–1999.)*

least 10 years' experience are selected from a panel of examiners. These examiners then observe a clinical perfusionist in training carrying out a clinical perfusion and assess the candidate on his or her practical ability.

3 Viva voce examination. This follows the same process as the practical examination; however, the candidate is assessed orally to assess his or her theoretical and cognitive skills.

On successful completion of this examination process, clinical perfusionists in training are deemed competent to practise clinical perfusion and are awarded the accreditation certificate of the Society of Clinical Perfusionists of Great Britain and Ireland. This accreditation process enabled the profession to measure the quality of clinical perfusion being delivered to patients undergoing cardiac surgery. It also laid the foundation for the first voluntary register of accredited clinical perfusionists within the UK and Ireland.

In 1986, the Society, with prominent surgeons, anaesthetists and academics, formed the Board of the School of Clinical Perfusion Sciences. The role of this Board was to establish through training, education and examination standards of clinical knowledge and clinical practice. The Board introduced a postgraduate diploma in clinical perfusion science, the first postgraduate course in clinical perfusion in Europe. Successful candidates of this two-year course, validated by the Open University, were also recognized by the Society with the award of the Advanced Certificate in Clinical Perfusion.

Clinical perfusion education was now flourishing within the UK and Ireland. In 1989, British and Irish perfusionists, with senior surgeons, recognized the need to establish standardized education for clinical perfusionists across Europe; they developed and founded the European Board of Cardiovascular Perfusion. Bringing together clinical perfusionists and surgeons across Europe, this Board was established in 1991.

The need for safety

Mortality and morbidity directly related to clinical perfusion is well documented. Stoney *et al.* (1980) and Wheeldon (1981) recorded accidents of just over three per 1000 perfusions for both the UK and USA for the period 1972–1979. Mortality for the same period was recorded as 0.42 per 1000 and 0.70 per 1000 perfusions for the UK and USA, respectively.

With increasing advances in the complexity and sophistication of surgical and perfusion techniques, representations from senior surgeons for the statutory regulation of the profession of clinical perfusion science were being made to the British government. At the 1994 annual general meetings of the Society of Cardiothoracic Surgeons of Great Britain and Ireland and the Association of Cardiothoracic Anaesthetists, the following resolution was passed:

> [The two Associations] wish the National Health Service Management Executive to know that they unanimously expect that any mechanical perfusion used in the management of a patient undergoing a surgical procedure in the United Kingdom or Ireland should be undertaken by a Perfusionist who has been accredited by the Society of Clinical Perfusionists of Great Britain and Ireland, or by a trainee under the direct supervision of an accredited Clinical Perfusionist.

Education revisited

In answer to increasing responsibility placed upon clinical perfusionists, and advice from our surgical colleagues, in 1995 the Society and the Board of the school of clinical perfusion sciences realized that the base level of education for clinical perfusionists was no longer suitable and proposed to raise the basic qualification to degree standard. A working group was formed, consisting of clinical perfusionists, surgeons and anaesthetists, and in 1997 a four-year part-time Bachelor of Science honours degree in clinical perfusion science was introduced as the basic educational standard for all clinical perfusionists practising within the UK and Ireland. Successful completion of this qualification would now lead to accreditation in clinical perfusion.

Around this time it was becoming apparent that the work of the Society was increasingly focused on political issues. The profession needed an independent body whose sole responsibility would be to oversee the standards of education and the profession as a whole. In 1998 the Board of the school of clinical perfusion science was dissolved and replaced by the College of Clinical Perfusionists of Great Britain and Ireland. In addition to this, and as a result of a gracious offer from our surgical colleagues, the central offices of the Society and the

newly formed College of Clinical Perfusionists of Great Britain and Ireland would now be based at the prestigious Royal College of Surgeons of England.

The primary objectives for which the College was established were:

- To liase with and consult with the Society of Clinical Perfusionists of Great Britain and Ireland on all matters of training and education of clinical perfusion scientists. To advance education in the knowledge and practice of perfusion and related studies for the benefit of the public. To liase with and consult with other professional bodies and institutions deemed necessary in pursuing these objectives.
- The accreditation and maintenance of a register of clinical perfusionists.
- The accreditation of training centres.
- The accreditation of trainers.
- The accreditation of external assessors for training centres and trainers.
- The award of the following Letters Designate: Licentiate member of the College (LCCP) and Fellow of the College (FCCP).
- To provide arbitration in matters of dispute on the relevance of other perfusion-related qualifications.
- To provide a disciplinary mechanism.
- To provide an appeals procedure.
- To advance continuing professional development.
- To provide courses of education, both full- and part-time, for students at all levels.
- To define a code of practice, the objective of which is to give guidance on good practice to which all registered clinical perfusionists should adhere.
- The implementation of a re-certification programme.

It was important that the College council membership should be representative of the field of cardiac surgery with university academic representation as well as representing clinical perfusion. Hence the composition of the council board was formed as follows: President; Vice-President; Secretary or Treasurer; Registrar; Society of Perfusionists Representatives; the Society of Cardiothoracic Surgeons Representatives; the Association of Cardiothoracic Anaesthetists Representatives; Academic Clinician.

Since its inception, the College has been responsible for the publication of the following important guidelines for the practice of clinical perfusion: recommendations for standards of monitoring and alarms during cardiopulmonary bypass; codes of ethical conduct; and standards of practice.

In 1999, The Department of Health issued a circular entitled 'Good Practice Guidelines' to all NHS hospitals. This document would now recommend that the employment of clinical perfusionists within the NHS would be restricted to those whose names appeared on the voluntary register held by the College of Clinical Perfusionists of Great Britain and Ireland. This was to be an interim arrangement until statutory regulation of clinical perfusionists was achieved via parliament. With a form of regulation for clinical perfusionists now in place, the College swiftly introduced recertification for clinical perfusionists practising within the UK and Ireland. Recertification would now ensure that practising clinical perfusionists would be responsible for demonstrating continuing perfusion education and perfusion practice. The requirements of recertification would charge each and every practising clinical perfusionist to demonstrate, on an annual basis, that they had achieved the following criteria.

Each accredited clinical perfusionist must acquire 135 recertification points in a three-year period, with 15 points for professional activity and 120 points for clinical activity (40 points per year). They must file a Clinical Activity Report every year, and a Professional Activity Report every third year. The values of the proposed activities are:

- Clinical activity (40 points required per annum): clinical perfusions – one point per clinical perfusion; supervising students – 0.5 points per clinical perfusion (10 points maximum).
- Postgraduate education (15 points over a three-year period): in-house workshop, seminar or meeting – one point (plus two points for presenting); one-day congress – four points (plus five points for presenting); congress of two days or more – eight points (plus five points for presenting); teaching on a recognized course (under-/postgraduate) – two points per hour.
- Publications: journal without editorial policy (excluding letters) – two points; journal with editorial policy (excluding letters) – 10 points.

SCIENTIFIC DEVELOPMENT

To stay with Kirklin's (1980) description of the three-phase development process, the third phase is that of scientific development. The profession of clinical perfusion in the UK and Ireland, with the help of the Society of Clinical Perfusionists of Great Britain and Ireland, the College of Clinical Perfusionists of Great Britain and Ireland, and the respective societies and associations of cardiac surgeons and anaesthetists, has matured over the last 40 years. It is clear that the profession has gained a high level of autonomy and responsibility through striving for and achieving a body of specialist knowledge, which has been accepted and respected by the medical profession.

The College of Clinical Perfusionists of Great Britain and Ireland developed and will now offer the first Master of Science Degree in Clinical Perfusion Science in Europe. The creation of this postgraduate degree was as a result of the demand from an increasing number of clinical perfusionists who have engaged themselves in postgraduate studies and research at masters and doctorate levels of education.

At the beginning of the new millennium, the Society, College and its members agreed to rename the profession 'Clinical Perfusion Scientist'. This change of name and identity, which has now been adopted throughout the health services in North and Southern Ireland, Scotland, Wales and England, reflects the perseverance and achievements of what is now known as the Society of Clinical Perfusion Scientists of Great Britain and Ireland, and the College of Clinical Perfusion Scientists of Great Britain and Ireland, whose motto remains the same today as it did all those years ago, 'education, education, education'.

REFERENCES

Cleland, W.P., Goodwin, J.F., Bentall, H.H., Oakley, C.M., Melrose, D.G., Hollman, A. 1968: A decade of open heart surgery. *Lancet* **1**, 191–8.

Kirklin, J.W. 1990: The science of cardiac surgery. *European Journal Cardiothoracic Surgery* **4**, 63–71.

Stoney, W.S., Alford, W.C., Burrus, G.R., Glassford, G.M., Thomas, C.S. 1980: Air embolism and other accidents using pump-oxygenators. *Annals of Thoracic Surgery* **29**, 336–40.

Wheeldon, D.R. 1981: Can cardiopulmonary bypass be a safe procedure? In: Longmore, D.B., ed. *Towards safer cardiac surgery*. Lancaster: MTP Press: 427–46.

FURTHER READING

Department of Health. 1999: *Guidance on best practice for the employment of clinical perfusionists in the NHS.* (http://tap.ccta.gov.uk/doh/coin4.nsf)

Society of Clinical Perfusion Scientists of Great Britain and Ireland and the College of Clinical Perfusion Scientists of Great Britain and Ireland. 1999: *Code of ethical conduct.* (www.sopgbi.org)

Society of Clinical Perfusion Scientists of Great Britain and Ireland and the College of Clinical Perfusion Scientists of Great Britain and Ireland. 1999: *Standards of practice.* (www.sopgbi.org)

Society of Clinical Perfusion Scientists of Great Britain and Ireland, Association of Cardiothoracic Anaesthetists and the Society of Cardiothoracic Surgeons of Great Britain and Ireland. 2001: *Recommendations for standards of monitoring and alarms during cardiopulmonary bypass.* (www.sopgbi.org)

Wheeldon, D.R. 1981: Safty during cardiopulmonary bypass. *Proceedings of the First World Congress on Open-Heart Technology.* London: Franklin Scientific Projects: 27–9.

Standards, guidelines and education in clinical perfusion: the European perspective

LUDWIG K VON SEGESSER

INTRODUCTION

In the early 1950s, the introduction of cardiopulmonary bypass into clinical practice not only triggered the development of true open heart surgery but also brought along a new science that is now known as 'clinical perfusion'. For clinical perfusion science, the main concern in the early days was the development of a technology that not only allowed reliability but also provided adequate delivery of blood flow as well as gas and heat transfer. Early 'biological' attempts at clinical perfusion were based on perfusion techniques using patients' own lungs for oxygenation (Potts *et al.*, 1952) as well as homologous cross-circulation (Lillehei *et al.*, 1955). Although the proof of principle had been provided for both of these techniques, they were soon abandoned in favour of mechanical, so-called 'pump oxygenators'.

Following the introduction of true cardiopulmonary bypass into clinical practice by Gibbon in 1953 (Gibbon, 1954) a number of reusable pump oxygenator systems were developed in the leading centres performing open heart surgery. The basic principle that was applied for gas transfer was so-called 'film oxygenation', where the blood was spread out on a large surface as a thin film in an oxygen-saturated atmosphere in such a way that the gas diffusion distance could be kept at a minimum. This is similar to the concept already proposed by von Frey and Gruber (1885) for isolated organ perfusion.

Although the operation and maintenance of pump oxygenators was very demanding time-wise as well as knowledge-wise, it was also an essential part of training and development as most of the experts (surgeons and technicians) were in-house (von Segesser, 1997). Improved maintenance and serviceability were major goals in the later pumps built on the same principles. The Livio pump was a good example of a second-generation pump oxygenator based on the thin film principle. Relatively easy to clean flat disks, a corrosion-resistant housing (made from aluminium alloy) and improved reliability and serviceability, that is, overdimensioned high torque electric motors with self-adjusting V-belt drives are just some examples of the refinements made in those days. Still, the disassembly, cleaning and reassembly of the improved pump oxygenators remained a time-consuming procedure that generally took longer than the actual pump run time during its clinical application in open heart surgery.

The advent of disposable oxygenators (Rygg and Kyvsgaard, 1956) completely changed not only perfusion but open heart surgery as a whole. Despite the fact that some components, like heat exchangers (in general made from stainless steel) and connectors were still reused and had therefore to be cleaned, the most tedious part – cleaning the 'artificial lung' – disappeared. Suddenly, the most time-consuming activity linked to an open heart procedure had vanished and therefore the caseload a given cardiac unit could cope with increased dramatically. As a result the number of 'pump cases' rose in an unprecedented fashion and open heart surgery was booming all over the world.

For clinical perfusion, daily practice did not change that fast because the increased caseloads were initially compensated for by the reduced time needed for pump oxygenator preparation. Similarly, many experts in charge of reusable film oxygenators stayed in place and therefore the basic knowledge of pump oxygenator preparation and maintenance was still readily available in many units for a long time. However, with the rapid growth of open heart procedures, and the consecutive rise in the number of new heart surgery units that were opened, the relative density of perfusion experts decreased. In addition, more and more perfusionists were trained 'on the job' and now worked exclusively with disposable oxygenators. Hence, the basic perfusion technology knowledge that was originally intrinsic to all cardiac surgery units that built and serviced their own pump oxygenators in the hospital machine shop shifted gradually to the oxygenator and pump console manufacturers, who provided the necessary equipment on an industrial basis. Most heart surgeons, who had originally been the driving force for the development of the pump oxygenators for open heart surgery, changed their focus and so the expertise in perfusion technology available in many clinical units further decreased. A typical example of a development in perfusion technology that disappeared for many years is the concept of surface modification for improved biocompatability of synthetic surfaces exposed to the blood. The benefits of heparin surface bonding were reported by Gott et al. (1963). However, it took almost 30 years to bring this knowledge back into routine clinical practice (von Segesser et al., 1994, 1999) where it is now used in almost all arterial line filters.

In addition to the 'brain drain' in pump oxygenator technology, 'full-range' cardiac surgical units with sufficient numbers of trained perfusionists in all clinically relevant branches (including coronary, valve and congenital surgery in all sizes as well as aneurysms, transplantation, mechanical circulatory support and perfusion for oncological problems) are nowadays a minority. It can no longer be taken for granted that perfusionists trained on the job in a cardiac surgical programme selected at random have participated in the perfusion procedures of most clinically relevant operations; that they are aware of all serious adverse events (Stoney et al., 1980, Kurusz et al., 1995); or that they can automatically manage all relevant failures of the heart–lung machine within a useful time.

As a result, standards and guidelines had to be developed for training and education in clinical perfusion. This task, which is an ongoing process, has to take into account technological and scientific as well as demographic and social changes, and has been taken over by the professionals interested in the future development of perfusion.

EUROPEAN BOARD OF CARDIOVASCULAR PERFUSION

The European Board of Cardiovascular Perfusion was founded in 1991 (similar organizations exist for North America and Australasia) by the national delegates of perfusion societies in the member states of the European Community and the European Free Trade Association, on the one hand, and representatives of the European Association of Cardiothoracic Surgery, the European Society of Cardiovascular Surgery and the European Association of Cardiothoracic Anaesthesiologists, on the other. The Board is organized in a democratic fashion with a legislative power (the general assembly of the national delegates and the representatives of the related societies of surgeons and anaesthesiologists mentioned above) for its members, an executive power (chairman, general secretary and treasurer) and a judicative power (appeals). In addition, there is an academic committee proposing the educational goals, a certification sub-committee that is in charge of certification of individual perfusionists and an accreditation committee that is in charge of accreditation of perfusion schools and training programmes, both in accordance to the rules set by the European Board.

The objectives of the European Board of Cardiovascular Perfusion are to:

- establish, monitor and maintain equality of standards in education and training
- set out essentials and guidelines for training programmes
- set a common examination
- issue a European Certificate in Cardiovascular Perfusion
- establish a common certification and recertification process in Europe.

GUIDELINES FOR THE EDUCATION OR ACCREDITATION OF PERFUSION SCHOOLS AND TRAINING PROGRAMMES

The European Board of Cardiovascular Perfusion has published essentials and guidelines for accreditation of education and training programmes. These are designed to give guidance to institutions seeking the European Board's accreditation for their education and training programmes in perfusion sciences. The object is not to set a maximum level for programmes to attain, but to set minimum criteria. These criteria must be achieved by the institution, that is, the school of perfusion, hospital or university where the programme is being offered, before the European Board will grant accreditation. Criteria are set to define a suitable establishment, a programme director, a board of management, an academic committee, supervising perfusionists, a budget, equipment and facilities, a library, teaching standards, students' awareness, students' welfare and liability. Entry requirements for students wishing to enter a programme include school-leaving certificates in physics, chemistry, biology, mathematics and the national language (course duration two or three years). A science degree is required for schools offering a programme of short duration (minimum one year).

The syllabus for the programme must be clearly detailed in writing and adhered to. It must be included in the application for accreditation, and any alterations must be resubmitted. The syllabus must include: teaching of basic sciences (e.g. anatomy, physiology, pharmacology, pathology, haematology, microbiology, immunology, cardiopulmonary and vascular pathology, embryology, basic anaesthesia, instrumentation or basic electronics, computer studies, materials science and resource management). The clinical programme must include perfusion management, haemofiltration, haemodilution, haemodialysis, hypothermia, autotransfusion, extracorporeal membrane oxygenation, paediatric perfusion, intra-aortic balloon counterpulsation, blood gas analysis, fluid and electrolyte balance, coagulation, blood pressure monitoring, electrocardiogram, cardiac catheterization, myocardial preservation, organ preservation, ventricular assist devices, transplantation, cardiac surgery, cardiac investigation techniques, the basics of anaesthesia, cardiac anaesthesia and post-operative care. Student rotation through other cardiac units is encouraged. A logbook, in which is kept a record of the student's progress and achievements, is also mandatory.

The programme has to be reassessed constantly in conjunction with prospective employers to ensure that the students are taught all new advances in the technology. In addition, representatives of the academic committee of the European Board will perform site visits of the individual perfusion schools or programmes in order to ensure proper compliance with the rules.

CERTIFICATION OF CLINICAL PERFUSIONISTS GRADUATING FROM AN ACCREDITED PERFUSION SCHOOL OR TRAINING PROGRAMME

The European Board organizes examinations (von Segesser, 1995) for practising clinical perfusionists on a

yearly basis throughout Europe. Successful candidates receive the European Certificate for Cardiovascular Perfusion. Applicants wishing to sit the Board's examination must meet the following criteria:

- Applicants must have graduated from a training programme accredited by the Board and present their log books with their application.
- Applicants must have practised clinical perfusion for a minimum of two years.
- Applicants must be currently practising clinical perfusionists.
- Applicants must submit a logbook in which it is certified that: the applicant has conducted a minimum of 100 clinical perfusions; the applicant is fully versed and is competent in the avoidance and management of perfusion accidents; the applicant can set up and operate a wide range of commonly used equipment for cardiopulmonary bypass and support.

The examination is in three parts – written, practical and oral – and will be set in the European language used by the accredited programme of the candidate's choice. The written examination covers anatomy, pathology, physiology, pharmacology and perfusion technology. The practical examination is designed to assess candidates' ability to handle safety techniques, and the avoidance as well as the management of perfusion accidents. The oral examination covers perfusion equipment and technique. Candidates who successfully complete the written, practical and oral examinations are awarded the European Certificate in Cardiovascular Perfusion.

RECERTIFICATION OF BOARD–CERTIFIED PERFUSIONISTS

If it is nowadays well accepted that a structured education and minimal standards are necessary for education of clinical perfusionists, it is much less so for continuing education. However, despite all the progress that was made, clinical perfusion remains a delicate procedure with an extremely high potential for lethal and disabling complications. Various perfusion accident surveys (Stoney et al., 1980, Kurusz et al., 1986, 1995) Jenkins et al.,1997; Svenmarker and von Segesser, 1999; Mejak et al., 2000) have demonstrated this unpleasant reality repeatedly.

There are a number of measures that can be taken to further improve the competence of clinical perfusionists that have been developed by and for other professional groups, such pilots and surgeons. For the latter, education instead of training, emphasis on content instead of time, and the systematic measurement of outcomes have been recognized as essential for future development

(Benfield, 1999). Systematic measurement of outcomes implies not only monitoring of adverse events but also assessment of so-called 'critical incidents' (near-misses) in clinical perfusion. Monitoring of critical incidences and, consequently, the development of preventative strategies are of growing importance in medicine in general (Brennan *et al.*, 1991; Leape *et al.*, 1991). Preventive strategies for clinical perfusion evolving from earlier failures include the systematic use of pre-bypass checklists (Svenmarker and von Segesser, 1999), optimized positioning of disposable spare parts (pump loop, oxygenator, etc.) in the operating theatre (within arm's reach) and continuous training for minimized handling time for critical incidents (such as oxygenator changeover). The fact that specialists achieve better outcomes than generalists for lung cancer surgery (Silvestri *et al.*, 1998) also suggests that a minimum 'pump caseload' and adequate continuing education are necessary for good clinical perfusion. Similarly, training courses for new procedures may be useful not only for surgeons (Whaba *et al.*, 1998) but also for perfusionists. Hence, by decision of the European Board of Cardiovascular Perfusion, a minimum number of clinical perfusion procedures per year as well as adequate continuing education will have to be validated before recertification of clinical perfusionists.

REFERENCES

Benfield, J.R. 1999: Surgical education in changing times. *European Journal of Cardiothoracic Surgery* **16** (Suppl.1), S6–10.

Brennan, T.A., Leape, L.L., Laird, N.M. *et al.* 1991: Incidence of adverse events and negligence in hospitalized patients: results of the Harvard medical practice, Study I. *New England Journal of Medicine* **324**, 370–6.

Gibbon, J.H. 1954: Application of mechanical heart and lung apparatus to cardiac surgery. *Minnesota Medicine* **37**, 171–85.

Gott, V.L., Whiffen, J.D., Datton, R.C. 1963: Heparin bonding on colloidal graphite surfaces. *Science* **142**, 1297–8.

Jenkins, O.F., Morris, F., Simpson, J.M. 1997: Australasian perfusion incident survey. *Perfusion* **12**, 279–88.

Kurusz, M., Conti, V.R., Arens, J.F., Brown, J.P., Faulkner, S.C., Manning, J.V. 1986: Perfusion accident survey. *Proc Am Acad Cardiovasc Perfusion* **7**, 57–65.

Kurusz, M., Butler, B.D., Katz, J., Conti, V.R. 1995: Air embolism during cardiopulmonary bypass. *Perfusion* **10**, 361–91.

Leape, L.L. *et al.* 1991: The nature of adverse events in hospitalized patients: results from the Harvard medical practice, Study II. *New England Journal of Medicine* **324**, 377–84.

Lillehei, C.W., Cohen, M., Warden, H.E., Varco, L. 1955: The direct vision intracardiac correction of congenital anomalies by controlled cross circulation. *Surgery* **38**, 11–29.

Mejak, B.L., Stammers, A., Rauch, E., Vang, S., Viessman, T. 2000: A retrospective study on perfusion incidents and safety devices. *Perfusion* **15**, 51–61.

Potts, W.J., Riker, W.L., DeBord, L., Andrews, C.E. 1952: Maintenance of life by homologous lungs and mechanical circulation. *Surgery* **31**, 161–6.

Rygg, I.H., Kyvsgaard, E. 1956: A disposable polythylene oxygenator system applied in the heart/lung machine. *Acta Chirurgica Scandinavica* **112**, 433–7.

Silvestri, G.A., Handy, J., Lackland, D. *et al.* 1998: Specialists achieve better outcomes than generalists for lung cancer surgery. *Journal of Thoracic and Cardiovascular Surgery* **114**, 675–80.

Stoney, W.S., Alford, W.C., Burrus, G.R., Classford, D.M., Thomas, C.S. 1980: Air embolism and other accidents using pump oxygenators. *Annals of Thoracic Surgery* **29**, 336–40.

Svenmarker, S., von Segesser, L.K. 1999: The European Board of Cardiovascular Perfusion pre-bypass checklist. *Perfusion* **14**, 165–6.

von Frey, M., Gruber, M. 1885: Untersuchungen uber den Stoffwechsel isolierter Organe. *Archiv fur Physiologie* **9**, 519–32.

von Segesser, L.K. 1995: European Board of Cardiovascular Perfusion. Announcement. *Perfusion* **10**, 0–1.

von Segesser, L.K. 1997: Perfusion education and certification in Europe. *Perfusion* **12**, 243–6.

von Segesser, L.K., Weiss, B.M., Pasic, M., Garcia, E., Turina, M.I. 1994: Risk and benefit of low systemic heparinization during open heart operations. *Annals of Thoracic Surgery* **58**, 391–8.

von Segesser, L.K., Westaby, S., Pomar, J., Loisance, D., Groscurth, P., Turina, M. 1999: Less invasive aortic valve surgery: rationale and technique. *European Journal of Cardiothoracic Surgery* **15**, 781–5.

Whaba, A., Phillip, A., Behr, R., Birnbaum, D.E. 1998: Heparin coated equipment reduces the risk of oxygenator failure. *Annals of Thoracic Surgery* **65**, 1310–12.

Perfusion education in the USA at the turn of the twentieth century

ALFRED H STAMMERS

INTRODUCTION

Perfusion education in the USA has undergone numerous changes in the 40 years since the first organized programme in cardiovascular perfusion was established (Lange, 1986). The effects of numerous influences have affected this evolution, which continues to change. The underlying principle has always been to assure that perfusionists entering the field possess both a fundamental scientific knowledge on extracorporeal flow, and a practical ability to provide clinically competent care to all those who require extracorporeal circulation (Dake and Taylor, 1996). No viable argument has ever existed that attempted to establish goals in conflict with these. However, the means by which the primary education in perfusion has been conducted has always been carefully evaluated. This chapter examines some of the factors that have influenced how the delivery of primary education in perfusion has developed, and presents the state of perfusion education in the USA today.

PROGRAMME EXPANSION 1963–2003

Formal perfusion education began at the Cleveland Clinic, Ohio, USA in 1963 (Stammers and Lange, 1992). The programme took approximately six months to complete and students primarily received a 'hands-on' education. By 1969 there was a handful of programmes educating students in the developing field of extracorporeal circulation. The first university-based educational programme started in 1969 at the Ohio State University. Through the 1970s a number of educational programmes were established both in hospital and university settings. In 1981 there were 15 accredited educational programmes accepting students. By 1984 that number had expanded to 26, which represented a growth rate of 3.3 programmes per year. From 1986 to 1992 nine new programmes were accredited, although there were also a number of programmes that ceased to exist (Stammers, 1999). The apex of perfusion education programmes occurred in 1994, when the Committee on Allied Health Education and Accreditation (CAHEA) of the American Medical Association officially recognized 35 programmes. Since that time there has been a decline in number of programmes in existence in America. In fact, since 1995, 14 programmes have either closed or moved to an 'inactive' status. In 2003 there were 21 programmes accredited by the Commission on Accreditation of Allied Health Education Programs (CAAHEP). CAAHEP has managed perfusion education since taking over from CAHEA in 1995. Currently, 21 of 23 accredited programmes are accepting students for 2003 academic year. Programme numbers in the USA between 1989 and 2003 are shown in Fig. 19C.1. The accrediting agency, the Accreditation Committee on Perfusion Education (AC-PE), is made up of representatives from seven member organizations. These organizations include the American Academy of Cardiovascular Perfusion, the American Association of Thoracic Surgery, the American

Board of Cardiovascular Perfusion, the American Society of Extracorporeal Technology, the Perfusion Program Director's Council, the Society of Cardiovascular Anesthesiologists and the Society of Thoracic Surgeons.

PERFUSION GRADUATES

Regulation of the number of new perfusionists entering the field has been of immense concern to those dependent upon their services. Cardiac surgeons and hospitals performing cardiac and vascular surgery have expected that a ready number of competent individuals performing perfusion would be available to meet clinical demands. Perfusion service companies have looked to the education programmes to provide a constant number of graduates to meet the market demand for perfusionists. These expectations, however, have not been consistently met over the past decade.

Manpower demands for perfusionists have followed the growth in cardiovascular surgery, and hence are also susceptible to market factors. Between 1985 and 2000, the expansion in cardiac surgery has been described as 'explosive'. Employment opportunities were very good for perfusionists in the 1970s and 1980s, but stabilized in the 1990s as shown in Fig. 19C.2. The demand for perfusionists outpaced supply, which led to shortages in the early and mid-1980s. This situation led to an increase in the number of schools, with the output of new graduates peaking in the early 1990s. During this time the yearly graduate number approached 250 individuals. At the same time, however, there was also a decrease in the overall need for perfusionists, which led to decreased employment opportunities and a stabilization of salaries. Many believe that the overabundance of perfusionists in the 1990s resulted from an expansion in perfusionist responsibilities. The increase in perfusion graduation rate was concurrent with an expansion of percutaneous transluminal angioplasty. Unfortunately, this followed a period where the shortage of qualified clinicians had forced perfusionists to alter their scope of practice by reducing the number of services provided to hospitals. As market forces shifted to take advantage of demand economies, perfusionists saw a decline in employment opportunities. Many perfusionists blamed perfusion education programmes, and their output of graduates, for these conditions. However, this proved to be an overly simplistic interpretation of the events that were complex and diverse.

Controlling the number of perfusion graduates output is not as simple as accepting more, or fewer, individuals (Riley, 1991). The start of a new programme is difficult, laborious and very expensive. It is not unreasonable to expect start up cost to exceed $200,000 (USA) in the first year alone. It may take up to four years for a perfusion education programme to begin graduating students. The steps are vast and include programme planning, accreditation, acceptance of students, and graduation. The factors that were used to support the development of a programme may no longer exist by the time the programme graduates its first class. Few, if any, programmes are financially self-sufficient. Furthermore, the ability of a programme to meet the requirements of state education commissions imposes further demands. This may result in programmes seeking sponsorship in hospitals, where revenues from clinical enterprises can be used to offset educational expenses. The costs of beginning new college or university-based programmes may be prohibitive for perfusionists, since the number of graduates in most institutions is low by post-secondary education standard.

EDUCATIONAL LEVELS

Primary education in perfusion is performed in two distinct types of institutions: hospitals or universities (Hedzik and Larrick, 1992). The delineation between them is not clear, since university settings all use teaching in hospitals in some phase of their educational process. Instructors at hospital-based programmes also use pedagogic teaching principles based upon those found in higher level learning facilities. These may be the same principles utilized in university settings. Clearly, delineation of the

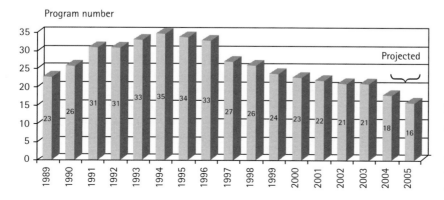

Program number

Figure 19C.1 *Perfusion education programme numbers in the United States, 1989–2003. Data modified from Stammers, A.H. 1999: Perfusion education in America at the turn of the century. J. Extracorp. Tech. 31, 112–7.*

quality of education based upon the type of institution at which it is delivered is not possible, and continues to be debated in the field.

There are three types of awards that are presently given to graduates of perfusion education programmes. These include certificates, baccalaureate and masters degrees. The type of award that students are given depends upon a number of factors and is usually related to the sponsoring institution. There are a number of programmes that are based in university systems that offer certificates of completion upon graduation. There are also programmes that are listed as baccalaureate programmes in promotional literature, but which offer this level of degree only to students who do not already possess a degree. Those that do will, instead, be given a certificate upon graduation.

As of 1994 all individuals who graduate from a USA CAAHEP-accredited programme must possess a minimum of a baccalaureate degree to enter the profession. Therefore, programmes that offer certificate of completion must require that students possess baccalaureate degrees before matriculation. In 2003 there were four programmes that offered masters degrees in perfusion, and a fifth that offered a certificate in perfusion, with optional masters degree in pharmacology. If one considers that the certificate programmes are all post-baccalaureates, then the majority of perfusion education in the USA is performed at the postgraduate level. Since only seven of the 21 programmes are at the undergraduate level it seems likely that the future of perfusion education will involve graduate-type education. This trend has also occurred in other allied health specialties such as physician assistants and certified registered nurse anaesthetists.

educational programme closure is financial. Like most post-secondary educational institutions, perfusion programmes receive the majority of their revenue from tuition. Even state-funded programmes receive a portion of their operating revenue from student tuition. The mean number of graduates per programme in 2003 is approximately six, which is an increase over the previous five years of approximately one additional individual (range 2–20 per annum). It is evident from this low number of perfusion graduates that the financial support for perfusion education programmes must be supplemented by alternate sources.

The primary administrative position for each programme is the programme director, who usually serves as the key faculty person. Of the 21 currently accredited programmes, 19 have programme directors who are certified (American Board of Cardiovascular Perfusion) cardiovascular perfusionists. In most cases financial support for these positions comes either partially, or entirely, from clinical enterprises. Although this may seem like a desirable means of bridging the gap between theoretical and applied perfusion education, it places significant challenges on directors. Their responsibility is to assure that the quality of education, both didactic and clinical, received by students is commensurate with the expectations of all stakeholders. The stakeholders include students, faculty, potential employers and, ultimately, patients. Balancing these needs demands that directors devote a significant part of each working day to meeting programme responsibilities, while at the same time balancing the demands of the clinic (Plunkett, 1993). Educational quality may be affected by such requirements and compromise the goals of both responsibility centres.

COSTS OF EDUCATION

The most significant expense related to perfusion education is the cost of personnel. The challenges faced by each programme in hiring and retaining qualified faculty are only one aspect of the financial challenges faced by education programmes. The most-often stated reason for

ASSESSMENT OF QUALITY

The measuring tools used to assess the quality of education programmes are influenced by a number of factors (Ferries, 1994). Determining clinical competence is elusive and challenging, yet remains the pinnacle of academic

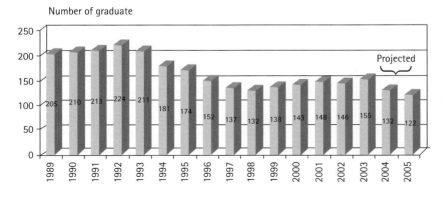

Number of graduate

Figure 19C.2 *Perfusion education programme graduates in the United States, 1989–2003. Data modified from Stammers, A.H. 1999: Perfusion education in America at the turn of the century.* J. Extracorp. Tech. *31, 112–7.*

achievement. Efforts have been made to classify education programmes according to either their sponsoring institution (hospital or academic) or the type of award granted (degree or certificate). Neither classification has been shown to reflect issues of educational quality and this is a moving target since programmes change both personnel and requirements. An effort to improve measures of quality for programmes was undertaken by the organization charged with maintaining the series of operational guidelines for perfusion education. These are termed the *Standards and Guidelines for an Accredited Educational Program for the Perfusionist* and are generated and approved through organized efforts of both the AC-PE and CAAHEP. These were initially adopted in 1980, and were revised in 1989, 1994 and most recently in 2001. All education programmes are reviewed periodically to ensure that they adhere to statutes for perfusion education. This periodic assessment includes written documentation, outcomes analysis, and an on-site review of resources, if deemed necessary. The standards, however, are deemed by most individuals to be a minimum set of operational guidelines. It always behoves a programme to improve its function in providing an education that is commensurate with the needs of employers and, ultimately, patients. It is through the review of outcomes that programme administrators and faculty members embark upon quality management processes for self-improvement.

Quantitative indicators of programme quality can be split into two categories: academic and clinical. Academic indicators for quality include results of programme graduates on the American Board of Cardiovascular Perfusion national board examinations, student selection for national scholarships, student publication and presentation rates at regional and national meetings and employment rates at graduation. Clinical quality indicators include the type and breadth of clinical experience, the total number of cases conducted by the student, and the level of competence of programme graduates (Stammers, 1999). The latter indicator is achieved only through review of prior student performance from employers. Such an assessment, therefore, comes from word-of-mouth discussions with perfusionist employers, and is quite subjective. The suggestion to use electronic simulators to test clinical acumen has been raised, and is under discussion in various councils involved in education. The lack of a reproducible measure of clinical skill is a deficiency that needs addressing. The measure of success for a clinical perfusionist is ultimately related to his/her ability to support the clinical function of the institution where they are employed. Achievement of these goals supercedes other responsibilities of the clinician. The total number of clinical practitioners is relatively small, and the experiences of one employer with a particular graduate may influence, positively or negatively, the employability of further graduates of that programme with that employer.

SUMMARY

The state of education for American perfusionists in the twenty-first century is one of turmoil. We have seen the closure of 40 per cent of perfusion education programmes in the past seven years, and undoubtedly this trend will continue. The interpretation of these closures must be considered from a critical perspective devoid of emotional influences, and with a discriminating eye on the future. The financial constraints facing hospitals and educational institutions continue to negatively impact the delivery of education. Educators from abroad have often used the model of American perfusion education as a template for the development of educational systems in their countries. What may be deemed 'good' for an individual may not be what is appropriate for a profession or a society. The challenges faced by the perfusion community include defining what indicators of quality are necessary to judge the performance of programme graduates. Once these are established, programme officials need to incorporate these requirements as benchmarks for self-evaluation. Changes to curricula, and most importantly ideologies, need to be made to ensure that programme graduates are prepared not only to find fruitful employment upon graduation but also to perform with a level of confidence commensurate with their skills. It is only through such dedication that perfusionists can continue to control the criteria for entry into the profession. Failing to look proactively at the factors influencing basic education in perfusion will undermine the advances that have occurred in education over the past 40 years, and suppress future initiatives. The demise of education shakes the foundation upon which perfusion has been established, which ultimately will affect patient care.

REFERENCES

Dake, S.B., Taylor, J.A. 1996: Meeting student differences in learning as a strategy for improving the quality of perfusion education. *Journal of Extra Corporeal Technology* **28**, 27–31.

Ferries, L. 1994: Perfusion schools and new graduates: quality versus quantity. *Perfusion Life* **11**, 8–[[CLOSING PAGINATION]].

Hedzik, K., Larrick, K. 1992: Hospital-based perfusion education versus academic institution-based perfusion education. *Perfusion Life* **9**, 8–11.

Lange, J. 1986: *The history of perfusion education in the United States*. Proceedings of the Mechanisms Meeting. Orlando, FL. October.

Plunkett, P. 1993: Perfusionist education in the United States: a future perspective. *Perfusion* **8**, 359–70.

Riley, J.B. 1991: Market forces affecting all levels of perfusion. *Perfusion Life* **8**, 6–9.

Stammers, A.H. 1999: Perfusion education in America at the turn of the century. *J Extra Corp Tech* **31**, 112–17.

Stammers, A.H., Lange, J. 1992: Controversies in perfusion education. Where do we go from here? *Perfusion Life* **9**, 10–19.

Index